MOSBY'S ORTHODONTIC REVIEW

MOSBY'S ORTHODONTIC REVIEW

Jeryl D. English, DDS, MS
Professor, Chairman and Program Director
Department of Orthodontics
The University of Texas Dental Branch at Houston
Houston, Texas

Timo Peltomäki, DDS, MS, PhD
Professor and Chairman
Clinic for Orthodontics and Pediatric Dentistry
Center for Dental and Oral Medicine
University of Zürich
Zürich, Switzerland

Kate Pham-Litschel, DDS, MS
Research Associate
Clinic for Orthodontics and Pediatric Dentistry
Center for Dental and Oral Medicine
University of Zürich
Zürich, Switzerland

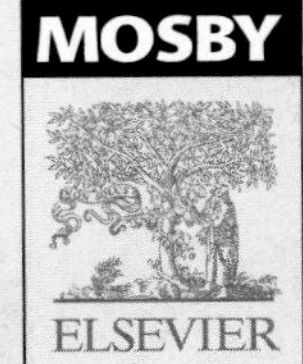

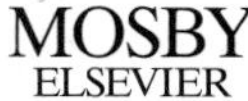

11830 Westline Industrial Drive
St. Louis, Missouri 63146

MOSBY'S ORTHODONTIC REVIEW

ISBN: 978-0-323-05007-4

NOTICE

Orthodontics is an ever-changing field. Standard safety precautions must be followed, but as new research and clinical experience broaden our knowledge, changes in treatment and drug therapy may become necessary or appropriate. Readers are advised to check the most current product information provided by the manufacturer of each drug to be administered to verify the recommended dose, the method and duration of administration, and contraindications. It is the responsibility of the licensed prescriber, relying on experience and knowledge of the patient, to determine dosages and the best treatment for each individual patient. Neither the publisher nor the author assumes any liability for any injury and/or damage to persons or property arising from this publication.

978-0-323-05007-4

Vice President and Publisher: Linda Duncan
Senior Editor: John Dolan
Developmental Editor: Courtney Sprehe
Publishing Services Manager: Patricia Tannian
Project Manager: John Casey
Designer: Andrea Lutes

Printed in China

Last digit is print number: 9 8 7 6 5 4 3 2

Contributors

Burcu Bayirli, DDS, MS, PhD
Associate Professor
Department of Orthodontics
School of Dentistry
University of Detroit Mercy
Detroit, Michigan

Barry S. Briss, DMD
Professor and Chairman
Department of Orthodontics
Tufts University
School of Dental Medicine
Boston, Massachusetts

Peter H. Buschang, PhD
Professor and Director of Orthodontic Research
Department of Orthodontics
Baylor College of Dentistry
Dallas, Texas

David A. Covell, Jr., DDS, PhD
Associate Professor and Chair
Department of Orthodontics
Oregon Health and Science University
Portland, Oregon

G. Fräns Currier, DDS, MSD, MEd
Professor, Program Director and Chair
Department of Orthodontics
University of Oklahoma
Adjunct Professor of Pediatric Dentistry
Chair, Division of Developmental Dentistry
Department of Orthodontics and Pediatric Dentistry
University of Oklahoma
Oklahoma City, Oklahoma

Cheryl A. DeWood, DDS, MS
Assistant Professor
Department of Graduate Orthodontics
University of Tennessee
Memphis, Tennessee

Thuy-Duong Do-Quang, DDS, MS
Clinical Assistant Professor
Department of Orthodontics
The University of Texas Dental Branch at Houston
Houston, Texas

Jeryl D. English, DDS, MS
Professor, Chairman and Program Director
Department of Orthodontics
The University of Texas Dental Branch at Houston
Houston, Texas

Jaime Gateno, DDS, MD
Professor
Department of Surgery, Oral and Maxillofacial Surgery
Weill Medical College
Cornell University
New York, New York;
Chairman
Department of Oral and Maxillofacial Surgery
The Methodist Hospital Research Institute
Houston, Texas

Peter M. Greco, DMD
Associate Clinical Professor
Department of Orthodontics
University of Pennsylvania
Adjunct Instructor
Department of Oral and Maxillofacial Surgery
Thomas Jefferson University of Hospital
Philadelphia, Pennsylvania

André Haerian, DDS, MS, PhD
Adjunct Clinical Assistant Professor
Department of Orthodontics and Pediatric Dentistry
University of Michigan
Ann Arbor, Michigan

Brody J. Hildebrand, DDS, MS
Assistant Clinical Professor
Department of Graduate Prosthodontics
Baylor College of Dentistry
Dallas, Texas;
International Team for Implantology (ITI)
Basel, Switzerland

Frank Tsung-Ju Hsieh, DDS, MSD
Assistant Professor
Department of Orthodontics
Oregon Health and Science University
Portland, Oregon

Hitesh Kapadia, DDS, PhD
Clinical and Research Assistant Professor
Department of Orthodontics
The University of Texas Dental Branch at Houston
Houston, Texas;
Assistant Professor
Department of Biomedical Sciences
Baylor College of Dentistry
Dallas, Texas

Sunil Kapila, DDS, MS, PhD
Robert W. Browne Endowed Professor and Chair
Department of Orthodontics and Pediatric Dentistry
The University of Michigan
Ann Arbor, Michigan

Chung How Kau, BDS, MScD, MBA, PhD, Morth, RCS (Edin), DSC, RCPS, FFD RCSI (Ortho), FAMS (Ortho)
Associate Professor and Director of the Facial Imaging Facility
Department of Orthodontics
The University of Texas Dental Branch at Houston
Houston, Texas

Richard Kulbersh, DMD, MS
Chairman and Program Director
Department of Orthodontics
School of Dentistry
University of Detroit Mercy
Detroit, Michigan

Steven D. Marshall, DDS, MS
Visiting Associate Professor
Department of Orthodontics
University of Iowa
College of Dentistry
Iowa City, Iowa

Kathleen R. McGrory, DDS, MS
Clinical Director and Clinical Assistant Professor
Department of Orthodontics
The University of Texas Dental Branch at Houston
Houston, Texas

James A. McNamara, Jr., DDS, MS, PhD
Thomas M. and Doris Graber Endowed Professor of Dentistry
Department of Orthodontics and Pediatric Dentistry
School of Dentistry
Professor of Cell and Developmental Biology
School of Medicine
Research Professor
Center for Human Growth and Development
The University of Michigan
Ann Arbor, Michigan

Laurie McNamara, DDS, MS
Adjunct Clinical Lecturer
Department of Orthodontics
University of Michigan
Ann Arbor, Michigan

Peter Ngan, DMD
Professor and Chair
Department of Orthodontics
West Virginia University
Morgantown, West Virginia

Valmy Pangrazio-Kulbersh, DDS, MS
Professor
Department of Orthodontics
School of Dentistry
University of Detroit Mercy
Detroit, Michigan

Timo Peltomäki, DDS, MS, PhD
Professor and Chairman
Clinic for Orthodontics and Pediatric Dentistry
Center for Dental and Oral Medicine
University of Zürich
Zürich, Switzerland

Kate Pham-Litschel, DDS, MS
Research Associate
Clinic for Orthodontics and Pediatric Dentistry
Center for Dental and Oral Medicine
University of Zürich
Zürich, Switzerland

Stephen Richmond, BDS, MScD, PhD, DOrth, RCS (Edin), FDS, RCS (Eng), FDS, MILT
Professor
Department of Dental Health and Biological Sciences
University Dental Hospital
Cardiff University
South Glamorgan, Wales

Christopher S. Riolo, DDS, MS, PhD
Private Practice
Ypsilanti, Michigan

Michael L. Riolo, DDS, MS
Adjunct Professor
Department of Orthodontics
School of Dentistry
University of Detroit Mercy
Detroit, Michigan

P. Emile Rossouw, BSc, BChD, BChD (Hons-Child-Dent), MChD (Ortho), PhD, FRCD(C)
Professor and Chairman
Department of Orthodontics
Baylor College of Dentistry
The Texas A&M University System Health Science Center
Dallas, Texas

Anna Maria Salas-Lopez, DDS, MS
Clinical Associate Professor
Department of Orthodontics
The University of Texas Dental Branch at Houston
Houston, Texas

Marc Schätzle, DDS, MS, PhD
Assistant Professor, Dr. med. dent.
Specialist in Orthodontics
Department of Orthodontics and Pediatric Dentistry
Center for Dental and Oral Medicine
and Cranio-Maxillofacial Surgery
University of Zürich
Zürich, Switzerland

Kirt E. Simmons, DDS, PhD
Assistant Professor of Surgery
Department of Otolaryngology
University of Arkansas for Medical Sciences
Director, Craniofacial Orthodontics
Department of Pediatric Dental Department
Arkansas Children's Hospital
Little Rock, Arkansas

Karin A. Southard, DDS, MS
Professor
Department of Orthodontics
University of Iowa
Iowa City, Iowa

Thomas E. Southard, DDS, MS
Professor and Chair
Department of Orthodontics
University of Iowa
Iowa City, Iowa

John F. Teichgraeber, MD, FACS
Professor
Division of Pediatric Plastic Surgery
Department of Surgery
Medical School
The University of Texas Health Science Center
at Houston
Houston, Texas

Michelle Thornberg, DDS, MS
Adjunct Professor
Department of Orthodontics
School of Dentistry
University of Detroit Mercy
Detroit, Michigan

Angela Marie Tran, DDS, MS
Department of Orthodontics
The University of Texas Dental Branch at Houston
Houston, Texas

Orhan C. Tuncay, DMD
Professor and Chairman
Department of Orthodontics
Kornberg School of Dentistry
Temple University
Philadelphia, Pennsylvania

James L. Vaden, DDS, MS
Professor and Chairman
Department of Orthodontics
University of Tennessee
Memphis, Tennessee

Sam A. Winkelmann, Jr., DDS, MS
Associate Clinical Instructor
Department of Orthodontics
The University of Texas Dental Branch at Houston
Houston, Texas

James J. Xia, MD, PhD, MS
Associate Professor
Department of Surgery, Oral and Maxillofacial
Surgery
Weill Medical College
Cornell University
New York, New York;
Director, Surgical Planning Laboratory
Department of Oral and Maxillofacial Surgery
The Methodist Hospital Research Institute
Houston, Texas

To my orthodontic family—faculty, colleagues, residents, and alumni—for their assistance and encouragement. To my family and especially to my wife, Kathy, whose love, encouragement, and support have helped make this book a reality. JE

I want to thank my wife, Sari, and my children Tuomo, Anna, and Saara for reminding me that there are values more precious than the field of orthodontics. TP

This book is dedicated to my husband and son, Ralph and Erik Litschel.
I am thankful everyday that you are in my life. KL

Preface

As the scope of orthodontics continues to change, so does the knowledge necessary for both the student and the practicing professional. Orthodontics is a clinically driven practice, with the mentorship model using case studies being one of the best ways to learn. *Mosby's Orthodontic Review* seeks not only to answer questions, but also to provide the reader with the knowledge and clinical expertise to achieve successful results for the patient. The reader should understand that there are no "secrets" that make orthodontics easy. Malocclusion presents as a complexity of problems in three tissues and three dimensions. By collecting and analyzing the appropriate data and establishing a correct diagnosis, orthodontists can focus their resources on the correct treatment plan to resolve a patient's malocclusion. We believe this book provides an excellent review of orthodontic concepts, diagnosis, treatment planning, and clinical treatment, as well as providing an update of current clinical information.

WHO IS THE INTENDED AUDIENCE FOR THIS BOOK?

We have written this book for three different segments of the orthodontic community: students and residents, general dentists, and orthodontists.

First, we are targeting senior dental students as they prepare for Part II of the National Board Dental Exam and for their entry into the profession of dentistry. We are also addressing orthodontic residents and recent orthodontic graduates as they prepare for the American Board of Orthodontics (ABO) written and clinical examinations. Second, we intend this book to be helpful for general dentists in their clinical practices and in their discussion of cases with orthodontists. We have included basic cephalometrics so that discussions are easily understood and communicated. Third, the experienced orthodontist who is interested in the scientific advances in orthodontics will find this review text helpful.

WHAT IS UNIQUE ABOUT THE FORMAT OF THIS BOOK?

We have chosen to use a question-answer format for each chapter. With this format, the reader can quickly focus on a specific area of interest to answer a question, such as the indication for removal of third molars, interpretation of 3D images, or how long to wear a bonded lingual 3-3 retainer. Each chapter on treatment or treatment planning is subjective; we wanted expert clinicians to share their thoughts and treatment experiences when correcting various malocclusions. Numerous clinical case reports are presented, incorporating learning around real patient scenarios.

HOW IS THIS BOOK ORGANIZED?

In organizing this book, we begin with basic foundational information first and then delve into more subjective areas of treatment planning and clinical treatment in the later chapters.

Chapter 1 is a review of craniofacial growth and development with current updates based on clinical research. Chapter 2 is a review of the development of the occlusion with a focus on arch development and eruption sequence. Chapter 3 focuses on the indications for orthodontic treatment from the primary dentition to permanent dentition. Chapter 4 addresses orthodontic records and case review. Chapter 5 discusses 3D imaging. Chapter 6 emphasizes the diagnosis of orthodontic problems in three tissues (dental, skeletal, and soft tissue) and in three planes of space (anteroposterior, transverse, and vertical). We have included a 3D-3T Diagnostic Grid to aid in creating a problem list. Diagnosis is objective, but all problems must be listed to avoid something being overlooked. Misdiagnosis is costly when one overlooks or ignores a patient's problem such as periodontal disease.

In Chapters 7 and 8, basic concepts in orthodontic appliances and biomechanics are discussed. The remaining 17 chapters focus on specific areas of orthodontic treatment; these areas are subjective and depend on both the training and experience of the clinician. Areas addressed in these chapters include the Invisalign system, minor tooth movement, implants, hygiene, craniofacial deformities, and more.

WHAT IS ON THE ACCOMPANYING CD-ROM?

Included on the accompanying CD-ROM are six sample orthodontic cases treated by orthodontic residents and written in the format required by the ABO for the Initial Clinical Examination using the required ABO forms (i.e., Discrepancy Index, Cast-Radiograph Evaluation, and Case Management Forms).

Although these cases have not been endorsed by the ABO and are not part of the ABO Clinical Examination, they reflect examples that compare to the requirements for a six-case Initial Clinical Exam or First Recertification Exam. We recommend residency programs use these forms on exit cases and mock board exams given to graduating residents to familiarize them with the required ABO format. These forms can be downloaded from the ABO website, www.americanboardortho.org

Also included is a practice exam taken directly from *Mosby's Review for the NBDE, Part II*. This exam is composed of 70 multiple-choice questions, and rationales are provided with the correct answers. This practice exam is designed to familiarize the student with the format of the NBDE, Part II exam.

WHO ARE THE CONTRIBUTORS, AND WHY WERE THEY ASKED TO PARTICIPATE?

As we are targeting both general dentists and orthodontists for this book, we asked some of the very best clinicians/educators to write chapters. We also included younger faculty members so that their perspectives could be included. These authors understand the needs of prospective students and residents, as well as what information the practicing professional will find useful.

It has been challenging to select the chapter topics and sequence them in a meaningful manner. Writing a book or a chapter in a book demands a great deal of time from the contributors. We appreciate their hard work, especially when faced with publisher deadlines. We are extremely pleased with the contributions to this book. We expected more than was reasonable and got more than we expected. The efforts of these authors are clear in their dedication to clinical excellence.

Note from the editor

I would be remiss if I did not thank Gloria Bailey for her help in typing and formatting the chapters. I would also like to thank the people at Elsevier, especially Courtney Sprehe for her advice and professionalism. This book would not have come to fruition without the contributions and support of my coeditors, Drs. Peltomäki and Pham-Litschel.

I am dedicated to contributing to the education of dental students, orthodontic residents, general dentists, and orthodontists, and I am confident that this book will serve as an excellent teaching resource on orthodontic diagnosis and treatment.

Jeryl D. English

Contents

MOSBY'S ORTHODONTIC REVIEW

Craniofacial Growth and Development

CHAPTER 1

Peter H. Buschang

Clinicians require a basic understanding of growth and development in order to properly plan treatments and evaluate treatment outcomes. As determined by the World Health Organization, growth and development provides one of the best measures available of individuals' health and well-being. Knowledgeable clinicians understand that general somatic growth provides important information about their patients' overall size, maturity status, and growth patterns. Because the timing of maturity events, such as the initiation of adolescent or attainment of peak growth velocity, is coordinated throughout the body, information derived from stature or weight can be applied to the craniofacial complex. In other words, the timing of peak height velocity (PHV)—a noninvasive and relatively easily obtained measure—can be used to determine the timing of peak mandibular growth velocity. Knowledge of general somatic growth is also useful when evaluating the sizes of patients' craniofacial dimensions. An individual's height and weight percentiles provide a measure of overall body size, against which craniofacial measures can be compared. For example, excessively small individuals (i.e., below the 5th percentiles in body size) might also be expected to exhibit a small craniofacial complex. Finally, the reference data available for somatic growth and maturation are based on large representative samples, making them more generally applicable and more precise at the extreme percentiles than available craniofacial reference data.

Postnatal craniofacial growth is a complex, but coordinated, ongoing process. The cranial structures are the most mature and exhibit the smallest relative growth rates, followed by the cranial base, and then the maxillary and mandibular structures, which are the least mature and exhibit the greatest growth potential. Knowledge about a structure's relative growth is important because it serves, along with heritability, as an indicator of its response potential to treatment and other environmental influences. It is essential that clinicians understand that the maxilla and mandible, the two most important skeletal determinants of malocclusion, follow similar growth patterns. Both are displaced anteriorly and, especially, inferiorly; both tend to rotate forward or anteriorly; both rotate transversely; and both respond to displacement and rotation by characteristic patterns of growth and cortical drift. It is also useful to understand that patients should be expected to adapt skeletally to orthodontic, orthopedic, and surgical interventions and that the adaptations mimic growth patterns exhibited by untreated patients. Perhaps most importantly, clinicians must understand the tremendous therapeutic potential that the eruption and drift of teeth provide. The maxillary molars and incisors, for example, undergo more eruption than inferior displacement of the maxilla, making them ideally suited for controlling vertical and AP growth.

Clinicians also often do not appreciate that adults show many of the same growth patterns exhibited by children and adolescents, simply in less exaggerated forms. It has been well established that craniofacial growth continues though the 20s and 30s, and perhaps beyond. Skeletal growth of adults appears to be predominately vertical in nature, with forward mandible rotation in males and backward rotation in females. The teeth continue to erupt and compensate depending on the individual's growth patterns. Adults also exhibit important soft tissue changes; the nose grows disproportionately and the lips flatten. Vertical relationships between the incisors and lips should also be expected to change with increasing age.

Finally, malocclusion must be considered as a multifactorial developmental process. Although genes have been linked with the development of Class III and perhaps Class II division 2 malocclusions, the most prevalent forms of malocclusions are largely environmentally determined. Equilibrium theory and the notion of dentoalveolar compensations provide the conceptual basis for understanding how closely linked tooth positions are with the surrounding soft tissues. They also make it possible to predict the type of compensations that should be expected. For example, they explain why the development of malocclusion is associated with various habits, assuming the habits occur regularly and are of long enough duration. In fact, anything that alters mandibular posture might be expected to elicit skeletal and dentoalveolar compensations. This explains why individuals with chronic airway obstructions develop skeletal and dental malocclusions that are phenotypically similar to malocclusions associated with weak craniofacial musculature; both populations of patients posture their mandibles similarly and undergo similar dentoalveolar and skeletal compensations. Based on the foregoing, the following questions are intended to provide a basic—although only partial—understanding of growth and development and its application to clinical practice.

1. At what ages do most children enter adolescence, and when do they attain PHV?

The adolescence growth spurt starts when decelerating childhood growth rates change to accelerating rates. During the first part of the growth spurt, statural growth velocities increase steadily until peak height velocity (PHV) is attained. Longitudinal assessments provide the best indicators of when adolescence is initiated and PHV is attained. Longitudinal studies pertaining to North American and European children[1] show that girls are advanced by approximately 2 years compared with boys in the age of initiation of adolescence and age of PHV. Based on the 26 independent samples of girls and 23 samples of boys, the average ages of PHV are 11.9 and 14.0 years, respectively. Girls and boys initiate adolescence at 9.4 years and 11.2 years, respectively. Maximum adolescent growth velocity in body weight usually occurs 0.3 to 0.5 year after PHV (Fig. 1-1).

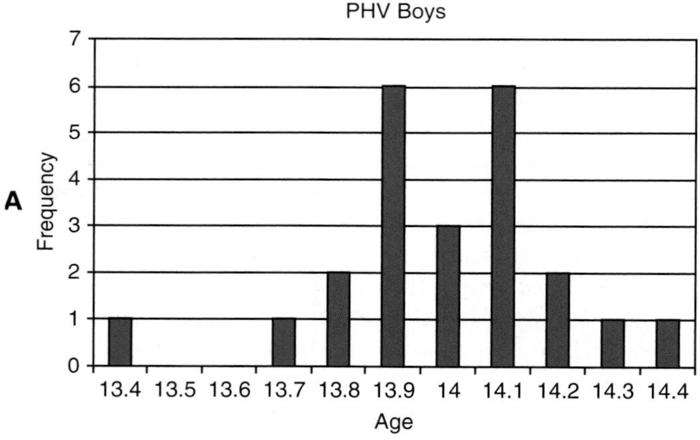

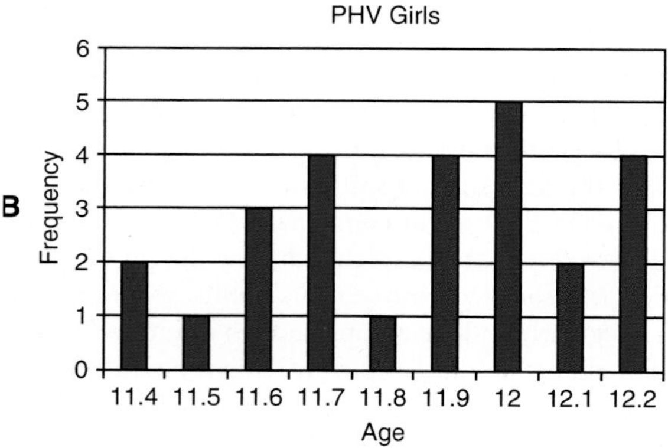

FIG 1-1 Frequency distribution of 26 sample ages of PHV for boys **(A)** and girls **(B)**. (From Malina RM, Bouchard C, Beunen G. *Ann Rev Anthropol* 1988;17:187-219.)

2. What is the mid-growth spurt, and how does it apply to craniofacial growth?

The mid-growth spurt refers to the increase in growth velocity that occurs in some, but not all, children several years before the initiation of the adolescent growth spurt. Mid-growth spurts in stature and weight have been reported to occur between 6.5 and 8.5 years of age; they tend to occur more frequently in boys than girls.[2,3] Based on yearly velocities, mid-growth spurts have been demonstrated for a variety of craniofacial dimensions—also between 6.5 and 8.5 years of age—occurring simultaneously or slightly earlier for girls than boys.[4-7] Applying mathematic models to large longitudinal samples, Buschang and colleagues[8] reported mid-growth spurts in mandibular growth for subjects with Class I and Class II molar relationships at approximately 7.7 years and 8.7 years of age for girls and boys, respectively.

3. Which skeletal indicators are most closely associated with PHV?

According to Grave and Brown,[9] PHV in males and females occurs slightly after the appearance of the ulnar sesamoid and the hooking of the hamate, and slightly before capping of the third middle phalanx, the capping of the first proximal phalanx, and the capping of the radius. According to Fishman's[10] skeletal maturity indicators, capping of the distal phalanx of the 3rd finger occurs less than 1 year before PHV, capping of the middle phalanx of the 3rd finger occurs just after PHV, and capping of the middle phalanx of the 5th finger occurs less than one half year after PHV. Based on the cervical vertebrae, PHV occurs between the development of the concavity on the inferior borders of the 2nd and 3rd vertebrae (CVMS II) and development of a concavity on the inferior borders of the 2nd, 3rd, and 4th vertebrae (CVMS III).[11]

4. What is the equilibrium theory of tooth position?

Although Brodie[12] was among the first to identify the relationship between muscles and tooth position, it was Weinstein and colleagues[13] who experimentally established that the teeth are maintained in a state of equilibrium between the soft tissue forces. Based on a series of experiments, they concluded that:

1. The forces (produced naturally or by orthodontic appliances) exerted on the crowns of teeth are sufficient to cause tooth movements
2. Each tooth may have more than one stable state of equilibrium
3. Even small forces (3–7 gm), if applied over a long enough period, can cause tooth movements

Proffit,[14] who revisited the equilibrium theory 15 years later, noted that the primary factors involved were:

1. The resting pressures of the lips, cheeks, and tongue
2. The eruptive forces produced by metabolic activity within the periodontal membrane

He further noted that extrinsic pressures, such as habits and orthodontic forces, can alter equilibrium, provided that they are sustained for at least 6 hours each day. Proffit[14] also identified head posture and growth displacements/rotations as secondary factors determining equilibrium. As the mandible rotates, the incisors move as dental equilibrium is reestablished. Björk and Skieller,[15] for example, have shown an association between changes in lower incisor angulation and true mandibular rotation.

5. What is the prevalence of Class II dental malocclusion among adolescents and young adults living in the United States?

The best direct epidemiologic evidence comes from the National Health Survey,[16,17] which evaluated approximately 7400 children between 6 and 11 years of age and over 22,000 youths 12 to 17 years of age. Unilateral and bilateral distoclusion occurs approximately 16.1% and 22.7% of the time among Caucasian children and 7.6% and 6.0% of the time among African-American children, respectively. Comparable incidences among Caucasian youths were 17.8% and 15.8% and 12.0% and 6.0% among African-American youths. Based on overjet provided by the NHANES III, Proffit and associates[18] estimated that the prevalence of Class II malocclusion (overjet ≥ 5 mm) decreases from over 15.6% between 12 and 17 years of age to 13.4% for adults. They also showed that Class II malocclusion is more prevalent among African-Americans (16.5%) than Caucasians (14.2%) and Hispanics (9.1%).

6. What is the prevalence of incisor crowding among individuals living in the United States, and how does it change with age?

According to the initial NHANES III data,[19] incisor irregularities increase from an average of 1.6 mm for children 8 to 11 years, to 2.5 mm for youths 12 to 17 years, to 2.8 mm for adults 18 to 50 years of age. Although incidences are similar at the youngest age, African-American youths and adults show significantly less crowding than Caucasians and Hispanics. Based on the complete NHANES data set, including 9044 individuals between 15 and 50 years of age, approximately 39.5% of U.S. adults have mandibular incisor irregularities ≥ 4 mm and 16.8% have irregularities ≥ 7.[20] Adult males tend to show greater crowding than females; Hispanics show greater crowding than Caucasians, who in turn display greater crowding than African-Americans. Based on the available data for untreated subjects followed longitudinally, rates of crowding increase precipitously between 15 and 50 years of age, especially during the late teens and early 20s (Fig. 1-2).[20]

7. Do the third molars play a role in determining crowding?

Although third molars have been related with crowding,[21-24] most contemporary studies show little or no relationship. A NIH conference in 1979 came to the consensus that there is little or no justification for extracting third molars solely to minimize present or future crowding of the lower anterior teeth.[25] Ades and co-workers[26] found no difference in subjects whose third molars were impacted, erupted in function,

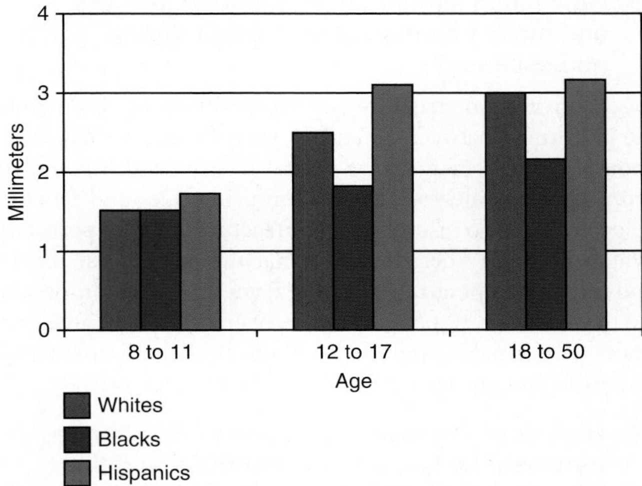

FIG 1-2 Average mandibular alignment scores, U.S. persons, 1988-1991. (Adapted from Brunelle JA, Bhat M, Lipton JA. *J Dental Res* 1996;75[special issue]:706-713.)

congenitally absent, or extracted at least 10 years before post-retention records were taken. Sampson and colleagues[27] also showed no difference in crowding between subjects whose third molars have erupted completely or partially, remained impacted, or were missing. A randomized controlled trial based on 77 patients followed for 66 months showed a 1.0 mm difference in anterior crowding between patients whose third molars had and had not been removed; the authors concluded that removal of third molars to reduce or prevent late crowding cannot be justified.[28] Based on the NHANES data, individuals who had erupted third molars displayed significantly less crowding than those who did not have erupted third molars.[20]

8. How does horizontal and vertical mandibular growth affect crowding?

Vertical growth makes the maintenance of lower incisor alignment after orthodontic treatment more problematic. Based on the notion that the lower incisors are carried into the lower lip as the mandibula grows anteriorly or rotates downwards, late mandibular growth has been suggested as a major contributor to post-retention crowding.[29] Although incisor compensation to backward mandibular rotation has been demonstrated,[15] crowding as a result of anterior growth displacements remains to be established. However, changes in lower incisor crowding have been shown to be related to vertical growth. Both treated and untreated patients who undergo greater inferior growth displacements of the mandible and associated greater eruption of the lower incisors show greater crowding than those who undergo less vertical growth and less eruption.[30,31] Since vertical mandibular growth continues well beyond the teen years, patients would be well advised to wear their retainers into their early and mid-20s.

9. How much should the mandibular incisors and molars be expected to erupt during adolescence?

Based on natural structure superimpositions of the mandible performed between 10 and 15 years of age, McWhorter[32] showed that the mandibular central incisors and first molars erupt approximately 4.3 and 2.5 mm in males and females, respectively. Also using natural structure superimpositions, Watanabe et al.[33] demonstrated that the mandibular molars and incisors erupt at rates ranging from 0.4 to 1.2 mm/yr and 0.3 to 0.9 mm/yr, respectively. Rates of eruption were greater in males than females, attaining peak velocities at approximately 12 and 14 years of age for females and males, respectively.

10. How does untreated arch perimeter change between the late primary dentition and the permanent dentition?

Computed based on a centenary curve extending from the mesial of the first molar to mesial of first molar,[34] arch perimeter increases during the early mixed dentition and decreases during and after the transition to the permanent dentition. Maxillary perimeter increases 4 to 5 mm between 6 and 11 years of age and decreases 3 to 4 mm between 11 and 16 years. In contrast, mandibular arch perimeter increases approximately 2 to 3 mm initially and then decreases 4 to 7 mm, with greater decreases in females than males (Fig. 1-3).

11. How do untreated maxillary and mandibular intermolar widths change during childhood and adolescence?

Bishara and colleagues[35] reported that intermolar widths increase 7 to 8 mm between the deciduous dentition (5.0 yrs of age) and the early mixed (8.0 yrs of age) dentitions and an additional 1 to 2 mm between the early mixed and early permanent (12.5 yrs of age) dentitions. Between 6 (first molar fully erupted) and 16 years of age, Moyers and colleagues[34] showed greater increases for males than females for both maxillary (4.1 versus 3.7 mm) and mandibular (2.6 versus 1.5 mm) intermolar widths. Based on a sample of 26 subjects followed longitudinally between 12 and 26 years of age, DeKock[36] reported no significant change for females and only slight increases (1.4 and 0.9 mm for maxilla and mandible, respectively) in intermolar width for males (Fig 1-4).

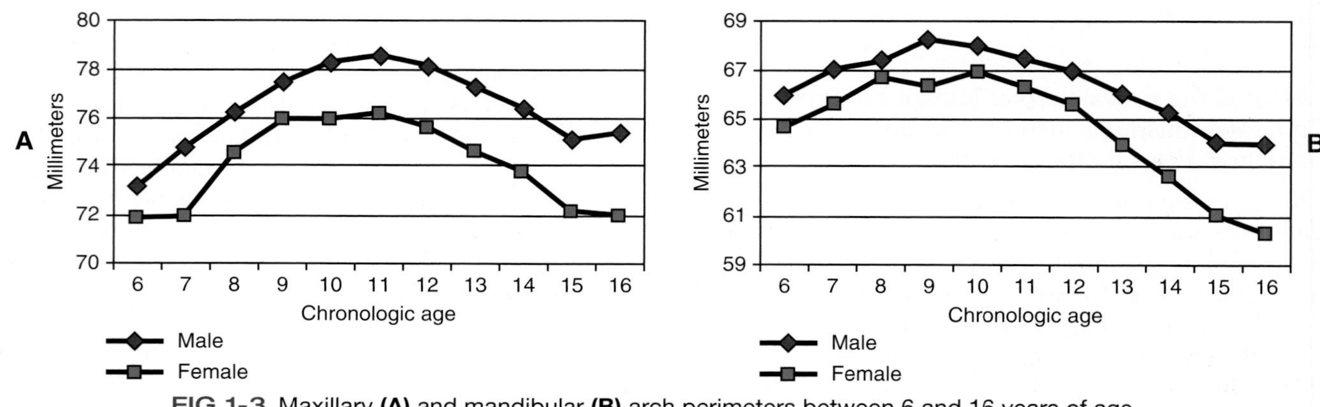

FIG 1-3 Maxillary **(A)** and mandibular **(B)** arch perimeters between 6 and 16 years of age. (Adapted from Moyers RE, van der Linden FPGM, Riolo ML, McNamara JA Jr. Standards of human occlusal development. Monograph #5, Craniofacial Growth Series, Center for Human Growth and Development, University of Michigan, Ann Arbor, Michigan, 1976.)

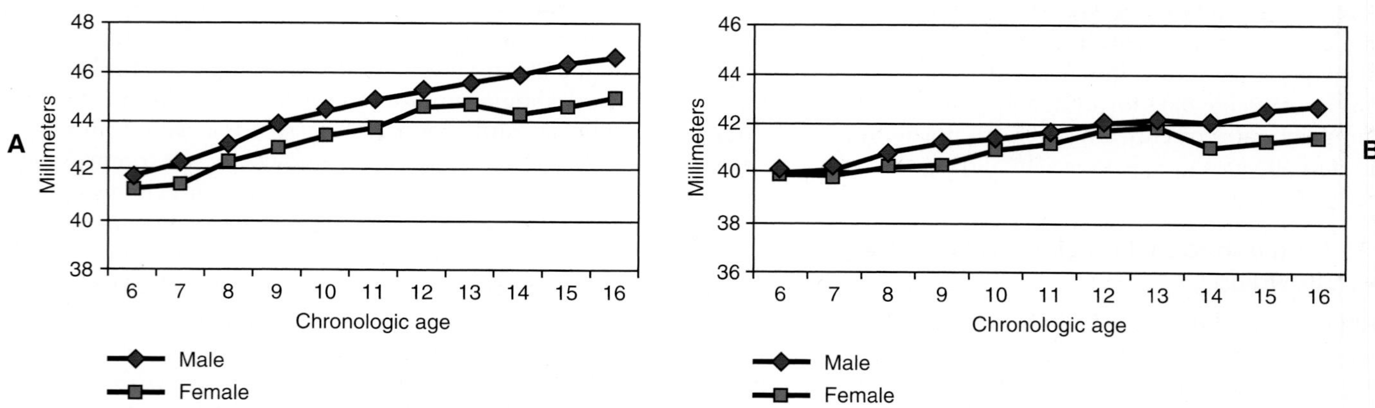

FIG 1-4 Maxillary **(A)** and mandibular **(B)** intermolar widths between 6 and 16 years of age. (Adapted from Moyers RE, van der Linden FPGM, Riolo ML, McNamara JA Jr. Standards of human occlusal development. Monograph #5, Craniofacial Growth Series, Center for Human Growth and Development, University of Michigan, Ann Arbor, Michigan, 1976.)

12. Without treatment, how do maxillary and mandibular arch depths change during childhood and adolescence?

Maxillary and mandibular arch depths, midline distances between a line tangent to the incisors, and a line drawn tangent to the distal crown of the deciduous second molars or their permanent successors show different patterns of growth changes. Maxillary arch depth increases 1.4 and 0.9 mm in males and females, respectively, during the eruption of the permanent incisors.[37] Mandibular arch depth shows little change over the same period. With the loss of the deciduous molars, maxillary arch depth decreases 1.5 and 1.9 mm, while mandibular arch depth decreases 1.8 and 1.7 mm in males and females, respectively.[37] DeKock[36] reported decreases (approximately 3.0 mm) in arch depth between 12 and 26 years of age, with rates diminishing over time. Based on subjects with normal occlusion, Bishara and co-workers[35] showed increases (1.1–1.8 mm) in arch depth between the deciduous and early mixed dentitions; between the mixed and early permanent dentition, maxillary arch depths increased only slightly (0.5–0.7 mm) and mandibular depths decreased 2.6 to 3.3 mm (Fig. 1-5).

13. How do untreated maxillary and mandibular intercanine widths change over time?

During the transition from the deciduous to permanent incisors, intercanine width increases approximately 3 mm.[37] Maxillary intercanine width shows a second phase of increase (approximately 1.5 mm) with the emergence of the permanent canines; mandibular intercanine widths decrease slightly after the emergence of the permanent canine.[37] Bishara and co-workers[35] also reported increases in maxillary and mandibular intercanine widths between the deciduous and early mixed dentition; mandibular intercanine widths increased or decreased slightly between the early mixed and early permanent dentitions. Intercanine widths of children followed by the University School Growth Study, Michigan,[34] increased approximately 3.0 mm between 6 and 9 years of age; maxillary widths increased an additional 2.5 mm with the emergence of the permanent canine (Fig. 1-6).

14. What differences exist in arch widths between subjects with normal and Class II malocclusion?

Lux and colleagues[38] reported that maxillary and mandibular arch intermolar widths are significantly smaller in subjects with Class II division 1 malocclusion than subjects with Class I

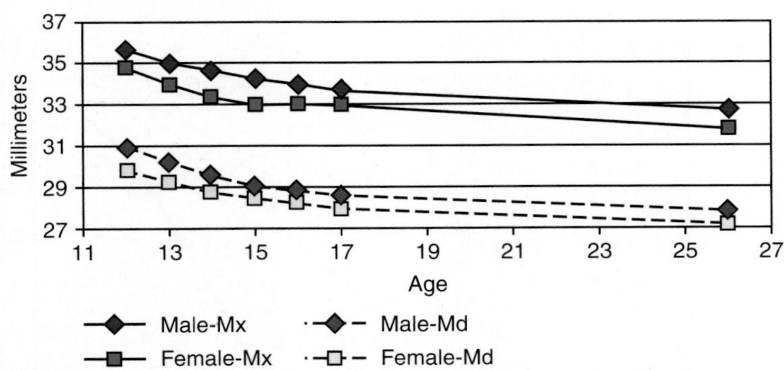

FIG 1-5 Maxillary *(Mx)* and mandibular *(Md)* molar arch depths between 11 and 27 years of age. (Adapted from DeKock WH: *Am J Orthod* 1972;62:56-66.)

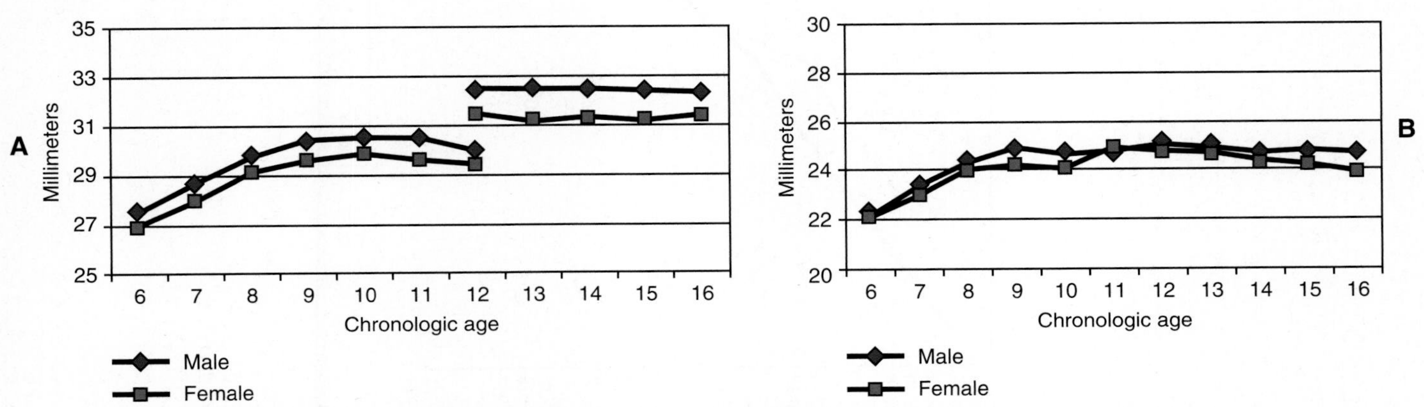

FIG 1-6 Maxillary **(A)** and mandibular **(B)** intercanine width between 6 and 16 years of age. (Adapted from Moyers RE, van der Linden FPGM, Riolo ML, McNamara JA Jr. Standards of human occlusal development. Monograph #5, Craniofacial Growth Series, Center for Human Growth and Development, University of Michigan, Ann Arbor, Michigan, 1976.)

malocclusion and normal occlusion; arches of subjects with Class II division 2 malocclusion were narrower than widths of subjects with normal occlusion and closely approximate subjects with Class I malocclusion. The group differences were apparent at 7 years of age and persistent through 15 years of age. Bishara and co-workers'[35] cross-sectional comparisons also showed that maxillary and mandibular intermolar widths were significantly larger in males with normal occlusion than in males with malocclusion. Comparing arch shape of subjects with Class I and Class II malocclusions, Buschang et al.[39] showed that subjects with Class II division 2 malocclusion have the shortest and widest maxillary arches, whereas subjects with Class II division 1 have the longest and narrowest maxillary arches.

15. Which craniofacial structures might be expected to be the least mature and show the greatest relative growth between 5 and 17 years of age?

Differences in the relative growth of the craniofacial structures have long been established. Hellman,[40] who was among the first to quantify relative growth, showed that at any given age, cranial widths are more mature than cranial depths, which are in turn more mature than cranial heights. Until the 1970s, growth of the splanchnocranium and neurocranium was categorized based on Scammon's[41] typology and was thought to follow either a general (i.e., somatic) or neural pattern. Baughan and co-workers[42] introduced three distinct growth patterns: a cranial pattern for the cranium and cranial base, a facial pattern for the maxilla and mandible, and a general pattern for the long bones of the body. Buschang and colleagues[43] demonstrated that the craniofacial complex is actually intergraded between Scammon's neural and general growth curves. Accordingly, relative craniofacial growth and maturation cannot be neatly categorized; it follows a developmental gradient moving from the more mature measures, such as head height (b-br; the most mature that they evaluated) through anterior cranial base (S-N), posterior cranial base (S-B), maxillary length (Ans-Pns), upper facial height (N-Ans), corpus length (Go-Gn), and ramus height (Ar-Go). After 9 to 10 years of age, ramus height is actually less mature than stature; it has approximately 10% of its growth remaining in boys 15.5 years of age (Fig. 1-7).

16. What sex differences exist in facial heights during childhood and adolescence?

Facial heights are 1% to 10% larger in males than females during childhood and adolescence. Sex differences during childhood are small but statistically significant.[44,45] Differences decrease slightly as females enter their adolescent phase of growth and then increase substantially after males enter adolescence. Male and female ratios

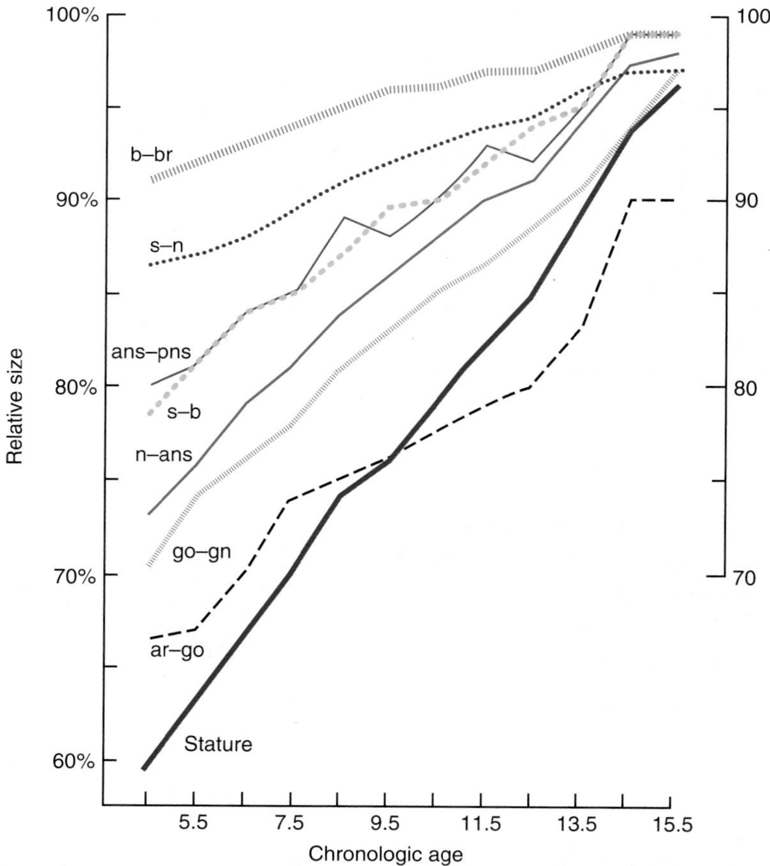

FIG 1-7 Relative (percentage of adult) size of seven craniofacial measures and stature for boys 4.5 to 15.5 years of age. (Adapted from Buschang PH, Baume RM, Nass GG: *Am J Phys Anthrop* 1983;61:373-381.)

of total anterior facial height to total posterior facial height remain similar throughout childhood and adolescence (Fig. 1-8).

17. What sex differences exist in mandibular size and position during childhood and adolescence?

During childhood, males exhibit significantly larger overall mandibular size (Co-Pg) than females, primarily due to increased corpus length (Co-Pg). Sex differences in ramus height (Co-Go) are small and do not become statistically significant until adolescence.[44,45] Sex difference in the Y-axis (N-S-Gn), the gonial angle (Co-Go-Me) and mandibular plane angles (S-N/Go-Me) are not statistically significant during childhood or adolescence (Fig. 1-9).

18. What craniofacial features characterize the morphology of hyperdivergent (skeletal open-bite) patients?

Compared with patients with Class I normal occlusion, hyperdivergent patients display decreased posterior-to-anterior face heights ratios, smaller upper-to-lower facial height ratios, and increased mandibular, gonial and palatal planes.[46-50] Associated with increased lower face heights and steeper mandibular plane angles, patients with hyperdivergent tendencies demonstrate excessive dentoalveolar heights in both the maxilla and mandible.[22,48,49,51,52] Children 6 to 12 years of age with high mandibular plane angles undergo significantly less true and apparent forward rotation than children with low MP-SN angles.[53]

19. How much change is expected in AP maxillomandibular relationships of Caucasians during adolescence?

The University of Michigan's mixed-longitudinal study of 83 untreated subjects[45] showed a 1- to 1.1-degree decrease of the ANB angle and a 3- to 3.1-degree decrease in N-A-Pg between 10 and 15 years of age. Adolescents followed by the Philadelphia Center for Research in Child Growth[54] demonstrated a decrease of 1.3 and 3.6 degrees for ANB and N-A-Pg angles, respectively, in males; these two measures decreased less than a degree in females between 10 and 15 years of age. The growth study conducted by King's College School of Medicine and Dentistry in London[44] showed a 0.5- to 0.8-degree decrease

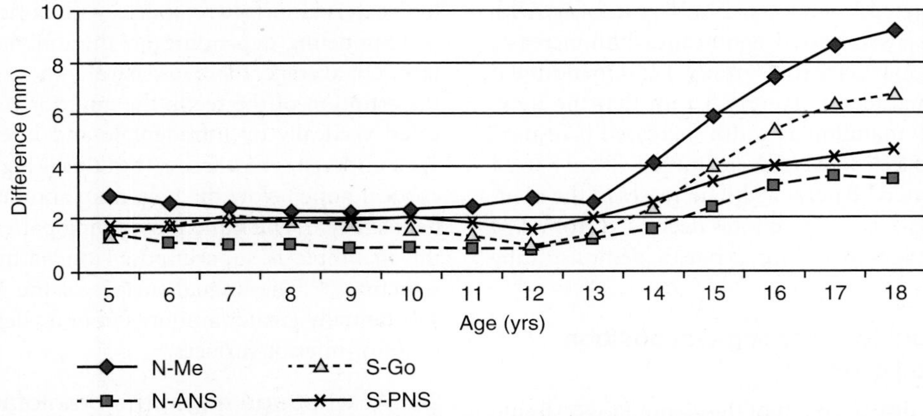

FIG 1-8 **Sex differences (male minus female) in facial heights.** (Modified from Bhatia SN, Leighton BC. *A manual of facial growth: a computer analysis of longitudinal cephalometric growth data.* New York: Oxford University Press, 1993.)

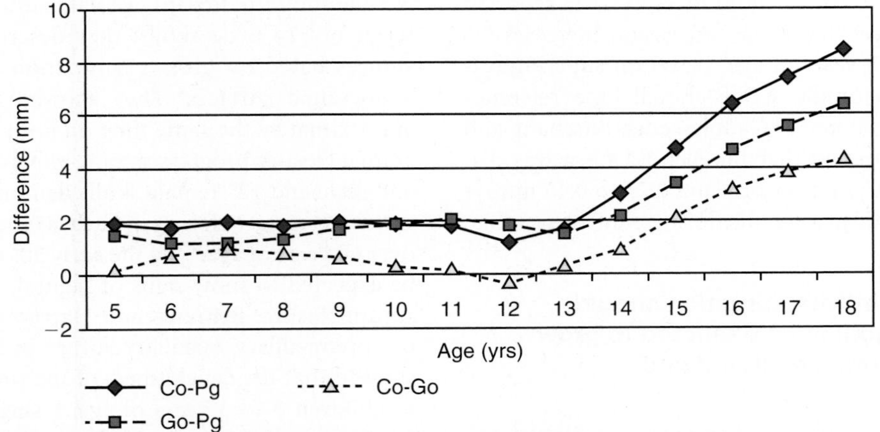

FIG 1-9 **Sex differences (male minus female) in mandibular size.** (Modified from Bhatia SN, Leighton BC. *A manual of facial growth: a computer analysis of longitudinal cephalometric growth data.* New York: Oxford University Press, 1993.)

of ANB and 2 to 3 degrees of decrease of N-A-Pg between 10 and 15 years of age. Untreated French-Canadian males and females between 10 and 15 years show 0.6- and 0.2-degree decreases of the ANB angle, respectively.[55] Although the average changes are small, individual variation is large, with approximately 30% and 26% of 10-year-olds classified as prognathic and retrognathic, respectively, changing to orthognathic by 15 years of age. Similarly, approximately 30% who are orthognathic at 10 years of age become either prognathic or retrognathic at 15 years.[55]

20. Does the mandible undergo transverse rotation like the maxilla? If so, how are the two related?

Björk and Skieller[56] showed that posterior maxillary implant widths increased approximately 0.4 mm/yr between 4 and 20 years of age. This compares well with the findings of Korn and Baumrind,[57] who reported increases of 0.43 mm/yr in the posterior-most region of the maxilla for children 8.5 to 15.5 years of age. Korn and Baumrind[57]were also the first to document transverse widening of the mandible based on metallic bone markers; they showed that the mandible widened 0.28 mm/yr or approximately 65% as much as the maxillary. Gandini and Buschang,[58] who evaluated 25 subjects 12 to 18 years of age with bone markers in both jaws, showed significant width increases between the posterior maxillary (0.27 mm/yr) and mandibular (0.19 mm/yr) bone markers. For every 1 mm that the maxillary width increased, mandibular width increased 0.70 mm. Iseri and Solow,[59] who followed children annually from 8 to 16 years of age, also reported bilateral width increases of the mandibular body in all subjects. Annual rates decreased from 0.34 mm/yr at the younger ages to 0.11 mm/yr at 15, demonstrating a clear age effect.

21. Does the glenoid fossa change its position during postnatal growth?

Inferior and posterior displacement of the glenoid fossa should be expected to occur along with growth at the spheno-occipital synchondrosis, elongation of the posterior cranial base, and associated displacement of the temporal bone.[60] Using articulare as a surrogate measure of the glenoid fossa, Björk[61] reported that the distance between the fossa and nasion increases 7.5 mm between 12 and 20 years of age. Based on superimpositions performed on naturally stable cranial base reference structures of 118 children and 155 adolescents, Buschang and Santos-Pinto[62] demonstrated that the glenoid fossa was displaced 0.45 to 0.53 mm/yr posteriorly and 0.25 to 0.45 mm/yr inferiorly, with greater displacements during adolescence than childhood.

22. How much and in what direction should condylion and gonion be expected to grow and remodel during childhood and adolescence?

The condyle grows superiorly and slightly posteriorly, whereas gonion drifts superiorly and posteriorly in approximately equal amounts. Björk and Skieller's[15] implant studies showed that, depending on the type of true rotation that occurs, the condyle is capable of growing in both anterior (forward rotators) and posterior directions (backward rotators). Also using metallic implants for superimposing, Baumrind and colleagues[63] demonstrated that the condyle grows predominately in a superior (2.5 mm/yr) and slightly posterior (0.3 mm/yr) direction between 8.5 and 15.5 years of age; gonion drifts superiorly (0.9 mm/yr) and posteriorly (1.0 mm/yr) at similar rates. Using naturally stable mandibular reference structures for superimpositions, Buschang and Santos-Pinto[62] reported 2.3 to 2.7 mm/yr superior and 0.2 to 0.3 mm/yr posterior growth of the condyle for large samples of children 6 to 15 years of age. Peak adolescent condylar growth velocities approximated 3.1 mm/yr (at 14.3 years) and 2.3 mm/yr (at 12.2 years) for males and females, respectively.[64]

23. How does the bony chin remodel during childhood and adolescence?

Relative to metallic bone markers inserted into the mandible, each of the 21 cases evaluated by Björk and Skieller[15] demonstrate stability (i.e., lack of remodeling) of the cortical region located slightly above pogonion. The remainder of the mandible's external surface remodels, with both the type and amount of remodeling depending on the individual's rotational pattern. On average, there is vertical bone growth associated with the eruption of the teeth; the anterior cortical region demarcated vertically by infradentale and inferiorly by the incisor apex undergoes resorption (but this is highly variable), and the cortical bone below the pogonion and below the symphysis is depository.[63] The same remodeling patterns are evident when the mandible is superimposed on naturally stable reference structures.[65] The lingual surface of the symphysis undergoes substantially greater amounts of bony deposition than the anterior or inferior surfaces.

24. At what age might the craniofacial sutures be expected to start closing?

The age at which sutural closure begins is variable and depends largely on how closure is measured. Todd and Lyon[66] were among the first to evaluate sutural closure. Based on a series of 514 male skulls, they described the closure of the sutures based on gross examination of the ectocranial and endocranial surfaces. They showed that closure begins at approximately the same time on both surfaces, but that ectocranial closure progresses more slowly. Gross examination of 538 male and 127 female skulls demonstrated that the cranial sutures can start closing as early as the late teens or as late as over 60 years of age.[67] By the early 30s or 40s, most people can be expected to show signs of sagittal, coronal, and lambdoid suture closure. Behrents and Harris[68] identified remnants of the premaxillary-maxillary suture in 50 subadult skulls and showed that the facial aspect of the suture was already closed in children 3 to 5 years of age. Using stained sections from 24 subjects, Persson and Thilander[69] reported that closure of the midpalatal and transverse sutures can begin as early as 15 years of age but can be delayed in some individuals into the late 20s or early 30s. Based on histological and microradiographic evaluations of growth activity, Melsen[70] showed that the midpalatal sutures showed evidence of growth through 16 years of age in girls and 18 years of age in boys. Kokich's[71] histological, radiographic, and gross examinations of 61 individuals showed no evidence of bony union of the frontozygomatic suture before 70 years of age (Table 1-1).

25. How much does lip length and thickness change during childhood and adolescence?

Subtelny[72] showed that upper and lower lip lengths increase similarly (approximately 4.5 mm) and progressively between 6 and 15 years of age. After full eruption of the central incisors, the vertical relationship of the maxillary incisor and upper lip is maintained through 18 years of age. Vig and Cohen,[73] who measured upper and lower lip heights relative to the palatal and mandibular planes, respectively, reported increases of approximately 5 mm for the upper and 9 mm for the lower lip between 5 and 15 years of age. Subtelny[72] also showed that increases in lip thickness were considerably greater in the vermilion regions than in the regions overlying skeletal structures. During the first 18 years of life, upper lip thickness at Point A increased approximately 7.8 and 6.5 mm in males and females, respectively. Nanda et al.[74] showed that upper lip length ($Sn\text{-}Sto_{upper}$) increased 2.7 mm (males) and 1.1 mm (females) between 7 and 18 years of age; lower lip length ($ILS\text{-}Sto_{lower}$) increased 4.3 mm in males and 1.5 mm in females.

26. Does the soft-tissue facial profile change during childhood and adolescence?

The changes that occur depend on whether or not the nose is included when measuring the soft-tissue profile. Subtelny[72] reported that total facial convexity (N′-Pr-Pog′) decreased 5 to 6 degrees between 6 and 15 years of age; soft-tissue profile (N′-Sn-Pog′) showed little or no change over the same time period. Bishara et al.[75] showed that the angle of total facial convexity (Gl′-Pr-Pog′) decreased approximately 7 degrees between 6 and 15 years of age. In contrast, the angle of facial convexity, which does not include the nose, maintained or increased slightly.

27. How does the nose change shape during childhood and adolescence?

It was originally reported that the "hump" on the nasal dorsum develops during the adolescent growth spurt,[72] and that nasal shape changes were due to the elevation of the nasal bone.[76] Similar types of shape changes actually take place during childhood (6–10 yrs) and adolescence (10–14 yrs).[77] The upper portion of the dorsum rotates upward and forward (counterclockwise) approximately 10 degrees between 6 and 14 years of age. The lower dorsum shows both downward and backward (clockwise) and upward and forward (counterclockwise) rotation, depending on the relative vertical/horizontal growth changes of the midface.[77] Changes in the nasal dorsum are more closely associated with angular changes of the lower dorsum than of the upper dorsum.

28. According to present evidence, when does growth of the craniofacial skeleton cease?

Behrents[78] reported both size and shape changes in adults. Based on 70 distances and 69 angular measures, he showed growth changes after 17 years of age for 91% of the distances and 70% of the angular measures evaluated. 80% of the distances and 41% of the angles showed growth changes after 30 years of age; 61% and 28% of the distances and angles, respectively, showed growth changes after 35 years of age. Lewis and Roche,[79] who evaluated 20 adults followed between 17 and 50 years of age, showed that cranial base lengths (S-N, Ba-N, Ba-S) and mandibular lengths (Ar-Go, Go-Gn, Ar-Gn) attained their maximum lengths between 29 and 39 years of age, after which they shortened slightly.

29. How does the mandible rotate during adulthood?

Behrents[78] reported that the mandible rotates in a counterclockwise manner in adult males and clockwise in adult females, with associated compensatory alterations of the dentition. He also showed that the Y-axis (N-S-Gn) decreases slightly in males and does not change in females. Relative to the PM vertical, the mandible comes forward in adult males (approximately 2 mm), but not in females. The mandibular plane angle (S-N/Go-Gn) decreases in males and increases in females. Behrents also showed

TABLE 1-1 Estimated Ages for the Initiation of Sutural Closure

REFERENCES	SUTURE	MALES	FEMALES
Todd and Lyon[66]	Sagittal & sphenofrontal	22	N/A
Todd and Lyon[66]	Coronal	24	N/A
Todd and Lyon[66]	Lambdoidal & occiptomastoid	26	N/A
Todd and Lyon[66]	Sphenoparietal	29	N/A
Todd and Lyon[66]	Sphenotemporal, maso-occipital	30–31	N/A
Todd and Lyon[66]	Squamosal, parietomastoid	37	N/A
Sahni et al.[67]	Sagittal	31–35	41–45
Sahni et al.[67]	Coronal	31–35	31–35
Sahni et al.[67]	Lambdoid	41–45	31–35
Behrents and Harris[68]	Premaxillary-maxillary	3–5	3–5
Persson and Thilander[69]	Midpalatal & transpalatal	20–25	20–25
Melsen[70]	Midpalatal & transpalatal	15–16	17–18
Kokich[71]	Frontozygomatic	80s	80s

greater posterior vertical development of the mandible in adult males than adult females. Bishara et al.[80] showed that adult males 25 to 46 years of age undergo greater increases of SNB and S-N-Pg than females, whereas females undergo significant increases of N-S-Gn. Forsberg et al.[81] reported an increase (0.3 mm) of the mandibular plane angle in males and females between 25 and 45 years of age.

30. What generally happens to the nose during adulthood?

The nose develops substantially during adulthood, with the tip growing forward and downward an average of 3 mm after 17 years of age.[78] Individual adults can exhibit much greater amounts of nasal growth. Males display significantly more nasal growth than females. Formby et al.[82] showed that nose height increases 0.6 mm, nose length increases 1.7 mm, and nose depth increases 2.3 mm between 18 and 42 years of age. Between 21 and 26 years of age, Sarnas and Solow[83] demonstrated 0.8- to 1.0-mm increases in nose length.

31. What generally happens to the upper lip length during adulthood?

Upper lip length increases 0.5 to 0.6 mm between 21 and 26 years of age.[83] Over the same period, upper incisor display (Sto-OP_{max}) decreases slightly (0.3 mm) in males and does not change in females. Formby et al.[82] showed that upper lip length increases 0.8 to 1.7 mm and upper incisor display (lip to incisal edge) decreases 1.0 mm between 18 and 42 years of age. Behrents[78] demonstrated that upper lip length (ANS-Sto) increases significantly in both males (2.8 mm) and females (2.2 mm), whereas the maxillary incisor to palatal plane distance increases only 0.06 to 0.08 mm after 17 years of age, thereby supporting an even greater decrease in upper incisor display.

32. How does the soft-tissue profile change during adulthood?

Sarnas and Solow[83] showed that the soft-tissue profile angle (including the nose) increased (0.3 degree) in males and decreased (0.4 degree) in females between 21 and 26 years of age. Behrents[78] provides the best longitudinal data demonstrating a straightening and flattening of the soft-tissue lip profile during adulthood. The lips become substantially less pronounced with increasing age.[78,80,81] The perpendicular distances of the upper and lower lips relative to the soft tissue plane (SLS-ILS) decreased approximately 1 mm in adults; angular changes indicate approximately 4 to 6 degrees flattening of the lips.[78]

REFERENCES

1. Malina RM, Bouchard C, Beunen G: Human growth: selected aspects of current research on well-nourished children. *Ann Rev Anthropol* 1988;17:187-219.
2. Tanner JM, Cameron N: Investigation of the mid-growth spurt in height, weight and limb circumference in single year velocity data from the London 1966-67 growth survey. *Ann Human Biol* 1980;7:565-577.
3. Gasser T, Muller HG, Kohler W, et al: An analysis of the mid-growth and adolescent spurts of height based on acceleration. *Ann Human Biol* 1985;12:129-148.
4. Nanda RS: The rates of growth of several facial components measured from serial cephalometric roentgenograms. *Am J Orthod* 1955;41:658-673.
5. Bambha JK: Longitudinal cephalometric roentgenographic study of the face and cranium in relation to body height. *J Am Dent Assoc* 1961;63:776-799.
6. Ekström C: Facial growth rate and its relation to somatic maturation in healthy children. *Swedish Dent J Suppl* 11, 1982.
7. Woodside DG, Reed RT, Doucet JD, Thompson GW: Some effects of activator treatment on the growth rate of the mandible and position of the midface. Trans 3rd Inter Orthod Congress. St Louis: Mosby; 1975;459–480.
8. Buschang PH, Tanguay R, Demirjian A, et al: Mathematical models of longitudinal mandibular growth for children with normal and untreated Class II, division 1 malocclusion. *Eur J Orthod* 1988;10:227-234.
9. Grave KC, Brown T: Skeletal ossification and the adolescent growth spurt. *Am J Orthod* 1976;69:611-624.
10. Fishman LS: Radiographic evaluation of skeletal maturation. *Angle Orthod* 1982;52:88-112.
11. Baccetti T, Franchi L, McNamara JA Jr: An improved version of the cervical vertebral maturation (CVM) method for the assessment of mandibular growth angle. *Orthodontics* 2002;72: 316-323.
12. Brodie AG: Muscular factors in the diagnosis, treatment and retention. *Angle Orthod* 1953;23:71-77.
13. Weinstein S, Haack DC, Morris LY, et al: On an equilibrium theory of tooth position. *Angle Orthod* 1963;33:1-26.
14. Proffit WR: Equilibrium theory revisited: Factors influencing position of the teeth. *Angle Orthod* 1978;48:175-186.
15. Björk A, Skieller V: Facial development and tooth eruption: An implant study at the age of puberty. *Am J Orthod* 1972;62: 339-383.
16. Kelly JE, Sanchez M, Van Kirk LE: An assessment of occlusion of the teeth of children 6-11 years. DHEW publication no. (HRA) 74-1612. Washington, DC: National Center for Health Statistics; 1973.
17. Kelly JE, Harvey C: An assessment of the teeth of youths 12 to 17 years. DHEW publication no. (HRA) 77-1644. Washington, DC: National Center for Health Statistics; 1977.
18. Proffit WR, Fields HW Jr., Moray LJ: Prevalence of malocclusion and orthodontic treatment need in the United States: Estimates from the NHANES III survey. *Int J Adult Orthod* 1998;13:97-106.
19. Brunelle JA, Bhat M, Lipton JA: Prevalence and distribution of selected occlusal characteristics in the US population, 1988-1991. *J Dental Res* 1996;75(special issue):706-713.
20. Buschang PH, Schulman JD: Incisor crowding in untreated persons 15-50 years of age: United States, 1988-1994. *Angle Orthod* 2003;73:502-508.
21. Bergstrom K, Jensen R: Responsibility of the third molar for secondary crowding. *Sven Tandlak Tidskr* 1961;54:111-124.
22. Janson GR, Metaxas A, Woodside DG: Variation in maxillary and mandibular molar and incisor vertical dimension in 12 year old subjects with excess, normal, and short lower anterior facial height. *Am J Orthod* 1994;106:409-418.
23. Vego L: A longitudinal study of mandibular arch perimeter. *Angle Orthod* 1962;32:187-192.
24. Kaplan RG: Mandibular third molars and postretention crowding. *Am J Orthod* 1974;66:411-430.
25. Judd WV: Consensus development conference at the National Institutes of Health. *Indian Health Service Dental Newsletter* 1980;18:63-80.

26. Ades AG, Joondeph DR, Little RM, Chapko MK: A long-term study of the relationship of third molars to changes in the mandibular dental arch. *Am J Orthod Dentofac Orthop* 1990;97: 323-335.
27. Sampson WJ, Richards LC, Leighton BC: Third molar eruption patterns and mandibular dental arch crowding. *Austr Orthod J* 1983;8:10-20.
28. Harradine NW, Pearson MH, Toth B: The effect of extraction of third molars on late lower incisor crowding: a randomized controlled trial. *Br J Orthod* 1988;25:117-122.
29. Proffit WR, Fields HW Jr: *Contemporary orthodontics*, ed 3. St Louis: Mosby; 2000.
30. Alexander JM: A comparative study of orthodontic stability in Class I extraction cases. Thesis Baylor University; Dallas, Texas, 1996.
31. Driscoll-Gilliland J, Buschang PH, Behrents RG: An evaluation of growth and stability in untreated and treated subjects. *Am J Orthod Dentofacial Orthop* 2001;120:588-597.
32. McWhorter K: A longitudinal study of horizontal and vertical tooth movements during adolescence (age 10 to 15). Thesis, Baylor College of Dentistry, Dallas, Texas, 1992.
33. Watanabe E, Demirjian A, Buschang PH: Longitudinal post-eruptive mandibular tooth movements of males and females. *Eur J Orthod* 1999;21:459-468.
34. Moyers RE, van der Linden FPGM, Riolo ML, McNamara JA Jr: *Standards of human occlusal development. Monograph #5, Craniofacial Growth Series, Center for Human Growth and Development,* University of Michigan, Ann Arbor, Michigan, 1976.
35. Bishara SE, Bayati P, Jakobsen JR: Longitudinal comparisons of dental arch changes in normal and untreated Class II, Division 1 subjects and their clinical implications. *Am J Orthod Dentofacial Orthop* 1996;110:483-489.
36. DeKock WH: Dental arch depth and width studied longitudinally from 12 years of age to adulthood. *Am J Orthod* 1972;62:56-66.
37. Moorrees CFA, Reed RB: Changes in dental arch dimensions expressed on the basis of tooth eruption as a measure of biologic age. *J Dent Res* 1965;44:129-141.
38. Lux CJ, Conradt C, Burden D, Domposch G: Dental arch widths and mandibular-maxillary base widths in Class II malocclusions between early mixed and permanent dentitions. *Angle Orthod* 2003;73:674-685.
39. Buschang PH, Stroud J, Alexander RG: Differences in dental arch morphology among adult females with untreated Class I and Class II malocclusion. *Eur J Orthod* 1994;16:47-52.
40. Hellman M: The face in its developmental career. *Dent Cosmos* 1935;77:685-699, 777-787.
41. Scammon RE: The measurement of the body in childhood. *The measurement of man.* University of Minnesota Press, 1930.
42. Baughan B, Demirjian A, Levesque GY, La Palme-Chaput L: The pattern of facial growth before and during puberty as shown by French-Canadian girls. *Ann Hum Biol* 1979;6:59-76.
43. Buschang PH, Baume RM, Nass GG: A craniofacial growth maturity gradient for males and females between four and sixteen years of age. *Am J Phys Anthrop* 1983;61:373-381.
44. Bhatia SN, Leighton BC: *A manual of facial growth: a computer analysis of longitudinal cephalometric growth data.* New York: Oxford University Press, 1993.
45. Riolo ML, Moyers RE, McNamara JA, Hunter WS: An atlas of craniofacial growth. Monograph #2, Center for Human Growth and Development, The University of Michigan; Ann Arbor, Michigan,1974.
46. Sassouni V: A classification of skeletal types. *Am J Orthod* 1969;55:109-123.
47. Bell WB, Creekmore TD, Alexander RG: Surgical correction of the long face syndrome. *Am J Orthod* 1977;71:40-67.
48. Cangialosi TJ: Skeletal morphologic features of anterior open-bite. *Am J Orthod* 1984;85:28-36.
49. Fields H, Proffit W, Nixon W: Facial pattern differences in long-faced children and adults. *Am J Orthod* 1984;85:217-223.
50. Nanda SK: Patterns of vertical growth in the face. *Am J Orthod Dentofacial Orthop* 1988;93:103-106.
51. Subtenly JD, Sakuda M: Open-bite: Diagnosis and treatment. *J Dent Child* 1964;60:392-398.
52. Isaacson JR, Isaacson RJ, Speidel TM: Extreme variation in vertical facial growth and associated variation in skeletal and dental relations. *Angle Orthod* 1971;41:219-229.
53. Karlsen AT: Association between facial height development and mandibular growth rotation in low and high MP-SN angle faces: A longitudinal study. *Angle Orthod* 1997;67:103-110.
54. Saksena SS, Walker GF, Bixler D, Yu P: *A clinical atlas of roentgeno-cephalometry in norma lateralis.* New York: Alan R. Liss. 1987.
55. Roberts RO: Adolescent maxillomandibular relationships: Growth pattern, inter-individual variability, and predictions. Thesis, Baylor College of Dentistry, Dallas, Texas, 2006.
56. Björk A, Skieller V: Growth of the maxilla in three dimensions as revealed radiographically by the implant method. *Br J Orthod* 1977;4:53-64.
57. Korn EL, Baumrind S: Transverse development of the human jaws between the ages of 8.5 and 15.5 years, studied longitudinally with the use of implants. *J Dent Res* 1990;69:1298-1306.
58. Gandini LG, Buschang PH: Maxillary and mandibular width changes studied using metallic implants. *Am J Orthod Dentofacial Orthop* 2000;117:75-80.
59. Iseri H, Solow B: Change in the width of the mandibular body from 6 to 23 years of age: an implant study. *Eur J Orthod* 2000;22:229-238.
60. Baumrind S, Korn EL, Issacson RJ, et al: Superimpositional assessment of treatment-associated changes in the temporomandibular joint and the mandibular symphysis. *Am J Orthod* 1983;84:443-465.
61. Björk A: Cranial base development. *Am J Orthod* 1955;41: 198-225.
62. Buschang PH, Santos-Pinto A: Condylar growth and glenoid fossa displacement during childhood and adolescence. *Am J Orthod Dentofacial Orthop* 1998;113:437-442.
63. Baumrind S, Ben-Bassat Y, Korn EL, et al: Mandibular remodeling measured on cephalograms. 1. Osseus changes relative to superimposition on metallic implants. *Am J Orthod Dentofacial Orthop* 1992;102:134-142.
64. Buschang PH, Santos-Pinto A, Demirjian A: Incremental growth charts for condylar growth between 6 and 16 years of age. *Eur J Orthod* 1999;21:167-173.
65. Buschang PH, Julien K, Sachdeva R, Demirjian A: Childhood and pubertal growth changes of the human symphysis. *Angle Orthod* 1992;62:203-210.
66. Todd TW, Lyon DW Jr: Endocranial suture closure: Its progress and age relationship. *Am J Phys Anthrop* 1924;7:325-384.
67. Sahni D, Jit I, Neelam S: Time of closure of cranial sutures in northwest Indian adults. *Forensic Science Inter* 2005;148: 199-205.
68. Behrents RG, Harris EF: The premaxillary-maxillary suture and orthodontic mechanotherapy. *Am J Orthod Dentofac Orthop* 1991;99:1-6.
69. Persson M, Thilander B: Palatal suture closure in man from 15 to 35 years of age. *Am J Orthod* 1977;72:42-52.
70. Melsen B: Palatal growth studied on human autopsy material: A histologic microradiographic study. *Am J Orthod* 1975;68;42-54.
71. Kokich VG: Age changes in the human frontozygomatic suture from 20-95 years. *Am J Orthod* 1976;69:411-430.
72. Subtelny JD: A longitudinal study of soft tissue facial structures and their profile characteristics. *Am J Orthod* 1959;45:481-507.
73. Vig PS, Cohen AM: Vertical growth of the lips—a serial cephalometric study. *Am J Orthod* 1979;75:405-415.

74. Nanda RS, Meng H, Kapila S, Goorhuis J: Growth changes in the soft-tissue profile. *Angle Orthod* 1991;60:177-189.
75. Bishara SE, Hession TJ, Peterson LC: Longitudinal soft-tissue profile changes: a study of three analyses. *Am J Orthod* 1985;88:209-223.
76. Posen JM: A longitudinal study of the growth of the noses. *Am J Orthod* 1969;53:746-755.
77. Buschang PH, De La Cruz R, Viazis AD, Demirjian A: Longitudinal shape changes of the nasal dorsum. *Am J Orthod Dentofac Orthop* 1993;103:539-543.
78. Behrents RG: Growth in the aging craniofacial skeleton. Monograph #17, Craniofacial Growth Series, Center for Human Growth and Development, University of Michigan, Ann Arbor, Michigan, 1985.
79. Lewis AB, Roche AF: Late growth changes in the craniofacial skeleton. *Angle Orthod* 1988;58:127-135.
80. Bishara SE, Treder JE, Jakobsen JR: Facial and dental changes in adulthood. *Am J Orthod Dentofacial Orthop* 1994;106:175-186.
81. Forsberg CM, Eliasson S, Westergren H: Face height and tooth eruption in adults—a 20 year follow-up investigation. *Eur J Orthod* 1991;13:249-254.
82. Formby WA, Nanda RS, Currier GF: Longitudinal changes in the adult facial profile. *Am J Orthod Dentofac Orthop* 1994;105:464-476.
83. Sarnas KV, Solow B: Early adult changes in the skeletal and soft-tissue profile. *Eur J Orthod* 1980;2:1-12.

Development of the Occlusion

CHAPTER

2

Timo Peltomäki

Development of the occlusion, in other words, eruption of the teeth and formation of the interrelationship between the teeth of the upper and lower jaws, is a genetically and environmentally regulated process. Coordination between tooth eruption and facial growth is essential to achieve a functionally and esthetically acceptable occlusion. Most orthodontic problems arise through variations in the normal tooth eruption/occlusal developmental process. Therefore, every developing malocclusion and dentofacial deformity must be evaluated against normal development.

In this chapter, normal eruption timing and sequence of primary and permanent teeth is discussed. Since occlusion is regarded as a dynamic rather than a static structure, changes in the dental arch dimensions are then discussed. Finally, various common deviations in the occlusal development are addressed.

1. What are the stages of tooth development?

Tooth development is a genetically regulated process characterized by interactions between the oral epithelium and the underlying mesenchymal tissue.[1] During the first stage of tooth development, called the initiation stage, a plate-like thickening of the oral epithelium (dental placodes) can be seen in histological examination. This is followed by the bud stage with epithelial ingrowth and formation of bud-shaped tooth germs. Next, the mesenchymal tissue condenses around the epithelial buds and progressively forms the dental papilla. Gradually the dental epithelial tissue grows to surround the dental papilla.

From this stage the epithelium can be called the enamel organ. It gains a concave structure; therefore, this stage is called the cap stage. A third structure, the dental follicle, originates from the dental mesenchyme and surrounds the developing enamel organ. During this stage the shape of the crown becomes evident, but the final shaping of a tooth occurs during the next stage, called the bell stage. During the bell stage cytodifferentiation begins and tooth-specific cell populations are formed. Some of these cells differentiate into specific dental tissue-forming cells. During the secretory stage the differentiated cells start to deposit the specific dental matrix and minerals. Once the dental hard tissue in the crown has been formed and completely calcified, tooth development continues with the root formation and tooth eruption.

Root formation takes place concomitantly with the development of the supporting structures of the teeth (periodontal ligament, cement, alveolar bone). The epithelial buds of the permanent teeth (except permanent molars) develop from the dental lamina of the primary teeth.

2. What are the stages of tooth eruption?

Eruption of teeth can be divided into different stages.[2] The first stage is called preemergent eruption when the developing tooth moves inside the alveolar bone but cannot yet be seen clinically. This movement begins once the root formation has started. Resorption of bone, and in the case of a permanent tooth, resorption of the roots of the primary teeth, is necessary to allow preemergent eruption. In addition, an eruption force (origin still unknown) must exist to move the tooth. Emergence, the moment when a cusp or an incisal edge of a tooth first penetrates the gingiva, usually occurs when 75% of the final root length is established. Next, postemergent eruption follows and a tooth erupts until it reaches the occlusal level (Fig. 2-1). Eruption speed is faster during this stage and therefore the stage term *postemergent spurt* is sometimes used. Eruption does not stop once the tooth has come to occlusion, but continues to equal the rate of the vertical growth of the face. On average a molar tooth erupts about 10 mm after having reached the occlusal contact. It is also important to know that eruption of a tooth causes the alveolar bone to grow. In other words, each tooth makes its own alveolar bone. This has a clinical bearing: if a tooth fails to erupt, no alveolar bone will develop; if a tooth is lost, alveolar bone is also gradually lost.

Recent studies have shown that short-term eruption of teeth follows day-night (circadian) rhythm.[3] Eruption occurs mainly during early hours of sleep, although some intrusion can happen during the day, particularly after meals. Furthermore, it has been found that tooth eruption and secretion of growth and thyroid hormones have a similar circadian pattern.[3]

3. What is the eruption timing and sequence of primary teeth?

There is a large individual variation in the eruption schedule of both primary and permanent teeth. Delay or acceleration of 6 months from the average eruption timetable is still within the normal range. Despite variation in the eruption schedule, the eruption sequence of teeth is usually preserved.

Generally the first primary teeth to erupt are the lower central incisors (on average at 7 months), followed soon by the upper central incisors (on average at 10 months). Thereafter, the upper and lower lateral incisors emerge (on average at 12 months), then the upper and lower first molars (on average at 16 months). Primary canines erupt on average at 20 months and finally the second molars on average at 28 months. Primary dentition is thus fully formed by the age of 2½ years with calcification of the roots of the primary teeth completed a year later (Table 2-1).

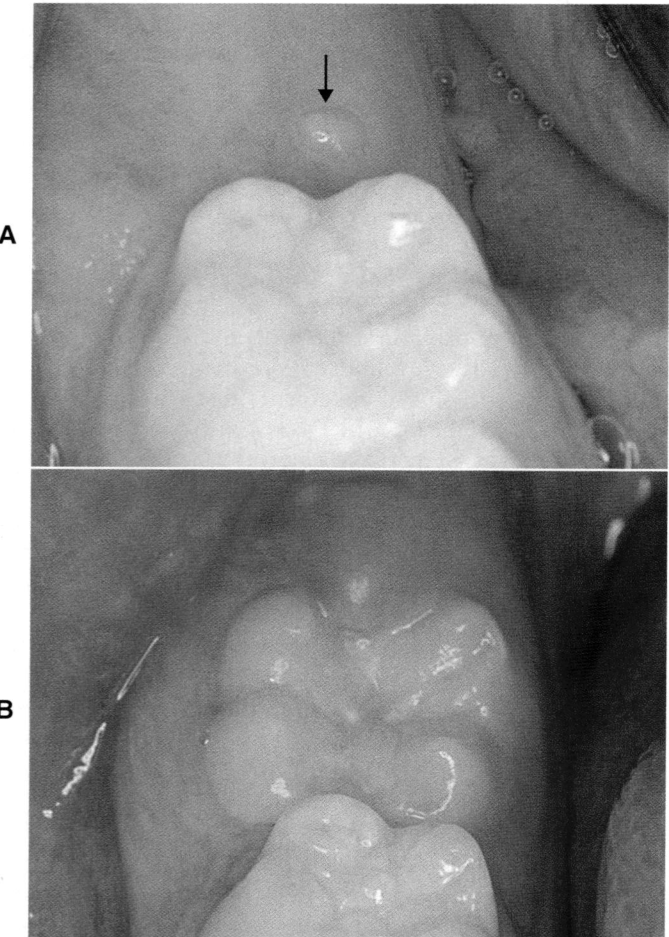

FIG 2-1 **A,** The mesiolingual cusp of the lower right first permanent molar *(arrow)* has emerged. **B,** Two months later the occlusal surface can be seen. Next, postemergent eruption follows and a tooth erupts until it reaches the occlusal level.

TABLE 2-1 Average Eruption Timing and Sequence of Primary Teeth

TOOTH	TIME (IN MONTHS)
Lower central incisors	7
Upper central incisors	10
Upper and lower lateral incisors	12
Upper and lower 1st molars	16
Upper and lower canines	20
Upper and lower 2nd molars	28

4. What are typical features of primary dentition?

Spacing in the primary dentition is a typical feature and a requirement to secure space for the larger permanent incisors (Fig. 2-2, *A*). About 70% of children have spaces in the front area of primary teeth. The largest spaces, called primate spaces, are located between the upper primary laterals and canines and between the lower primary canines and first molars. It is estimated that if the total amount of spaces per dental arch is 0 to 3 mm, there is 50% probability of crowding in the permanent dentition. If there are no spaces or even crowding in the primary dentition, crowding is inevitable in the permanent dentition (Fig. 2-2, *B*).[4] During the full primary dentition stage (3-6 years), not much happens in the dimensions of the dental arches; however, overjet and overbite may decrease.[5]

5. What is the terminal plane and what are the different terminal plane relationships in the primary dentition?

Terminal plane denotes the anteroposterior relationship (discrepancy) between the distal surfaces of the upper and lower second primary molars. It can be a flush terminal plane or there may be a mesial or a distal step (Fig. 2-3). Occurrence of different terminal planes differs greatly according to the method used to define terminal plane and the population studied. In the Caucasian (European descent) population, about 60% of children exhibit mesial step (in about 40% the mesial step is less than 2 mm and in 20% more than 2 mm), about 30% exhibit flush terminal plane, and about 10% distal step.[6] In children of African-American descent, the prevalence of distal step is lower (5%) and mesial step higher (89%).[7]

6. What does the terminal plane relationship of the primary second molars predict on the permanent molar relationships?

The terminal plane relationship determines the anteroposterior position of the permanent first molars at the time of their eruption. Differential forward drift of the lower and upper first permanent molars (generally more forward drift of the lower molar) and differential maxillary and mandibular forward growth (generally more forward growth of the mandible) play a role in this transition. In about 80% of the individuals with mesial step less than 2 mm, Angle's Class I molar relationship will result. If the mesial step is more than 2 mm, Class III molar relationship will result in 20% of the subjects. The flush terminal plane will result in either Class I (56% of subjects) or Class II (44% of subjects) molar relationship, depending on the amount of mandibular anterior growth and forward drift of the lower first primary molars in relation to the upper ones.

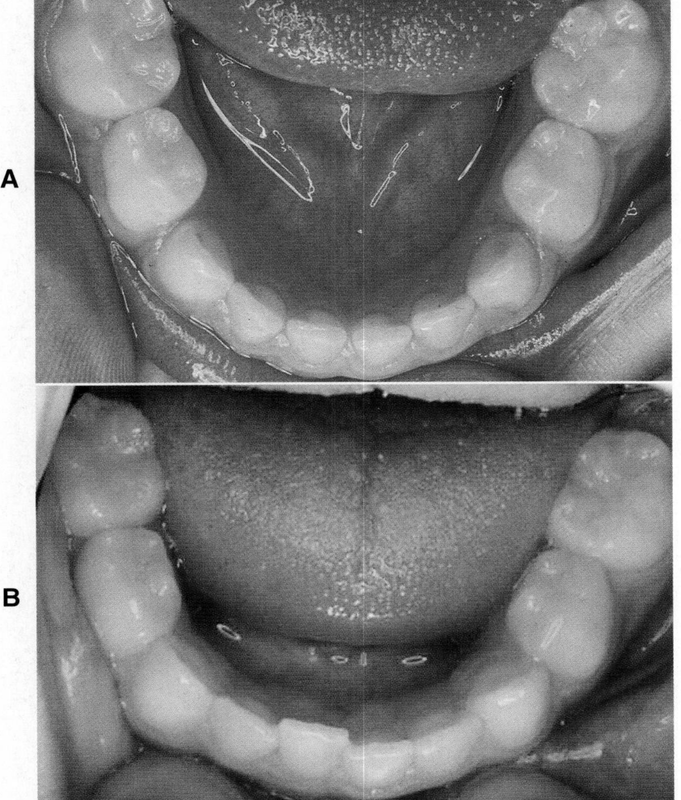

FIG 2-2 **A,** Spacing in the primary dentition is a typical feature and is a requirement to secure space for the larger permanent incisors. **B,** If there is crowding in the primary dentition, crowding is inevitable in the permanent dentition.

Distal step of the primary second molars almost invariably results in a Class II molar relationship in the permanent dentition.[6]

7. How is Angle's classification of occlusion defined?

Angle's original classification of occlusion is based on the anteroposterior relationship between the upper and lower first permanent molars. In Class I occlusion, the mesiobuccal cusp of the upper first molar occludes with the buccal groove of the lower first molar. Class I occlusion can further be divided into normal occlusion and malocclusion. Both subtypes have the same molar relationship but the latter is also characterized by crowding, rotations, and other positional irregularities.

Class II occlusion is when the mesiobuccal cusp of the upper first molar occludes anterior to the buccal groove of the lower first molar. Two subtypes of Class II occlusion exist. Both have Class II molar relationship, but the difference lies in the position of the upper incisors. In Class II division 1 malocclusion, the upper incisors are labially tilted, creating significant overjet. On the contrary, the upper central incisors are lingually inclined and the lateral incisors are labially inclined in Class II division 2 malocclusion. When measured from the first incisors, overjet is within normal limits in individuals with Class II division 2 malocclusion.

Class III malocclusion is opposite to Class II: the mesiobuccal cusp of the upper first molar occludes more posterior than the buccal groove of the lower first molar.

8. What is the eruption timing and sequence of permanent teeth?

The eruption sequence can be checked with the help of eruption charts and is a useful tool for the orthodontist to assess the dental age of a patient (Table 2-2). As a general rule, a tooth should erupt once two thirds of its root is formed.

Permanent teeth erupt in two different stages. The first transitional period occurs between the ages of 6 and 8 and is followed by approximately a 2-year intermediate period. The second transitional period starts on average at the age of 10

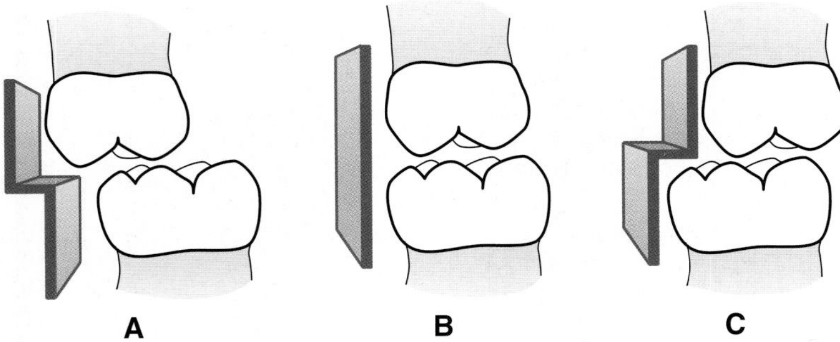

FIG 2-3 Terminal plane denotes the anteroposterior relationship between the distal surfaces of the upper and lower second primary molars. In the Caucasian population about 60% of children exhibit mesial step **(A),** about 30% flush terminal plane **(B),** and about 10% distal step **(C).** (From Bath-Balogh M, Fehrenbach MF: *Illustrated dental embryology, histology, and anatomy,* ed 2, St Louis, 2006, Saunders.)

years and lasts around 2 years. In general, teeth erupt earlier in girls than in boys. As in the primary dentition, there is a great individual variation in the eruption timing of permanent teeth. Delay or acceleration of 12 months from the average eruption timetable is still within the normal range.

The first transitional period, between 6 and 8 years, can be divided further into three yearly stages. At 6 years the upper and lower first molars (also called 6-year molars) and the permanent lower central incisors erupt (Fig. 2-4). At 7 years the upper central and the lower lateral incisors emerge and erupt. The first transitional period is completed by the eruption of the upper lateral incisors at the age of 8 years. By this time all the permanent upper and lower incisors and first molars have erupted, for a total of 12 permanent teeth. The term *mixed dentition* is used to describe a dentition containing both primary and permanent teeth.

The second transitional period can also be divided into three yearly stages. The first period is characterized by the eruption of the lower canines and lower and upper first premolars within the same time frame at about 10½ years of age. This is followed soon by the eruption of the upper and lower second premolars and usually somewhat later by the upper canines (at the age of 11 years). The second molars (12-year molars) complete the second transitional period at the age of 12 years.

Eruption of the third molars occurs much later with large individual variation (range, 17-25 years).

9. When does the mineralization of the permanent teeth occur?

Radiologically visible mineralization of the permanent first molars starts approximately at the time of birth and is followed 6 months later by the upper and lower central and lower lateral incisors. The long canines require a long time to become fully mineralized and therefore start the mineralization early (at 12 months) despite late eruption. Upper lateral incisors have an opposite mineralization/eruption pattern: a fairly late start of mineralization at 18 months and much earlier eruption than canines. The mineralization of premolars and second molars begins between ages 2½ and 3½ years. Signs of mineralization of the third molars can be seen at approximately 10 years, with particularly large variation. As a general rule, completion of crown formation (mineralization) takes 4 years and the root formation another 5 years ±1 year, depending on the size of the tooth.

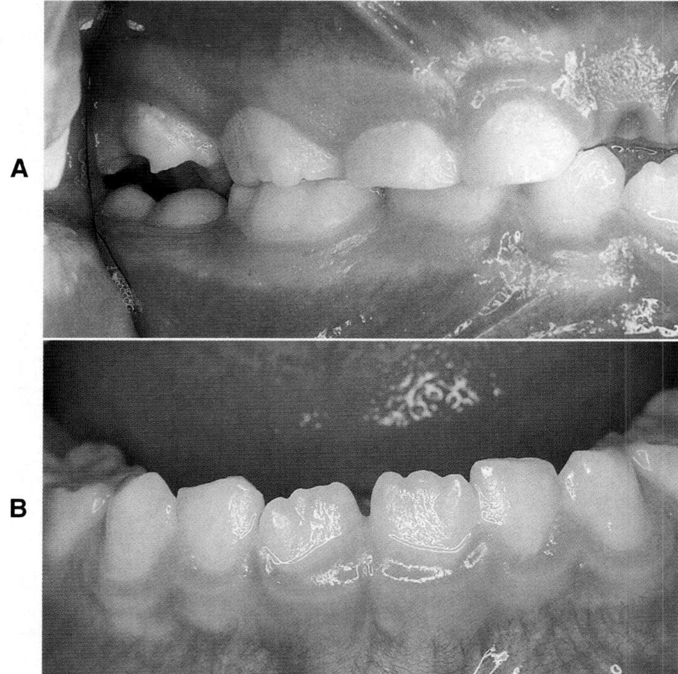

FIG 2-4 The first transitional period starts at approximately the age of 6 years with the eruption of the upper and lower first molars **(A)** and the lower central incisors **(B).**

TABLE 2-2 Average Eruption Timing and Sequence of Permanent Teeth

TRANSITION PERIOD	AGE	TEETH	FEMALE (TIME IN YEARS)	MALE (TIME IN YEARS)
First				
	6 yrs	Lower 1st molars	5.9	6.2
		Upper 1st molars	6.2	6.4
		Lower central incisors	6.3	6.5
	7 yrs	Upper central incisors	7.2	7.5
		Lower lateral incisors	7.3	7.7
	8 yrs	Upper lateral incisors	8.2	8.3
Second				
	10 yrs	Lower canines	9.9	10.8
		Upper 1st premolars	10.0	10.4
		Lower 1st premolars	10.2	10.8
	11 yrs	Upper 2nd premolars	10.9	11.2
		Lower 2nd premolars	10.9	11.5
		Upper canines	11.0	11.7
	12 yrs	Lower 2nd molars	11.7	12.1
		Upper 2nd molars	12.3	12.7
		Upper and lower 3rd molars	17-25	17-25

10. How do the initial location and size of the permanent incisors compare with the primary teeth?

In the maxilla and mandible the permanent incisors develop on the palatal/lingual side of the roots of the primary incisors with considerable crowding. Upper lateral incisors are located even more palatally than the central ones. Total mesiodistal dimension of the upper permanent incisors is about 8 mm larger than that of the primary incisors. In other words, in the upper front area there is lack of space, approximately the size of an upper lateral incisor. In the lower arch, the difference is less (5-6 mm), approximately the mesiodistal dimension of a lower incisor.

11. How is the space deficit between the primary and permanent incisors solved?

For the upper permanent incisors, several factors are available to regain this 8 mm or so space deficit. First, the upper incisors generally erupt to a wider dental arch circumference than the primary incisors, which is the most effective way to gain space for these teeth. Second, when the central permanent incisors erupt, they push the primary lateral incisors distally. The same "pushing effect" repeats when the permanent laterals erupt and push the primary canines distally. With this "pushing effect" the existing spaces of primary dentition are also closed and used for the larger permanent incisors to accommodate. Another mechanism of space-gaining in the permanent dentition is the transverse growth of the maxilla at its midpalatal suture. Thus, despite the initial lack of space in the maxillary anterior area, space conditions are generally resolved for the permanent incisors. Naturally, if the above factors are not available or working, crowding and/or cross-bite, particularly of the upper laterals, can be seen.

In the mandibular anterior area, comparable pushing takes place as in the maxillary anterior area to make space for the erupting permanent incisors. However, lower anterior teeth do not generally erupt to a wider dental arch circumference than the primary ones, and no transverse growth can take place in the anterior area of the mandible. If considerable spacing in the primary dentition (> 5-6 mm) does not exist, crowding is commonly seen once the permanent lower incisors have erupted. This is called *physiological crowding*.

12. Is anterior spacing common once permanent incisors have erupted?

Despite the initial crowding of the permanent incisors in the maxillary bone, spacing is a common finding in the upper anterior area once the incisors have erupted. A large space (> 2 mm) between the upper central incisors, called *midline diastema*, may exist due to a strong labial frenum. Upper lateral incisors may be inclined distally due to the pressure of the erupting canines on their roots. This normal spacing condition in the upper front area is called *ugly duckling*. Once the permanent canines erupt, upper spaces usually close and uprighting of the lateral incisors can be seen. On the other hand, spacing in the mandibular anterior area is very seldom seen. Rather, some crowding is typical for this developmental stage.

13. What are nonsuccedaneous teeth and how is space secured for them?

Nonsuccedaneous teeth are teeth that do not succeed deciduous teeth (i.e., all permanent molars). In the upper dental arch, space is created for the molars by bone apposition at the free posterior border of the maxilla. Also, the transverse palatal suture may make a contribution. For the lower molars bone apposition occurs on the posterior side of the mandibular ramus, and bone resorption occurs on the anterior portion of the ramus. During normal occlusal development, upper and lower first molars usually drift forward because of excess space due to the leeway space. This anterior drift of the first molars opens up space for the second molars to erupt.

14. What is leeway space and what is its importance?

The space occupied by the primary canines and molars is greater than that required for the corresponding permanent teeth. This size difference of the primary and permanent teeth is known as the *leeway space*. On average, 1 to 1.5 mm of excess space exists in each upper quadrant and 2 to 2.5 mm in the lower quadrants with large individual variation. A significant contribution of the leeway space comes from the difference in the second primary molars and their counterparts. The primary molars are on average 2 mm larger than the second premolars. During normal occlusal development, about 2 mm of the leeway space is used by the anterior drift of the molars. Lower molars usually drift more mesially than the upper ones, which often strengthens the Class I molar relationship. Physiological crowding in the lower front area may also be reduced from the leeway space, allowing the permanent canines to drift distally.

15. Is the eruption sequence of teeth important?

The eruption sequence presented in Question 8 is the most optimal one for a proper occlusion to develop. However, variations from this normal sequence are frequently seen during the second transitional period, and these variations may have clinical significance.

Sometimes the lower second molars erupt before the second premolars. This may cause anterior drift of the first permanent molars too early and, as a consequence, space loss for the second permanent premolars. Therefore, it is preferable that the second premolars erupt before the second permanent molars.

Since the leeway space provides the space needed by the upper canines, they should erupt after the permanent premolars. If not, lack of space may cause the upper canines to erupt too labially.

16. What changes occur in the dental arch length during occlusal development?

Dental arch length has a special meaning in orthodontics. Arch length denotes the distance from the most labial surfaces of the central incisors to the line connecting the mesial (or distal) points of the first permanent molars in the midsagittal plane.

Measurements and changes in the dental arch dimensions are largely based on the studies of Moorrees.[5] Changes in the arch length occur in two different phases during occlusal development. During the first transitional period, upper dental arch length increases slightly (on average 0.5 mm) because of the more labial eruption of the upper permanent central incisors. Essentially, this eruption pattern creates a larger dental arch circumference compared with the positions of the primary incisors. An additional increase of approximately 1 mm can be seen when the permanent lateral incisors erupt. During the second transitional period, arch length commonly decreases because the leeway space allows permanent premolars and first molars to drift forward. Therefore, the average upper dental arch length is slightly longer or the same at 3 years than at 15 years.

In the lower dental arch, no clinically significant changes occur in the arch length during the first transitional period because lower permanent incisors erupt into the same arch circumference as the primary incisors. A considerable shortening of the lower dental arch length takes place during the second transitional period. As discussed earlier, larger leeway space in the lower compared with the upper dental arch allows more anterior migration of the premolars and molars, which leads to the shortening of the arch length. The average lower dental arch length is thus slightly longer at 3 years than at 15 years. According to Moorrees,[5] 2- to 3-mm shortening of the lower dental arch length can be seen from the full primary dentition to the permanent dentition.

17. What changes occur in the dental arch width during occlusal development?

During the eruption of the maxillary permanent incisors, intercanine dimension (measured between primary canines) increases on average by 3 mm. Before or at the time of eruption of the permanent canines, another increase of approximately 2 mm takes place in canine to canine distance. The increase in the upper intercanine distance may be caused by the distalizing pressure of the erupting permanent incisors on the permanent canines and growth in width of the maxilla at the midpalatal suture. A steady increase (total 4-5 mm) in the distance between the upper first permanent molars can be seen after their emergence.

In the lower dental arch, a comparable increase of the intercanine distance as in the upper arch occurs during the eruption of the permanent incisors (3 mm on average). However, unlike in the upper arch, no additional increase in the canine-canine distance takes place in the lower arch during the later stages of dental development. This early establishment of the lower intercanine distance has an important clinical bearing in that attempts to increase lower intercanine distance by orthodontic means usually leads to relapse.[8] After the emergence of the molars, the distance between the lower first molars increases steadily corresponding to the upper arch.

There are two ways to measure dental arch width. The more common method is to measure the distance between the corresponding contralateral teeth at the cusp tips (e.g., intercanine or intermolar width). Another measurement can be made at the palatal/lingual gingival level of the teeth; this measurement describes the width of the bony arch.[5] The increase in the intercanine distance is greater when measured from the cusp tips of the teeth than at the gingival level, particularly in the upper dental arch. This may be because the labio-lingual crown diameter of the permanent canine is greater than that of the primary canines.

18. What changes occur in the dentition once permanent teeth (excluding wisdom teeth) have erupted?

Appearance of, or actual increase of, already existing crowding, called *late* or *secondary crowding,* in the lower anterior area is a typical finding in late dental development in the late teens and early 20s. This crowding occurs before or simultaneously with the emergence of wisdom teeth and may take place both in orthodontically untreated or treated subjects. Several factors are thought to play a role in this crowding in the lower anterior area.[9] Maxillary and mandibular differential growth is considered to have an effect on the late crowding. Growth of the maxilla ceases earlier than growth of the mandible. Because of overbite, lower anterior teeth cannot move forward to the extent of the lower jaw growth but tilt lingually to a smaller circumference, which results in crowding. In addition, the maturation of soft tissues that occurs during the teenage period may increase the pressure from lips, causing crowding. More forward drift takes place in the lower dentition than in the upper, which also increases crowding.

19. Do wisdom teeth play a role in the lower anterior crowding?

Eruption of wisdom teeth often occurs simultaneously with the appearance or increase in lower anterior crowding. It is a common belief that this is because of pressure created by the erupting wisdom teeth. However, current evidence suggests that wisdom teeth play a minor role, if any, in the late lower incisor crowding. Individuals with congenitally missing third molars may also have this crowding. Thus, there is no evidence to support a recommendation to extract third molars in order to prevent late incisors crowding.[10]

20. What are the most common reasons for interference with normal tooth eruption?

As stated earlier, great individual variation occurs in the timing of eruption of permanent teeth. Premature tooth eruption is possible, but delayed tooth eruption is more common. This may occur only on one side or on both sides of the dental arch.

Reasons for the delayed tooth eruption may be divided into rare systemic factors and more frequent local factors.[11] Systemic factors usually involve a disease process with the whole dentition commonly affected. Bone metabolism for necessary resorption of the alveolar bone and/or roots of the primary tooth may be disturbed, and eruption may therefore be delayed or even hindered. If a permanent tooth fails to fully or partially move from its crypt position in the alveolar process into the oral cavity without evident cause (presumably due to malfunction of the eruption mechanism), this condition is called "primary failure of tooth eruption."[12]

Local factors that delay tooth eruption may be mechanical in nature, and once the obstruction is eliminated, further tooth eruption may take place. Local factors include supernumerary teeth, heavy fibrous gingival tissue because of premature loss of a primary tooth, crowding, and sclerotic alveolar bone. Ankylosis of a tooth also causes delay or prevention of a tooth eruption. As a rule of thumb, if a permanent tooth has erupted but its counterpart does not within 6 months, an eruption problem is evident and further investigation is recommended.

21. What is tooth ankylosis and what is its clinical significance?

Ankylosis of a tooth is defined as the union/fusion between a tooth and alveolar bone. This means that the periodontal ligament is obliterated in one or more locations, and there is contact between the cementum of a tooth and alveolar bone. Ankylosis is more common in the primary, particularly primary molars, than in the permanent dentition (Fig. 2-5). Prevalence of primary molar ankylosis is 5% to 10%. Ankylosis is thought to be related to the noncontinuous resorption process of the roots of the primary teeth. In other words, during the resorption phase of the root, there are periods of rest and reparation. During the reparative phase, fusion of the cement and alveolar bone may develop. Causative factors for ankylosis are currently unknown.

An ankylosed tooth cannot erupt; consequently, the tooth appears to submerge with continued alveolar growth. In reality, an ankylosed tooth does not submerge, but when it fails to erupt, a vertical deficiency in the occlusal level will develop as the adjacent teeth continue erupting. The term *infraocclusion* is used to describe this condition and the amount of infraocclusion of an ankylosed tooth depends on when the ankylosis occurred. It is known that a molar erupts on average 1 mm yearly. This means that if the vertical defect is large, one may speak about *early ankylosis*. On the other hand, *late ankylosis* denotes infraocclusion as minor (1-2 mm), and ankylosis had evidently occurred near the time of exfoliation of a primary molar.

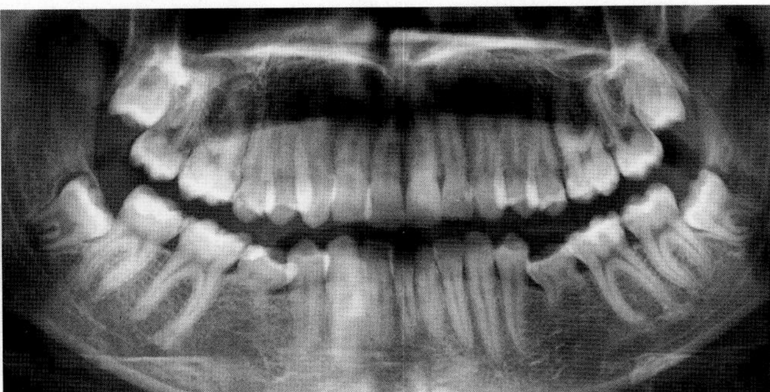

FIG 2-5 Because of ankylosis of the lower primary second molars on both sides, a vertical deficiency in the occlusal level developed since the ankylosed teeth could not erupt and the adjacent teeth continued erupting. Note also congenital missing lower second permanent premolars, which are the most commonly missing permanent teeth.

22. What is ectopic eruption?

Ectopic eruption of a tooth means that the tooth erupts away from the normal position. This condition can have a multifactorial underlying etiology. Sometimes a tooth erupts ectopically because of an abnormal initial position of the tooth bud. Upper first molars and canines are most commonly observed to erupt ectopically, followed by lower canines, upper premolars, lower premolars, and upper lateral incisors. In the permanent dentition, the upper first molars erupt most commonly ectopically (prevalence approximately 4%) (Fig. 2-6). The molar may then erupt too far anteriorly and make contact with the distal root of the second primary molar. As a consequence, the first permanent molar may fail to erupt on both sides or only on one side. It may also happen that an ectopically erupting first permanent molar causes severe resorption (called undermining resorption) to the roots of the second primary molar, leading to early exfoliation of that primary molar. This causes a more anterior eruption of the first permanent molar, resulting in space loss and future crowding of that quadrant. Because of insufficient space, the upper and lower lateral incisors may also erupt ectopically and too distally. The clinical significance of this may be an early loss of the primary canines from undermining resorption.

23. What are eruption problems of the upper permanent canines?

Canines, particularly maxillary canines, have the longest way of all teeth to erupt from their initial position to the occlusion. Initially the upper canines are located high in the maxilla, in the canine fossa, close to the base of the nose. In pre-emergent eruption, they move downward along the distal aspect of the roots of the lateral incisors. When the child is 9 to 10 years

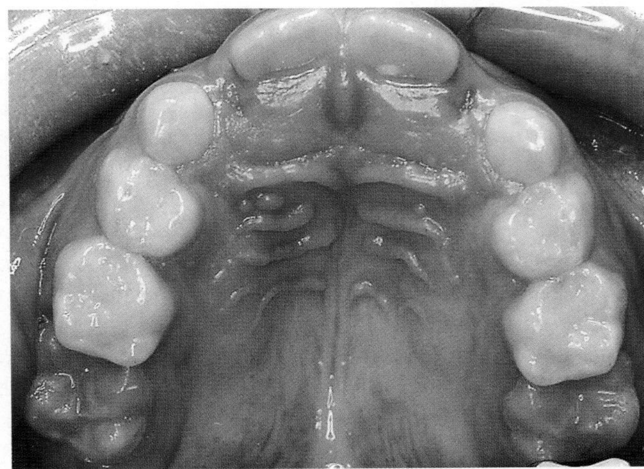

FIG 2-6 Both upper first molars have erupted ectopically, too far anteriorly. This may lead to early exfoliation of the upper second primary molars by undermining resorption and space loss in these quadrants.

old, these teeth should be palpable in the fornix between the permanent lateral incisor and the primary first molar. If not, ectopic eruption or impaction may be expected. Maxillary canines are the last teeth to erupt and are therefore strongly influenced by spacing conditions. The canines' long path of eruption, coupled with their late emergence timing, causes their high prevalence of impaction (about 2%).

Most of the impacted upper canines are palatally located. Interestingly, nearly 50% of patients with palatally located upper canines present with anomalous (peg shaped) or congenitally missing upper lateral incisors. Because of this clinical link, it has been proposed that a common genetic etiology may be responsible for canine impaction and hypodontia.[13,14] Another explanation of this observation could be that a guiding structure for the proper eruption of canine is missing, and, therefore, the canine is palatally displaced.

In a computed tomography (CT) study, researchers found that even in cases of normal eruption of upper canines, the continuity of the periodontal ligament of the lateral incisor may be temporarily lost with no resorption sign in the root.[15] When the path of eruption abnormally diverges so that the canines make contact with the roots of the lateral incisors, resorption of the incisor may be expected unrelated to the size of the dental follicle of the canine.[15]

24. What is a typical eruption problem of the second permanent molars?

If space is not adequate for the upper second permanent molars, they will often tilt buccally and distally before their emergence and eventually erupt too buccally. On the contrary, the lower second permanent molars tend to tilt lingually because of insufficient space. When the second molars erupt like this, they may not occlude properly and a scissor-bite or buccal cross bite may develop. In the scissor-bite, the upper second molar is positioned too far to the buccal and the lower second molar is too far to the lingual.

25. Which factors have an effect on tooth position?

When a tooth is erupting, it is affected by two forces that dictate its vertical position; a force causing eruption brings a tooth to the oral cavity, but a force from the occlusion has an opposing effect. In addition, external forces from the cheeks and lips and internal forces from the tongue play a role in the buccolingual position of a tooth. According to Proffit,[16] forces from the cheeks, lips, and tongue are not in balance; however, periodontally healthy teeth do not move. The balancing factor is probably the periodontal ligament, an active element capable of stabilizing tooth position. On the other hand, if support from alveolar bone and periodontal ligament is reduced, teeth are prone to move.

Light but long-lasting forces (force from the soft tissues at rest, periodontal ligament, and gingival fibers) are more important than heavy but short-lasting forces (biting, swallowing) to cause a tooth to move or to maintain its position.

26. What is the relationship between occlusal development and facial growth?

Eruption of permanent teeth does not stop once a tooth has reached occlusion. Eruption of teeth causes an elongation of dentoalveolar processes that continues at a rate that parallels the rate of vertical growth of the face, and vertical growth of the mandibular ramus in particular. In an optimally growing individual, growth of the anterior and posterior face height is approximately equal. This means that the amount of eruption of the anterior and posterior teeth that have already reached the occlusal contact is in balance. During the period between 8 and 18 years of age, anterior and posterior face heights increase about 20 mm.[17,18] At the same time, each tooth erupts about 10 mm (1.0 mm/yr) to keep contact with its opposing tooth. In some individuals, however, growth of the anterior and posterior face is not in balance, and either anterior or posterior growth rotation of the mandible occurs. This is followed by overeruption of posterior or anterior teeth in posterior rotation pattern versus anterior rotation pattern, respectively.

27. Can individuals be found with variations in the number of teeth?

Variation in the number of teeth is a frequent finding in any patient population. Instead of the normal 20 primary teeth and 32 permanent teeth, individuals with excessive or reduced numbers of teeth can be seen. In the permanent dentition, one or two teeth are often congenitally missing. This condition is called *hypodontia* or *agenesis of teeth.* If more than six permanent teeth are missing, the condition is called *oligodontia. Anodontia,* which is characterized by complete failure of tooth development, is extremely rare. If supernumerary teeth are present, it is called *hyperdontia.*

28. How common is hypodontia, and which teeth are most often affected?

Based on epidemiological studies worldwide, the prevalence of congenitally missing permanent teeth has been found to vary according to the population studied as well as to gender. Studies from Europe and Australia show prevalence of hypodontia ranging between 5.5% and 6.3%, whereas in North America (both Caucasians and African Americans), the prevalence is 3.9%.[19] These numbers exclude the third molars, but when they are included the prevalence is considerably higher, since one or more wisdom teeth are missing in about 20% to 25% of the subjects. On the other hand, prevalence of congenitally missing primary teeth is only 0.1% to 0.4%. The prevalence of hypodontia is significantly higher (1.37 times) in girls than in boys.[19]

Hypodontia commonly runs in families, an indication that genetic factors are involved. Missing teeth can be inherited as part of a syndrome or isolated in an autosomal-dominant or autosomal-recessive way. Several gene defects have been found to be associated with hypodontia. The main genes known today to be involved in hypodontia are MSX1, PAX9, and AXIN2.[1]

Individuals who are missing several teeth often have disturbances in other organs of ectodermal origin (e.g., a condition called ectodermal dysplasia).

The most commonly missing permanent teeth are the lower second premolars (more than 40% of the missing teeth), followed by the upper laterals and upper second molars. The number of other congenitally missing teeth is considerably lower. As a general rule, the last tooth within its dental group is the one most likely to be congenitally missing. In other words, third molars are more likely to be missing than the first and second molars, second premolars more often than the first ones, and lateral incisors more often than the central incisors.

29. How common is hyperdontia?

Prevalence of hyperdontia is lower than that of hypodontia. In the primary dentition the prevalence of hyperdontia is about 0.5% and in the permanent dentition about 1%. Supernumerary teeth are most often (85%) located in the upper jaw, particularly in the premaxilla area. A supernumerary tooth may be typical or atypical in shape. An atypical supernumerary tooth is often found in the midline of the premaxilla and is called a mesiodens (Fig. 2-7). Overall, mesiodens is the most prevalent supernumerary tooth, followed by extra molars, and lower second premolars. Hyperdontia may also be associated with generalized syndromes, such as cleft palate, Apert, cleidocranial dysplasia, Gardner, Down, Crouzon, Sturge-Weber, orofacial-digital, and Hallermann-Steiff; these syndromes are linked to hyperactivity of the dental lamina.

30. Does variation in tooth size have an effect on occlusion?

Variation in tooth size is a relatively common finding and may have an effect on occlusion. It is estimated that the prevalence of "tooth size discrepancy" (also called "Bolton discrepancy"[20]) is about 5%.[21] Upper permanent lateral incisors show the largest variation in size. If they are significantly smaller or larger than average, ideal occlusion is difficult to establish. As a general rule, if the mesiodistal dimension of an upper lateral incisor is smaller than that of a lower incisor, normal overjet and overbite is difficult to obtain.

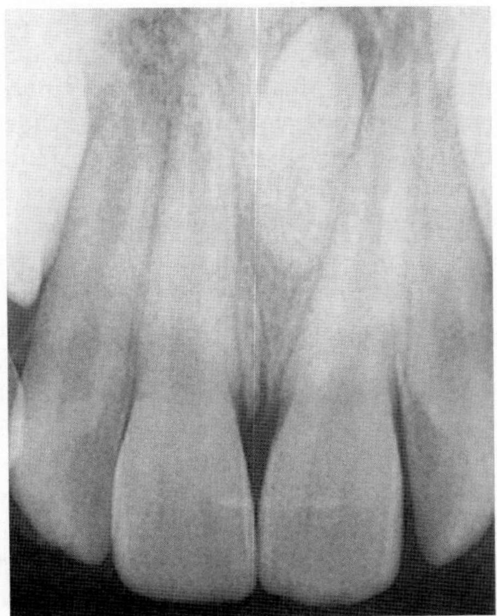

FIG 2-7 Supernumerary teeth are most often located in the upper jaw. A supernumerary tooth is seen in the midline of the premaxilla and is called a mesiodens.

REFERENCES

1. Thesleff I: Epithelial-mesenchymal signalling regulating tooth morphogenesis. *J Cell Sci* 2003; 116:1647-1648.
2. Lee CF, Proffit WR: The daily rhythm of tooth eruption. *Am J Orthod Dentofacial Orthop* 1995; 107:38-47.
3. Risinger RK, Proffit WR: Continuous overnight observation of human premolar eruption. *Arch Oral Biol* 1996; 41:779-789.
4. Leighton BC: The early signs of malocclusions. *Trans Eur Orthodon Soc* 1969, 353-368.
5. Moorrees CFA: *The dentition of the growing child. A longitudinal study of dental development between 3 and 18 years of age.* Cambridge, Massachusetts: Harvard University Press, 1959.
6. Bishara SE, Hoppens BJ, Jakobsen JR, Kohout FJ: Changes in the molar relationship between the deciduous and permanent dentitions: A longitudinal study. *Am J Orthod Dentofacial Orthop* 1988; 93:19-28.
7. Anderson AA: Occlusal development in children of African American descent. Types of terminal plane relationships in the primary dentition. *Angle Orthod* 2006; 76:817-823.
8. Bishara SE, Ortho D, Jakobsen JR, et al: Arch width changes from 6 weeks to 45 years of age. *Am J Orthod Dentofacial Orthop* 1997; 111:401-409.
9. Richardson ME: The etiology of late lower arch crowding alternative to mesially directed forces: A review. *Am J Orthod Dentofacial Orthop* 1994; 105:592-597.
10. Southard TE, Southard KA, Weeda LW: Mesial force from unerupted third molars. *Am J Orthod Dentofacial Orthop* 1991; 99:220-225.
11. Suri L, Gagari E, Vastardis H: Delayed tooth eruption: Pathogenesis, diagnosis, and treatment. A literature review. *Am J Orthod Dentofacial Orthop* 2004; 126:432-445.
12. Proffit WR, Vig KWL: Primary failure of eruption: A possible cause of posterior open-bite. *Am J Orthod* 1981; 80:173-190.
13. Pirinen S, Arte S, Apajalahti S: Palatal displacement of canine is genetic and related to congenital absence of teeth. *J Dent Res* 1996; 75:1742-1746.
14. Baccetti T: A controlled study of associated dental anomalies. *Angle Orthod* 1998; 68:267-274.
15. Ericson S, Bjerklin C, Falahat B: Does the canine dental follicle cause resorption of permanent incisor roots: A computed tomographic study of erupting maxillary canines. *Angle Orthod* 2002; 72:95-104.
16. Proffit WR: Equilibrium theory revisited: Factors influencing position of teeth. *Angle Orthod* 1978; 48:175-186.
17. Bishara SE: Facial and dental changes in adolescents and their clinical implications. *Angle Orthod* 2000; 70:471-483.
18. Thilander B, Persson M, Adolfsson U: Roentgen-cephalometric standards for a Swedish population. A longitudinal study between the ages of 5 and 31 years. *Eur J Orthod* 2005; 27:370-389.
19. Polder BJ, Van't Hof MA, Van der Linden FPGM, Kuijpers-Jagtman AM: A meta-analysis of the prevalence of dental agenesis of permanent teeth. *Community Dent Oral Epidemiol* 2004; 32:217-226.
20. Bolton WA: The clinical application of a tooth-size analysis. *Am J Orthod* 1962; 48:504-529.
21. Proffit WR, Fields HW, Sarver DM: *Contemporary orthodontics*, ed 4. St Louis: Mosby, 2007.

CHAPTER

3 Appropriate Timing for Orthodontic Treatment

Kate Pham-Litschel

Our goal in orthodontic treatment is to provide the best possible outcome in the shortest possible time with the least biological, financial, and psychosocial cost to our patients. When those results are functionally necessary and beneficial to the psychosocial well-being of our patients, we would like to begin as soon as possible. However, if we think that beginning earlier extends the duration of treatment and increases costs without sufficient warrant, we would delay treatment. Deciding when to initiate treatment may be complicated, and this certainly has been debated in the orthodontic literature. In this chapter, we review the differing opinions of appropriate timing, discuss the research findings on this topic, and, based on these findings, formulate a guideline for various specific orthodontic problems.

1. What is the definition of early treatment and what does it involve?

Early treatment, or Phase I orthodontic treatment, is defined as "treatments started in either the primary or mixed dentitions that are performed to enhance the dental and skeletal development before the eruption of the permanent dentition. Its purpose is to either correct or intercept a malocclusion and to reduce the need or the time for treatment in the permanent dentition."[1]

As opposed to the conventional late orthodontic treatment, when orthodontic therapy is initiated on children in the late mixed dentition stage, early treatment is often a two-phased treatment. Phase I treatment typically begins when the child is about 8 years or younger and lasts about 6 to 12 months. This is followed by intermittent observation of transition from the mixed to the permanent dentition. Phase II treatment, usually with the fixed orthodontic appliances on permanent teeth, begins 6 to 9 months before the eruption of the second molars.[2] It has been estimated that one fourth of all patients, and one third of all children, are treated in a two-phase manner.[3,4]

Single phase treatments have gained popularity in contemporary orthodontics.[2] Here early treatment is initiated in the late mixed dentition, just before the loss of the deciduous second molars, and is followed immediately by banding and bonding of the permanent teeth. Reduction in the total treatment time and better control of the leeway spaces in the transitional dentition are some advantages of this methodology.

2. What are some perceived advantages of early treatment?

In 2001, the Diplomates of the American Board of Orthodontics were asked about their perception of early treatment. The following points were listed[1]:

Ability to modify skeletal growth is one of the strongest perceived benefits of early treatment.

Better and more stable treatment results are another presupposed advantage of early treatment. By correcting the malocclusion as soon as it develops, we are establishing more normal function and development.

Less iatrogenic tooth damage may be another benefit of early treatment. The less developed roots of permanent teeth may mean more favorable biologic responses to orthodontic forces.

Better cooperation is another possible justification for early treatment. Patients may be more cooperative if they are treated before they reach high school. Older children tend to have more outside interests or parental conflicts at home, making orthodontic treatment a lesser priority in their lives.[5] Earlier treatment can mean an earlier finish. Patients who begin orthodontic or orthopedic treatment in the second or third grade are likely to finish Phase II before high school. Furthermore, scheduling of appointments for these patients may be easier when they are in middle school as opposed to high school.

Improved patient self esteem and parental satisfaction are also listed as benefits of early treatment. There is a clear correlation between improved esthetics and psychosocial well-being. Malocclusion is listed as one of the most common reasons for teasing in children.[6] Moreover, parents, teachers, and peers are more likely to respond positively to attractive children. From this standpoint, early treatment is especially beneficial to children with debilitating malocclusions.

3. What are the perceived disadvantages of early treatment?

The Diplomates of the American Board of Orthodontics were also asked to list the perceived disadvantages of early treatment[1]:

Variation in results and stability is listed as a major disadvantage.

Increased financial cost to the patient is another drawback of a two-phase treatment.

Patient "burnout" from longer total treatment duration is a concern.

Iatrogenic problems may be more prevalent when starting treatment early. These problems may include dilacerations of roots, decalcification under bands, impaction of maxillary canines by prematurely up-righting the roots of the lateral incisors, and impaction of the maxillary second molars from the distalization of first molars.

Moreover, treatment of younger patients may be more uncertain because of the **unpredictable dynamics of growth**. Treatment goals can be more definitive in older children.[5]

4. What are the controversies concerning early treatment?

There have been many debates about the justifications of early treatment. Orthodontists have asked if early treatment is worth the extra cost, time, and energy involved. If early treatment is effective, just how early can treatment begin in the primary, early mixed, or late mixed dentition?

Interestingly, orthodontists are more likely to recommend Phase I if they are more experienced with early treatment, or if their practices have younger children.[5] Yet according to Johnston, clinicians "have a responsibility, individually and collectively, to sift through and evaluate the available evidence with an eye toward the delivery of 'evidence-based' treatment."[7] The early treatment proposals should be based less on perceived benefits or personal experiences and more on current research findings.

So what are the scientific studies suggesting about early treatment? The following questions are reviews of studies on treatment timing, as well as suggestions of when to begin.

5. What are the problems that can be treated in the primary dentition?

DIGITAL AND PACIFIER HABITS

In most cases, treatment for a prolonged digital or pacifier habit should be initiated between the ages of 4 and 6 years, before the eruption of the permanent incisors. Keep in mind that anteroposterior dental and skeletal changes are less likely to self-correct than are the vertical dental changes.[8] Anterior open bites resulting from digital sucking do not generally need to be treated because they will likely correct spontaneously if the habit ceases before 9 years of age.[8] Skeletal open bite and distal step molar relationship, on the other hand, may worsen unless treated early.

POSTERIOR CROSSBITE WITH A FUNCTIONAL SHIFT

It is important that a posterior crossbite with the presence of a functional shift be treated as soon as it is diagnosed to prevent the asymmetrical positioning and growth of the condyles.[9] The true cause of such a crossbite is a bilateral constriction of the maxillary arch. In order to have at least one side of functioning posterior occlusion, the condyles are positioned asymmetrically within their respective fossae, resulting in the characteristic midline discrepancy in centric occlusion. If left untreated, this condition can lead to asymmetrical growth of the mandible and possible remodeling of the glenoid fossa.[10] A permanent facial asymmetry may result and persist, even though the constricted maxillary arch is corrected at a later date.[9]

SPACE MANAGEMENT

Although traditionally not considered active orthodontic treatment, space maintainers are important appliances in some conditions of the primary dentition. Whether a space resulting from the premature loss of a tooth needs to be maintained depends on the following three factors[8]:

1. **Root development:** A tooth erupts when its root is 75% developed. The less developed the permanent root, the stronger the recommendation for space maintenance.
2. **Distance between the permanent tooth and the alveolar crest:** The amount of bone overlying the succedaneous tooth also predicts the timing of the tooth's eruption.
3. **Type of tooth prematurely lost:** When primary incisors are lost, space maintenance is not necessary as long as the primary canines have already erupted into occlusion. With the loss of a primary canine, the extraction of the contralateral canine and placement of a lower lingual holding arch are necessary to prevent the undesirable drifting of the midline. With the loss of a primary first molar, a band and loop space maintainer helps prevent the unfavorable mesial drifting of the second primary molar. This forward sliding of the second primary molar would reduce the space available for the unerupted first premolar. Finally, a space maintainer is always recommended when the primary second molar is lost before the eruption of the first permanent molar.

It seems logical that use of space maintainers would reduce the prevalence and severity of crowding. However, the existing studies in literature do not have enough scientific weight for one to recommend for or against the use of space maintainers to prevent or reduce the severity of malocclusion in the permanent dentition.[11] Yet one may argue that the roles of space maintainers are so intuitive that waiting for evidence of their effectiveness may impede the benefits to the patients.

6. When should a posterior crossbite *without* a functional shift be treated?

A maxillary constriction without a lateral shift does not carry the same urgency as one with a shift; it can be treated in the early mixed dentition or even closer to adolescence.[10,12] Maxillary expansion involves manipulation of the sutures within and surrounding the maxilla. This procedure should precede the ossification of these sutures, most likely before the onset of puberty. Once the circummaxillary sutures fuse, correction of this skeletal crossbite may require surgical intervention. However, there is no evidence to suggest that expansion in the primary dentition is more stable than in the early-to-late transition dentition.[12]

7. When is the best time to treat crowding?

According to Gianelly,[4,13] the best time to start treatment of cases with mild to moderate crowding is in the late mixed dentition, after the eruption of the first premolars. At this stage, alignment can be achieved in about 73% of the patients primarily by preserving and using the leeway space. Immediately after the placement of a lower lingual arch, fixed appliances can be placed to direct the permanent teeth into the newly created space. For the cases that need extractions, the timing of late mixed dentition is suitable because the first premolars are already erupted for extraction.[4,13]

Serial extraction is a viable treatment for early diagnosis of severe crowding. The purpose of serial extractions of primary teeth is to encourage the early eruption of permanent premolars, which themselves would be extracted. This allows for the remaining teeth to erupt within the alveolus, and thus simplifies later orthodontic treatment.[10] Serial extraction is best done for a severely crowded malocclusion with a normal overbite.

8. Is the early treatment of open-bite malocclusion effective?

Various studies of dentoskeletal open bite treatments suggest that early functional therapy is able to intercept the malocclusion to reduce the need for treatment during adolescence. This is especially true in the cases of open bite caused by sustained oral habits. However, when these studies are reviewed for statistical quality, no evidence-based conclusion can be drawn.[14]

9. Is the early treatment of Class II malocclusion effective?

The results of recent randomized clinical trials (RCTs) have brought new perspectives to this debate. One of the RCTs, performed at the University of North Carolina (UNC), addressed the benefits of early treatment on Class II division I malocclusions.[18-20] In the first part of this study, patients in the mixed dentition with moderate to severe overjet were randomly assigned to three groups:

1. Early treatment with headgears
2. Early treatment with a bionator
3. Observation only

The findings of this study confirm the conventional belief that early treatment with either headgears or functional appliances improves the skeletal relationships of Class II malocclusions, with 75% of the patients showing significant improvements. A headgear produces greater changes in the maxilla, whereas a bionator brings about more mandibular changes.[18,20]

The second part of this study asks whether these differences in outcome are sustained over time.[19] This time, the same group of patients was again randomly assigned to Phase II fixed appliance therapies. An evaluation of the results at the completion of treatment suggests that skeletal effects of early treatment generally are not sustained. There is no significant difference among the three group's skeletal relationships. The apparent improvement in jaw relationship in the first part of the study may be due to acceleration in growth, rather than an actual increase of growth. The authors' message was that moderate to severe Class II malocclusions do not benefit more from two-phased treatment than from a conventional one-phase treatment.

Independently, University of Florida (UF) underwent similar examination of Class II early treatment.[15-17] With slight variations on treatment mechanics and duration, UF also compared an observation group and a headgear/bionator group after the completion of Phase II therapy. Its results closely matched that of UNC's showing that despite the significant skeletal and dental improvements between the groups after Phase I treatment, by the end of Phase II, the differences between those who had received Phase I and those who had not was indistinguishable. Furthermore, the range of changes in the two groups was similar, with each group having extremes of great improvement to severe worsening of the Class II relationship. UF also invalidated Phase I treatment to reduce the incidence of incisor trauma in children. After 3 years of follow up, there were no significant correlations with new incisal injury and years in treatment. In addition, no significant difference was found in the post-treatment stability at 3 years.

Another RCT was performed by the University of Pennsylvania using headgears and Frankel appliances.[21] The researchers asked the same question of whether early treatment for Class II malocclusion is effective, and if so, when intervention should begin. The results of the study suggested that headgears and functional regulators are both effective in correcting Class II division I malocclusions in children. Similar to the North Carolina study, this study also suggested that the appliances' effects on each jaw differ. The headgear has a distal effect on the maxilla and first molars whereas the Frankel appliance restrains the maxilla, reclines the incisor, and advances the mandible. As for the question of the best time to initiate therapy, the conclusion was that treatment in the late mixed dentition is as effective as that in the early mixed dentition. They recommended starting treatment in the late mixed dentition as the first step of a one-phase treatment.

A group of researchers in Manchester, United Kingdom made a similar study using Twin Block.[22,23] As in the North Carolina study, the first part of this research was designed to address the effectiveness of early treatment for Class II division I malocclusions. The second part of the research analyzed the patients after completion of Phase II treatment to see if the differences are sustained. The results showed that early treatment with Twin Block appliances resulted in favorable dentoalveolar changes, such as reduction in overjet and correction of molar relationships. Furthermore, the Manchester group considered the sociopsychological benefits of early treatment and found that early treatment increased the patient's self-esteem as well as reduced negative social experiences. However, measurements after the completion of Phase II showed there is no difference

TABLE 3-1 Chapter Summary of Appropriate Treatment Timing

DECIDUOUS DENTITION 4-6 YEARS	EARLY MIXED 6-8 YEARS	LATE MIXED 8-11 YEARS	PERMANENT (GROWING)	PERMANENT (NON-GROWING)
Digital and pacifier habits	Posterior crossbite without functional shift			Surgical Class II
Space management	Severe crowding leading to serial extractions	Moderate to severe mandibular crowding		Surgical Class III
Posterior crossbite with functional shift		Class II malocclusions		
	Class III malocclusions: facemask therapy			

between the orthodontic results of the early treatment group and the control group. As for the issue of self-esteem, both groups at the end of Phase II treatment showed similar improvements in sociopsychological well-being. Thus, aside from an earlier improvement in self-esteem, it seems that early orthodontic treatment of Class II malocclusion does not offer an advantage over a later treatment. At least for Class II division I malocclusions, the orthodontic pendulum has swung far to the side of delaying treatment until late mixed dentition, or even eliminating early treatment altogether. Whether it stays there indefinitely will depend on future studies.

10. When should Class III early treatment start?

Protraction facemask therapy, with or without maxillary expansion, is the most common early treatment for Class III malocclusion. Initiated at the early mixed dentition stage, the justification for this treatment is that the application of prolonged force on the circummaxillary sutures may stimulate the formation of new bone, resulting in the forward and downward movement of the maxilla. Clinical reports suggest that this early treatment results in skeletal and soft tissue correction, leading to improved profiles.[24-27]

Skeletal changes are primarily the result of anterior and vertical movement of the maxilla. Mandibular movement was directed downward and backward accompanied by a slight increase in lower facial height. Therefore, a Class III malocclusion with a deep bite is much easier to treat than one with an open bite because of the increase in anterior lower facial height. The facemask and expansion therapy can also be a viable option for older children, although it is not as effective as it is with younger children and results in more dental rather than skeletal changes.[28]

11. What is the appropriate time for orthognathic surgery?

It may be difficult to determine the appropriate time for orthognathic surgery for patients who are still growing at the time of their presurgical orthodontic treatment. The rule of thumb is to operate excesses late and deficiencies early.[8] Mandibular prognathism cases should be treated after the cessation of mandibular growth. This is generally around 18 years of age for males and 16 years for females. Early surgery on growing patients with mandibular prognathism will risk outgrowth of the surgical correction and require retreatment.

For patients with growth deficiencies, surgery can be considered earlier, but rarely before the adolescent growth spurt. Maxillary vertical excesses may be treated at age 14 or later since vertical growth is generally completed at this time. Superimpositions of serial cephalograms can more accurately determine the appropriate time to send a patient to surgery. Surgery should be delayed until good superimposition supports that deceleration of growth has occurred (see Chapter 4). Problems of maxillary deficiencies may be treated earlier than problems of excess because the growth in these patients does not substantially alter the surgical correction. Table 3-1 provides a summary of the suggested treatment timing of the various orthodontic problems that have been discussed in this chapter.

REFERENCES

1. Bishara SE, Nemeth R: Current challenges and future dilemmas facing the orthodontic profession. Proceedings of a Workshop, The College of Diplomates of the American Board of Orthodontics. Sun Valley, Idaho, July 21-25, 2001. *Angle Orthod* 2002;72:88-90.
2. Ghafari JG: Emerging paradigms in orthodontics—an essay. *Am J Orthod Dentofacial Orthop* 1997;111:573-580.
3. Gottlieb EL, Nelson AH, Vogels DS III: 1990 JCO study of orthodontic diagnosis and treatment procedures. 2. Breakdowns of selected variables. *J Clin Orthod* 1991;25:223-230.
4. Gianelly AA: Crowding: timing of treatment. *Angle Orthod* 1994;64:415-418.
5. Yang EY, Kiyak HA: Orthodontic treatment timing: a survey of orthodontists. *Am J Orthod Dentofacial Orthop* 1998;113:96-103.
6. Mohlin B, Kurol J: To what extent do deviations from an ideal occlusion constitute a health risk? *Swed Dent J* 2003;27:1-10.
7. Johnston LE Jr: Early treatment 2005: deja vu all over again. *Am J Orthod Dentofacial Orthop* 2006;129(4 Suppl):S45-46.
8. Kanellis MJ: Orthodontic treatment in primary dentition. In Bishara SE, ed: *Textbook of orthodontics*, Philadelphia: Saunders, 2001, pp 248-255.
9. Pirttiniemi P, Kantomaa T, Lahtela P: Relationship between craniofacial and condyle path asymmetry in unilateral cross-bite patients. *Eur J Orthod* 1990;12:408-413.
10. Kluemper GT, Beeman CS, Hicks EP: Early orthodontic treatment: what are the imperatives? *J Am Dent Assoc* 2000;131: 613-620.
11. Brothwell DJ: Guidelines on the use of space maintainers following premature loss of primary teeth. *J Can Dent Assoc* 1997;63(10):753-766.
12. Petren SL, Bondemark L, Soderfeldt B: A systematic review concerning early orthodontic treatment of unilateral posterior crossbite. *Angle Orthod* 2003;73(5):588-596.
13. Gianelly AA: One-phase versus two-phase treatment. *Am J Orthod Dentofacial Orthop* 1995;108:556-559.

14. Cozza P et al: Early orthodontic treatment of skeletal open-bite malocclusion: a systematic review. *Angle Orthod* 2005;75(5):707-713.
15. Wheeler TT et al: Effectiveness of early treatment of Class II malocclusion. *Am J Orthod Dentofacial Orthop* 2003;121:9-17.
16. Dolce C et al: Centrographic analysis of 1-phase versus 2-phase treatment for Class II malocclusion. *Am J Orthod Dentofacial Orthop* 2005;128:195-200.
17. King GJ et al: Comparison of peer assessment ratings (PAR) from 1-phase and 2-phase treatment protocols for Class II malocclusions. *Am J Orthod Dentofacial Orthop* 2003;123:489-496.
18. Tulloch JF et al: The effect of early intervention on skeletal pattern in Class II malocclusion: a randomized clinical trial. *Am J Orthod Dentofacial Orthop* 1997;111(4):391-400.
19. Tulloch JF, Phillips C, Proffit WR: Benefit of early Class II treatment: progress report of a two-phase randomized clinical trial. *Am J Orthod Dentofacial Orthop* 1998;113(1):62-72.
20. Tulloch JF, Proffit WR, Phillips C: Influences on the outcome of early treatment for Class II malocclusion. *Am J Orthod Dentofacial Orthop* 1997;111(5):533-542.
21. Ghafari J et al: Headgear versus function regulator in the early treatment of Class II, division 1 malocclusion: a randomized clinical trial. *Am J Orthod Dentofacial Orthop* 1998;113(1):51-61.
22. O'Brien K et al: Effectiveness of early orthodontic treatment with the Twin-block appliance: a multicenter, randomized, controlled trial. 1. Dental and skeletal effects. *Am J Orthod Dentofacial Orthop* 2003;124(3):234-243.
23. O'Brien K: Is early treatment for Class II malocclusion effective? Results from a randomized controlled trial. *Am J Orthod Dentofacial Orthop* 2006;129(4 Suppl):S64-65.
24. Takada K, Petdachai S, Sakuda M: Changes in dentofacial morphology in skeletal Class III children treated by a modified maxillary protraction headgear and a chin cup: a longitudinal cephalometric appraisal. *Eur J Orthod* 1993;15(3):211-221.
25. Ngan P et al: Effect of protraction headgear on Class III malocclusion. *Quintessence Int* 1992;23(3):197-207.
26. Ngan P et al: Cephalometric and occlusal changes following maxillary expansion and protraction. *Eur J Orthod* 1998;20(3):237-254.
27. Ngan P et al: Treatment response and long-term dentofacial adaptations to maxillary expansion and protraction. *Semin Orthod* 1997;3(4):255-264.
28. Kapust AJ, Sinclair PM, Turley PK: Cephalometric effects of face mask/expansion therapy in Class III children: a comparison of three age groups. *Am J Orthod Dentofacial Orthop* 1998;113(2):204-212.

CHAPTER 4

Orthodontic Records and Case Evaluation

Jeryl D. English • Thuy-Duong Do-Quang • Anna Maria Salas-Lopez

In a problem-oriented approach to diagnosing and treatment planning of patients with malocclusions, it is necessary to gather relevant information in a consistent manner in order to start a comprehensive database of information for each patient.

First, the orthodontist must establish a case history of each patient, noting the chief concerns, including medical and dental history. Second, a thorough clinical examination of the patient should be conducted to obtain accurate measurements and objective findings, which are the basis of the orthodontic diagnosis. This clinical examination should include a facial evaluation, both in the frontal and profile views, as well as an examination of the patient's extraoral and intraoral soft tissue. The clinical examination should also contain an assessment of the dentition and a functional analysis of the temporomandibular joint (TMJ). Finally, complete orthodontic records should be taken, which consist of digital or plaster of Paris study models, panoramic and cephalometric radiographs, bitewing and periapical radiographs of the anterior teeth in adults, and extraoral and intraoral photographs. Any additional records that the orthodontist deems necessary should be included. In general, these orthodontic records document the patient's initial condition and supplement the diagnostic information obtained through the patient interview and examination. The orthodontist can now analyze the collected data for problems in the areas of clinical examination, study casts analysis, radiographic analysis, and photographic analysis (Box 4-1).

After completion of the analysis, a list of problems in each of these areas can be developed and prioritized. In addition, a 3D-3T diagnostic grid is recommended as an aid in ensuring that all three dimensions (3D) of a malocclusion as well as all three tissues (3T) are evaluated. The three dimensions include sagittal, transverse, and vertical plane; the three tissues include skeletal, soft tissue, and dental structures. It is critical to understand that incorrect diagnosis is usually related to lack of information.

Box 4-1

Data Areas Used for Analyses

- Clinical examination
  - Case history
  - Chief complaint
  - TMJ function analysis
  - Periodontal and caries analyses
- Study casts analysis
- Radiographic analysis
  - Panoramic x-ray
  - Lateral cephalometric and posterior-anterior x-rays
  - Periapical and bitewings
- Photographic analysis

A comprehensive diagnosis will provide a summary of the most important problems from each of the four areas listed above.

CLINICAL EXAMINATION

1. Which key points should be clarified in the patient's medical and dental history?

It is important to note the patient's chief concern and specify whether treatment is sought for functional reasons, esthetic improvement, or both.[1] Medical conditions, diseases, hospitalizations, and current medications should be recorded. Drugs that may trigger hyperplastic gingival response such as phenytoin, calcium channel blockers, and immunosuppressives[2] as well as medications that may inhibit orthodontic tooth movement, such as bisphosphonates[3] or prostaglandin-inhibitors,[4] are important to document on the patient's problem list.[5] Allergies, especially to nickel or latex, should be noted by the orthodontist. Any facial or dental trauma, extractions, and habits should be listed and the oral hygiene regimen assessed. Possible familial patterns of malocclusion should be explored by collecting information about whether parents or siblings have undergone orthodontic treatment.[6] Finally, voice change in boys and menarche in girls can be used to assess the stage of the patient's development.[7]

2. Which aspects should be covered in the clinical examination?

In general, the face, oral cavity, and surrounding areas (including dentition) and TMJs should be examined. This specifically includes assessment of asymmetries, lip position in closure and repose, classification of the perioral musculature, and measurement of the incisor display at rest (see following cephalometric and photographic analysis questions). The health of all oral tissues and the patient's periodontal status, especially in adults, should be evaluated. Periapical and bitewing radiographs are essential in evaluating all adult patients.[8] It is imperative to test probing depths for adult patients and document a periodontal screening index (PSI) to document the status of the periodontium prior to any orthodontic treatment.[9] The condition of the teeth with detailed recording of caries as well as dental and occlusal anomalies in the transverse, sagittal, and vertical plane should be noted along with assessment of the maxillary and mandibular apical bases, determination of facial and dental maxillary and mandibular midlines, and palpation of unerupted teeth.

3. Which aspects of jaw and occlusal function should be evaluated?

There are five main areas of interest to the orthodontist: mastication, speech, breathing mode, orofacial dysfunctions, and TMJ function. Mastication, including swallowing patterns as well as the presence of speech problems such as articulation distortion, stuttering, or dyslexia, requires evaluation. Depending on the severity, this may necessitate referral to a specialist. The patient should also be asked about the prevalent respiration mode, mouth versus nasal breathing, and possible sleep disorders or problems with restricted airways, such as snoring. These may be associated with such conditions as tonsillar or adenoid enlargement, nasal obstruction, allergies, and retruded mandible. However, the etiologic significance of respiration mode in relationship to facial growth and development of malocclusions remains controversial throughout the literature.[10,11] Deleterious habits (i.e., lip biting or thumb or finger sucking [Fig. 4-1, *A*]), cheek biting, bruxism, nail biting, and tongue thrusting [Fig. 4-1, *B*]) are imperative to document. They might be partially etiologic to open bite[12] and posterior crossbite[13] or, in case of tongue thrusting, compensatory factors of a presenting malocclusion.[14]

4. How is the TMJ function examined?

The patient should be initially questioned about existing TMJ problems and the history of symptoms verified through manipulation and auscultation of the TMJ for sounds such as clicking, popping, or crepitus. Palpation of the TMJ and masticatory muscles is necessary to detect tenderness or pain. In addition, the patient's range of motion (ROM) should be recorded by observing and measuring maximal mouth opening, right and left lateral excursions, and protrusive movement.[15] Ideally, mandibular movements should be painless and, for adults, within a normal range of 50 mm maximal opening and 10 mm lateral excursions. The amount of maximal mouth opening is age related and therefore generally less than 50 mm for children. Functional shifts between centric occlusion (CO) and centric relation (CR) outside the normal range of 1.5 mm need to be recorded, since they have been correlated with increased temporomandibular disorders (TMDs).[16] CO-CR discrepancy may result in a false bite commonly referred to as *Sunday bite,* which is the forward postural position of the mandible adopted by patients with Class II profiles in order to enhance their appearance. Shifts can also be related to occlusal interferences, requiring posturing into pseudo Class III malocclusions.[17] TMD is subdivided into true pathologies of the TMJ (TMJ disorders) and myofacial pain dysfunction (MPD),[18] which affects masticatory and cervical muscles.[19] Any clinical diagnosis should be substantiated by radiographic evidence, as well as CT and/or MRI scans as needed. However, most patients presenting with MPD usually lack clinical or radiographic evidence of pathologic TMJ changes.[18]

5. Which areas should be explored in the patient's social and behavioral evaluation?

The patient's motivation to seek orthodontic treatment should be assessed, since attitude and expectations concerning treatment are closely related to motivation. In general, internally as opposed to externally motivated patients show better cooperation.[20] Progress in school and reaction to past medical or dental treatment may also be indicative of the patient's compliance

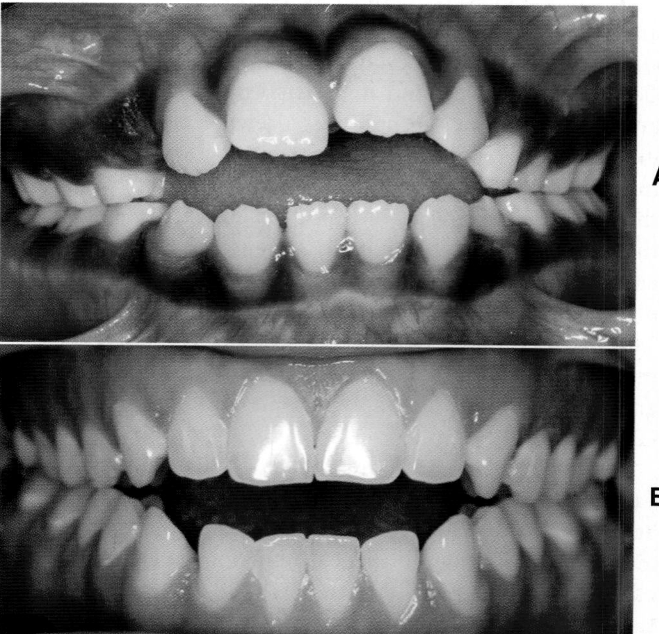

FIG 4-1 **A,** Open bite malocclusion caused by a thumb-sucking habit. **B,** Malocclusion caused by a tongue-thrusting habit.

level. A history of prolonged sucking habits, poor educational advancement, sleepwalking in younger children, and enuresis in older children may be related to emotional problems. In addition, patients affected by conditions such as autism and attention deficit disorder (ADD)/attention deficit hyperactivity disorder (ADHD) should be identified to determine the best mode of treatment.

6. What are the ages that need to be considered in orthodontic care?

Chronologic, skeletal, dental, mental, and emotional age are differentiated in the assessment of the development of a patient. Chronologic age does not correlate well with the other ages; thus, assessment of the skeletal or physiologic age helps to determine the biologic age.[21] This is most commonly done by evaluation of a hand-wrist radiograph of the non-working hand or both hands in children under 6 years of age.[22] It is indicated in children above the 95th or under the 5th percentile of somatograms and prospective orthognathic surgery patients. The method determines developmental and somatic maturity with a variability of ± 1 year, although in patients less than 10 years of age, poor correlation to chronologic, dental, or mental age has been observed. Understanding the timing and sequence of formation of both the primary and permanent dentition is essential for diagnosis of the dental age. It is best determined by the stages of individual tooth mineralization, since this process is not affected by early tooth loss. Various tests have been developed to assess the mental and emotional age of a patient that may not closely correlate with the developmental age. The latter can be roughly determined by evaluation of the secondary sexual characteristics. A child is considered an early or late developer if a difference of ± 2 years is found between chronologic and dental age.

7. What methods can be applied to assess the physical growth and maturation status of an individual?

Evaluation of the skeletal maturity of a patient is important to maximize efficiency and effectiveness of orthodontic treatment through proper timing. If a treatment plan demands a skeletal dentofacial orthopedic modification, the patient should be treated as close as possible to the peak velocity of growth.[23] The use of headgear or functional appliances, like the Twin Block or Herbst appliance, appears more effective if applied at or slightly after the onset of the pubertal growth spurt in the late mixed dentition.[24,25] Information regarding active growth cessation is crucial, especially in patients undergoing orthognathic surgery. Gender-specific growth curves classify a child under a height and weight percentile to establish norms for chronologic age. Currently, hand-wrist radiographs are the gold standard of growth assessment. The skeletal age is evaluated by analysis of a predictable ossification sequence of long bones of the wrist and carpal bones of the hand in children up to 9 years and metacarpals after 9 years of age.[26,27] Specific skeletal maturational events can then be linked to identify the patient's progression on the pubertal growth curve.[28] Application of this method is indicated in orthognathic surgery patients ranging in age from 16 to 20 years and in patients with marked discrepancy between chronological and dental age.

More recently, it has been shown that the peak pubertal growth can also be estimated by evaluation of the maturation level of the cervical vertebrae pictured on a cephalographic radiograph.[29,30] Shape as well as concavity of the inferior border of C2 through C6 is sequentially assessed in this method,[31] thereby eliminating the need for an additional hand-wrist radiograph, since a cephalogram is routinely taken for every prospective orthodontic patient.[32-34]

8. How is the malposition of individual teeth classified?

A malposed tooth can be inclinated, centrically or eccentrically malpositioned, totally displaced, rotated, transposed, or localized by various combinations thereof. According to Liescher's nomenclature, the malposition of a tooth is termed *mesioversion* if it is displaced toward the facial midline (Fig. 4-2, *A*); it is classified as *distoversion* if it is located further away from the midline (Fig. 4-2, *B*).

If an incisor or canine is misplaced outside the arch form toward the lip, this is described as *labioversion* (Fig. 4-2, *C*); if a posterior tooth is dislocated toward the cheek, it is described as *buccoversion*. A tooth is known to be *linguoverted* if it is inclined toward the tongue (Fig. 4-2, *D*). The term *infraversion* is applied if a tooth is not erupted to the occlusal plane (Fig. 4-2, *E*) whereas *supraeruption* describes an overerupted tooth. A tooth rotated on its own axis is classified as *torsiversion*. Transposition or *transversion* denotes a positional interchange of two adjacent teeth,[35] which is found most commonly in the maxilla with an incidence described as high as 1 in 300 patients.[36,37] The transposition of an upper canine with the first premolar is shown in Fig. 4-2, *F*.

9. Which tooth most often displays an anomaly?

In general, third molars are most commonly affected by size and shape variations, followed by upper lateral incisors and lower second premolars. Anomalies can result from genetic factors as well as environmental influences such as nutrition or diseases during the prenatal period of tooth development. Upper lateral incisors have been described as absent, peg-shaped, hypoplastic, dens evaginatus or invaginatus. Peg-shaped laterals are found in 1% to 2% of the population and are characterized as being small, conical, and tapered toward the incisal (Fig. 4-3, *A*).

Shovel-shaped incisors mark another morphological variant. These teeth show pronounced lingual ridges and cingula and are more common in the Asian, Eskimo, and Native American populations.[38] In contrast, cusps of Carabelli on permanent molars have the greatest incidence among Caucasians (Fig. 4-3, *B*).[39]

The term *taurodontia* describes a tooth whose crown and pulp chamber is elongated with little or no constriction at the cementoenamel junction (CEJ), resulting in a short root. The

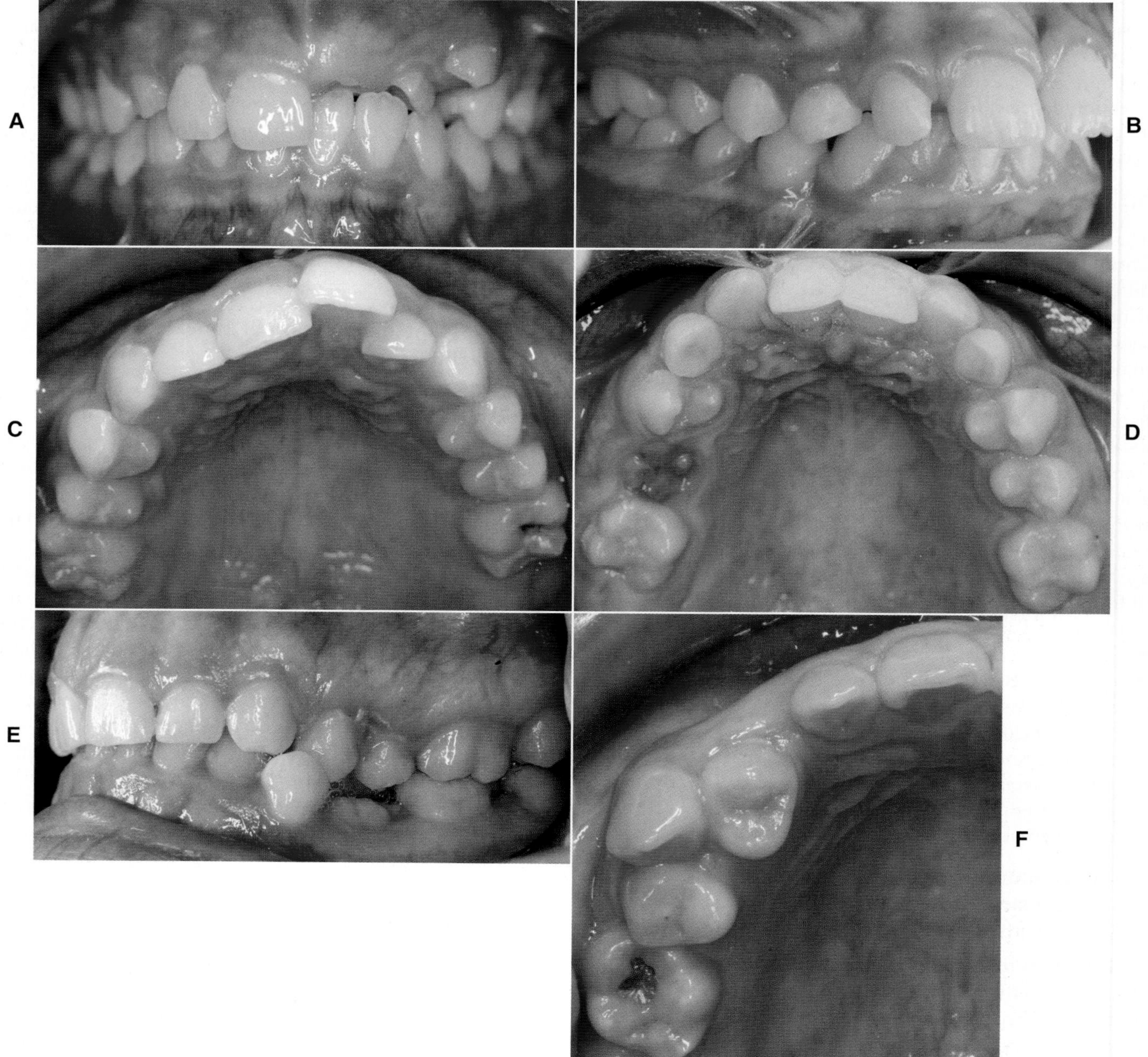

FIG 4-2 **A,** Mesioversion of maxillary right central incisor. **B,** Distoversion of maxillary right lateral incisor. **C,** Labioversion of maxillary left central incisor. **D,** Linguoversion of maxillary central incisors. **E,** Infraversion of mandibular left second deciduous molar. **F,** Transposition of maxillary right cuspid and first premolar.

incomplete division of a single tooth germ is known as *gemination* (Fig. 4-3, *C*).

These teeth clinically appear as fused with a notch in the crown but generally display a single root and pulp chamber. Truly fused teeth, however, result from union of the dentin of two adjacent tooth buds. Consequently, tooth count will normally reveal one less individual tooth in the affected arch. *Twinning* is the complete division of one tooth germ into two teeth, resulting in one more individual tooth than the normal complement. If two adjacent teeth are joined only at the cementum, they are described as being *concrescent*.

A dens evaginatus is characterized by a talon cusp (Fig. 4-3, *D*). Invagination of the enamel organ into the crown, thereby extending into the dentin and root of a tooth, is known as *dens invaginatus* or *dens in dente*. It is more common in the permanent dentition with an incidence of about 2% and usually affects the upper lateral incisor.[40]

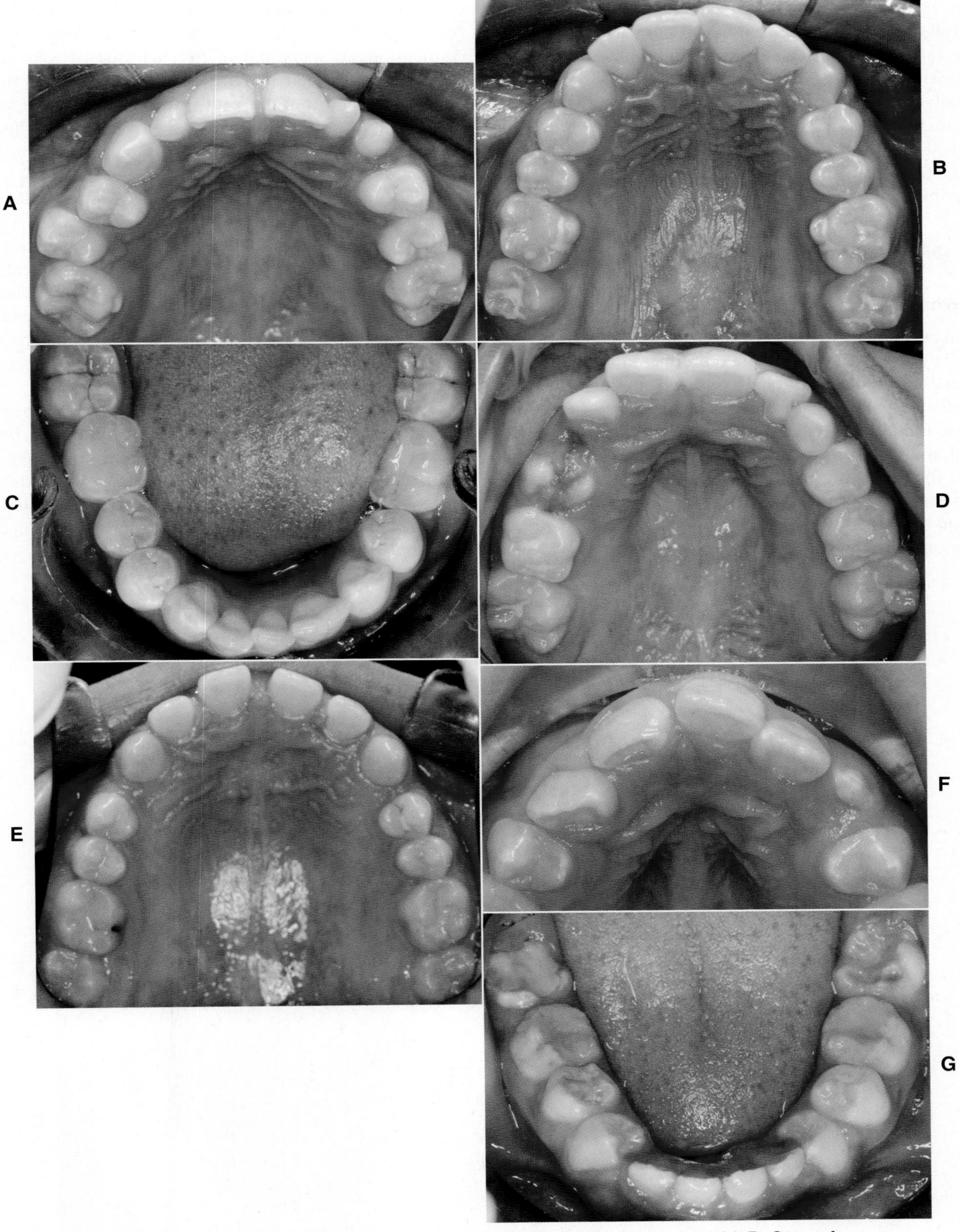

FIG 4-3 **A,** Maxillary peg lateral incisors and retained left deciduous cuspid. **B,** Cusp of Carabelli on maxillary first molars. **C,** Gemination of mandibular central and lateral incisors. **D,** Dens in dente with talon cusp. **E,** Microdontia of maxillary tooth with generalized spacing. **F,** Macrodontia of maxillary lateral incisors. **G,** Amelogenesis imperfecta.

The teeth can be hypoplastic (microdontia) (Fig. 4-3, *E*) or hyperplastic (macrodontia) (Fig. 4-3, *F*) in size, and discolorations can be of intrinsic or extrinsic origin.

Mineralization abnormalities can also be observed sporadically or as part of a syndrome such as dentinogenesis and amelogenesis imperfecta (Fig. 4-3, *G*), characterized by deficient calcification as in hypermineralization or deficient matrix formation as in hyperplasia of the affected tooth component.

ORTHODONTIC MODELS

10. What are the significant areas of cast analysis?

Dental casts obtained from impressions that extend far enough into the sulcus to allow accurate reproduction of the soft tissue anatomy should accurately represent the dentition and immediate supporting structures. The objective of study cast analysis is the 3D assessment of the maxillary and mandibular dental arches and their occlusal relationships. This encompasses the metric analysis of arch width, length, symmetry, and palatal height as well as tooth size and space analysis in relation to the apical bases and examination of the interarch occlusion. The apical base arch is the area of alveolar bone on the level of the root apices of the teeth, whereas the basal arch is formed by the maxillary and mandibular corpus. Its dimensions are stable and unaffected by tooth loss or alveolar resorption. The dental arch perimeter is measured through the contact points of the teeth and ideally should be congruent to the sizes of the alveolar and basal arches. It should be noted that the mandibular arch is often referred to as the *diagnostic arch* because of the cortical bone on the facial and lingual surfaces. In contrast to the intermolar width, which significantly increases in the maxillary arch between 3 and 13 years of age, the mandibular intercanine distance increases during the transition of primary to permanent dentition[41] (see Chapter 2), then decreases slightly until adulthood.

As part of the cast analysis, the individual arch shape should be appreciated. It has been shown that the most common arch form is the ovoid arch, followed by tapered and squared arch shapes (Fig. 4-4).[42]

Arch length discrepancy, also referred to as *arch circumference discrepancy,* is identified as the difference between the available arch length and the required arch length. It is determined by measuring the mesiodistal tooth widths of the permanent teeth from the mesial of the permanent mandibular first molars for the mandibular arch and permanent maxillary first molars for the maxillary arch.

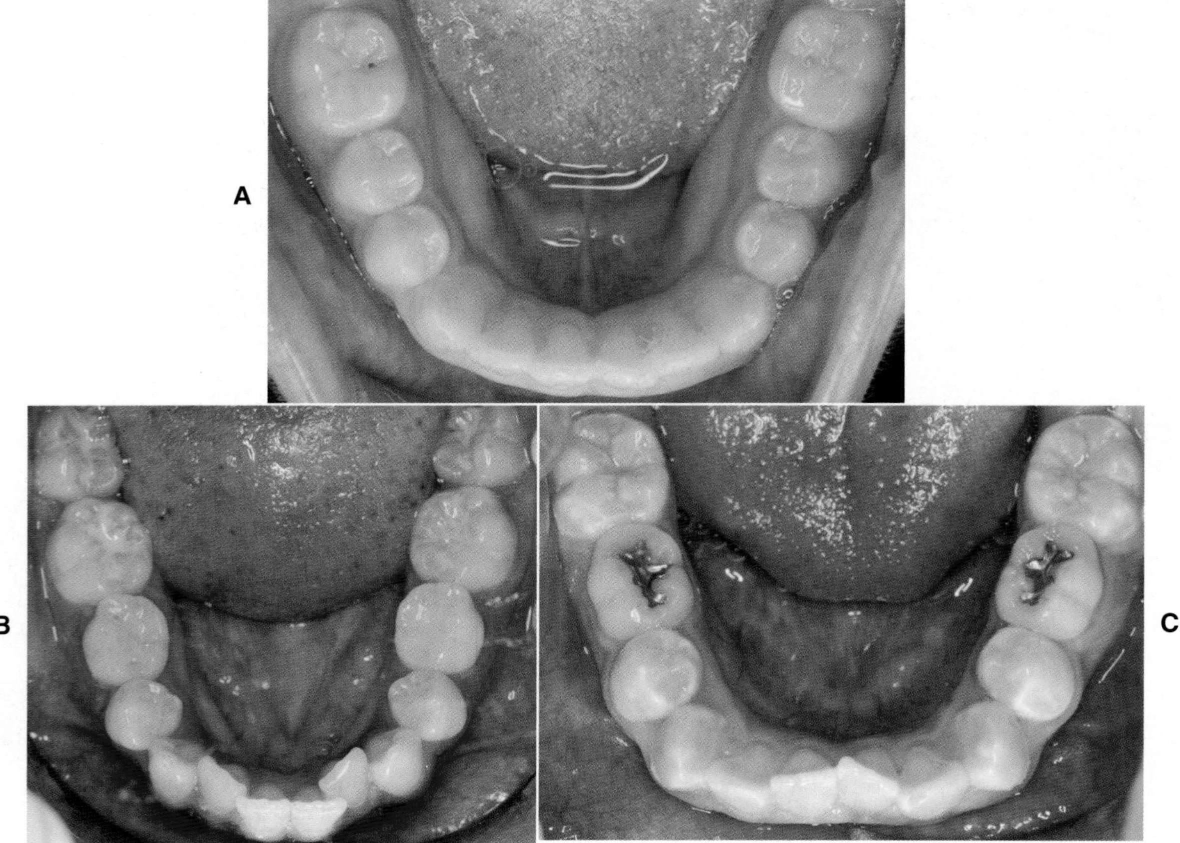

FIG 4-4 Arch forms. **A,** ovoid; **B,** tapered; **C,** square.

11. What is the Bolton analysis?

The Bolton analysis offers a method to determine the ratio of the mesiodistal widths of the maxillary versus the mandibular permanent teeth, also known as *tooth size discrepancy,* and its interarch effects. When looking at interarch relationships, it is essential to treat the anterior teeth separately from the posterior units. Tooth size discrepancies in the anterior region can be corrected only with compensations in the anterior region and not through treatment changes in the posterior teeth. Thus, the Bolton analysis consists of an anterior ratio analysis, designed to identify incompatibilities in anterior teeth, or a whole dentition ratio, which, when compared to the anterior ratio, determines the discrepancies of the posterior teeth. The anterior ratio is calculated by dividing the sum of the mesiodistal widths of the mandibular six anterior teeth by the sum of the mesiodistal widths of the maxillary anterior teeth and then multiplying the result times 100. The mean anterior ratio is 77.2, whereas the mean overall ratio is 91.3. The latter is calculated according to the same principle as the anterior ratio but is calculated by dividing the sum of the mesiodistal widths of the mandibular right first molar tooth to the left first molar tooth by the sum of the mesiodistal widths of the maxillary first molar to first molar teeth.[43,44] Studying the Bolton ratios using standardized tables for comparison of the anterior and overall ratio relationship helps to estimate the overbite and overjet relationship that will likely be obtained through orthodontic treatment as well as to identify occlusal discrepancies produced by interarch tooth size incompatibilities. It has been found that there is a high incidence of tooth size discrepancies throughout all malocclusion groups.[45] Statistically, about 5% of the population display some disproportion among individual tooth sizes, with the upper lateral incisor being most commonly affected. However, application of the Bolton analysis should be handled with care, since arch length discrepancies seem to be specific for gender and ethnicity.[46]

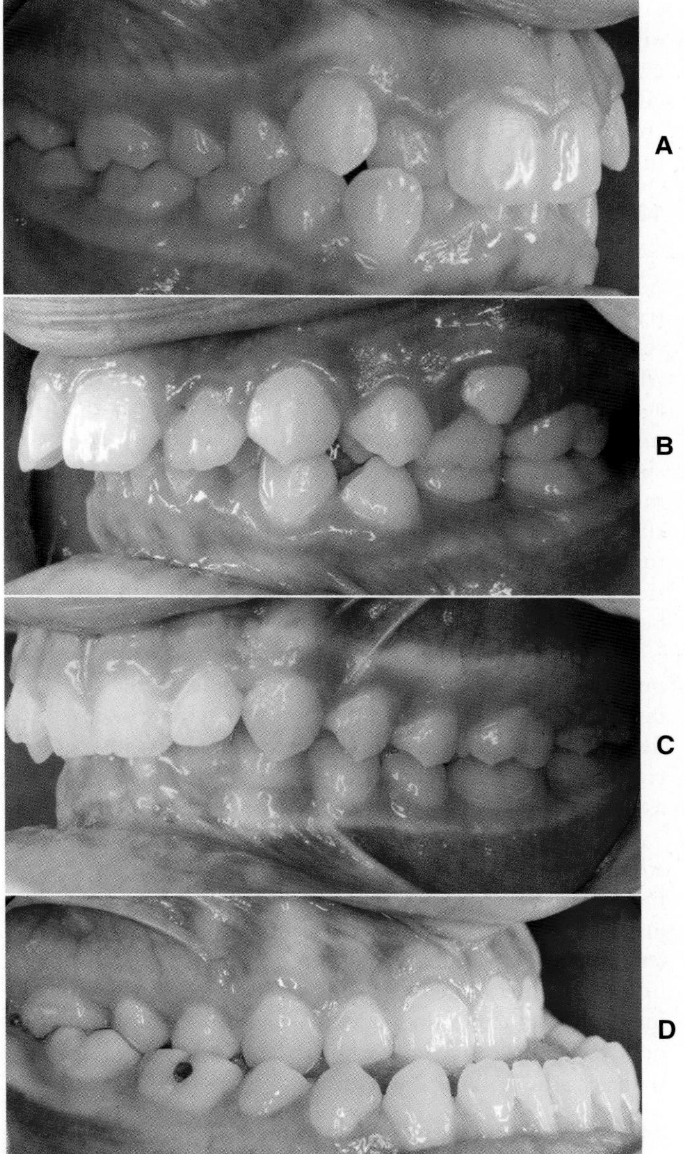

FIG 4-5 **A,** Angle's Dental Class I malocclusion. **B,** Angle's Dental Class II, division 1 malocclusion. **C,** Angle's Dental Class II, division 2 malocclusion. **D,** Angle's Dental Class III malocclusion.

12. What represents the basis for Angle's dental classification?

The Angle classification, first published in the 1890s, is based on the anteroposterior occlusal relationship of the permanent first molar that was termed the key to occlusion. According to Angle, a Class I normal occlusion is defined by the interlocking of the mesiobuccal cusp of the upper first molar into the mesiobuccal groove of the lower first molar (Fig. 4-5, *A*).

A Class II malocclusion is defined by the buccal groove of the mandibular first molar being distally positioned when in occlusion with the mesiobuccal cusp of the upper first molar. If the maxillary anterior teeth are also proclined with a large overjet, the resulting malocclusion is classified as Class II division 1 (Fig. 4-5, *B*).

If a patient presents with retroclined maxillary incisors often in combination with a deep overbite, the malocclusion is termed Class II division 2 (Fig. 4-5, *C*).

A Class III malocclusion is diagnosed when the buccal groove of the mandibular first molar is mesially positioned to the mesiobuccal cusp of the upper first molar in occlusion (Fig. 4-5, *D*).[47] According to the NHANES III study, 30% of the U.S. population present with a normal occlusion and 50-55% with a Class I malocclusion. The prevalence of Class II malocclusion is 15-20%, whereas less than 1% of the population is affected by a Class III malocclusion.[48] It has often been criticized that the Angle classification only addresses malocclusions in the sagittal dimension without evaluation of dental alignment and amount of crowding.

Only dentoalveolar relationships are described without any further skeletal or dentoskeletal evaluation, and even here, the system fails to address all possible malocclusion groups such as subdivisions that represent the condition of a unilateral malocclusion (also see questions in Chapter 2).[49]

13. How are asymmetric occlusal relationships classified?

Asymmetric occlusal relationships can result from asymmetry within an individual arch or from asymmetric skeletal relationships. If the center of the mandible is not aligned with the facial midline in rest position as well as occlusion, a true asymmetry is present and termed *laterognathy*. If a midline shift of the mandible is discernible only in occlusion within a symmetrical skeleton, a functional shift is most likely the cause of this phenomenon called *laterocclusion* (Fig. 4-6). If this patient's posterior crossbite with functional shift is not treated early with a maxillary expansion appliance and equilibration, the facial asymmetry will become permanent.

The relative contributions of skeletal and dental components to occlusal asymmetries must be distinguished in order to develop treatment plans that will achieve skeletal and dental symmetry.[50] It should be noted that mandibular and/or condylar trauma may contribute to the development of skeletal asymmetries.

Ankylosis of primary molars with resultant tipping of the adjacent teeth into the space as well as ectopic eruption of maxillary permanent first molars that often leads to premature loss of the primary second molar and subsequent loss of arch length may contribute to dental arch asymmetry. Congenitally missing or supernumerary teeth as well as space loss caused by interproximal caries or premature loss of primary or permanent teeth can result in asymmetric occlusal relationships as well as dental midline shifts.[51]

A

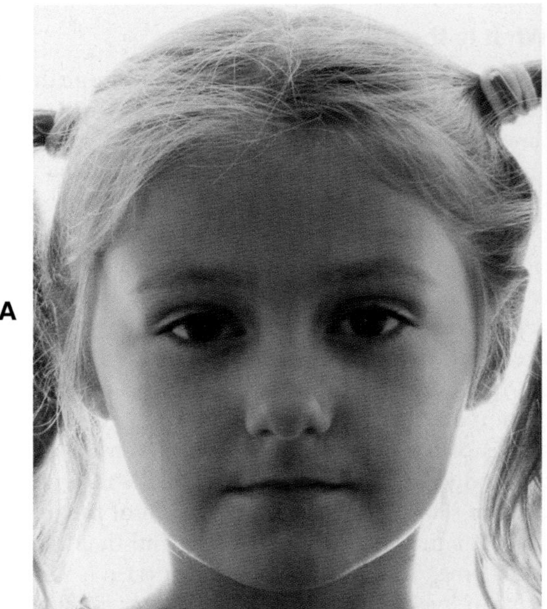

B

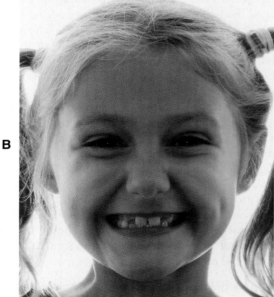

FIG 4-6 Functional shift. **A,** Patient is relaxed in centric relation. **B,** Patient is biting in centric occlusion with obvious mandibular functional shift.

14. Are digital models as reliable for diagnosis as plaster of Paris models?

OrthoCAD or e-models for 3D study cast analysis have been shown to reproduce the dentition with an accuracy of ± 0.01 mm, thus rendering a reliable tool for assessment of a patient's occlusal relationships.[52] These programs also quickly provide several tools to aid diagnosis and treatment planning such as Bolton and space analysis as well as occlusograms. In addition to improving acquisition, storage, and retrieval of the study models, the digital representation facilitates communication with other practitioners.[53,54]

15. When would a diagnostic set-up be useful?

A prognostic or diagnostic set-up is a technique that involves cutting teeth off a working cast and resetting them into a more desirable position to visualize space concerns and ascertain amount and direction of tooth movement before treatment is initiated. This may be especially helpful in interdisciplinary cases or cases using osseointegrated implants, unusual extraction patterns as well as prediction of treatment outcomes. Digital models, however, offer a less time-consuming tool to address the previously described issues.

16. What are indications for mounting orthodontic casts on the articulator?

Advocates of mounted orthodontic study casts stress the importance of this technique in revealing determinants of CO-CR discrepancy such as anteroposterior changes, vertical discrepancies, occlusal plane cants, and functional shifts caused by premature tooth contacts,[55] especially since a study revealed that 34% of adolescents and 66% of adults present with CO-CR discrepancies greater than 2 mm.[56] However, there is no evidence to support the need to mount orthodontic models.[57,58] The key assumption of articulator mounted models (i.e., that the relative position of the condyle to the occlusion will remain stable) is never met in growing patients. Considering CR registration and transferring as another potential error source,[17] it can be concluded that mounted casts do not enhance the diagnostic profile of children and adolescents. Mounted models are indicated in treatment planning and splint fabrication for orthognathic surgery patients, especially those undergoing a bimaxillary procedure, as well as recording of excursive movements in interdisciplinary cases when restorative dentistry is planned, or if a CO-CR shift greater than 2 mm is present.[17,55]

ORTHODONTIC RADIOGRAPHS

17. What are the advantages of a panoramic radiograph over a series of intraoral periapical radiographs?

Some patients can be diagnosed with missing teeth (Fig. 4-7, *A*) or supernumerary teeth (Fig. 4-7, *B* and *C*) at the clinical examination without radiographs. However, panoramic radiographs offer a broader view of the entire maxillary and mandibular arch including the TMJ (Fig. 4-7, *D*). Thus it is more likely to show any pathological lesions and mandibular asymmetries as well as supernumerary or missing teeth, variations in development or eruption timing, impaction, and deviations in tooth morphology while offering limited information about gross periodontal health, sinuses, and root parallelism.[59] It is also a useful tool in assessing quality and quantity of alveolar bone for implant or temporary anchorage device (TAD) placement and their proximity to vital structures such as the mandibular canal. Although exposing the patient to much lower radiation doses than a full mouth series, a disadvantage of the rotary panoramic radiograph technique is possible distortion of the x-ray in the anterior region.

18. When are supplemental intraoral periapical films indicated?

Whereas panoramic radiographs offer a reliable screening tool for detection of dental abnormalities,[60] additional periapical x-rays are needed if the panoramic radiograph suggests a pathologic condition that requires depiction in greater detail for more accurate evaluation.[59] It is also indicated to assess the periodontal status in adult patients as well as for the evaluation of root morphology and length in cases of root resorption[61] and appreciation of the periodontal ligament (PDL) space to rule out possible ankylosis.

19. What is the primary rationale for taking a posteroanterior cephalometric film?

It is indicated in patients with significant clinical facial asymmetries who display a large discrepancy of the border of the mandible in the lateral cephalogram as well as for evaluation of

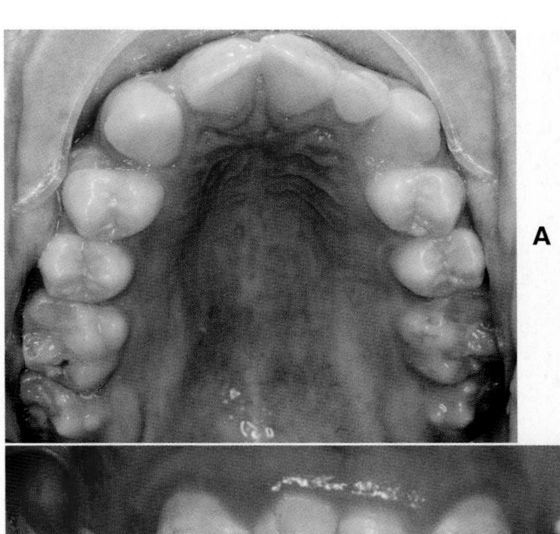

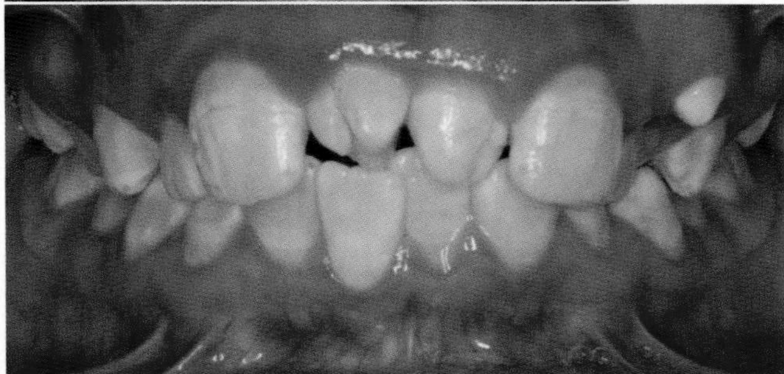

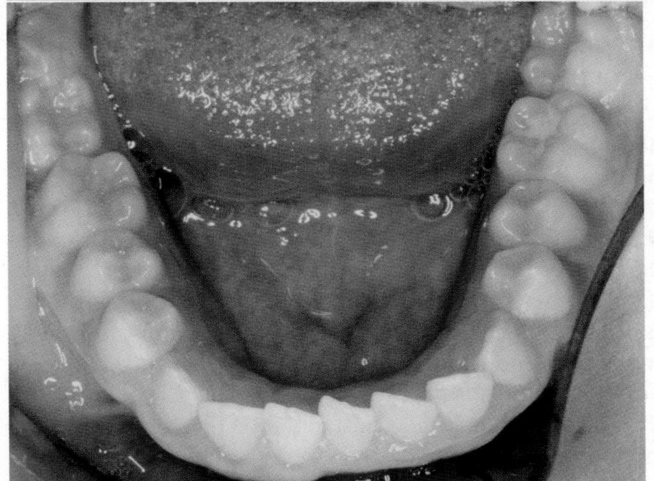

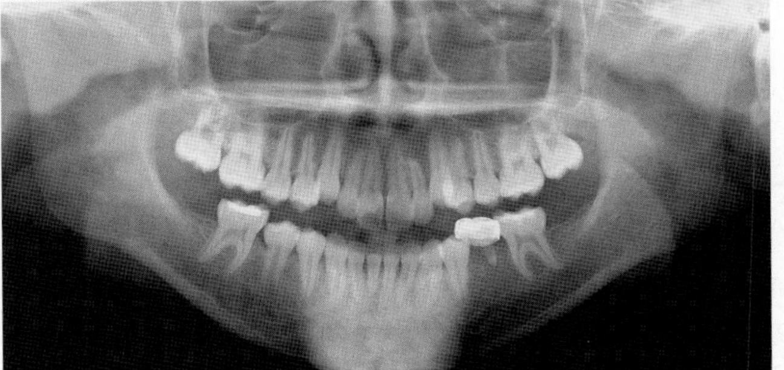

FIG 4-7 **A,** Congenitally missing maxillary lateral incisors. **B** and **C,** Supernumerary teeth: two maxillary mesiodens **(B)** and five mandibular incisors **(C)**. **D,** Panoramic radiograph demonstrating tooth agenesis.

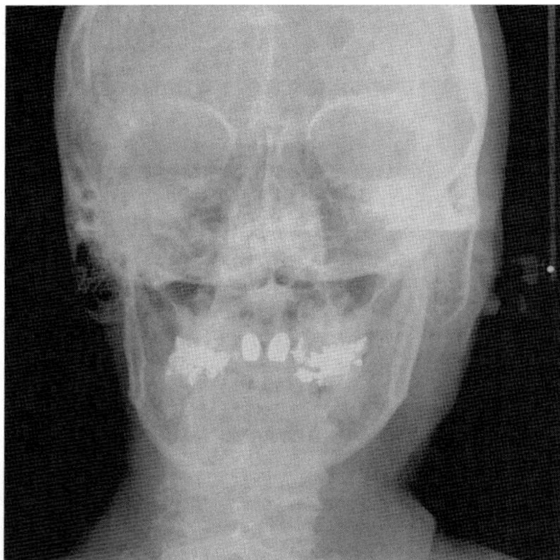

FIG 4-8 Posteroanterior cephalometric film for asymmetry.

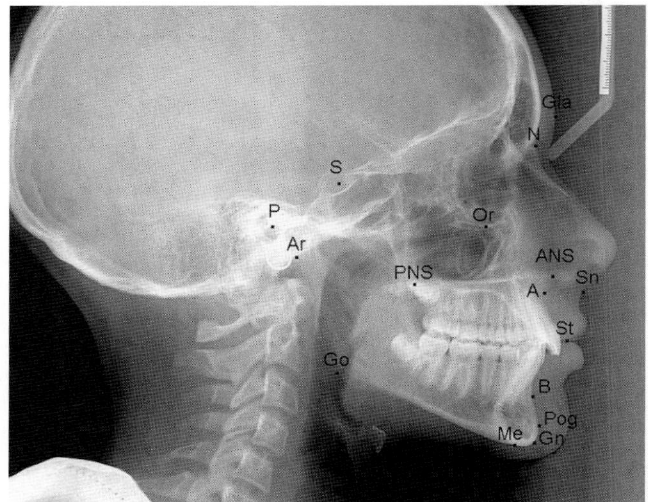

FIG 4-9 Cephalometric radiograph showing the landmarks.

severe dental midline discrepancies (Fig. 4-8). The horizontal symmetry of the mandible as well as angulation of its condyles and craniofacial anomalies can also be further explored via a submento-vertex cephalogram as needed.[62]

20. What are the different applications of a lateral cephalometric radiograph?

With the introduction of cephalometric analysis in 1931 by Hofrath[63] in Germany and Broadbent[64] in the United States, the orthodontist was given a tool to accurately evaluate the underlying anatomical basis for malocclusion and reveal details of skeletal and dental relations. Information from assessment of the configuration of the facial skeleton, relation of the jaw bases, axial inclination of the incisors, as well as soft tissue morphology, growth pattern and direction can be used in diagnosis and treatment planning, as well as prediction and recapitulation of treatment responses.[65,66] Critical limitations of the cephalogram lie foremost in the 2D representation of 3D structures. Therefore, advances in craniofacial imaging techniques will overcome these restrictions.[67]

21. What are the important hard and soft tissue points in cephalometric analysis?

LANDMARKS

Landmarks describe anatomic points that are used in measuring a cephalogram for analysis (Fig. 4-9). When these measurements are compared with "normals," they aid in diagnosis and treatment decision to correct the underlying problems. Cephalometric landmarks are divided into two types: anatomic and derived. Anatomic landmarks are those representing actual anatomical structures of the skull. Derived landmarks are constructed points from anatomical structures. Certain structures fall in the midsagittal plane and are therefore identified as a single point. Many other structures occur on both sides of the face, resulting in two radiographic points that are not coincident because of enlargement by the x-ray beam. To obtain a single, measurable point, these points are "bisected,", thereby taking an average of the two points.[68]

Hard Tissue Landmarks

Midsagittal Landmarks

Sella (S): Center of the hypophyseal fossa (sella turcica).

Nasion (N): Most anterior point of the junction of the nasal and frontal bones (frontonasal suture).

Anterior nasal spine (ANS): Most anterior bony point on the maxilla at the base of nose.

Posterior nasal spine (PNS): Posterior limit of the bony palate, radiologically constructed at the intersection of the continuation of the anterior wall of the pterygomaxillary fissure and the nasal floor.

"A" point or subspinale (A): Innermost arbitrary measure point on the curvature from the maxillary ANS to the crest of the maxillary alveolar process. "A" point is the most anterior point of the maxillary apical base and is usually located at the level of the maxillary central incisor root tip.

"B" point or supramentale (B): Deepest arbitrary measure point on the anterior bony curvature of the mandible. It is usually located at the level of the root tip of the lower central incisor representing the most anterior point of the mandibular apical base.

Pogonion (Pog): Most anterior point on the contour of the bony chin (mandibular symphysis).

Menton (Me): Most inferior point on the mandibular symphysis.

Gnathion (Gn): Most anterior inferior point on the curvature of the symphysis of the mandible. It is usually located halfway between pogonion and menton.

Bilateral Landmarks

Orbitale (Or): Lowest point on the inferior margin of the orbit.

Porion (P): Most superior point on the anatomical external auditory meatus (mechanical porion *not* used).

Articulare (Ar): A point midway between the two posterior borders of the left and right mandibular ramus at the intersection with the basilar portion of the occipital bone.

Gonion (Go): Midpoint of the curvature at the angle of the mandible. Represents junction of the ramus and body of the mandible at its posterior inferior aspect.[68]

Soft Tissue Landmarks

Glabella (Gla): Most anterior midsagittal point on the prominence of the forehead.

Subnasale (Sn): Point at which the nasal columella merges with the upper lip integument in the midsagittal plane.

Stomion (St): Located at the junction of the upper and lower lip. If lip incompetence in rest position is present, the most inferior point on the upper lip should be used to represent stomion.[68]

22. What are the important diagnostic reference planes?

Reference lines connecting two landmarks are constructed before angular, linear, and proportional measurements are made. SN is the major horizontal cranial reference plane, whereas the Frankfort horizontal (FH) forms the reference to the face and the Y-axis determines the growth pattern. Lateral cephalograms should be taken in the natural head position (NHP) that is registered when the patient looks at a mirror in front of himself or herself at eye level (Fig. 4-10). Since the NHP is not affected by intracranial landmarks and is more accurately reproducible, true vertical and horizontal reference lines can be traced.[68]

ANATOMIC PLANES

Sella-nasion (SN): Plane formed by connecting S point to N point. It represents a relatively stable anatomic structure known as the anterior cranial base. During growth and treatment, the SN plane remains relatively constant and can be used as a reference point to measure positional change of the maxilla and mandible.

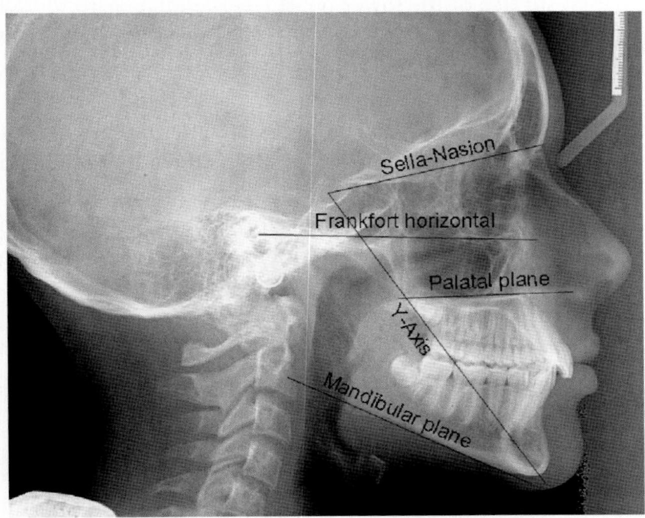

FIG 4-10 A cephalometric radiograph showing the diagnostic reference planes and measurements.

Frankfort horizontal (FH): Formed by connecting porion and orbitale.

Palatal plane (PP): Formed by a line connecting ANS to PNS. Palatal plane and FH are usually nearly parallel.

Mandibular plane (MP): A line drawn from menton to gonion. The inferior border of the mandible may vary somewhat from the line drawn through gonion, especially in cases with steep (high) mandibular plane angles. Drawing the line through bisected gonion is the most reproducible representation of MP.

Y-Axis (S-Gn): The line from sella to gnathion. It is used as an indicator for facial growth tendency by measuring the angle formed between SGn and FH.

23. Which linear and angular values are essential for both the general dentist and orthodontist to know and characterize the three different planes of space in orthodontic diagnosis?

ESSENTIALS OF THE CEPHALOMETRIC ANALYSIS

Table 4-1 provides a summary of the following findings.[68]

Anteroposterior Skeletal Measurements

SNA angle: Draw a line from nasion to A point, measure the angle formed between this line and the SN plane.

$$\text{Norm} = 82° \pm 3$$

SNB angle: Draw a line from nasion to B point and again measure the angle formed with the SN plane. The SNB angle represents the anteroposterior position of the mandible to the cranial base.

$$\text{Norm} = 80° \pm 3$$

SNA and SNB angles indicate the anteroposterior position of the maxilla and mandible relative to the cranial base. Values higher than the norms indicate prognathism for that particular jaw and lower values indicate retrognathism. However, these measurements can be erroneously affected by the shape or flexure of the cranial base: A more horizontal SN line gives a different value than a more divergent SN line. An SNA of 88 degrees would indicate maxillary prognathism, whereas the maxilla may actually be in a normal spatial relationship. Because of excessive cranial base flexure, it may only appear to be prognathic. Therefore, the relative relationship of the maxilla to the mandible determined by measuring the ANB angle is a more significant measurement.

ANB angle: Subtract the angle SNB from SNA. Measurement of ANB furnishes a relative determination of the relationship of the maxilla to the mandible.

$$\text{Norm} = 2° \pm 2$$

An ANB in the range of 0.5 to 4.5 degrees indicates a Class I skeletal pattern. Positive numbers indicate that the maxilla is ahead of the mandible. A negative angle represents

TABLE 4-1 Cephalometric Analysis Summary

PATIENT	CAUCASIAN
AP SKELETAL MEASUREMENTS	**MEAN/S.D.**
SNA	82° ± 3
SNB	80° ± 3
ANB	2° ± 2
Vertical skeletal measurements	
SN-MP	32° ± 5
SGn-FH (Y-axis)	59° ± 3
Incisor measurements	
U1-SN	103° ± 5
U1-NA	+3 mm ± 2
L1-MP	93° ± 7
L1-NB	+3 mm ± 2
U1-L1	130° ± 2
Soft tissue measurements	
Pog-NB	+3 mm ± 2
E plane	−2 mm ± 2

a mandible that is more anteriorly positioned than the maxilla. ANB has a negative value if SNB is greater than SNA. An ANB value greater than 4.5 degrees indicates an anteroposterior skeletal problem with a Class II skeletal pattern. An ANB of 0 degrees or less indicates a Class III skeletal pattern.

Vertical Skeletal Measurements

SN-MP: The mandibular plane angle is measured between SN and MP.

Norm = 32° ± 5

It is a measure for vertical growth patterns. SN-MP can be erroneously affected by excess cranial base flexure. A steep mandibular plane angle may appear normal if the anterior cranial base is flexed more anteriorly.

SGn-FH (Y-axis): Anteroinferior angle formed by the intersection of a line drawn from sella to gnathion and the Frankfort horizontal.

Norm = 59° ± 3

The Y-axis determines the overall growth pattern of the face. A patient with a vertical growth tendency would have a high Y-axis value and exhibit a "long face" tendency.

Incisor Measurements

U1-SN (upper incisor to SN): Line through the long axis of the upper incisors forms an angle with the SN plane horizontal.

Norm: 103° ± 5

Measures the inclination of the upper incisors to the SN plane. It aids in the decision whether to extract to reduce incisor proclination and crowding or to expand to resolve crowding if the upper incisors are retroclined.

U1-NA (upper incisor to NA line): Determines the anteroposterior position of the upper central incisors by the most labial surface of the upper incisor perpendicular to the NA line.

Norm: +3 mm ± 2

Positive values are recorded if the incisor is located anteriorly to the NA; negative values are recorded if the incisor is posterior to it.

L1-MP (lower incisor to mandibular plane): Line through the long axis of the most proclined lower central incisor forms an angle with MP.

Norm: 93° ± 7

It is used as a treatment goal: The more the lower incisor is flared, the greater the angle. If L1-MP is greater than 100 degrees, further labial movement of the lower incisors should be avoided. Abnormal vertical relationships will result in erroneous values of this angle.

L1-NB (lower incisor to NB line): The anteroposterior position of the lower incisor relative to the mandible can be determined by measuring the linear distance from the most labial surface of the lower incisor perpendicular to the NB line.

Norm: +3 mm ± 2

Positive values are recorded if the lower central incisor is anteriorly positioned to this line; negative values are recorded if it is posterior to it.

U1-L1 (interincisal angle): Angle formed by intersection of the long axis of the most proclined upper and lower central incisors.

Norm: 130° ± 2

Used as a treatment goal, since normal incisor angulation is critical for anterior guidance and treatment stability.

Soft Tissue Measurements

Pog-NB (pogonion to NB line): The prominence of the chin is often an important diagnostic consideration in orthodontics, especially in regard to extractions. The millimetric distance of pogonion is measured perpendicular to the line NB.

Norm: +3 mm ± 2

The soft tissue covering of the bony chin can be relatively thick or thin. A thick soft tissue could exaggerate a bony chin or produce the appearance of a normal chin in a person with a deficient bony chin button. A thin soft tissue covering could give the appearance of normality in a case with a prominent bony chin or could exaggerate a "weak" chin, resulting in an unbalanced profile.

E plane (esthetic line): The distance between the most protrusive point of the lower lip and the esthetic line (tip of nose to tip of chin).

Norm: −2.0 mm ± 2

This line indicates the soft tissue balance between lips and profile. Protrusive upper and/or lower incisors will cause a protrusive lower lip (positive values beyond the esthetic plane).

24. Which predictive analysis is a mandatory part of the diagnostic process in orthognathic surgery cases?

The visual treatment objective (VTO) is a tool to predict desirable anteroposterior and vertical changes that will occur as a result of changes in the denture bases and tooth position caused by growth, orthodontic treatment, and orthognathic surgery. It is used in the development of the treatment plan as well as to present anticipated treatment results for different treatment options of orthodontic camouflage or orthognathic surgery to a prospective patient.[69] Since the growth prediction is based on average changes, this method is more reliable in adults or late adolescents with little or no remaining growth. In summary, the accuracy of the prediction is dependent on the accuracy of the treatment effect and future growth.[70]

25. Why do orthodontists superimpose serial cephalograms?

Superimpositions are used to retrospectively study changes in jaw and tooth positions brought about through orthodontic treatment and growth.[71] To study maxillary changes, pre-treatment and post-treatment cephalograms are superimposed on the lingual curvature of the palate.[72] The mandibular composite is registered on the internal cortical outline of the symphysis with best fit on the mandibular canal to assess mandibular tooth movement as well as incremental growth of the lower jaw.[73,74] Superimposition of the cephalometric records on sella enables the evaluation of overall growth and treatment changes.[75] This technique is also used in orthognathic surgery cases to confirm growth cessation in the craniofacial region by superimposing two sequential cephalograms taken within a 6- to 12-month interval. The lack of bony changes affirms that no further growth has taken place in that time interval.

ORTHODONTIC PHOTOGRAPHS

26. What are the views captured in orthodontic photographs?

For evaluation of the craniofacial and soft tissue relationships, a facial profile view, a frontal view, and a smiling frontal photograph should be routinely taken for each prospective patient. The photos should be oriented to the FH and taken with relaxed lips and exposed ears. In addition, they should be one-quarter life size from top of the head to the bottom of the chin. Moreover, a sequence of intraoral photographs at 1:1 ratio to life size should be recorded in centric occlusion consisting of a frontal view with the teeth in maximal intercuspation, as well as right and left lateral views. The picture series should be completed with maxillary and mandibular occlusal views that show a clean dentition free from saliva or bubbles. These intraoral photographs are an important aspect in the documentation of existing dental conditions such as tooth discoloration and oral hygiene status at initiation of treatment. In addition, the frontal photograph can be used to identify the patient's facial type (Fig. 4-11, *A-C*) and lip competency (Fig. 4-11, *D* and *E*), whereas the profile view can be helpful in determining the patient's profile (Fig. 4-11, *F-I*).

In evaluation of the buccal corridors, the smiling photograph can prove to be helpful (Fig. 4-11, *J* and *K*). Dark buccal corriders may be indicative of a maxillary transverse deficiency, and intermolar width may need to be increased with an expansion appliance.

To compare the relation of dental midlines to the facial midline, have the patient sit upright and facing the orthodontist. Dental floss placed along the facial skeleton, from soft tissue glabella through the philtrum to soft tissue pogonion, can be used to identify deviations of the dental midlines (Fig. 4-11, *L-N*). Achieving upper and lower dental midlines with each other and with the facial midline is an esthetic goal for every orthodontic patient. In addition, coincident midlines serve a functional purpose to assist in establishing good buccal interdigitation.

27. Which aspects should be noted in the diagnosis of frontal photographs?

The symmetry of the face should be evaluated by dividing the face into vertical thirds measured from trichion to glabella, glabella to subnasale, and subnasale to menton. This is known as the Rule of Thirds (Fig. 4-12, *A*).

The evaluation of the lower third is especially important since it is most profoundly affected by orthodontic treatment. It can be further divided into one third from subnasale to stomion and two thirds from stomion to soft-tissue menton.

The Rule of Fifths (Fig. 4-12, *B*) describes the ideal transverse relations of the face. For this assessment, the face is divided into a centered fifth bordered by vertical lines through the inner canthi of the right and left eye. Ideally, it should be coincident with the alar base of the nose. The medial fifths represent the width of the eyes and should be coincident with

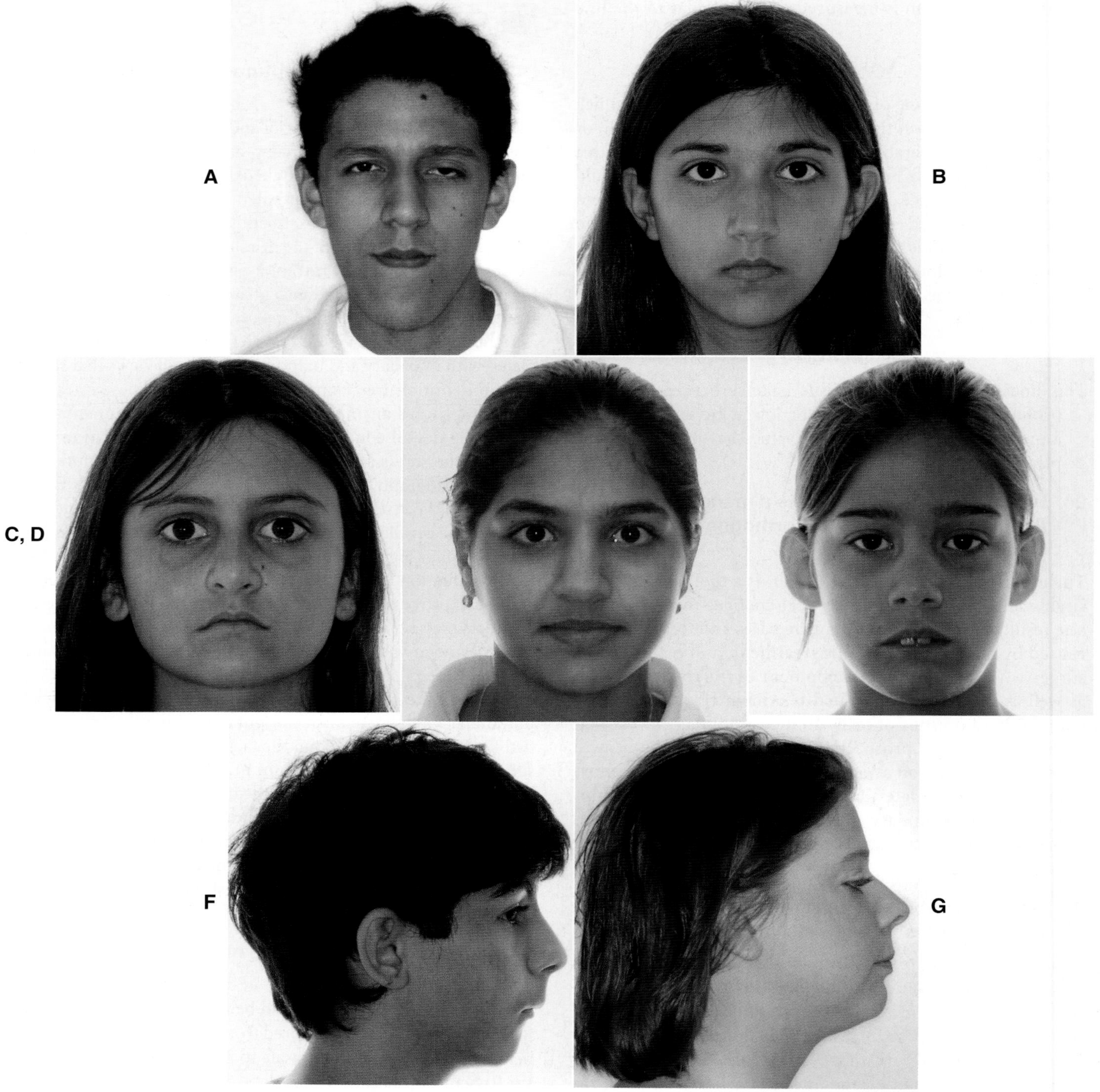

FIG 4-11 Frontal facial photographs: dolichofacial **(A),** mesofacial **(B),** and brachyfacial **(C);** lips: competent **(D)** and incompetent **(E);** profile photographic analysis: convex **(F),** straight **(G).**

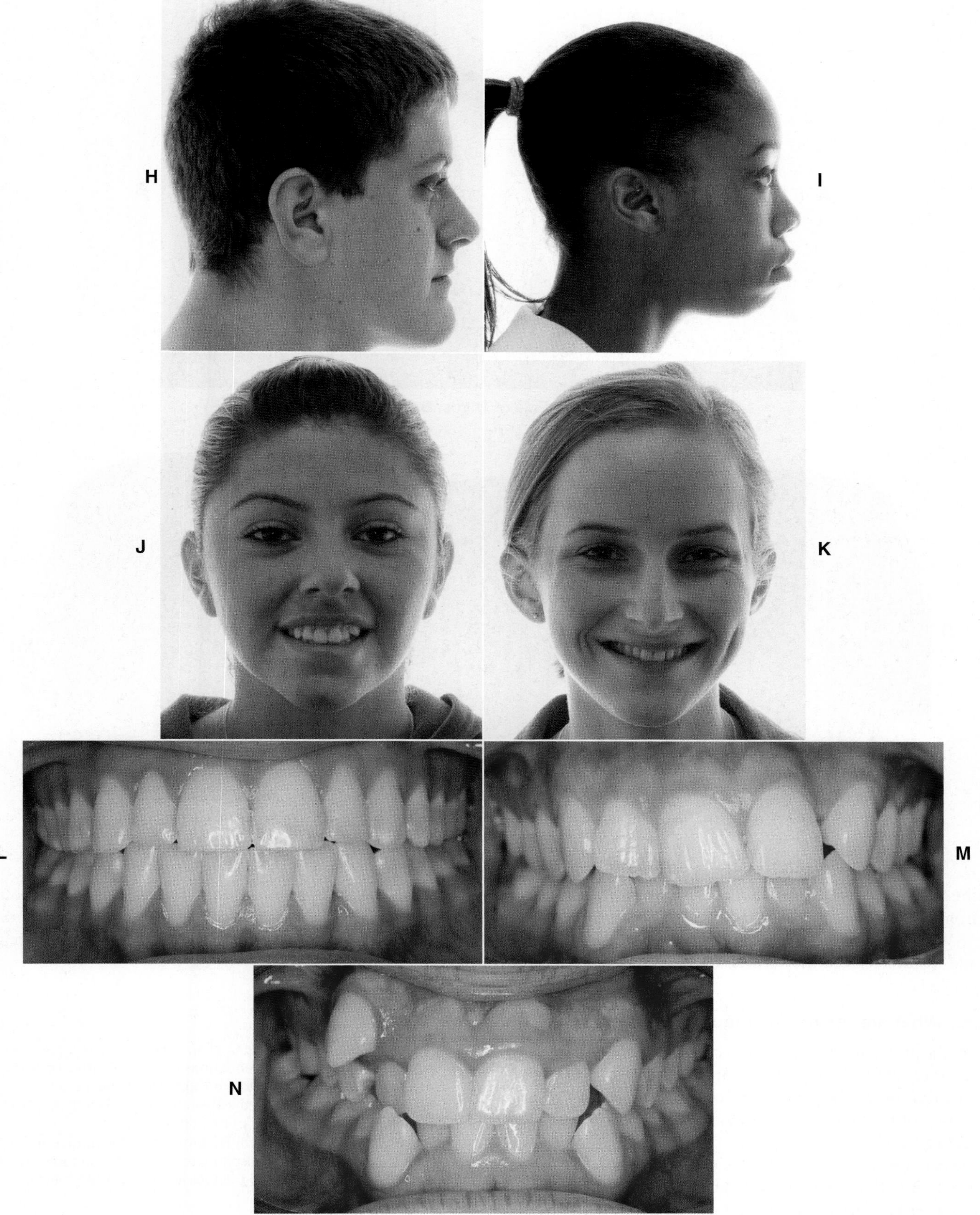

FIG 4-11—cont'd, Profile photographic analysis: concave **(H)** and bimaxillary protrusion **(I);** buccal corridors: normal **(J)** and dark **(K);** midlines: coincident **(L),** UDML shift to left **(M),** and UDML shift to right **(N).**

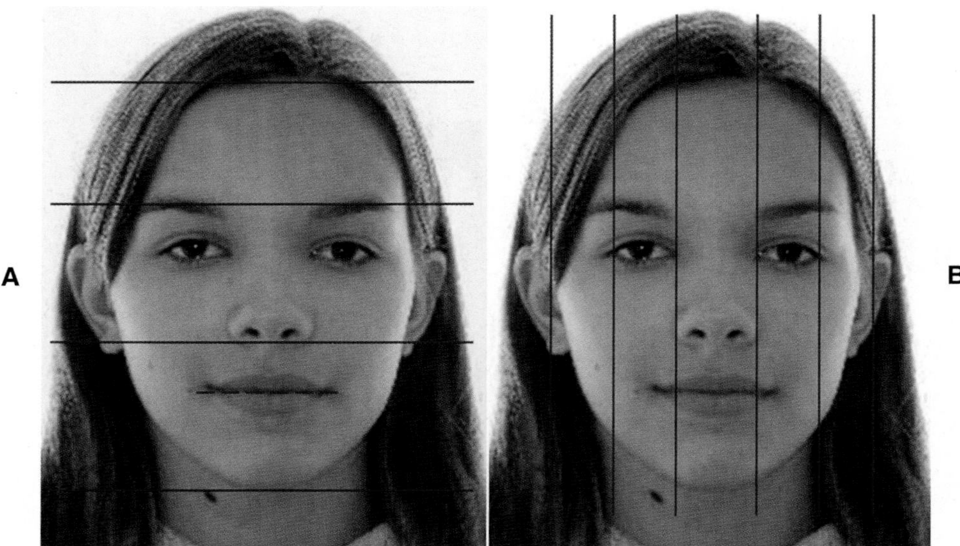

FIG 4-12 **A,** The Rule of Thirds. **B,** The Rule of Fifths.

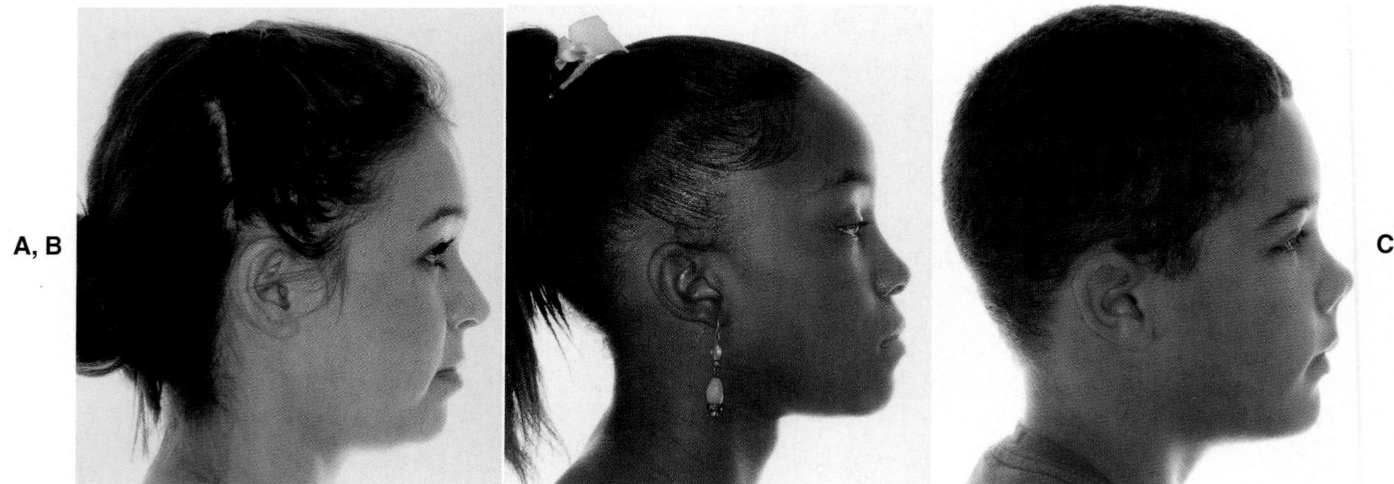

FIG 4-13 Profile analysis—nasolabial angle: normal **(A)**, acute **(B)**, and obtuse **(C)**.

the gonial angles of the mandible. The outer fifths are measured from the outer canthus to the helix of the ear on each side.

With the aid of these reference lines, facial disproportions and asymmetries in the vertical and transverse planes can be appreciated.[76,77]

28. What are the goals of facial profile analysis?

On the profile photograph, facial convexity and the anteroposterior position of the jaws should be evaluated. Furthermore, attention should be paid to lip posture and tonicity as well as incisor prominence with the nasolabial angle as an excellent reference. The nasolabial angle (NLA) is very important in the decision to extract teeth (Fig. 4-13). In the patient with an acute NLA, the extraction would be beneficial to the facial profile. However, extraction in a patient with an obtuse NLA would be detrimental to facial esthetics.

The overall facial proportions and mandibular angle should be assessed. It is important to take into consideration that mentioned characteristics are influenced by race and ethnicity, as well as gender.[76,78]

REFERENCES

1. Rivera SM, Hatch JP, Dolce C, et al: Patients' own reasons and patient-perceived recommendations for orthognathic surgery. *Am J Orthod Dentofacial Orthop* 2000;118(2):134-141.
2. Meraw SJ, Sheridan PJ: Medically induced gingival hyperplasia. *Mayo Clin Proc* 1998;73(12):1196-1199.
3. Igarashi K, Mitani H, Adachi H, Shinoda H: Anchorage and retentive effects of a bisphosphonate (AHBuBP) on tooth movements in rats. *Am J Orthod Dentofacial Orthop* 1994;106(3): 279-289.

4. Arias OR, Marquez-Orozco MC: Aspirin, acetaminophen, and ibuprofen: their effects on orthodontic tooth movement. *Am J Orthod Dentofacial Orthop* 2006;130(3):364-370.
5. Tyrovola JB, Spyropoulos MN: Effects of drugs and systemic factors on orthodontic treatment. *Quintessence Int* 2001;32(5):365-371.
6. Mossey PA: The heritability of malocclusion: part 2. The influence of genetics in malocclusion. *Br J Orthod.* 1999;26(3):195-203.
7. Hägg U, Taranger J: Menarche and voice change as indicators of the pubertal growth spurt. *Acta Odontol Scand* 1980;38(3):179-186.
8. Mathews DP, Kokich VG: Managing treatment for the orthodontic patient with periodontal problems. *Semin Orthod* 1997;3(1):21-38.
9. Zachrisson BU: Clinical implications of recent orthodontic-periodontic research findings. *Semin Orthod* 1996;2(1):4-12.
10. Kluemper GT, Vig PS, Vig KW: Nasorespiratory characteristics and craniofacial morphology. *Eur J Orthod.* 1995;17(6):491-495.
11. Vig KW: Nasal obstruction and facial growth: the strength of evidence for clinical assumptions. *Am J Orthod Dentofacial Orthop* 1998;113(6):603-611.
12. Cozza P, Baccetti T, Franchi L, et al: Sucking habits and facial hyperdivergency as risk factors for anterior open bite in the mixed dentition. *Am J Orthod Dentofacial Orthop* 2005; 128(4):517-519.
13. Larsson E: Sucking, chewing, and feeding habits and the development of crossbite: a longitudinal study of girls from birth to 3 years of age. *Angle Orthod* 2001;71(2):116-119.
14. Fraser C: Tongue thrust and its influence in orthodontics. *Int J Orthod* 2006;17(1):9-18.
15. Laskin DM: The clinical diagnosis of temporomandibular disorders in the orthodontic patient. *Semin Orthod* 1995;1(4): 197-206.
16. Fu AS, Mehta NR, Forgione AG, et al: Maxillomandibular relationship in TMD patients before and after short-term flat plane bite plate therapy. *Cranio* 2003;21(3):172-179.
17. Clark JR, Hutchinson I, Sandy JR: Functional occlusion: II. The role of articulators in orthodontics. *J Orthod* 2001;28(2):173-177.
18. Laskin DM: Etiology of the pain-dysfunction syndrome. *J Am Dent Assoc* 1969;79(1):147-153.
19. Griffiths RH, Laskin DM: The President's Conference on the Examination, Diagnosis and Management of Temporomandibular Disorders. Anonymous American Dental Association; 1983.
20. Mehra T, Nanda RS, Sinha PK: Orthodontists' assessment and management of patient compliance. *Angle Orthod* 1998; 68(2):115-122.
21. Hunter CJ: The correlation of facial growth with body height and skeletal maturation at adolescence. *Angle Orthod* 1966;36(1):44-54.
22. Fishman LS: Chronological versus skeletal age, an evaluation of craniofacial growth. *Angle Orthod* 1979;49(3):181-189.
23. Malmgren O, Omblus J, Hägg U, Pancherz H: Treatment with an orthopedic appliance system in relation to treatment intensity and growth periods. A study of initial effects. *Am J Orthod Dentofacial Orthop* 1987;91(2):143-151.
24. Pancherz H: The effects, limitations, and long-term dentofacial adaptations to treatment with the Herbst appliance. *Semin Orthod* 1997;3(4):232-243.
25. Baccetti T, Franchi L, Toth LR, McNamara JA, Jr: Treatment timing for Twin-block therapy. *Am J Orthod Dentofacial Orthop* 2000;118(2):159-170.
26. Fishman LS: Maturational patterns and prediction during adolescence. *Angle Orthod* 1987;57(3):178-193.
27. Fishman LS: Radiographic evaluation of skeletal maturation. A clinically oriented method based on hand-wrist films. *Angle Orthod* 1982;52(2):88-112.
28. Moore RN: Principles of dentofacial orthopedics. *Semin Orthod* 1997;3(4):212-221.
29. Hassel B, Farman AG: Skeletal maturation evaluation using cervical vertebrae. *Am J Orthod Dentofacial Orthop* 1995;107(1):58-66.
30. Baccetti T, Franchi L, McNamara JA, Jr: An improved version of the cervical vertebral maturation (CVM) method for the assessment of mandibular growth. *Angle Orthod* 2002;72(4): 316-323.
31. Lamparski DG: Skeletal age assessment utilizing cervical vertebrae, master's thesis, Pittsburgh, University of Pittsburgh, 1972.
32. Franchi L, Baccetti T, McNamara JA, Jr: Mandibular growth as related to cervical vertebral maturation and body height. *Am J Orthod Dentofacial Orthop* 2000;118(3):335-340.
33. Flores-Mir C, Burgess CA, Champney M, et al: Correlation of skeletal maturation stages determined by cervical vertebrae and hand-wrist evaluations. *Angle Orthod* 2006;76(1):1-5.
34. Kucukkeles N, Acar A, Biren S, Arun T: Comparisons between cervical vertebrae and hand-wrist maturation for the assessment of skeletal maturity. *J Clin Pediatr Dent* 1999;24(1):47-52.
35. Lischer BE: *Principles and methods of orthodontics.* Philadelphia: Lea & Febiger, 1912.
36. Thilander B, Jakobsson SO: Local factors in impaction of maxillary canines. *Acta Odontol Scand* 1968;26(2):145-168.
37. Shapira Y, Kuftinec MM: Maxillary tooth transpositions: characteristic features and accompanying dental anomalies. *Am J Orthod Dentofacial Orthop* 2001;119(2):127-134.
38. Kharat DU, Saini TS, Mokeem S: Shovel-shaped incisors and associated invagination in some Asian and African populations. *J Dent* 1990;18(4):216-220.
39. Tsai SJ, King NM: A catalogue of anomalies and traits of the permanent dentition of southern Chinese. *J Clin Pediatr Dent* 1998;22(3):185-194.
40. Hülsmann M: [Dens invaginatus–its etiology, incidence and clinical characteristics (I). A review]. *Schweiz Monatsschr Zahnmed* 1995;105(6):765-776.
41. Ward DE, Workman J, Brown R, Richmond S: Changes in arch width. A 20-year longitudinal study of orthodontic treatment. *Angle Orthod* 2006;76(1):6-13.
42. Nojima K, McLaughlin RP, Isshiki Y, Sinclair PM: A comparative study of Caucasian and Japanese mandibular clinical arch forms. *Angle Orthod* 2001;71(3):195-200.
43. Bolton WA: The clinical application of a tooth-size analysis. *Am J Orthod* 1962;48(7):504-529.
44. Bolton WA: Disharmony in tooth size and its relation to the analysis and treatment of malocclusion. *Angle Orthod* 1952;28:113.
45. Crosby DR, Alexander CG: The occurrence of tooth size discrepancies among different malocclusion groups. *Am J Orthod Dentofacial Orthop* 1989;95(6):457-461.
46. Smith SS, Buschang PH, Watanabe E: Interarch tooth size relationships of 3 populations: "does Bolton's analysis apply?" *Am J Orthod Dentofacial Orthop* 2000;117(2):169-174.
47. Angle EH: Classification of malocclusion. *Dent Cosmos* 1899;41(2):248-264.
48. Proffit WR, Fields HW, Jr, Moray LJ: Prevalence of malocclusion and orthodontic treatment need in the United States: estimates from the NHANES III survey. *Int J Adult Orthod Orthognath Surg* 1998;13(2):97-106.
49. Siegel MA: A matter of Class: interpreting subdivision in a malocclusion. *Am J Orthod Dentofacial Orthop* 2002;122(6):582-586.
50. Burstone CJ: Diagnosis and treatment planning of patients with asymmetries. *Semin Orthod* 1998;4(3):153-164.
51. Kronmiller JE: Development of asymmetries. *Semin Orthod* 1998;4(3):134-137.
52. Costalos PA, Sarraf K, Cangialosi TJ, Efstratiadis S: Evaluation of the accuracy of digital model analysis for the American Board of Orthodontics objective grading system for dental casts. *Am J Orthod Dentofacial Orthop* 2005;128(5):624-629.
53. Marcel TJ: Three-dimensional on-screen virtual models. *Am J Orthod Dentofacial Orthop* 2001;119(6):666-668.

54. Zilberman O, Huggare JAV, Parikakis KA: Evaluation of the validity of tooth size and arch width measurements using conventional and three-dimensional virtual orthodontic models. *Angle Orthod* 2003;73(3):301-306.
55. Cordray FE: Centric relation treatment and articulator mountings in orthodontics. *Angle Orthod* 1996;66(2):153-158.
56. Agerberg G, Sandström R: Frequency of occlusal interferences: a clinical study in teenagers and young adults. *J Prosthet Dent* 1988;59(2):212-217.
57. Rinchuse DJ, Kandasamy S: Articulators in orthodontics: an evidence-based perspective. *Am J Orthod Dentofacial Orthop* 2006;129(2):299-308.
58. Ellis PE, Benson PE: Does articulating study casts make a difference to treatment planning? *J Orthod* 2003;30(1):45.
59. Quintero JC, Trosien A, Hatcher D, Kapila S: Craniofacial imaging in orthodontics: historical perspective, current status, and future developments. *Angle Orthod* 1999;69(6):491-506.
60. Ferguson JW, Evans RI, Cheng LH: Diagnostic accuracy and observer performance in the diagnosis of abnormalities in the anterior maxilla: a comparison of panoramic with intraoral radiography. *Br Dent J* 1992;173(8):265-271.
61. Sameshima GT, Asgarifar KO: Assessment of root resorption and root shape: periapical vs panoramic films. *Angle Orthod* 2001;71(3):185-189.
62. Forsberg CT, Burstone CJ, Hanley KJ: Diagnosis and treatment planning of skeletal asymmetry with the submental-vertical radiograph. *Am J Orthod* 1984;85(3):224-237.
63. Hofrath H: Die Bedeutung der Röntgenfern-und Abstandsaufnahme für die Diagnostik der Kieferanomalien. *J Orofacial Orthop/Fortschritte Kieferorthopädie* 1931;1(2):232-258.
64. Broadbent BH: A new X-ray technique and its application to orthodontia. *Angle Orthod* 1931;1(2):45-66.
65. Steiner CC: The use of cephalometrics as an aid to planning and assessing orthodontic treatment. *Am J Orthod* 1960;46(10): 721-735.
66. Ricketts RM: Perspectives in the clinical application of cephalometrics. The first fifty years. *Angle Orthod* 1981;51(2):115-150.
67. Harrell WE Jr, Hatcher DC, Bolt RL: In search of anatomic truth: 3-dimensional digital modeling and the future of orthodontics. *Am J Orthod Dentofacial Orthop* 2002;122(3):325-330.
68. Salas-Lopez A: Cephalometric Tracing Technique Manual, University of Texas Dental Branch at Houston, Department of Orthodontics, 2006.
69. Bench RW: The visual treatment objective: Orthodontic's most effective treatment planning tool. *Proc Found Orthod Res* 1971;4(2):165-194.
70. Toepel-Sievers C, Fischer-Brandies H: Validity of the computer-assisted cephalometric growth prognosis VTO (Visual Treatment Objective) according to Ricketts. *J Orofac Orthop* 1999;60(3):185-194.
71. Efstratiadis SS, Cohen G, Ghafari J: Evaluation of differential growth and orthodontic treatment outcome by regional cephalometric superpositions. *Angle Orthod* 1999;69(3):225-230.
72. Bjork A, Skieller V: Growth of the maxilla in three dimensions as revealed radiographically by the implant method. *Br J Orthod* 1977 Apr;4(2):53-64.
73. Björk A, Skieller V: Normal and abnormal growth of the mandible. A synthesis of longitudinal cephalometric implant studies over a period of 25 years. *Eur J Orthod* 1983;5(1):1-46.
74. Cook AH, Sellke TA, BeGole EA: The variability and reliability of two maxillary and mandibular superimposition techniques. Part II. *Am J Orthod Dentofacial Orthop* 1994;106(5):463-471.
75. Ghafari J, Engel FE, Laster LL: Cephalometric superimposition on the cranial base: a review and a comparison of four methods. *Am J Orthod Dentofacial Orthop* 1987;91(5):403-413.
76. Peck H, Peck S: A concept of facial esthetics. *Angle Orthod* 1970;40(4):284-318.
77. Morris W: An orthodontic view of dentofacial esthetics. *Compendium* 1994;15(3):378.
78. Bishara SE, Jakobsen JR, Hession TJ, Treder JE: Soft tissue profile changes from 5 to 45 years of age. *Am J Orthod Dentofacial Orthop* 1998;114(6):698-706.

Three-Dimensional Imaging in Orthodontics

CHAPTER 5

Chung How Kau • Stephen Richmond

The advances of three-dimensional (3D) technology have accelerated at a tremendous pace over the last two decades with newer machines and advanced software support. This now means that applications for the clinical settings can be created and used in routine diagnosis, treatment planning, and patient education. Orthodontists will find that these advances will also impact the profession, and this chapter aims to give the reader the basic foundation on which to understand this interesting and exciting topic.

1. Imaging techniques and devices—what do these mean to the orthodontist?

New technologies reach the commercial and clinical environments on a daily basis and filter through every aspect of the medical and dental field. Orthodontists too are exposed to this fast pace of change, and these advancements have allowed innovative methods for facial diagnosis, treatment planning, and clinical application.

With continuing innovations and the use of powerful computer software tools, the last two decades have seen a reintroduction of both hard and soft tissue imaging devices in rapid succession. The orthodontist needs to embrace these new methods of diagnosis and treatment planning, since the images produced add a new dimension to present day concepts and test the foundations of our knowledge.

2. What does it mean to have a three-dimensional image and how is it obtained?

Three-dimensional image reconstruction is a complex task using mathematical principles. The 3D image is essentially an object that appears to have an extension in depth. In photography, a 3D image is reconstructed by the principles of stereoscopic vision when two images are pieced together from two or more cameras at known distances and angles. In radiography, multi-slice or multi-views of an object are cleverly reconstructed using complex mathematical algorithms to produce a representation of the object.

3. What is a possible classification of these devices?

Three-dimensional images may be obtained in a variety of ways. A possible classification system is listed in Table 5-1.

4. What are some clinical applications?

There are a number of reported and possible clinical applications. These will be discussed under two main headings: surface imaging and hard tissue imaging.

SURFACE IMAGING

Facial Growth

Significant investigations have been done in the past on hard tissue growth of the cranial skeleton. However, reported studies focusing on and analyzing soft tissue morphology and growth are comparatively small in relation to the general orthodontic literature.[1] Yet the external profile is by far the most visible entity from which clinicians and lay people make perceptions and formulate judgments. In this current day and age, with a greater emphasis being placed on the balance between the hard and soft tissues, it is important to have reliable and readily available data on the external soft tissue profile. At present, there is a lack of emphasis on the longitudinal development of the soft tissues. Most of the available data on the changing soft tissue profile have been obtained from cephalometric data with an additional small number from limited 3D data. Soft tissue studies are difficult and the tissue structures are inevitably affected by movements and distortions. However, careful patient positioning and good technical detailing have allowed these images to be reproducible to a high level of clinical acceptability.

Early 3D imaging research has shown that the growth of facial structures broadly follows in line with gender and age. Growth is present in a number of facial structures and may be visualized as surface and volume changes (Fig. 5-1). Furthermore, the system is so sensitive that asymmetric growth is identified in 33% of 11- to 12-year-olds. In the vast majority of these cases, the asymmetrical growth levels out over 1 year of assessment. However, there are a small proportion of children who continue to grow asymmetrically (Fig. 5-2).

Average Faces and Superimposition

Average faces of 3D images from a cohort of same-age individuals may also be created.[2,3] This procedure involves prealignment of the images by determining their principal axes

TABLE 5-1 Tabular Representation of Surface Imaging Devices

METHOD	SOURCE	INDUSTRY EXAMPLES
Direct Contact	Manual Probe	a. Polhemus 3 Space Digitizer b. ELITE
Photo-grammetry	Conventional photography	a. Stereo-photogrammetry
Lasers	670–690 nm Class I or II FDA approved laser lights	a. Fixed Units • Medical Graphics and Imaging Group, UCL • Cyberware Laboratory 3030 / SP • Others
	670–690 nm Class I or II FDA approved laser lights	b. Portable and Mobile • Minolta Systems (Model versions 700, 900, 910, 9i) • Polhemus hand-held (FASTSCAN)
Structured Light	Distorted light patterns and photogrammetric light capture	a. Single Camera b. Multiple Camera • Moire patterns • OGIS Range Finder RFX-IV • CAM, three-dimensional Shape system • C3D-dimensional Stereo-photogrammetry (Glasgow)—Computer aided • 3dMD™ Face System • Others
Video-Imaging	Video sequencing	a. Motion-Analysis™
Radiation Sources	Radiation pulses	a. CT Scans b. Cone Beam CTs
Others		a. MRI b. Ultrasound

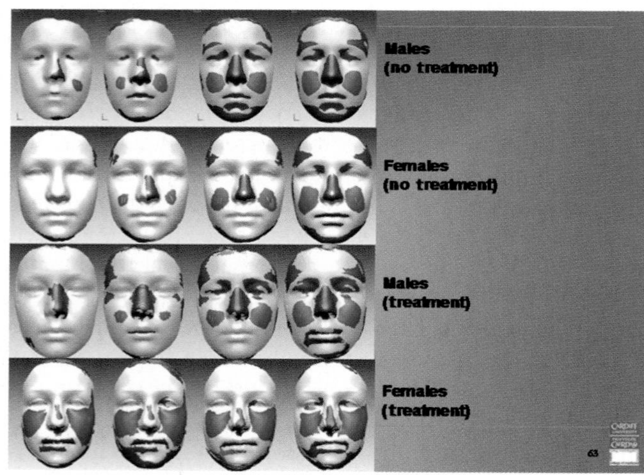

FIG 5-1 Facial growth as illustrated by average facial changes in males and females. Red areas indicate positive changes, whereas blue areas indicate negative changes.

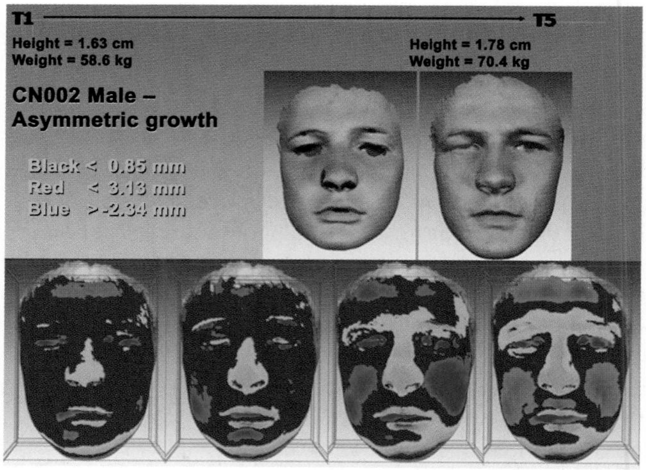

FIG 5-2 Asymmetrical growth of a child's face over a 2-year growth period. Note the asymmetrical shuffling of the mandible.

(based on computing the tensor of inertia of each 3D image) followed by best fit alignment of the images and then by averaging the image coordinates normally to the facial plane. For each point representing the obtained average facial plane, the standard deviations are calculated allowing construction of the "standard deviation" faces that indicate variation from the average face. The results obtained may be used for the identification of facial anomalies in patients (Fig. 5-3). The face examined is superimposed onto the average face using the best fit technique, and then a divergence map can be constructed showing the regions with abnormal deviations. The deviations can be identified and quantified in terms of linear, area, and volumetric measurements.

Surgical Evaluations

Patients are often anxious to know the treatment effects following orthognathic surgery, and current information available can only be extrapolated from research using 2D data. As a result, clinicians are not able to provide an accurate picture to the patient and to give advice regarding the morbidity involved. The successful application of 3D imaging technology provides a means for further analysis in clinical trials.[4] Initial

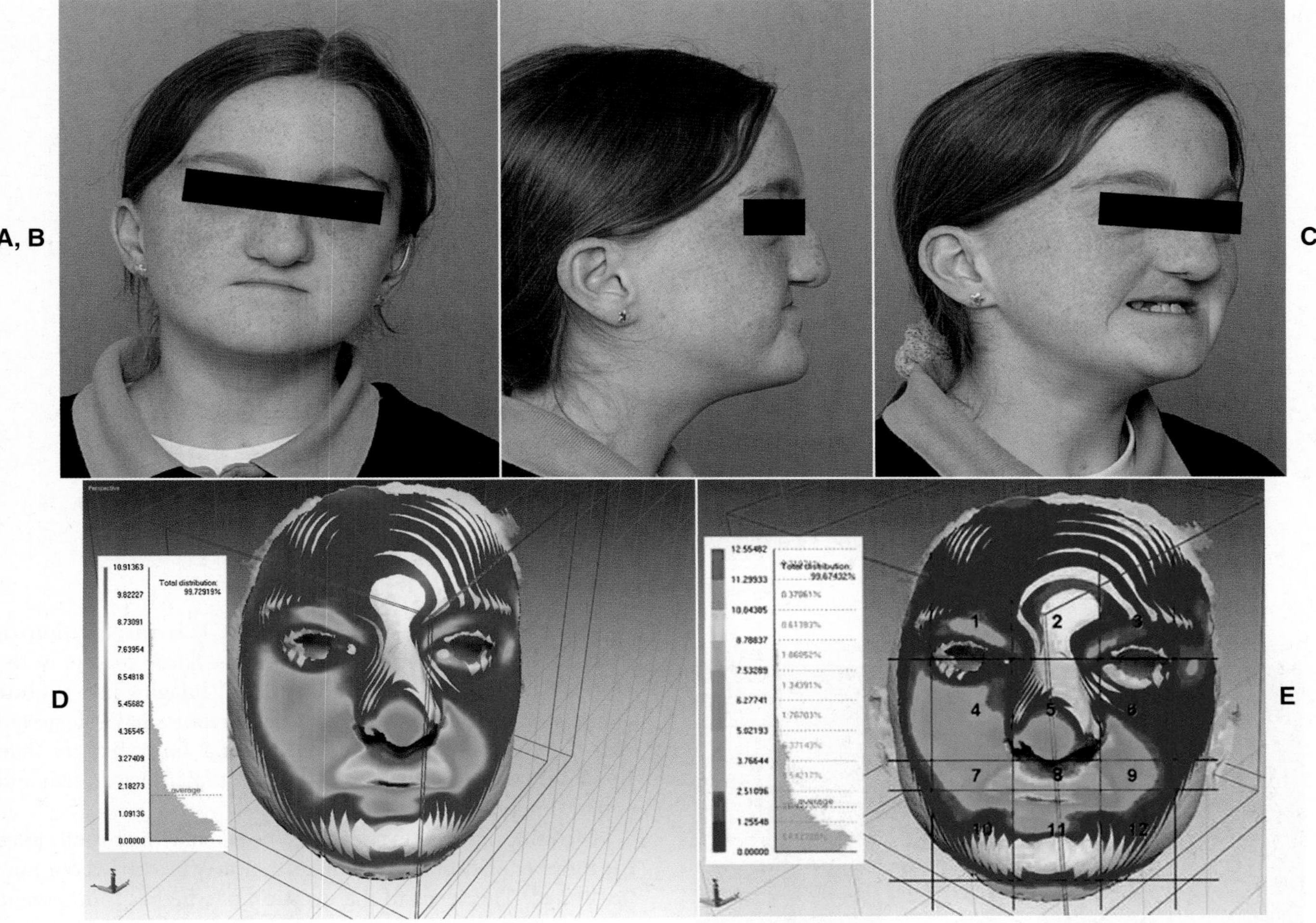

FIG 5-3 **A-C,** 11-year-old girl with right unilateral cleft lip and palate. **D,** Superimposition of patient on the average 11-year-old face; color map indicating the magnitude of deviation around the cleft region (red, 10.9 mm; green, 6.5 mm; cyan, 3.3 mm retrusive compared with the average face). **E,** Zonal method of evaluation, 12 zones indicating area and depth of deviation from the average face.

research data show that the amount of swelling is greatest 1 day after surgery but improves significantly with time. Two-jaw surgery produces a greater amount of swelling but reduces at a faster rate than single-jaw surgery. Furthermore, approximately 60% of the initial swelling is reduced after 1 month for both single and two-jaw orthognathic surgery. Fig. 5-4 depicts surgical examples.

HARD TISSUE IMAGING

Probably the greatest impact in 3D imaging techniques to both orthodontics and dentistry has been the introduction of cone beam technology. This relatively low-radiation technique permits all possible radiographs to be taken in under 1 minute. The orthodontist now has the diagnostic quality of periapicals, panoramic cephalograms, and occlusal radiographs, and TMJ series at their disposal, along with views that cannot be produced by regular radiographic machines like axial views and separate cephalograms for the right and left sides. A number of clinical applications have already been reported in the literature (Fig. 5-5).[5]

Impacted Teeth and Oral Abnormalities

The incidence of maxillary ectopic cuspids occurs in approximately 3% of the population. The distribution and location has been reported at 80% palatally and 20% buccally. The tube shift method (also known as the *parallax technique*) has been the traditional method of locating these cuspids and provides an arbitrary position and approximation of the level of difficulty for the management of the cuspid. This investigative

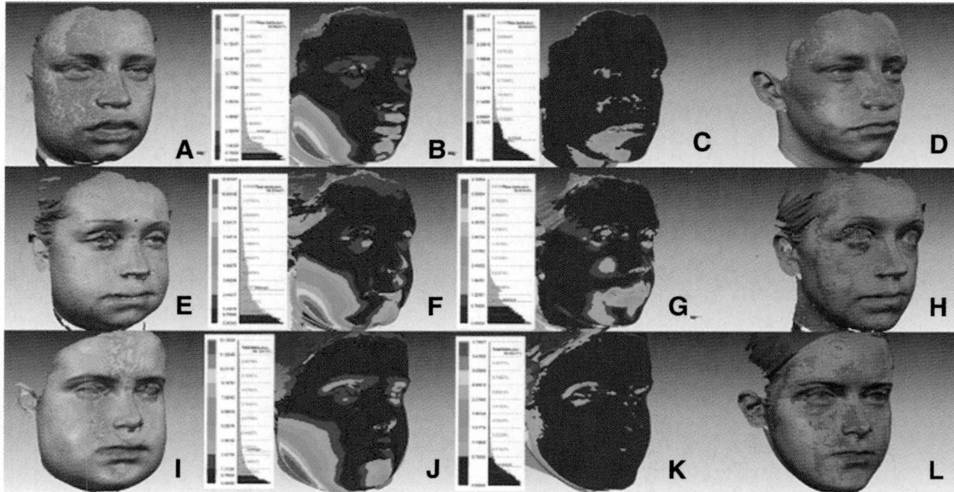

FIG 5-4 **A-D,** Facial swelling changes associated with a patient presenting with a Class II division 1 malocclusion. **E-L,** Facial swelling changes associated with patients with Class III malocclusions. Note that the swelling process is similar in all cases in the sub-masseteric region and improves with time.

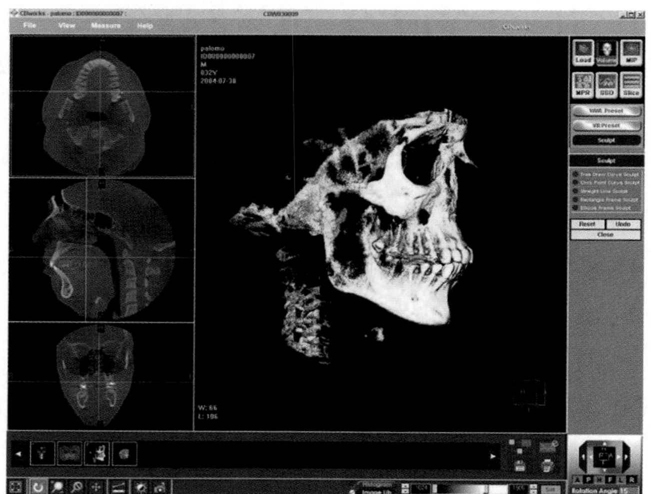

FIG 5-5 Cone Beam Image with traditional 3D views for evaluation. (Courtesy of Mr. Arun Singh, Imaging Sciences, US.)

technique uses two conventional radiographs and the location of the tooth identified by the movement of the objects respectively to the way in which the radiograph was taken. In addition, the extent of the pathology caused by the ectopic tooth and its surrounding structures has also been evaluated by these radiographs.[6] However, clinical reports using 3D conventional CT scans have shown that the incidence of root resorption to the adjacent teeth has been larger than previously thought.[7]

A recent report found that the use of cone beam CT (CBCT) technology could add value to the management of patients with such anomalies.[8] The authors used the technology to precisely locate ectopic cuspids and to design treatment strategies that allowed minimally invasive surgery to be performed and helped to design effective orthodontic strategies.

Another interesting use of the CBCT is the location of incidental oral abnormalities in patients. Some centers in the United States have begun to adopt CBCT imaging into routine dental examination procedures. Initial reports have suggested that there were higher incidences of oral abnormalities than previously suspected (e.g., oral cysts, ectopic/buried teeth and supernumeraries) (Fig. 5-6).

The value of these findings must be taken with caution, since the number of elective treatments that may be carried out may be limited. This leads to the question of whether to intervene in every abnormality located on these 3D images and the extent to which the patient needs to be informed. In the event that these abnormalities were to lead to pathological episodes, what responsibilities would the clinician and patient hold in the decision-making process? This could lead to a host of future medico-legal problems on how clinicians and patients manage the information.

Airway Analysis

The CBCT technology provides a major improvement in the airway analysis, allowing for its 3D and volumetric analysis. Airway analysis has conventionally been carried out using lateral cephalograms. A recent study on 11 subjects, using lateral cephalograms and CBCT imaging, found moderate variability in the measurements of upper airway area and volume.[9] Three-dimensional airway analysis no doubt will be useful in understanding the reasons why clinical conditions like sleep apnea and enlarged adenoids affect the way clinicians manage these complex conditions.

Assessment of Alveolar Bone Heights and Volume

Implantologists have long appreciated the third dimension in their clinical work. Conventional CT scans are used routinely to assess bone dimensions, bone quality, and the alveolar

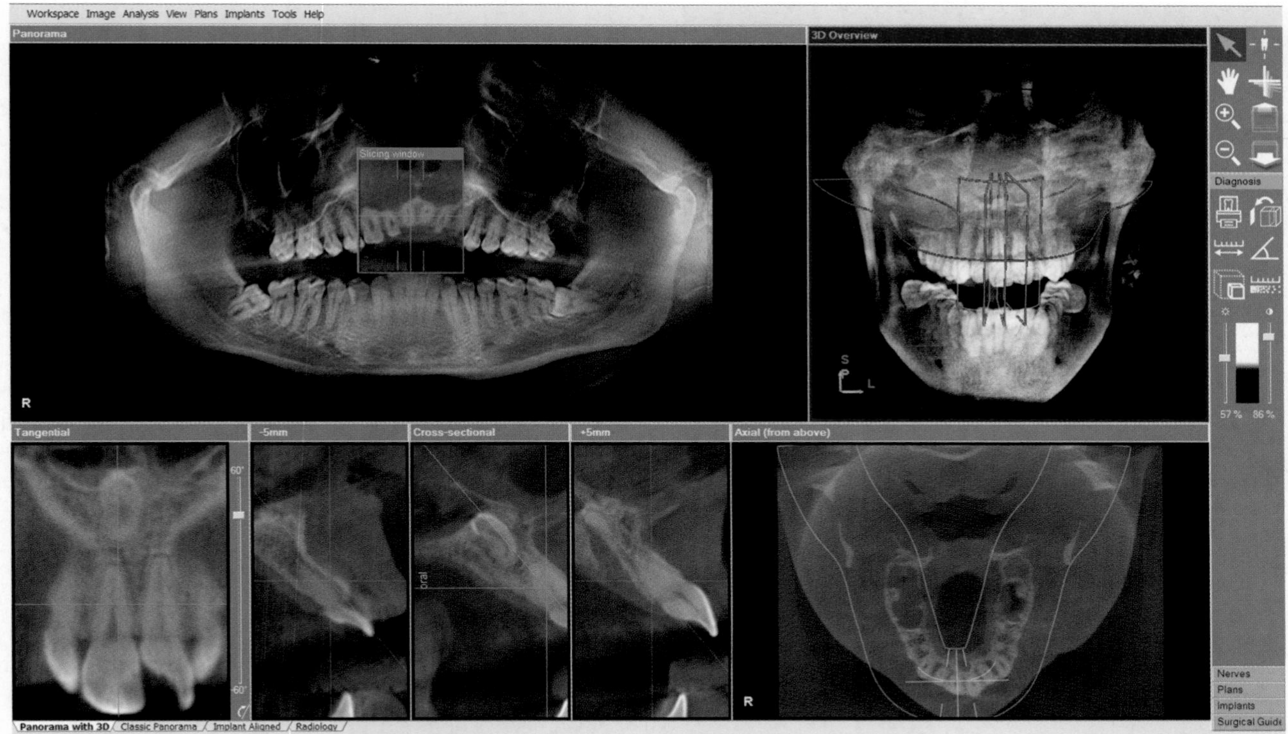

FIG 5-6 Assessment of impactions in the anterior maxillary region. (Courtesy of Dr. JE Zoller, University of Cologne.)

heights, especially when multiple units are proposed. This has improved the clinical success of the prosthesis and has led to more accurate and aesthetic outcomes in oral rehabilitation.

The introduction of CBCT technology means that both the cost and the effective radiation dose can be reduced, suggesting that its frequency of use may increase. The CBCT has already been in use in implant therapy[10] and may be useful in orthodontics for the clinical assessment of bone graft quality following alveolar surgery in patients with cleft lip and palate.[11] The images produced resulted in higher precision evaluation of bone sites and therefore gave the clinician a greater chance of restoring the site with implants as well as in the decision process of whether to move teeth orthodontically into the repaired alveolus (Fig. 5-7).

Temporomandibular Joint (TMJ) Morphology

Condylar resorption occurs in 5% to 10% of patients who undergo orthognathic surgery. Recent 3D studies have tried to understand how the condyle remodels, and preliminary data suggest that much of the condylar rotation resulting in remodeling is a direct result of the surgical procedures alone.[12] TMJ changes following distraction osteogenesis treatment and dento-facial orthopedics still need further study.

The quality of the images of the TMJ with CBCT machines is comparable to conventional CTs, but the image-taking is faster and less expensive and provides less radiation exposure. This has opened a new avenue for imaging the TMJ (Fig. 5-8).[13]

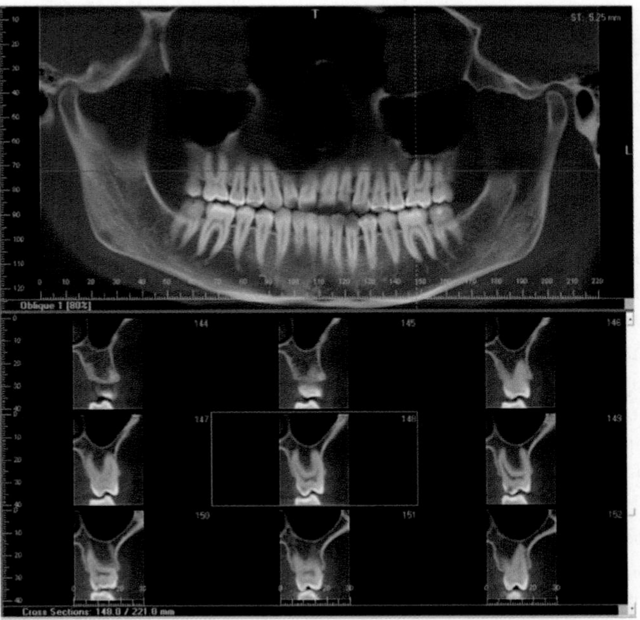

FIG 5-7 Assessment of buccal/lingual bone in the maxillary molar region. (Courtesy of Mr. Arun Singh, Imaging Sciences, US.)

5. What types of analysis are available?

A number of analyses have been reported in the literature. These techniques are often extensions from traditional methods of analysis using landmarks and points. Future analysis will

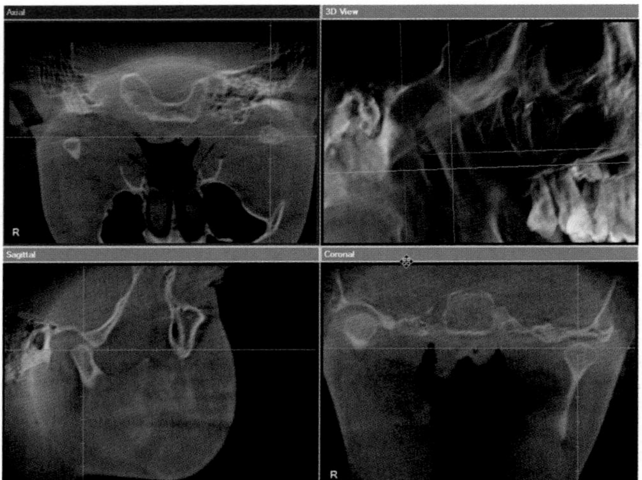

FIG 5-8 TMJ morphology. (Courtesy of Dr. JE Zoller, University of Cologne.)

focus on the use of surface areas and volumes for evaluation and quantification of diagnostic parameters and treatment changes.

6. Where are we with this technology?

Surface imaging and hard tissue imaging is revolutionizing the orthodontic specialty. To date, there are dozens of schools in the United States that possess both the surface imaging system and cone beam technology. In the next few years, there will be several papers in the literature discussing diagnostic and clinical outcomes and applications.

7. Are there limitations in the systems?

Yes, there are. Take the CBCT device, for example. It is excellent in imaging hard tissue structures and most soft tissue components; however, it does not have the ability to precisely map out the muscle structures and their attachments. These intricate structures would have to be imaged using conventional magnetic resonance imaging (MRI) technology, which incidentally does not predispose the patient to radiation exposure.

In addition, the CBCT soft tissue images do not capture the true color texture of the skin. Therefore, in order to obtain photograph-quality resolution, manipulation of the images is still required. Successful attempts to map tissue texture maps onto conventional CTs have been reported and may be similarly applied to this new technology.[14] When they become available, perhaps they can successfully replace the photographs taken during records. Another criticism made is the long capture time for a full view of a subject (scan time of 30–40 seconds), during which involuntary muscle movements (nostrils and breathing) lead to inaccuracies in soft tissue capture. These limitations mean that the 3D devices like stereo-photogrammetry and laser scanning are still better soft tissue alternatives for surface texture capture.

8. What are the costs involved?

These devices are expensive in the current market. A surface imaging device costs approximately $50,000, whereas the cone beam technology costs $200,000. The cost of a maintenance contract for each machine is often 10% of the retail price. Another substantial cost to consider is the need for someone to operate the machines as well as someone to interpret the results.

9. What is the best clinical setting for the different imaging devices?

At present, the best clinical setting is a pooled resource center. These centers often take the form of a designated imaging laboratory or faculty institution. Hard and soft tissue images can be imaged and transited to the doctor's office via weblink or CD-ROM.

10. Are there medico-legal issues with these devices?

Yes and no. It is less likely that surface capture systems will pose a problem unless the surface scans are used for advertisements or teaching; patient consent is required in such circumstances. The main problem arises when CBCT radiation technology is used. The issues of radiation protection and clinical diagnosis become more evident at this point. For example, is the orthodontist responsible for the diagnosis of pathology outside of the realms of his clinical responsibility? Some clinicians "get around" the problem by informing their patients in writing that they are responsible for only the orthodontic diagnosis. These patients are encouraged to seek the advice of other specialists.

At present there are no strict guidelines governing these issues, although in the future there most certainly will be regulations in these areas to protect both the clinician and the patient.

11. What does the future hold?

The future for orthodontists is promising and bright. The long-awaited incorporation of the third dimension to our soft tissue and radiographic records is now a reality. There is still room for improvement, but these technologies appear to be here to stay.

REFERENCES

1. Riolo ML, Moyers RE, TenHave TR, Mayers CA: Facial soft tissue changes during adolescence. In: Carlson DS, Ribbens KA, editors. Craniofacial growth during adolescence. Monograph 20. Ann Arbor: Center for Human Growth and Development, 1987.
2. Kau CH, Zhurov AI, Richmond S, et al: The 3-dimensional construction of the average 11-year-old child face- a clinical evaluation and application. *J Oral Maxillofac Surg* 2006;64(7):1086-1092.
3. Kau CH, Zhurov A, Richmond S, et al: Facial templates: a new perspective in three dimensions. *Orthod Craniofac Res* 2006;9(1):10-17.

4. Kau CH, Cronin A, Durning P, et al: A new method for the 3D measurement of postoperative swelling following orthognathic surgery. *Orthod Craniofac Res* 2006;9(1):31-37.
5. Blais F: Review of 20 years of range sensor development. *J Electro Imag* 2004;13(1):231-240.
6. Chaushu S, Chaushu G, Becker A: The role of digital volume tomography in the imaging of impacted teeth. *World J Orthod* 2004;5(2):120-132.
7. Ericson S, Kurol PJ: Resorption of incisors after ectopic eruption of maxillary canines: a CT study. *Angle Orthod* 2000;70(6): 415-423.
8. Mah J, Enciso R, Jorgensen M: Management of impacted cuspids using 3-D volumetric imaging. *J Calif Dent Assoc* 2003;31(11):835-841.
9. Aboudara CA, Hatcher D, Nielsen IL, Miller A: A three-dimensional evaluation of the upper airway in adolescents. *Orthod Craniofac Res* 2003;6 Suppl 1:173-175.
10. Hatcher DC, Dial C, Mayorga C: Cone beam CT for pre-surgical assessment of implant sites. *J Calif Dent Assoc* 2003;31(11): 825-833.
11. Hamada Y, Kondoh T, Noguchi K, et al: Application of limited cone beam computed tomography to clinical assessment of alveolar bone grafting: a preliminary report. *Cleft Palate Craniofac J* 2005;42(2):128-137.
12. Bailey LJ, Cevidanes LH, Proffit WR: Stability and predictability of orthognathic surgery. *Am J Orthod Dentofac Orthop* 2004;126(3):273-277.
13. Tsiklakis K, Syriopoulos K, Stamatakis HC: Radiographic examination of the temporomandibular joint using cone beam computed tomography. *Dentomaxillofac Radiol* 2004;33(3): 196-201.
14. Khambay B, Nebel JC, Bowman J, et al: 3D stereophotogrammetric image superimposition onto 3D CT scan images: the future of orthognathic surgery. A pilot study. *Int J Adult Orthod Orthognath Surg* 2002;17(4):331-341.

SUGGESTED READING

Kau CH, Zhurov AI, Bibb R, Hunter ML, Richmond S. The investigation of the changing facial appearance of identical twins employing a three-dimensional laser imaging system. *Orthodontics Craniofacial Research* 2005;8(2):85-90.

Kau CH, Richmond S, Savio C, Mallorie C. Measuring adult facial morphology in Three Dimensions. *Angle Orthodontist* 2006;76(5):771-776.

Aldridge K, Boyadjiev SA, Capone GT, DeLeon VB, Richtsmeier JT. Precision and error of three-dimensional phenotypic measures acquired from 3dMD photogrammetric images. *American Journal of Medical Genetics* 2005;138(3):247-253.

Harrison JA, Nixon MA, Fright WR, Snape L. Use of hand held laser scanning in the assessment of facial swelling: a preliminary study. *British Journal of Oral Maxillo-facial Surgery* 2004;42(1):8-17.

Mah J. 3D imaging in private practice. *Am J Orthod Dentofacial Orthop* 2002;121(6):14A.

Mah J, Bumann A. Technology to create the three-dimensional patient record. *Seminars in Orthodontics* 2001;7(4):251-257.

Mah J, Enciso R. The virtual craniofacial patient. In: *McNamara JA*, editor. Center for human growth and development, Craniofacial Growth Series; 2003.

Schulze D, Heiland M, Thurmann H, Adam G. Radiation exposure during midfacial imaging using 4- and 16-slice computed tomography, cone beam computed tomography systems and conventional radiography. *Dentomaxillofac Radiol* 2004;33(2):83-86.

Frederiksen NL. X rays: what is the risk? *Texas Dental Journal* 1995;112(2):68-72.

Kiefer H, Lambrecht JT, Roth J. [Dose exposure from analog and digital full mouth radiography and panoramic radiography]. *Schweiz Monatsschr Zahnmed* 2004;114(7):687-693.

Bottollier-Depois JF, Trompier F, Clairand I, et al. Exposure of aircraft crew to cosmic radiation: on-board intercomparison of various dosemeters. *Radiat Prot Dosimetry* 2004;110(1-4):411-415.

Bottollier-Depois JF, Chau Q, Bouisset P, Kerlau G, Plawinski L, Lebaron-Jacobs L. Assessing exposure to cosmic radiation on board aircraft. *Adv Space Res* 2003;32(1):59-66.

Brenner D, Elliston C, Hall E, Berdon W. Estimated risks of radiation-induced fatal cancer from pediatric CT. *AJR Am J Roentgenol* 2001;176(2):289-296.

Rogers LF: Radiation exposure in CT: why so high? *AJR Am J Roentgenol* 2001;177(2):277.

Isaacson KG, Thom AR, *editors*. Guidelines for the use of radiographs in clinical orthodontics. London: British Orthodontic Society; 2001.

Kau CH, Zhurov AI, Scheer R, et al. The feasibility of measuring three-dimensional facial morphology in children. *Orthodontics and Craniofacial Research* 2004;7(4):198-204.

Kau CH, Cronin AC, Durning P, Zhurov AI, Richmond S. A new method for the 3D measurement of post-operative swelling following orthognathic surgery. *Orthod Craniofac Res* 2005;In Press.

Kau CH, Richmond S, Zhurov AI, et al. Reliability of measuring facial morphology using a 3-dimensional laser scanning system. *American Journal of Orthodontics and Dento-facial Orthopedics* 2005;128(4):424-430.

Palomo JM, Subramanyan K, Hans MG. Creation of three dimensional data from bi-plane head x-rays for maxillo-facial studies. *Int Congress Series* 2004;1268C: 1253-1253.

Palomo JM, Hunt DW, Jr., Hans MG, Broadbent BH, Jr. A longitudinal 3-dimensional size and shape comparison of untreated Class I and Class II subjects. *Am J Orthod Dentofacial Orthop* 2005;127(5):584-591.

CHAPTER

6

Diagnosis of Orthodontic Problems

Kathleen R. McGrory • Jeryl D. English • Barry S. Briss • Kate Pham-Litschel

Carolus Linnaeus (1707-78), Swedish botanist and taxonomist, is considered to be the founder of the binomial system of nomenclature and the originator of modern scientific classification of plants and animals. To paraphrase a quote attributed to him: "Without classification there is only chaos."[1] In systems that are described as being in disorder, there is an underlying phenomenon whereby order can be found from seemingly random data.

Before Edward Hartley Angle devised his scheme of classification of malocclusion, there was no reliable or simple method to describe a malocclusion.[2] Thus, in a very real sense, he gave order to what otherwise might have been a chaotic situation in the fledgling specialty of orthodontics. His scheme worked because it was simple and reliable, and we still use it this very day. Similarly, we might look at diagnosis and treatment planning as bringing order to what, at first glance, seems to be chaotic random data. We look at the data and create order from it by developing a diagnosis, treatment objectives, treatment options, a treatment plan, and finally an appropriate treatment. This diagnostic roadmap should lead to successful treatment and results.

The second law of thermodynamics (law of entropy) was formulated in the middle of the nineteenth century by the earlier observations of Carnot and later by Clausius and Thomson.[3] Their key insight was that the world is inherently active and the spontaneous production of order from disorder is the expected consequence of basic laws (physics). The law of entropy, as it turns out, has a similar relationship to life itself, our biology, our evolution, and our ecological system. The major revolution in the last decade is the recognition of the "law of maximum entropy production" (MEP) and with it an expanded view of thermodynamics. This new idea shows that the spontaneous production of order from disorder is the expected consequence of basic laws.[3] Is there a commonality to these two concepts (chaos theory and the law of entropy) and with what we do? If so, what do they have to do with orthodontics? Although it may be a leap of faith to equate these rather esoteric and complicated concepts of science and nature to orthodontic diagnosis, it may not be as far fetched as one might think.

On a daily basis, we are all faced with patients who seek treatment for the correction of particular problems, some of which are relatively simple and some of which are rather complex. Certainly, the patients' reasons for seeking our help are multivariant. Nevertheless, no matter the reason, we are obliged to assess their problem, answer their questions, and provide them with information pertinent to their chief complaint. Thus, we perform a thorough diagnosis, create a list of problems, discuss treatment options, and then establish a treatment modality to achieve the goal. The sequencing of the previous sentence is logical and purposeful in its design. After all, it would make little sense to reverse its order and state it this way: "We achieve the goal, we treat the problem, we create treatment options, we set treatment objectives, and we diagnose."

Orthodontics is both art and science. By its very nature, there is more than one roadmap to a successful treatment for any particular problem, and each orthodontist may have a different approach. In the end, however, each of us must formulate that treatment based upon a sound diagnosis. Orthodontists, like physicians, develop what is frequently referred to as the *differential diagnosis*. What does this mean, and why is it different than the medical diagnosis? In medicine, a patient presents with certain symptoms. The physician, after interviewing the patient and making a preliminary examination, develops a hypothesis of what he thinks the problem is and develops a differential diagnosis, which is nothing more than a list of possible causes for the patient's complaint. Not until he performs a variety of tests is he able to narrow the list down and arrive at "the" single most likely definitive diagnosis (e.g., appendicitis). In orthodontics, however, the differential diagnosis represents a somewhat different concept. It is, in fact, a complete description of the malocclusion; it includes those multifactorial conditions that exist at a particular moment in time that make the malocclusion unique unto itself. In other words, we do not simply describe a malocclusion as Class II. Rather, we add to that basic Angle classification a description of all the salient entities that make the malocclusion different from others of the same classification, e.g., division 1, division 2, subdivision, crowding, deep bite, crossbite.

In this chapter the questions ask about the treatment of a particular malocclusion. Suggested treatment approaches are described in the answers and are meant to associate the treatment decision to an understanding of the underlying problem based upon a proper diagnosis. Because there are many ways to correct a particular problem, these suggested treatments are for illustrative purposes only. It is important to note that treatment (mechanotherapy) and diagnosis are entities that are joined at the hip and cannot be separated. A poor treatment result will most certainly result from a poor diagnosis.

As orthodontists, we acknowledge and understand that we treat in three planes of space: the sagittal, the vertical, and the transverse. Although these three dimensions can be thought of as three separate entities, they are not. Why? Treating one will most certainly have a separate or collective effect upon each of the others, either in a positive or a negative way. Therefore, having a complete understanding of all of them and how they interrelate and interact is important when formulating the treatment.

Let us consider, for example, the vertical dimension. The vertical dimension dictates many of the decisions made by the orthodontist when devising a treatment plan. In the case of a patient with a dolichofacial pattern, the comprehensive treatment goal often includes a plan to control the vertical dimension and to not make it worse.[4-7] The vertical dimension seems to be the one dimension that gives the orthodontist much cause for concern because, when presented with a patient with this pattern, all that we do for the patient seems to affect the vertical in a negative way. By the same token, in those cases that present with the opposite form of facial pattern (i.e. brachyfacial), the opposite seems to be the case. In these instances, increasing the vertical dimension is often one of the objectives of treatment. And yet, in patients who present with a Class II division 2 malocclusion and a 100% overbite, for example, the vertical dimension resists our attempt to increase it. To make the correct diagnosis, the orthodontist must consistently develop a diagnostic database.

DIAGNOSTIC DATABASE

1. What comprises the diagnostic database?

The diagnostic database is composed of multiple clinical, functional, and record analyses that allow the clinician to formulate a comprehensive diagnosis and begin to work toward a treatment plan that is most beneficial to the patient.[8]

CASE HISTORY

A thorough case history including family and patient history helps establish any pre-existing developmental problems. Medical conditions relating to orthodontic treatment and psychological aspects of treatment should be explored.

CLINICAL EXAMINATION

The most important diagnostic tool is the clinical examination of the patient. The general state of the patient in terms of growth and development should be assessed, along with the development and health of the dentition and surrounding structures. A frontal and profile analysis should be performed to discover any discrepancies that would fall into the problem list. The patient's chief complaint should be noted and evaluated.

FUNCTIONAL ANALYSIS

In the functional analysis, head posture and freeway space are evaluated. The dentition is evaluated for any discrepancies in function, such as functional shifts or pseudo-bites. Swallowing function should be explored to discover tongue-thrust habits that may lead to relapse after orthodontic treatment is completed. The temporomandibular joints (TMJs) are palpated and the patient is questioned concerning joint function and noise. Any discrepancies from normal should be further evaluated through clinical and radiographic examination as needed.

RADIOLOGIC EXAMINATION

Panoramic radiographs are useful in orthodontic diagnosis as a survey of the total dentition, the TMJs, and surrounding structures. Periapical radiographs or vertical bitewings should be taken on all adult cases to evaluate bone heights. Occlusal views or a cone beam scan may be beneficial in cases with impacted teeth to determine their three-dimensional (3D) location.

PHOTOGRAPHIC ANALYSIS

Profile and frontal photographs are taken to evaluate the relationship between the soft-tissue and the skeletal supporting structures. In the profile view, the patient's head is parallel to the Frankfort horizontal plane in the natural head position, the eyes are focused straight ahead, and the ear is visible.

CEPHALOMETRIC ANALYSIS

Cephalometric analysis is used to evaluate the formation of the facial skeleton, the relationship of the jaw bases, the axial inclination of the incisors, soft-tissue morphology, growth patterns, localization of malocclusion, and treatment limitations.

STUDY CAST ANALYSIS

The dentition and degree of malocclusion can be analyzed in three dimensions using study cast analysis. Analysis of the arch form can be subdivided into the sum of upper incisor widths, anterior arch width, posterior arch width, anterior arch length, and palatal height. Arch symmetry is evaluated using a perpendicular to the mid-palatal raphe. Space analysis is calculated by subtracting the total amount of tooth structure—or predicted tooth structure if the patient is in the mixed dentition—from the total space available. Incisor inclination, sagittal discrepancies, and depth of the curve of Spee may also influence the space available. Bolton analysis, a ratio of mandibular teeth width sum to maxillary teeth width sum, gives an index to determine how teeth will couple. The overall calculated ratio should be 91%; if the ratio is reduced, the maxillary teeth are relatively too large. The anterior ratio should be 77%. Finally, the occlusion can be studied and classification of the malocclusion can be made and overjet and overbite relationships determined.[8-10]

2. What is a prioritized problem list?

A prioritized problem list places the orthodontic/developmental problems into priority order to help evaluate the interaction, compromise, and cost/benefit of treatment for each of the problems in order to determine the appropriate course of action that maximizes benefit to the patient.[9] To create an orthodontic problem list, group all related findings into major categories (Box 6-1). For example, facial convexity, mandibular retrognathism, upper incisal protrusion and proclination, and an excessive overjet may all be manifestations of a skeletal Class II malocclusion.

3. What are the orthodontic problems in the 3 planes of space?

ANTEROPOSTERIOR PLANE

The anteroposterior (AP) plane passes through the body parallel to the sagittal suture, dividing the head and neck into left and right portions. The AP or sagittal dimension deals with maxillary and mandibular forward growth.[8-11] Cephalometric analysis is used to determine if the underlying skeletal bases are in harmony or if there is a significant deviation that warrants consideration. A determination is made about whether a patient is in skeletal Class I, II, or III function. Orthodontic profiles are examined in this plane as well as the dental and skeletal classification of malocclusions. Overjet would also be noted in the dental position. Soft tissue analysis is used to determine esthetics and facial balance of the patient.

TRANSVERSE PLANE

The transverse plane passes horizontally through the body, at right angles to the sagittal and vertical planes, dividing the body into upper and lower portions. The transverse dimension is evaluated skeletally by measuring the width of the posterior maxilla. Measurements less than 36 mm from the upper first molar mesiolingual gingival margins may indicate a skeletal discrepancy.[8-11] Dental transverse deficiencies are more commonly due to lingually tilted upper bicuspids and molars, or buccally tilted lower bicuspids and molars. The soft tissue is evaluated for deviations in alar base width and overall facial harmony. By looking at the diagnostic records in this plane, one may detect any problem relating to right and left asymmetries. The occlusal views of orthodontic models are in the transverse plane. Dental and skeletal posterior crossbites are noted in this dimension as well as intercanine and intermolar widths.

BOX 6-1

Orthodontic Problem List

1. Dental Class II division 1
2. Skeletal Class II malocclusion
   a. Facial convexity
   b. Maxillary incisal proclination/protrusion
   c. Overjet 6 mm
   d. Mandibular retrognathism
   e. Retrusive AP chin position
3. Posterior crossbite
   a. Unilateral (right side)
   b. Deviation of jaw towards affected side
   c. Presence of CO/CR shift
   d. Constricted maxillary dental arch relative to mandibular dentition
   e. Midline off center
4. Mild crowding
   a. Mandibular arch crowding 5 mm
   b. Rotated upper and lower incisors
5. Mandibular hypodivergence
   a. Normal cephalometric mandibular plane angle
   b. Anterior deepbite 5 mm

VERTICAL PLANE

The vertical plane passes longitudinally through the body from side to side, dividing the head and neck into front and back parts. Skeletal discrepancies in the vertical dimension may be determined by analysis of a lateral cephalometric radiograph in coordination with a clinical examination. Discrepancies can include increased or decreased facial height, extremely low or high mandibular plane angle (MPA), or skeletal open bite.[8-11] Dental analysis can reveal an open bite relationship, a deep impinging overbite, a deep curve of Spee, or non-erupting or ankylosed teeth. (Overbite is listed in the dental portion of the grid.)

4. What is included in the frontal analysis?

The frontal analysis allows evaluation of the overall relationship between the face and the dentition. The four main areas of interest when analyzing the face include: (1) midline, (2) lip posture, (3) buccal corridor space, and (4) smile.[4,12,13]

MIDLINES

When evaluating the midline of a patient, it is important to consider both the facial and dental midlines. An evaluation should be made to determine if the dental midlines are coincident with the facial midline and whether they are coincident with one another.[13] This is best accomplished by looking face-to-face with the patient in an upright portion. The relation of the contact point of the centrals to the facial midline should be considered to rule out a non-parallel dental-to-facial midline. If a facial midline deviation is determined, such as a deviation of the chin, additional radiographs may be required to establish the cause of the deviation. A posteroanterior cephalometric radiograph or a 3D scan can help determine if the problem is in the condyle, the ramus, or the body of the mandible. One must be careful to separate true skeletal deviations from functional deviations caused by occlusal discrepancies.

LIPS

The lip posture should be evaluated both at rest and with the lips lightly touching. Watch for evidence of lip strain on closure, which may indicate a need for extraction treatment.

Evaluate the upper lip length and the amount of tooth and gum display at rest and on full smile. If no amount of tooth is displayed at rest, the teeth may be dried, utility wax placed at the incisal edges, and the lip length indexed on the wax. The amount of vertical deficiency can then be read from the wax. Excessive gingival display on smiling can be due to short upper lip length, short clinical crowns from excess gum tissue, or vertical maxillary excess. In females, 3–4 mm of incisal display should be present at rest; at full smile, the upper lip should reach the height of the centrals or slightly above.[4]

BUCCAL CORRIDORS

Dark buccal corridor spaces can be due to lingually set or lingually tipped premolars. Indiscriminate expansion has questionable long-term stability and can create buccal root dehiscences.[14,15]Proper use of expansion requires careful treatment planning.

SMILE LINE

The relationship of the upper teeth to the lower lip should be evaluated for parallelism among their curvatures. Treatment should be aimed at keeping or creating parallelism and avoiding a flat or reverse smile line.

5. What is included in the profile view?

The profile view is used to evaluate the AP relationship of the maxilla and mandible to the overall face, the nose, lip posture, and vertical discrepancies. [8-11]

ANTEROPOSTERIOR

The relationship of the maxilla and the mandible to the overall face is evaluated. Deviations in midface projection and mandibular projection are noted.

NOSE

The nose plays an important part in facial balance. Note any morphological variations in shape and discuss any concerns with the patient. Upturned nasal tips tend to be more youthful in appearance but may require variations in treatment planning if extractions are being considered to eliminate crowding in the dentition.

LIPS

The lip posture should again be considered at rest and with lips lightly touching. The interlabial gap should be approximately 1–3 mm at rest posture. Evaluate the amount of incisor display at rest, as well as the inclination of the incisors in relation to facial balance. The nasolabial angle is an indication of upper lip inclination. The E-line proposed by Ricketts is influenced by the nose and chin but can aid in evaluating lip protrusion or retrusion.

VERTICAL

The height of the lower face, from subnasale to menton, can be further subdivided. One third of the distance is measured from subnasale to stomion and two thirds of the distance is measured from stomion to menton. Deviations from this ratio may indicate vertical maxillary excess, a short upper lip, a skeletal open bite, or an increase in anterior facial height. The normal ratio of the lower facial height to the posterior facial height is 0.69.[16] The general characteristics of a long face include increased anterior facial height relative to posterior facial height, steep MPA, possible lip incompetence, and a shallow mentolabial fold.

6. What is the 3D-3T diagnostic grid, and why is it important as a routine part of an orthodontic patient record?

The 3D-3T diagnostic grid represents a diagnostic summary of the findings in the three tissue categories: skeletal, soft tissue, and dental for the sagittal, transverse, and vertical planes of space (Table 6-1). With its systematic and comprehensive description of examination results, it offers a helpful tool to develop a prioritized problem list and facilitate treatment planning to correct the problems. Orthodontic diagnosis is an objective process with each practitioner developing the same measurements for the problem list. Once the list is completed, the treatment planning process begins with prioritized treatment objectives discussed with the patient. Treatment planning is a very subjective process and is individualized for each orthodontic patient.

7. What are the advantages of using the 3D-3T diagnostic grid in treatment planning?

Listing the examination and orthodontic analyses data in this format ensures that all factors and possibilities for a given case are considered before a treatment plan is established. Each box is designated for a specific problem type; thus, completion of the table ensures that all diagnostic records are carefully considered. In addition, the side effects of correcting one problem, which may help or worsen another problem, are more clearly evaluated before a list of objectives and the best possible treatment plan is selected. The immediate insight into the difficulty of a case is another advantage of this methodology. Understandably, cases with abnormalities involving all tissue categories or all three planes of space require more attention than a case having fewer dimensional problems. A malocclusion with problems in all three places of skeletal tissue will be very difficult to treat. The end result of such an approach is a comprehensive and effective treatment plan with concise and realistic goals.

8. What are the steps of the 3D-3T treatment plan method?

1. Creation of the 3D-3T grid
2. Creation of an orthodontic problem list
3. Listing of treatment objectives
4. Formation of a treatment plan

TABLE 6-1 3D-3T Grid with Common Findings

3D-3T	SAGITTAL (AP) PLANE	TRANSVERSE PLANE	VERTICAL PLANE
Skeletal Findings of Cephalometric Analysis and Model Analysis	Box 1 • Class I, II, or III skeletal malocclusion • Maxillary prognathism/ retrognathism • Mandibular prognathism/ Retrognathism • Incisal protrusion/retrusion • Anteroposterior position of chin	Box 2 • Constricted/wide maxillary arch • Constricted/wide mandibular arch • Intermolar width • Posterior skeletal crossbite	Box 3 • Posterior skeletal open bite/deep bite • Posterior facial height • Anterior facial height • Rotation of palatal plane • Mandibular plane angle • Mandibular hyper/hypodivergence
Soft Tissue Findings of Clinical Examination and Photographs	Box 4 • Facial profile: straight/convex/ concave • Lip protrusion/retrusion • Lip soft tissue thickness • Facial musculature: strong/weak masculatory muscles • Nasolabial angle	Box 5 • Facial asymmetry • Deviation of jaw to one side • Buccal corridors	Box 6 • Proportion of facial thirds: upper, middle, lower thirds • Lip competence/incompetence • Gummy smile (VME)
Dental Findings of Clinical Examination and Model Analysis	Box 7 • Angle's classification of molar relationship: Class I, Class II div. 1, Class II div. 2, Class III • Incisal proclination/retroclination • Overbite • Anterior crossbite	Box 8 • Asymmetries in the dental arch • Posterior dental crossbites —buccal or lingual • Bolton discrepancies • Congenitally missing teeth • Previous extractions • Blocked out teeth • Rotated teeth • Dental midline	Box 9 • Posterior dental open bite/deepbite • Occlusal cant • Overjet • Anterior open bite/deepbite

9. What information is contained within each box?

Table 6-1 shows a 3D-3T grid with some common findings listed in each box. As a rule of thumb, soft tissue problems are detected in the clinical examination and orthodontic photographs. Exceptions are soft tissue cephalometric analyses, which are also useful diagnostic tools for detecting soft tissue problems in all planes of space. Dental tissue findings are observed in the patient examination and by performing an orthodontic model analysis. Skeletal tendencies or problems are sometimes detected during the patient examination but are confirmed with a cephalometric analysis. A 3D-3T grid with various problems listed in each of the three planes and three tissues is presented (see Table 6-1).

10. What are treatment objectives?

After the review of all diagnostic findings and the formation of a problem list, the clinician forms a list of goals and treatment objectives listed in order of importance for each patient.[8-11,14] The patient's chief concern is always given high priority. Failure to accomplish correction of the patient's chief complaint will usually result in the patient being dissatisfied with the overall orthodontic treatment.

Ideally one would like to correct all existing malocclusions, and in many cases, this can be achieved without difficulty. However, there will be cases in which one or more limiting factors will force the clinician to limit the goals to those most beneficial to the patient. For example, when the patient is a non-grower, the complete correction of a skeletal Class II malocclusion is likely only with the assistance of orthognathic surgery. If the patient is opposed to correctional surgery, the only other realistic alternative, aside from no treatment, is an orthodontic treatment plan designed to camouflage the problem. When Class I molar correction is unlikely, a better aim may be to get the cuspids into a Class I relationship. In cases of upper premolar extractions (without extraction in the lower arch), the cuspids are positioned into a Class I relationship while the molars are kept at a full step Class II position. However, to establish an ideal occlusion, the normal molar 14-degree rotation must be corrected to 0 degrees if in a Class II molar relationship.

Although the treatment goals are made before the treatment plan is created, sometimes they are modified during the process of treatment planning.[8-11] Insights coming from closer attention to the case may cause one to switch goals or change their order of importance. At the end, one should be able to break down the treatment plan into the individual components that will address each of the goals. An orthodontist should be able to confidently predict the chances of reaching a goal. When the clinician anticipates that a goal will be difficult to achieve, the patient should be made aware of this to avoid false expectation at the end of treatment.

11. How does one form a treatment plan?

To form a treatment plan, one takes the treatment objective and then chooses a treatment modality that will achieve that desired result.[8-11] In orthodontics, a patient presents with symptoms and problems, the dentist and orthodontist engage in diagnosing these problems, and they finally agree on treatment options to correct the problems. Based on the collective data, one treatment choice may be more effective and advantageous than another. If the patient decides not to choose the ideal option for treatment, alternatives should be presented to meet the patient's desired needs, realizing it may be a compromised treatment plan. We have to be certain that we listen to what our patients perceive their problems to be and agree on a treatment strategy that is acceptable to both the patient and the orthodontist.

At times, an orthodontic tool designed to correct one problem may actually make another problem worse. For example, the correction of a posterior crossbite with a quad helix or "W" appliance, without exceptional control of upper molar eruption, is contraindicated for patients with mandibular hyperdivergence or anterior open bite. In cases like these, it may be better to use a rapid maxillary expander with bonded posterior occlusion to prevent excessive extrusion of the upper molars. Of course, if the patient is a non-grower with a profile that has excessive anterior facial vertical height, one may opt to correct the maxillary constriction at the time of the orthognathic surgical correction of the vertical problem. In order to easily go from a problem list to a concrete treatment plan, one has to know the many orthodontic treatment modalities, their main functions and side effects, advantages and disadvantages, and indications and contraindications.

To more clearly demonstrate how to formulate a treatment plan, refer back to the sample problem list of the patient J.S. in question 2. Based on knowledge of appropriate treatment timing, one should correct the transverse problem (the posterior crossbite) first. J.S.'s posterior crossbite is unilateral and deviates to the right-hand side, causing the jaw to deviate to the affected side. The presence of a CO/CR shift reveals that the posterior crossbite is a functional crossbite resulting from a constricted maxillary dental arch. J.S. is a growing individual, so one expects to be able to expand his maxillary arch with an expansion appliance without surgical assistance. The extrusion of the upper molars is a side effect of maxillary expansion, but in this case, it will help the patient's anterior deepbite and mandibular hypodivergence. This same extrusive effect, however, may cause the mandibular plane to rotate counterclockwise and worsen the patient's convexity.

The patient has a facial convexity with a retrognathic mandible and retrusive chin. He has protrusive and proclined maxillary teeth with a moderate overjet. Because of his age, the patient has an advantageous growth potential. There are a number of appliances designed to correct a skeletal Class II malocclusion in a growing patient: the headgear; the bionator and Twin Block (and other early treatment appliances); and the Herbst appliance, the MARA, and the Jasper Jumper, just to name a few. Treatment with headgear is eliminated because this appliance is indicated for skeletal Class II malocclusion with maxillary prognathism. All the early treatment appliances are ruled out because they are most effective (if effective at all; see Chapter 3) during the early mixed dentition stage. Now the choices are narrowed to the Herbst, the MARA, and the Twin Block, which are all appliances aimed at growing patients in the late mixed dentition stage. Refining these choices would have to depend on the patient's motivation and attitude and the doctor's own clinical skill and experience. For a non-compliant preadolescent male, a fixed Herbst appliance may be a wise choice. Remember, a treatment plan is subjective and will vary among orthodontists based on their expertise!

The minor crowding and rotations in this case will readily resolve with the fixed upper and lower orthodontic appliances. The mandibular arch may be stabilized with a fixed intercanine retainer, whereas the upper arch can be retained with a removable maxillary appliance.

The Following Questions Further Discuss Information in the 3D-3T Diagnostic Grid. The intention of this section is to encourage the diagnostic and treatment approach using the 3D-3T grid. It is beyond the scope of this section to encompass all aspects of orthodontic problems. The individual chapters in this book, as well as other orthodontic textbooks recommended in the reference list, provide further insights and knowledge of the related subjects.

12. What are the problems in the sagittal (A-P) plane of space?

AP orthodontic problems of all three tissue types are detected in the sagittal plane of space. A compilation of the data in this plane will result in a definitive classification of the patient's soft-tissue, dental, and skeletal malocclusion. The clinical examination of the patient's profile at the start of treatment gives the clinician an immediate impression of the patient's facial harmony and esthetics as well as the underlying dental and skeletal structure before taking any records. The succeeding orthodontic model analysis will give more insight to the patient's dental malocclusion, whereas the skeletal component data derived from the cephalometric analysis will give the clinician a complete picture of the sagittal malocclusion.

SKELETAL TISSUE IN THE SAGITTAL PLANE

Class I, II, or III Skeletal Malocclusion

There are numerous cephalometric methods to distinguish the skeletal relationship of the maxilla and the mandible to each other and to the cranial base. In the **Steiner's analysis**, the **ANB** angle (formed between the A-point, nasion, and B-point) indicates the AP position of the maxilla in relation to the AP position of the mandible. A comparison of the SNA and SNB angles from the norm further shows if the problem is a **maxillary** or **mandibular prognathism** or **retrognathism**. The **Wit's analysis,** using the difference between the projections of points A and B to the functional occlusal plane, is another common method to verify the relationship of the maxilla and the mandible.

SOFT TISSUE IN THE SAGITTAL PLANE

Evaluation of the Facial Profile

The soft tissue problems of the AP plane are best seen through a profile analysis of the patient. A proper analysis gives valuable information about the patient's esthetics and shows whether the jaws are proportionately positioned in this plane of space. With the patient sitting or standing in the upright position and looking at a distant object, an imaginary line connecting the bridge of the nose to the base of the upper lip and extending to the chin is evaluated.[8-11] When this line is straight, the soft tissue profile of the patent is **harmonious.** A disproportion in the size of the jaws, on the other hand, results in a profile convexity or concavity. A **convex** profile is indicative of a Class II jaw relationship, whereas a **concave** profile points to a Class III relationship. Since esthetics is a major reason for orthodontic treatment, a severe profile convexity or concavity points to more involved orthodontic treatment and possible orthognathic surgery. The non-harmonious profile by itself does not indicate which jaw is at fault. That information is derived from examining the skeletal tissue in this plane of space.

During the clinical examination of the soft tissue profile, it is also helpful to visualize the MPA. This can be accomplished by placing a mirror handle or other instrument along the border of the mandible.[9] When the mirror handle is angulated slightly below the ear, the MPA is predicted to be normal. Too steep an inclination indicates a high cephalometric mandibular plane value or **mandibular hyperdivergence;** too flat an inclination indicates a low MPA or **hypodivergence**. A hyperdivergent mandible is an indicator of a difficult malocclusion of increased vertical dimension. In general, a very steep mandibular angle coincides with a long and narrow face. The **facial musculature** of a dolichocephalic patient shows masseter muscles that are weak and hypotrophic. Strong hypertrophic masseter muscles are characteristic of a brachycephalic patient with mandibular hypodivergence. The facial form of this patient tends to be short in facial height and square in appearance.

Lip Protrusion/Retrusion

By looking at the lips' position in this plane, one gets a quick impression of the underlying dental position, such as maxillary dental protrusion or lack of upper lip support in cases of Class II division 2 malocclusion.[14] A determination of lip protrusion or retrusion also helps the clinician decide if extraction treatment is necessary.

One way to assess the AP position of the lip is through the **Ricketts' E-line** or **Esthetic line**. This line is drawn from the tip of the nose (point Pn) to soft tissue pogonion (Pog). Ideally, the upper lip should be approximately 4 mm behind the line, while the lower lip should be about 2 mm behind it. Another way to assess the position of the lips is by looking at the **lower facial plane**, created by connecting a point at the base of the nose (Subnasale or Sn) to soft tissue pogonion (Pog). The lips should appear relaxed in the repose position. Thin lips respond more readily than thick lips to orthodontic retraction of the incisors. Extractions followed by retraction of incisors behind the subnasale-pogonion line should be avoided.[14]

DENTAL TISSUE IN THE SAGITTAL PLANE

Interarch Molar and Incisal Relationships

Labeling the relationship of the first molars of each case according to **Angle's classification of malocclusions** is essential because the establishment of a normal Class I molar relationship is frequently a goal in orthodontics.

Overjet is also best studied in this plane. Normal **overjet** is the horizontal overlap of the upper incisors to the lower incisors. Ideally it is 2 mm. When there is negative overjet, or when the lower incisors are anterior to the upper incisors, the condition is called an **anterior crossbite.** To determine if this anterior crossbite has a skeletal component and not just a functional expression of a dental malocclusion, the orthodontist looks for the presence of an anterior CO/CR shift. When the malocclusion is a functional one, the incisors show negative overjet in centric occlusion but touch edge to edge in centric relation. An anterior dental crossbite tends to be easier than one with a functional shift or of a skeletal nature.

The evaluation of the inclination of the incisors is important to Angle's molar classification (distinguishing Class II division 1 from division 2) and the identification of an abnormal overjet relation. Excessive **incisal proclination** is related to crowding. This is further discussed in the section addressing findings of the transverse plane. The upper incisor should be proclined 103 degrees to the SN plane whereas the lower incisor should be proclined 93 degrees to the mandibular plane.

13. What are the problems in the vertical plane of space?

The scope of this question is a discussion of the proportions of the face as viewed in the vertical plane as well as posterior crossbite and open bite.

SKELETAL TISSUE IN THE VERTICAL PLANE OF SPACE

A general strategy of cephalometric analyses used to evaluate vertical problems is to compare the posterior to anterior facial heights. The more equal these measurements are, the more likely it is that the patient will display a short square facial type known as brachyfacial with low MPA, decreased anterior vertical dimension, and a deepbite. On the contrary, when the anterior facial height is excessively long compared with the posterior portion, a long and narrow facial type known as *dolichofacial* is evident.

COMPARISON OF THE POSTERIOR TO ANTERIOR FACIAL HEIGHT

In the Steiner's analysis, the **vertical position of the mandible** is measured by the relationship between the anterior cranial base (defined by the plane sella to nasion) and the mandibular plane (extending from points gonion to gnathion). The mean value is 32 degrees for SN-GoGo. An increase in this angle correlates with an increase in anterior facial height.[8-11,14]

The **mandibular plane angle** is helpful in locating the vertical chin. It is formed by the intersection between the Frankfort horizontal and the Go-Gn (gonion-gnathion) line and relates the cant of the mandibular plane to the Frankfort horizontal plane. The mean value for MPA is 25 degrees.

SOFT TISSUE IN THE VERTICAL PLANE OF SPACE

Proportion of the Facial Thirds

A well-proportioned face can be divided into approximately equal vertical thirds with the upper third extending from point **trichion (Tr)**, at the top of the forehead, to soft tissue **glabella (G),** the most anterior point of the forehead. The second vertical third extends from soft tissue glabella to the **subnasale (Sn),** or the point at which the columella of the nose merges with the upper lip in the midsagittal plane. The lower third begins with subnasale and ends with soft tissue **menton (Me),** the lowest point on the contour of the soft tissue chin, found by dropping a perpendicular line from a horizontal line through skeletal menton.[14]

It is important to evaluate middle and lower facial thirds. At the initial evaluation of the patient, a "sunken" appearance of the midface in the middle third may be an indication of a maxillary AP deficiency or **maxillary retrognathism** associated with skeletal Class III malocclusion. This finding should be confirmed with a cephalometric analysis.

The middle third to lower third vertical height of the face should have a 5:6 ratio.[14] The upper lip length should make up one third of the lower facial height and the distance from the lower lip to soft tissue menton should be two thirds. Aside from facial proportion, one should also examine the lips in this plane, since their harmonious position is essential to facial esthetics. When the upper and lower lips do not meet at rest, this is known as **lip incompetence.** When asked to close their lips, these patients may exhibit mentalis strain and display some lip strain. Lip incompetence is an association of an excessive AP discrepancy between the maxilla and mandible or an increased anterior vertical facial height.

DENTAL TISSUE IN THE VERTICAL PLANE OF SPACE

Overbite, or the vertical overlap of the upper and lower incisors, is normally 2 mm. When it is positive and excessive, an **anterior deep bite** exists. When there is a negative overbite and the incisors fail to overlap, an **anterior open bite** exists.

Open bites and **deep bites** are dental malocclusions in the vertical plane of space. Anterior open bites are the result of an under-eruption of the anterior teeth or an over-eruption of posterior teeth. Likewise, when the posterior teeth are under-erupted, the clinical observation will be an anterior deep bite. Anterior open bite and deep bite with differing etiologies warrant different treatments. If the anterior open bite is derived from an under-eruption of the anterior teeth themselves, this is indicative of a dental open bite due to a tongue or digit habit. The treatment aim is to extrude the anterior teeth. If the open bite is a result of an over-eruption of the posterior teeth, this is indicative of a skeletal open bite. The treatment mechanics should be aimed toward intruding these teeth and usually leaving the incisors in their original position. If one sees a greater underlying skeletal cause of the open bite (through a cephalometric analysis), it is more likely that the patient will need a combination of orthodontics and orthognathic surgery to correct the malocclusion. Precision in diagnosis allows the orthodontist the great advantage of treating the abnormal to the normal, ensuring the best chance of getting beautiful, healthy results.

14. What are the problems of the transverse plane of space?

Although no face is perfectly symmetrical, the absence of any obvious asymmetry is necessary for good facial esthetics. In order to assess **facial symmetry**, an imaginary line is drawn through the soft tissue glabella down the center of the face to the midpoint of the chin.[14] The maxillary and mandibular **dental midlines**, also known as *UDML* and *LDML*, should be assessed in relation to the facial midline. Some dental factors that may have caused midline shifts include crowding, rotations, and blocked-out teeth, as well as missing and irregularly sized teeth.

A facial asymmetry caused by a **mandibular lateral displacement** may be a sign of a posterior crossbite or of a more complicated skeletal disorder. A deviation of the mandible to one side, accompanied by a **cant of the occlusal plane**, can be detected as the patient bites on a wooden spatula, with his head positioned so that the projected interpupillary line is parallel to the floor. The parallelism of the wooden spatula is then evaluated to this interpupillary line.

A more common malocclusion that may involve a mandibular lateral displacement is a **posterior crossbite.** Viewing the intercuspation of the posterior occlusion in the coronal plane allows the best visualization of this malocclusion, described as when the mandibular teeth occlude in buccal version to the maxillary teeth. An infrequent reverse of this malocclusion is a complete lingual version of the posterior mandibular segments, often referred to as a *Brodie bite* or **scissor bite.**

A **posterior crossbite** may be bilateral or unilateral and can be dental or skeletal. As in the anterior crossbite, a unilateral dental posterior crossbite can often be distinguished from a skeletal crossbite by the presence of a posterior CO/CR shift. When the posterior crossbite exists in centric occlusion but disappears in centric relation, the bite is functional in nature, and often results from the combination of a constricted maxillary arch and a shift of the mandible to the affected side on closure. To find if the constricted maxilla is caused solely by a constricted dental arch, or also a narrow bony palate, one should measure the palatal transversal dimensions of the orthodontic study model. **Intercanine** and **intermolar widths** are measured and compared with a chart of norm for the patient's age and gender. When they are very narrow compared with the norm, most likely the crossbite is skeletal. A stronger skeletal problem mandates more aggressive treatment and is more sensitive to the developmental age of the patient.

Table 6-2 is an example of the Diagnostic Grid (3D-3T), which includes those areas and measurements that absolutely must be included.

15. What is the discrepancy index used by the American Board of Orthodontics (ABO)?

The ABO discrepancy index is a grading system used to assess the complexity of an orthodontic case.[17] There are 11 target disorders evaluated and scored depending on the severity of their manifestation: overjet, overbite, anterior and lateral open bite, crowding, occlusion according to the Angle classification, lingual crossbite or buccal crossbite, ANB angle, SN-GoGn angle, and U1-SN angle. Other features may add to the complexity of the case, such as congenitally missing teeth or supernumerary teeth, ectopy or ectopic eruption, transposition, impaction, anomalies of tooth size and shape (e.g., peg lateral incisors), significant skeletal asymmetries that require dental compensation, significant midline discrepancies or CO-CR shifts, and excessive curve of Wilson. Examples of the Discrepancy Index form used by the ABO can be seen on the CD-ROM that accompanies this book.

CASE EXAMPLES

It is impossible to list in this chapter all of the orthodontic malocclusions that could exist. Following are some case examples using the 3D-3T Grid for diagnosis and actual treatment.

Case 1: Headgear

(Fig. 6-1 and Table 6-3)

16. How does one decide what type of headgear to use?

To begin with, one must ask a series of questions. Is the patient a child or an adult? What sort of facial pattern does the patient have; is it hypodivergent or hyperdivergent? What sort of malocclusion exists; is it a dental problem or is it a skeletal problem? What is the soft tissue picture; is it characterized by a flat lip posture or are the lips full, protrusive, and convex? What are the anchorage requirements of the case once treatment is instituted? What are the treatment objectives for this case? Is the malocclusion a Class II and how is it to be corrected? The answers to these questions come only with a complete set of diagnostic records and a thorough understanding of an entire range of subjects.[8-11,18]

Assume, for the sake of this discussion, that the patient has a Class II division 1 malocclusion with bimaxillary crowding, bimaxillary protrusion, open bite tendency, a high MPA, and a slightly retrognathic mandible. Assume that the treatment requires more than simply minimum anchorage control. If a headgear was the anchorage mechanism of choice, then a decision must be made as to design and how it is to be used. Age of the patient certainly will play a major role in these decisions. In the case of an 11-year-old, the treatment might be considerably different than it would be for a 21-year-old. In the first instance, harnessing whatever horizontal growth might be available could help in gaining at least part of the Class II correction.[18] In the adult patient, however, growth is not a factor and Class II correction may have to be accomplished in an entirely different manner. Then again, while a headgear might be appropriate for the child, it may not be for the adult; microimplants might be more advisable. In the Class II adult, treatment options are usually limited to two choices: performing orthognathic surgery to advance the mandible or camouflaging this case with extraction of

TABLE 6-2 Diagnostic Grid (3D-3T)

	ANTEROPOSTERIOR	TRANSVERSE	VERTICAL
Skeletal	SNA	6-6 Width	SN-MP
	SNB		FMA
	ANB	6' to 6' Width	
Soft Tissue	Profile	Buccal corridor	Lips
	NLA		VME
	E-line		
Dental	Molar classification	UDML	OB
	OJ	LDML	Curve of Spee
	1 to NA	U-ALD	Incisor display
	1' to NB	L-ALD	
	1 to SN	3' to 3' Width	
	1' to MP		
Other Considerations	Mandibular arch form		
	Discrepancy Index (DI)		
	Perio status		

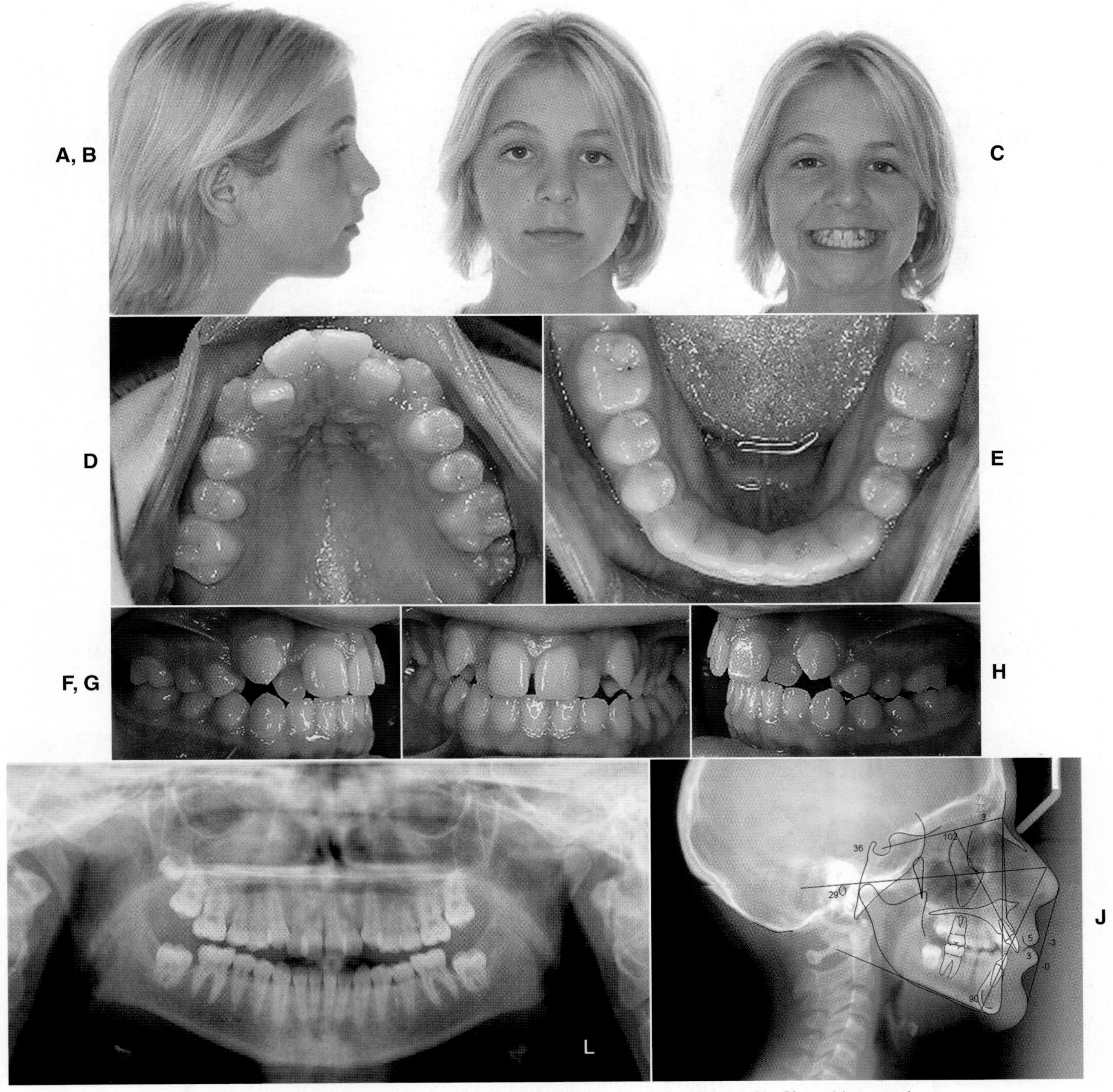

FIG 6-1 Case 1: Headgear. **A-H,** Composite initial photographs. Facial **(A-C)** and intraoral **(D-H)**. **I,** Initial panoramic radiograph. **J,** Initial cephalometric tracing.

Continued

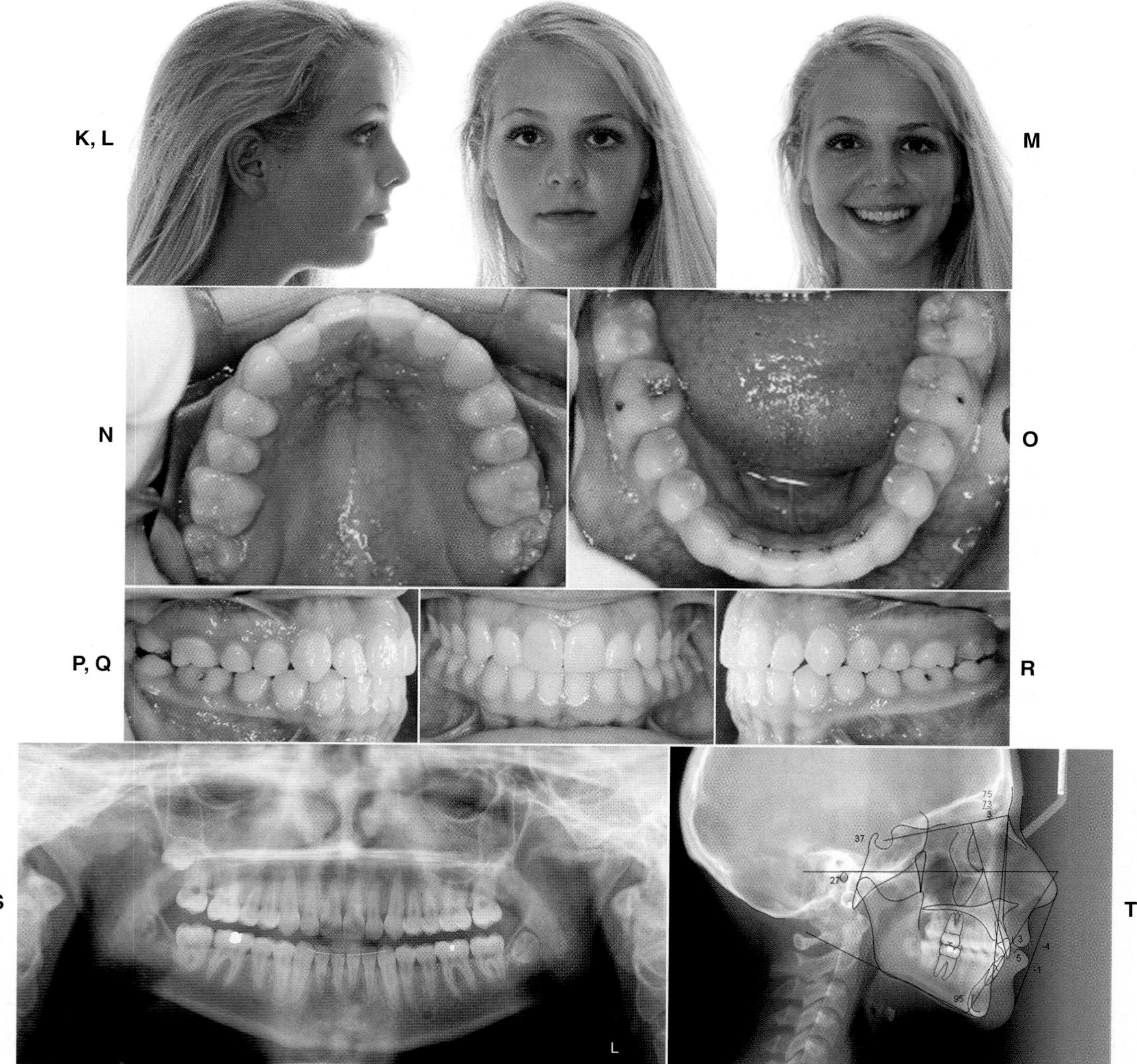

FIG 6-1—cont'd K-R, Composite final photographs. Facial **(K-M)** and intraoral **(N-R)**. **S,** Final panoramic radiograph. **T,** Final cephalometric tracing.

TABLE 6-3 Diagnostic Summary (3D-3T): Case 1—Headgear (M.B., 12 y 7m)

	ANTEROPOSTERIOR	TRANSVERSE	VERTICAL
Skeletal	SNA = **78°** SNB = **74°** ANB = **4°**	6-6 Width = **29.5 mm** 6' to 6' Width = **40.3 mm**	SN-GoGn = **35°** FMA = **27°**
Soft Tissue	Profile = **slightly convex** NLA = **obtuse** E-line = **- 3.4 mm**	Buccal corridors = **narrow**	Lips competent Thin upper lip Mesofacial
Dental	Molar: **Class II L, end on R** OJ = **4 mm** 1 to NA = **3.6 mm** 1' to NB = **2.8 mm** 1 to SN = **100°** 1' to GoGn = **90.2°**	UDML = **3 mm R** LDML = **coincident** U-ALD = **2 mm** L-ALD = **0 mm** 3' to 3' Width = **26.8 mm**	OB = **0.5 mm**
Other Considerations	Mand Arch Form = **Ovoid** DI = **17** Perio/OH = **Good oral hygiene**		

PRIORITIZED TREATMENT OBJECTIVES	TREATMENT PLAN
1. Establish Class I molar and cuspid 2. Correct maxillary dental midline 3. Improve facial esthetics 4. Maintain vertical control 5. Restrict maxillary growth in AP 6. Close diastema 7. Maintain oral hygiene	1. Deliver cervical-pull headgear 2. Full-time wear until molar correction; then night time only 3. Band and bond Mx/Mn 4. Level and align CCS to open space for U-2s and shift UDML 5. Detail occlusion 6. Class II elastics prn 7. Retain: Mx Wrap Mn 3-3

maxillary first bicuspids, leaving the first molars in a Class II. In either case, if extraction treatment is necessary, anchorage requirements must be established and decisions made relative to Class II molar correction.

If, as has been illustrated, the patient presents with a hyperdivergent facial pattern,the headgear of choice might very well be a high pull design.[6] If, on the other hand, this hypothetical patient had presented with a hypodivergent facial pattern, the headgear of choice might be a cervical pull design.[18]

In the end, factors such as anchorage requirements, patient age, facial pattern, and treatment objectives will help the orthodontist decide upon the appropriately designed appliance. In this present hypothetical example, if the patient was a child and if the molars were in a full-step Class II relationship, the facial pattern were hyperdivergent, the mandibular anchorage requirement were maximum, and the final treatment objective was to achieve Class I molar relationship, how many hours of headgear would be required to achieve the goal? Since, in this case, the Class II molar relationship will result without mesial movement of the mandibular molars (maximum anchorage), the Class I molar relationship will be achieved by some distalization of the maxillary molars and forward growth or repositioning of the mandible. Therefore, the number of hours required to wear a headgear to create the desired change—if, in fact, the objective could be reached at all—might be 14 hours/day or more. Of course, it is assumed that molar distalization with high pull headgear is not necessarily an appropriate expectation. In fact, in the case of a hyperdivergent patient, it is understood that distalization of molars could easily increase the anterior facial height as the molars "wedge" the mandible down and back in a clockwise direction.[6] This, in and of itself, is a limiting factor in the successful treatment of such a malocclusion. In the adult patient with a similar malocclusion, the treatment of choice might not include headgear; it also might not involve just orthodontics alone. It would be unrealistic to expect the adult to wear a headgear the required number of hours, if at all. In addition, with no growth potential available to help with the correction, microimplants might be a better option in correcting the dental malocclusion. As to the issue of the skeletal discrepancy, surgery might very well be the only choice for the adult.[9,10]

Case 2: Extraction vs. Non-Extraction (Fig. 6-2 and Table 6-4)

17. What factors can affect the decision to extract teeth when correcting a malocclusion?

Facial profile and soft tissue considerations have come to play a much more important role in terms of the method of treatment. A knowledge and understanding of the interplay and interrelationship of the soft tissue response to normal growth and tooth movement is critical to the success or failure in creating a pleasing soft tissue appearance. Studies have shown that people have difficulty in distinguishing between patients who have or

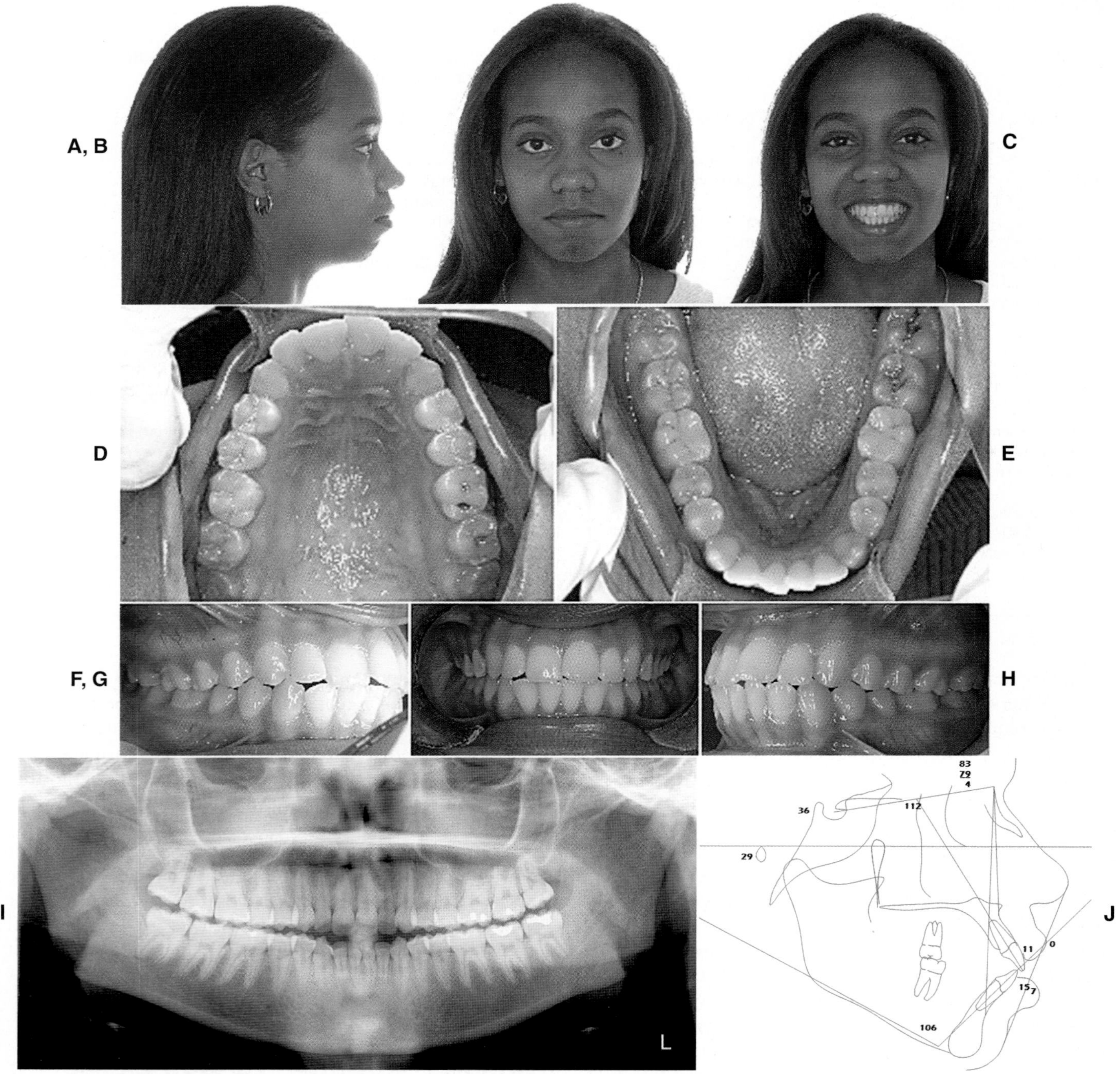

FIG 6-2 Case 2: Extraction. **A-H,** Composite initial photographs. Facial **(A-C)** and intraoral **(D-H)**. **I,** Initial panoramic radiograph. **J,** Initial cephalometric tracing.

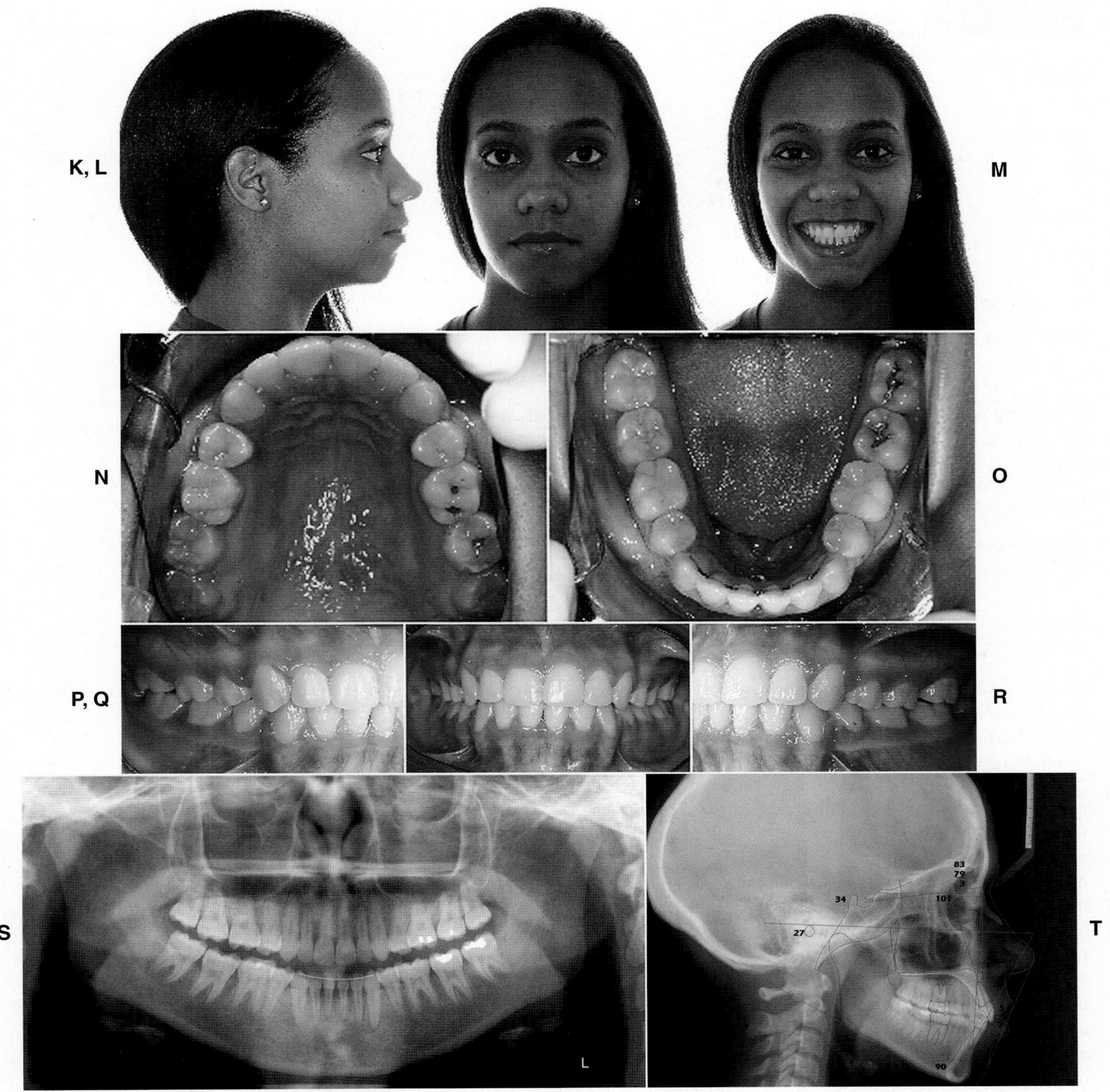

FIG 6-2—cont'd K-R, Composite final photographs. Facial **(K-M)** and intraoral **(N-R)**. **S,** Final panoramic radiograph. **T,** Final cephalometric tracing.

TABLE 6-4 Diagnostic Summary (3D-3T): Case 2—Extraction (J.M., 17 y 7 m)

	ANTEROPOSTERIOR	TRANSVERSE	VERTICAL
Skeletal	SNA = **83°** SNB = **79°** ANB = **4°**	6-6 Width = **32.5 mm** 6' to 6' Width = **40.6 mm**	SN-GoGn = **36°** FMA = **29°**
Soft Tissue	Profile = **convex** NLA = **Acute** E-line = **+ 7 mm** **Bi-dentoalveolar protrusion**	Buccal corridors = **normal**	Lips incompetent **Dolichofacial mentalis strain**
Dental	Molar: **Class I** OJ = **4 mm** 1 to NA = **11 mm** 1' to NB = **15 mm** 1 to SN = **112°** 1' to GoGn = **106°**	UDML = **on** LDML = **on** U-ALD = **–1 mm** L-ALD = **–1.5 mm** 3' to 3' Width = **26.8 mm**	OB = **1.5 mm**
Other Considerations	Mand Arch Form = **Tapered** DI = **15** Perio/OH = **Good oral hygiene**		

PRIORITIZED TREATMENT OBJECTIVES	TREATMENT PLAN
1. Reduce dentoalveolar protrusion	1. Extract all first bicuspids
2. Eliminate crowding in Mx/Mn	2. Band and bond Mx/Mn
3. Retract and upright Mx and Mn incisors	3. Level and align
4. Improve facial and dental esthetics	4. Close extraction spaces Detail occlusion
5. Establish ideal OB and OJ with coincident dental midlines	5. Class II elastics prn
6. Maintain oral hygiene	6. Retain: Mx Wrap Mn 3-3
7. Maintain Class I molar and cuspid	7. Crown lengthening UR1

have not had extractions when evaluating post-treatment soft tissue results.[19-21] Thus, it may be assumed that a proper diagnosis treatment plan and ultimate treatment approach should result in a patient who has a pleasing soft tissue appearance.

The degree of dental discrepancy and patient age play important roles in the decision to treat a malocclusion with or without the extraction of permanent teeth. For example, the patient who presents in the mixed dentition may be a candidate for a nonextraction approach if the orthodontist feels that it is possible to take advantage of growth and by developing increased arch length to accommodate the permanent teeth. In certain situations, one must decide if a combination of arch development and air rotor stripping (ARS) is sufficient to accomplish the treatment objectives.[22,23] Some suggest that a significant amount of mesio-distal tooth reduction can, in a significant number of cases, reduce the need for extraction of teeth. In the end, however, a patient who presents in the permanent dentition with a severe enough discrepancy in arch length might very well require extraction treatment.

Certain cephalometric findings might also tip the balance toward extraction treatment when these findings are superimposed upon other factors such as those mentioned previously. In a borderline extraction case, the orthodontist will tend not to extract in a low MPA case but will tend to extract in a high mandibular plane angle case.

For example, when the degree of protrusion, which may be considered a form of crowding, and the amount of retraction are combined with the desired change in soft tissue and the need for decrowding of the dentition, extraction may become the treatment of choice.[8-11]

Case 3: Maxillary Expansion

(Fig. 6-3 and Table 6-5)

18. What is the difference between the treatment approach of the adult or child who requires expansion of the maxillary arch?

As is the case in all other situations, a proper diagnosis is required in order to determine the nature of the problem.[24-27] If, for example, there is a posterior crossbite and it is determined that the transverse discrepancy is of dental origin, the correction of the malocclusion will be considerably different than if the problem is skeletal in nature. Aside from a clinical evaluation and a routine set of diagnostic records, the addition of an AP cephalogram would be an appropriate diagnostic tool for determining the nature of the problem. If the malocclusion is determined to be of dental origin, the correction may be similar for either the adult or the child patient in terms of mechanotherapy. If, on the other hand, the transverse discrepancy is due to a maxillary basal bone constriction, the treatment will be considerably different for the adult and the child.[28]

Let us first consider the treatment of a dental maxillary transverse discrepancy of dental origin in the child patient. In the mixed dentition, spontaneous correction is a possibility if the permanent teeth erupt in a more buccal position relative to the deciduous teeth. Failing that, however, mechanical expansion

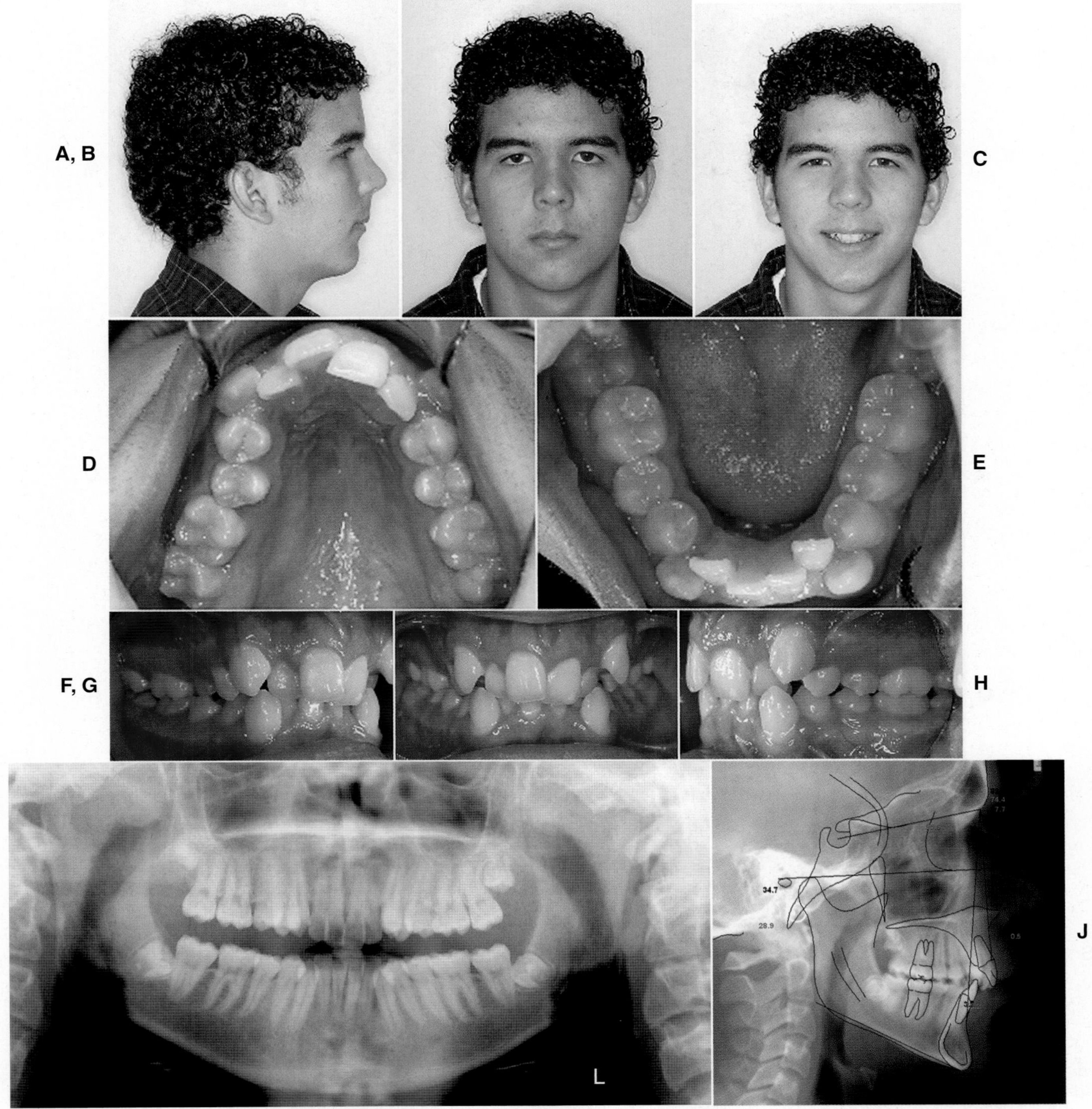

FIG 6-3 Case 3: Maxillary expansion. **A-H,** Composite initial photographs. Facial **(A-C)** and intraoral **(D-H)**. **I,** Initial panoramic radiograph. **J,** Initial cephalometric tracing.

Continued

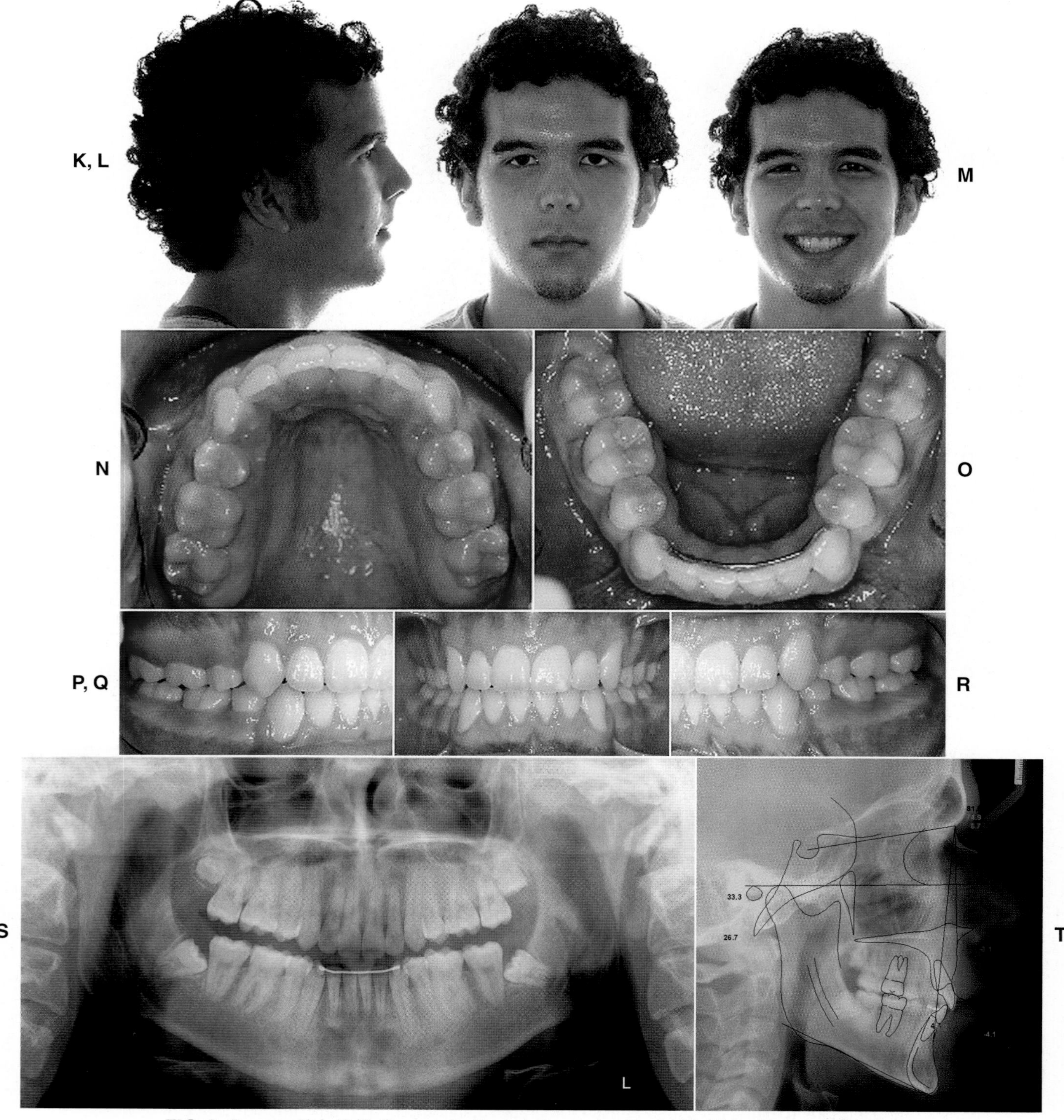

FIG 6-3—cont'd K-R, Composite final photographs. Facial **(K-M)** and intraoral **(N-R)**. **S,** Final panoramic radiograph. **T,** Final cephalometric tracing.

TABLE 6-5 Diagnostic Summary (3D-3T): Case 3—Maxillary Expansion (C.M., 15 y 6 m)

	ANTEROPOSTERIOR	TRANSVERSE	VERTICAL
Skeletal	SNA = **82°** SNB = **74°** ANB = **8°**	6-6 Width = **29 mm** 6' to 6' Width = **36.2 mm**	SN-GoGn = **35°** FMA = **29°**
Soft Tissue	Profile = **convex** NLA = **obtuse** E-line = **−0.4 mm**	Buccal corridors = **narrow**	Lips **Strain on closure** **Dolichofacial** **Long lower third**
	Molar: **Class II end on** OJ = **3 mm** 1 to NA = **0.5 mm** 1' to NB = **3.5 mm** 1 to SN = **96°** 1' to GoGn = **87°**	UDML = **on** LDML = **on** U-ALD = **−12 mm** L-ALD = **−9 mm** 3' to 3' Width = **25 mm**	OB **6 mm**
Other Considerations	Mand Arch Form = **Tapered** DI = **34** Perio/OH = **Good oral hygiene** **Crossbite– UR5, UL2**		

PRIORITIZED TREATMENT OBJECTIVES	TREATMENT PLAN
1. Eliminate ALD in both arches	1. Extract all first bicuspids
2. Expand the maxilla transversely	2. Banded RPE to expand approx 9 mm
3. Establish Class I molar and cuspid with cuspid and anterior guidance	3. Band and bond Mx/Mn
4. Establish ideal OB and OJ with coincident midlines	4. Level and align Close extraction spaces with reverse curve TMA CLAW
5. Decrease lip strain	5. Detail occlusion with seating elastics
6. Improve dental and facial esthetics	6. Retain: Mx Wrap Mn 3-3
7. Maintain oral hygiene	7. Refer for extraction of 8's

is likely the treatment of choice. Although certain constraints exist in terms of how much mechanical expansion can be done, this approach is certainly reasonable. If, however, the transverse discrepancy is due to a basal bony problem, the treatment of choice is rapid maxillary expansion. Naturally, an understanding of the timing of midpalatal suture closure is critical to the diagnosis and treatment planning for the maxillary expansion procedure.[9-11] At what age the midpalatal suture closes can vary from patient to patient, but certain general rules apply. If, however, the young patient has reached an age beyond which the orthodontist feels comfortable attempting a routine expansion, a surgically assisted procedure may be the treatment of choice.

In the adult patient who presents with a dental posterior crossbite, mechanical expansion is also an acceptable treatment, as it is in the child, but in adults it is important to include a periodontal evaluation prior to instituting expansion mechanics. In the presence of untreated mild to moderate periodontal disease, mechanical expansion may be somewhat risky and contraindicated. If, in the adult patient, the maxillary transverse problem is due to a narrowness of the basal bone, the treatment of choice is a surgically assisted rapid palatal expansion appliance (SARPE). Similar prerequisites apply in terms of overall periodontal health.

In the patient who presents with a hyperdivergent facial pattern, control of the vertical dimension is important when considering any form of posterior expansion therapy, whether it is mechanical or orthopedic in nature. During correction of a posterior crossbite, one might typically expect an increase in the anterior vertical dimension. This usually results as the buccal cusps of the maxillary teeth override the buccal cusps of the mandibular teeth. Under normal circumstances this phenomenon is of a temporary nature, since the cusps achieve a more normal bucco-lingual relationship. In circumstances in which the patient is a young growing individual, one might have an easier time controlling this problem with the use of various extra-oral appliances (e.g., vertical pull headgears/vertical pull chin cups) to redirect vertical growth. In the adult patient, however, controlling the vertical may be entirely different. Adult patients who present with these types of malocclusions often exhibit other characteristics of the so-called long face syndrome such as maxillary vertical excess. In cases like these, the treatment of choice is often orthognathic surgery with any number of different approaches to correcting the transverse and vertical discrepancies.[8-11]

Case 4: Impacted Cuspid

(Fig. 6-4 and Table 6-6)

19. In what instance(s) might one choose to extract an impacted cuspid rather than bring it into its normal position?

The diagnosis and treatment of impacted teeth, especially the maxillary cuspid, presents the orthodontist with a particularly difficult problem and a serious challenge.[29,30] For

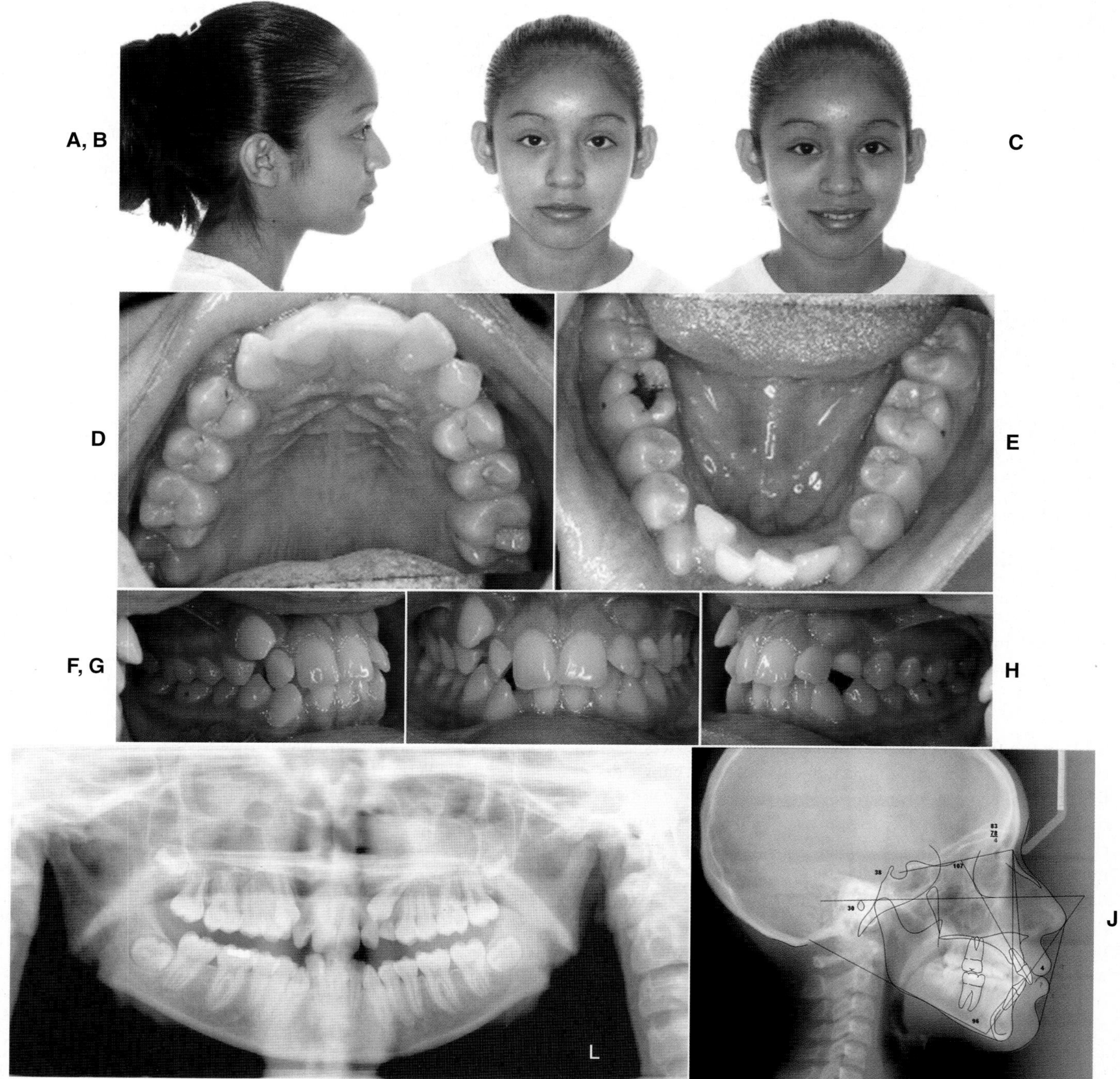

FIG 6-4 Case 4: Impacted cuspid. **A-H,** Composite initial photographs. Facial **(A-C)** and intraoral **(D-H)**. **I,** Initial panoramic radiograph. **J,** Initial cephalometric tracing.

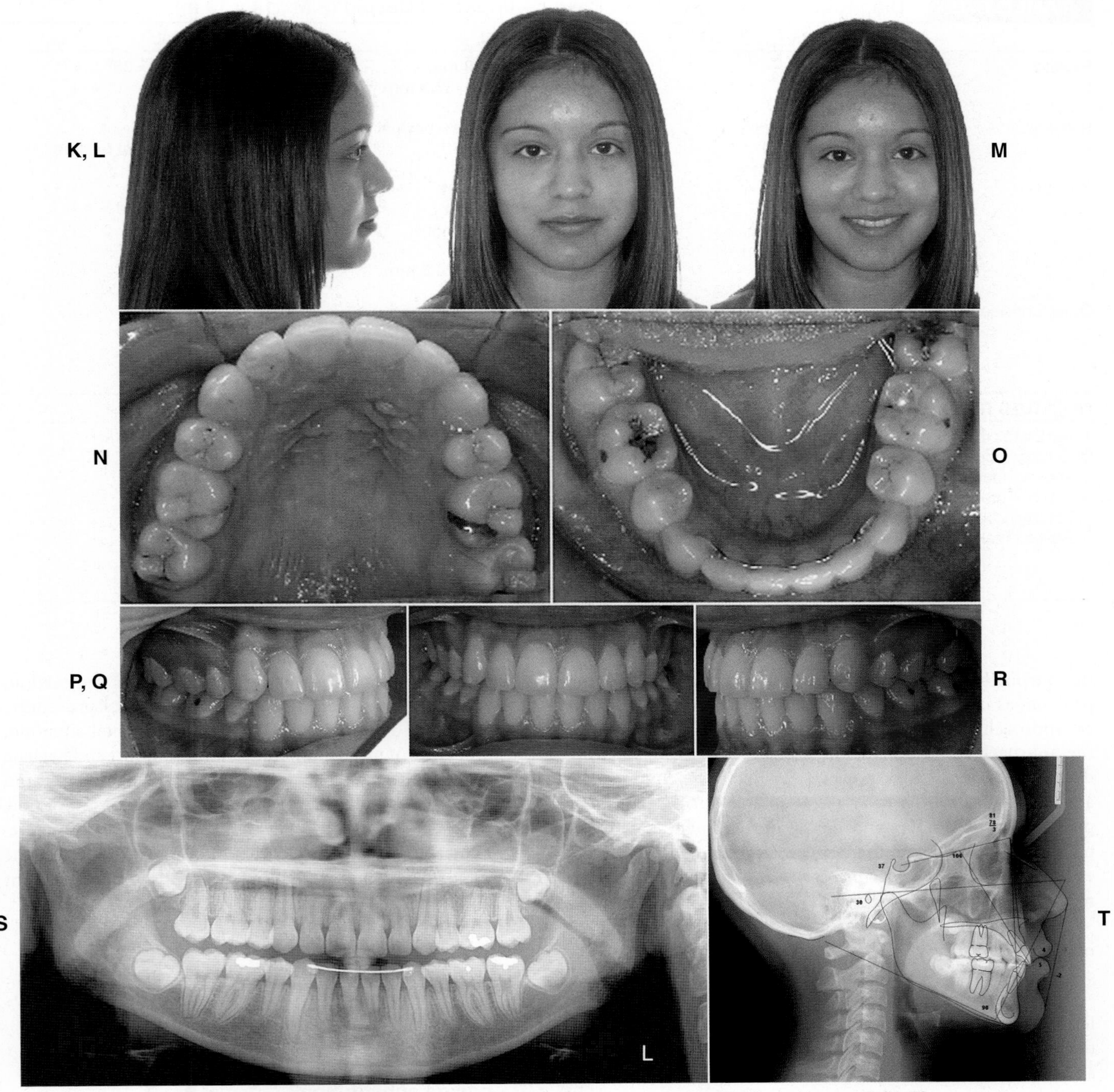

FIG 6-4—cont'd K-R, Composite final photographs. Facial **(K-M)** and intraoral **(N-R)**. **S,** Final panoramic radiograph. **T,** Final cephalometric tracing.

TABLE 6-6 Diagnostic Summary (3D-3T): Case 4—Impacted Cuspid (S.M., 14 y 10 m)

	ANTERIOR-POSTERIOR	TRANSVERSE	VERTICAL
Skeletal	SNA = **82°** SNB = **78°** ANB = **5°**	6-6 Width = **38 mm** 6' to 6' Width = **37.5 mm**	SN-GoGn = **38°** FMA = **30°**
Soft Tissue	Profile = **convex** NLA = **normal** E-line = **- 2 mm**	Buccal corridors = **normal**	Lips Competent **Dolichofacial full lips**
Dental	Molar: **Class I** OJ = **3 mm** 1 to NA = **4 mm** 1' to NB = **7 mm** 1 to SN = **107°** 1' Go-GA = **96°**	UDML = **3 mm Rt** LDML = **2 mm Rt** U-ALD = **−10.5 mm** L-ALD = **− 9 mm** 3' to 3' Width = **24.5 mm**	OB **2 mm**
Other Considerations	Mand Arch Form = **Ovoid** DI = **17** Perio/OH = **Fair oral hygiene but some decalcification present** **Maxillary left canine impacted facially**		

PRIORITIZED TREATMENT OBJECTIVES	TREATMENT PLAN
1. Eliminate crowding in Mx/Mn	1. Place Nance arch
2. Establish ideal OB/OJ with coincident midlines	2. Extract all first bicuspids and ULC
3. Improve facial and smile esthetics	3. Band and bond remaining teeth
4. Improve oral hygiene	4. Close extraction spaces
5. Establish Class I mutually protected occlusion	5. Detail occlusion
6. Restrict maxillary growth	6. Retain: Mx Wrap Mn 3-3

the purposes of this brief discussion, we will focus on the problem as it relates to the maxillary cuspid. There is a logical approach to the diagnosis of this particular problem, but the approach to treatment may not necessarily be so easily determined, and it may not be similar for the child vs. the adult patient. In order to arrive at an appropriate treatment plan, one must understand dental development, retention, biomechanics, mechanotherapy, periodontal considerations, esthetics, functional occlusion, and other topics before making the decision.

Although most orthodontists would prefer to bring an impacted maxillary cuspid into its normal position, there are certain circumstances that might preclude that decision.

Let's look at the following example. Assume that the maxillary left cuspid is palatally and somewhat horizontally impacted, that the left buccal occlusion is in Class II dental relationship, and that there is little or no space available for the cuspid in that quadrant. In addition, assume that the case requires extraction of permanent teeth in all four quadrants of the mouth. With a complete understanding of the treatment objective relative to establishing a final occlusion, it is determined that the maxillary left first bicuspid will finish in a Class I relation to the mandibular left cuspid. Thus, the question arises: "Does it make sense to extract the first bicuspid or the cuspid?" The decision to remove the cuspid in this instance may preclude establishing an ideal cuspid guided occlusion in favor of avoiding the risks or uncovering the cuspid and bringing it into place. This decision is predicated upon the orthodontist's ability to weigh the risk/reward benefits of erupting the cuspid as opposed to extracting the tooth. The inherent risks in the surgical procedure, the possibility of a compromised final periodontal situation, the difficulties of mechanotherapy, the discomfort and hygiene problems for the patient, and the chance of failure of the cuspid to erupt are all factors that contribute to the decision of how to treat the problem. A thorough radiographic, cephalometric, and clinical diagnosis coupled with an understanding of the factors just mentioned should lead to an appropriate treatment modality.[29]

Case 5: Missing Maxillary Laterals

(Fig. 6-5 and Table 6-7)

20. The congenitally missing maxillary lateral incisor presents the orthodontist with a true dilemma. What is one to do—implant or canine substitution?

There are few entities in orthodontics that challenge one's diagnostic skills more than that of a unilateral congenitally missing maxillary lateral incisor. The decision as to an appropriate treatment approach encompasses a whole range of options based upon the findings in the diagnostic records. A list of questions that must be answered might include, but are not limited to, any or all of the following:

- What is the morphology of the contralateral lateral incisor?
- What is the morphology of the cuspid on the side of the missing tooth?

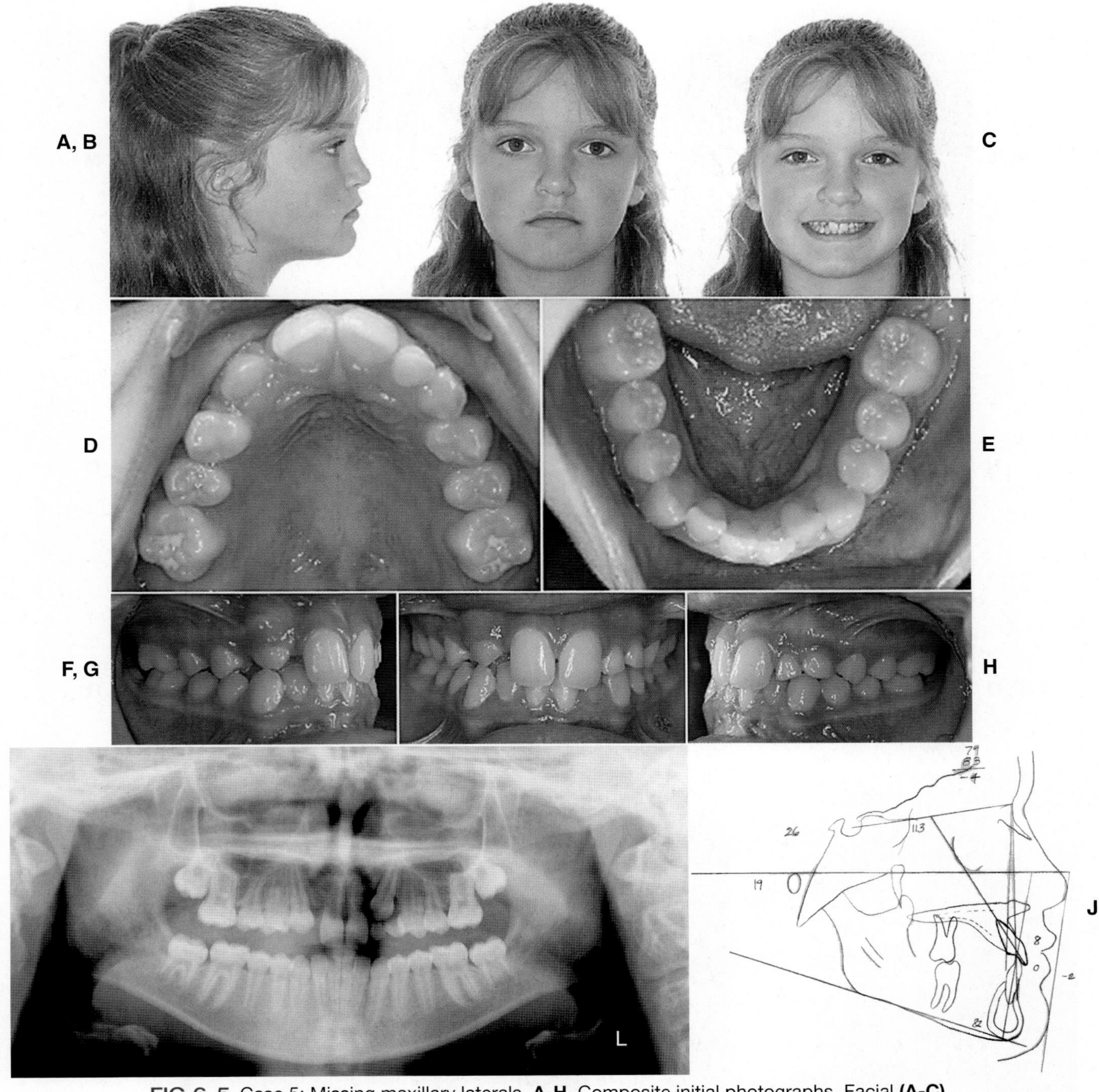

FIG 6-5 Case 5: Missing maxillary laterals. **A-H,** Composite initial photographs. Facial **(A-C)** and intraoral **(D-H)**. **I,** Initial panoramic radiograph. **J,** Initial cephalometric tracing.

Continued

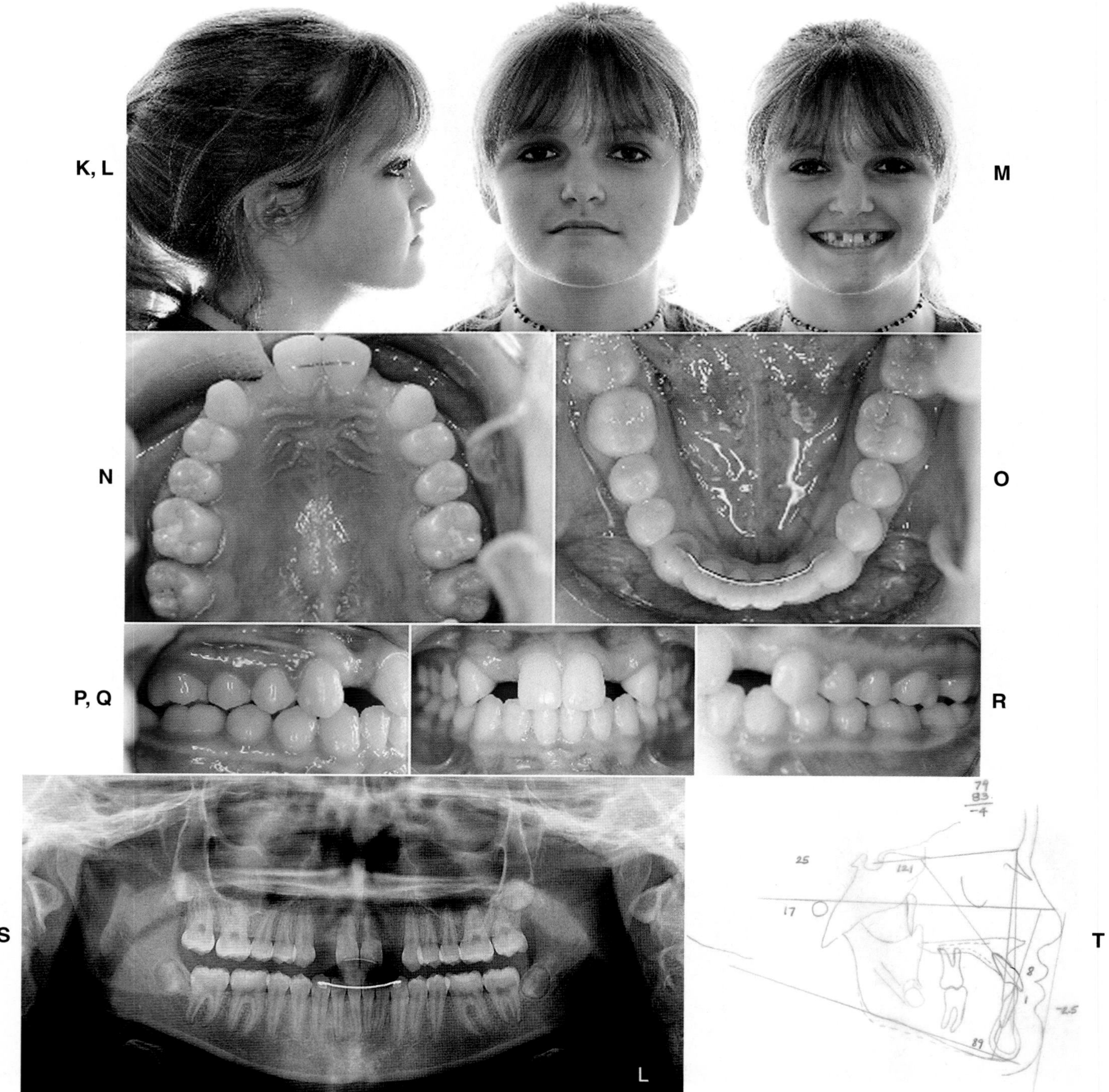

FIG 6-5—**cont'd K-R,** Composite final photographs. Facial **(K-M)** and intraoral **(N-R)**. **S,** Final panoramic radiograph. **T,** Final cephalometric tracing.

TABLE 6-7 Diagnostic Summary (3D-3T): Case 5—Missing Maxillary Laterals (B.B., 12 y 3 m)

	ANTERIOR-POSTERIOR	TRANSVERSE	VERTICAL
Skeletal	SNA = **79°** SNB = **83°** ANB = **−4°**	6-6 Width = **30 mm** 6' to 6' Width = **38 mm**	SN-GoGn = **26°** FMA = **19°**
Soft Tissue	Profile = **concave** NLA = **normal** E-line = **−2 mm**	Buccal corridors = **normal**	Lips Competent
Dental	Molar: **Class I** OJ = **2 mm** 1 to NA = **8 mm** 1' to NB = **0 mm** 1 to SN = **113°** 1' Go-GA = **82°**	UDML = **1 mm L** LDML = **coincident** U-ALD = **3 mm** L-ALD = **2 mm** 3' to 3' Width = **26 mm**	OB **5 mm**
Other Considerations	Mand Arch Form = **Ovoid** DI = **17** Perio/OH = **Fair oral hygiene but some decalcification present** **Maxillary left canine impacted facially**		

PRIORITIZED TREATMENT OBJECTIVES	TREATMENT PLAN
1. Improve dental & facial esthetics	1. Extract UL B, C
2. Establish ideal OB / OJ with coincident midlines	2. Band and bond U6-6, L6s
3. Correct transposition, rotations, and crowding	3. Band and bond U3s, L5-5 as available
4. Obtain Class I molar & cuspid, with cuspid guidance	4. Level and align
5. Improve oral hygiene	5. Place U2 pontics, as possible
6. Establish Class I mutually – protected occlusion	6. Detail occlusion
7. Retain	7. Retain: Mx Wrap with pontics Mn 3-3
	8. Lateral implants upon termination of growth

- How much space is available in the missing lateral position?
- What is the condition of the ridge in the missing lateral area?
- What is the buccal occlusion on both sides of the dentition?
- What sort of restoration will be planned for the missing tooth?

Assume, in just one scenario, that the occlusion on the side of the missing tooth is such that at least half the lateral space has been lost. Further assume that the patient has a high MPA and little or no overbite. Is it possible, or is it even advisable, to attempt space opening mechanics by distalizing the buccal segment? Given the difficulties of the scenario, one might decide to forgo the "ideal' plan and "settle for" the space closure in that quadrant, reshape the cuspid, and leave the left buccal occlusion in Class II. Given this situation, the decision must be made as to the disposition of the existing right lateral incisor. Is it desirable to retain the lateral and finish with an asymmetrical situation? Or is it better to remove the contralateral lateral incisor and close the space in order to maintain symmetry? In this particular situation, one must consider the anterior occlusion, the esthetics, the final functional occlusion, and the difficulties such mechanics might present given that there is little overjet.[31] The decision to place osseointegrated implants upon termination of growth was made for this patient.

Case 6: Ankylosis

(Fig. 6-6 and Table 6-8)

21. How does one treat an ankylosed tooth?

The diagnosis of an ankylosed tooth requires a combination of findings. Often the main finding on clinical examination is a tooth below the plane of occlusion of adjacent teeth (infraocclusion) in a patient with a previously level occlusion. The cessation of eruption is known as *ankylosis* and occurs when the cementum or dentin of the tooth fuses with alveolar bone. Percussion of the involved tooth may produce a sharp, solid sound, but only when more than 20% of the root is fused to bone.[32] The involved tooth may also radiographically show a loss of PDL space in areas where the tooth is fused to alveolar bone. If a determination cannot be made at the examination, an attempt to move the tooth with orthodontic traction will give a definitive answer.

When a tooth is determined to be ankylosed, there are three options for treatment, depending on the level of ankylosis and the tooth involved: (1) surgical removal of the tooth, (2) distraction osteogenesis of the tooth-bone segment, or (3) corticotomy of the surrounding bone and luxation of the tooth. Each option has its benefits and drawbacks, and each treatment for an ankylosed tooth should be determined on a case-by-case basis. Mandibular primary second molars are the most common ankylosed teeth, and treatment often involves

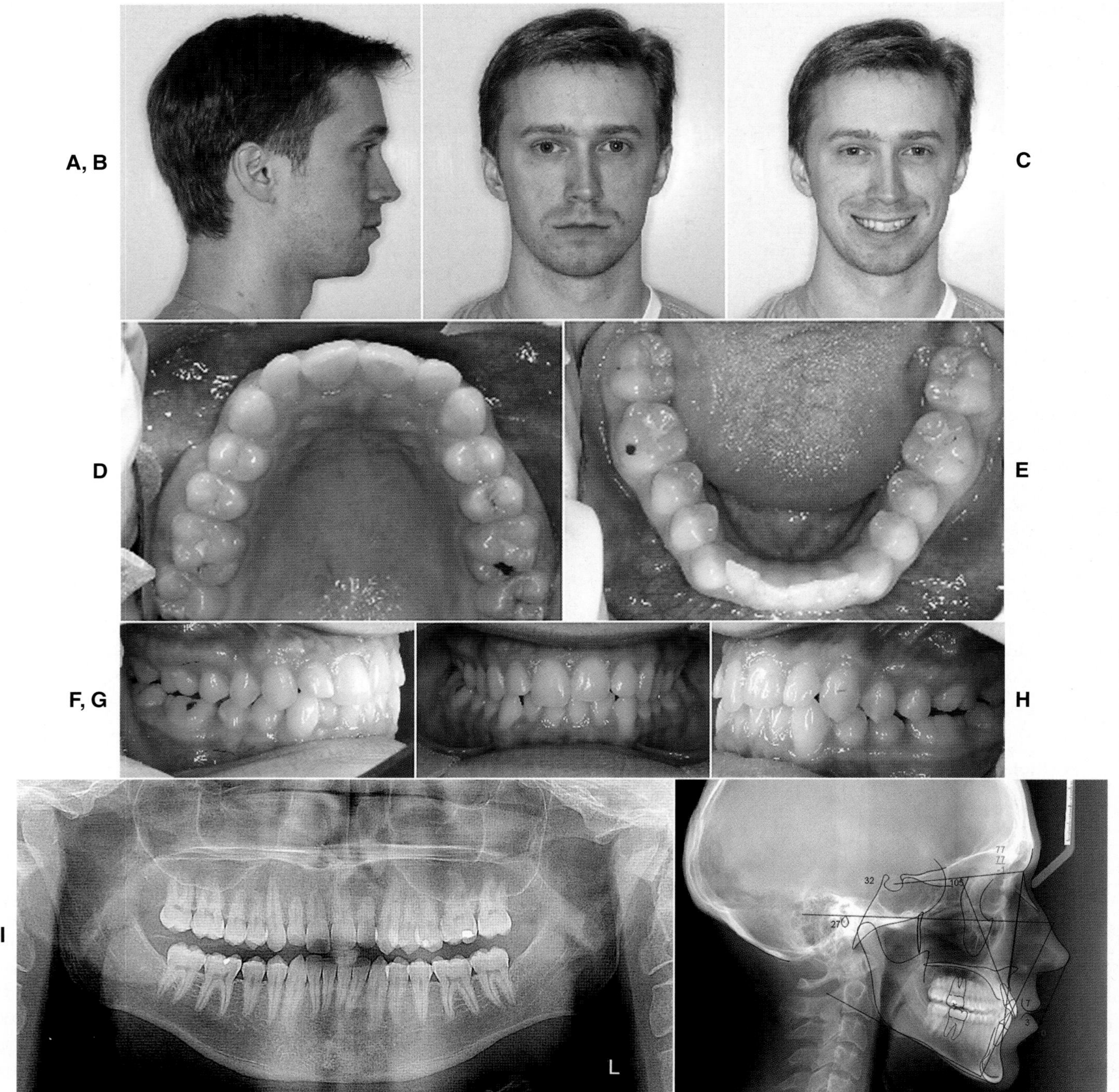

FIG 6-6 Case 6: Ankylosis. **A-H,** Composite initial photographs. Facial **(A-C)** and intraoral **(D-H)**. **I,** Initial panoramic radiograph. **J,** Initial cephalometric tracing.

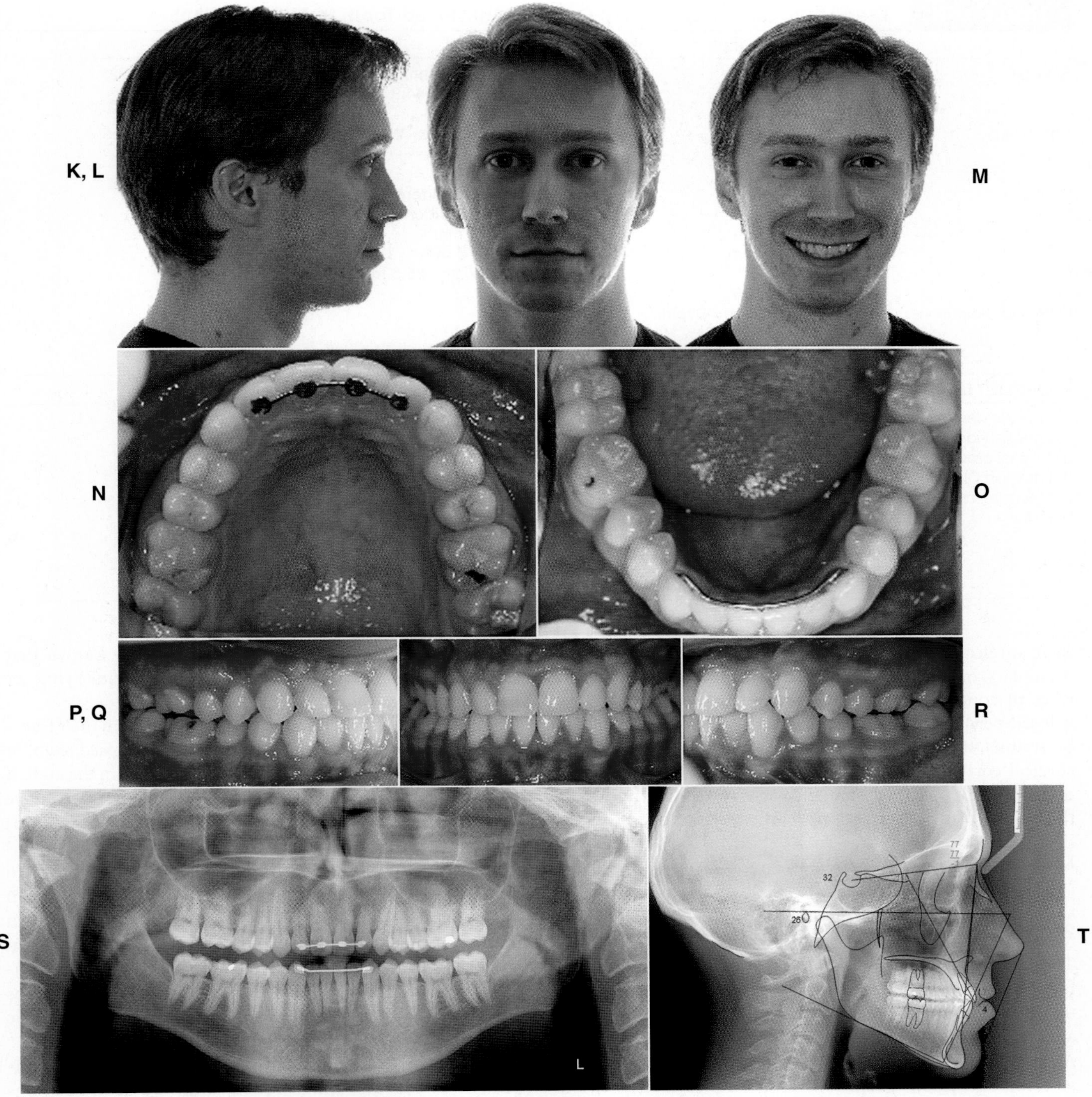

FIG 6-6—cont'd **K-R,** Composite final photographs. Facial **(K-M)** and intraoral **(N-R)**. **S,** Final panoramic radiograph. **T,** Final cephalometric tracing.

TABLE 6-8 Diagnostic Summary (3D-3T): Case 6—Ankylosed Tooth (K.M., 27 y 10 m)

	ANTEROPOSTERIOR	TRANSVERSE	VERTICAL
Skeletal	SNA = **77°** SNB = **77°** ANB = **−1°**	6-6 Width = **34mm** 6' to 6' Width = **44.9 mm**	SN-GoGn = **32°** FMA = **27°**
Soft Tissue	Profile = **straight** NLA = **normal** E-line = **0 mm**	Buccal corridors = **WNL**	Lips Competent Mesofacial
Dental	Molar: **Class I** OJ = **3 mm** 1 to NA = **7 mm** 1' to NB = **3 mm** 1 to SN = **105°** 1' to GoGn = **86°**	UDML = **coincident** LDML = **coincident** U-ALD = **1 mm** L-ALD = **4.5 mm** 3' to 3' Width = **25.5 mm**	OB = **4 mm**
Other Considerations	Mand Arch Form = **Ovoid** DI = **11** Perio / OH = **Good oral hygiene**		

PRIORITIZED TREATMENT OBJECTIVES	TREATMENT PLAN
1. Improve dental & facial esthetics 2. Establish ideal OB / OJ with coincident midlines 3. Correct crowding, rotations, and crossbite 4. Establish Class I molar and cuspid, with cuspid guidance 5. Maintain oral hygiene 6. Retain	1. Band and bond all teeth 2. Determine status of UL1 3. If ankylosed, decorticate or osteotomy 4. Level and align 5. ARS as needed 6. Detail occlusion 7. Retain: Mx 2-2, wrap Mn 3-3

their surgical removal to allow for eruption of the second premolars, or to allow space closure or tooth replacement in cases of congenitally missing lower second premolars. Ankylosed permanent teeth, especially those that were affected by trauma, are likely to require distraction osteogenesis or surgical corticotomy and luxation, with or without the addition of temporary anchorage devices to aid in eruption of the tooth.[33,34]

Case 7: Transposition

(Fig. 6-7 and Table 6-9)

21. Should a transposition be corrected?

Tooth transposition is a unique form of ectopic eruption that requires an intensive exploration of treatment options prior to treatment. *Tooth transposition* is a relatively rare dental anomaly term applied to extreme cases of ectopic eruptions. All transpositions are a form of ectopic eruptions, but not all ectopic eruptions qualify as transpositions. Transposition can be defined as the "positional interchange of two adjacent teeth, especially their roots, or the development or eruption of a tooth in a position occupied normally by a nonadjacent tooth."[35] Transposition is often accompanied by other dental anomalies. The most frequently reported of these include missing, small or peg-shaped laterals, congenitally missing teeth (excluding third molars), severe rotations or malpositions of adjacent teeth, retention of deciduous teeth, dilacerations of roots, or malformation of teeth. Although many originally thought that canine transposition was caused by overretention of a deciduous canine, it is now known that canine–first premolar transpositions have an underlying genetic basis.[35]

Treatment options include alignment of teeth in their transposed positions, extraction of one or both transposed teeth, or orthodontic movement to their proper positions in the arch. If probable transposition is detected early enough, interceptive orthodontics may be used with little disturbance to the supporting structures. Longer treatment time and possible gingival recession are drawbacks to correcting transpositions.[36] In cases of complete transposition, where the roots are parallel, an attempt to move the teeth to their correct position in the arch may be detrimental to the teeth or supporting structures.[37] In those cases it may be beneficial to the patient for the orthodontist to consider aligning the teeth in their transposed positions and reshaping their occlusal surfaces to enhance the esthetic outcome.[38]

In planning the treatment of transposition cases, it is important to consider initial root positions and inclinations and sufficiency of bone in which to move the transposed teeth. Tooth movement should be monitored closely while treatment is rendered. Tooth transpositions can be a challenge to the practitioner. Understanding how teeth can be transposed and the etiology behind the transposition can help the practitioner make an informed decision on treatment options. Transpositions must be carefully evaluated prior to beginning treatment so that the method of treatment will provide the most beneficial outcome to the patient.

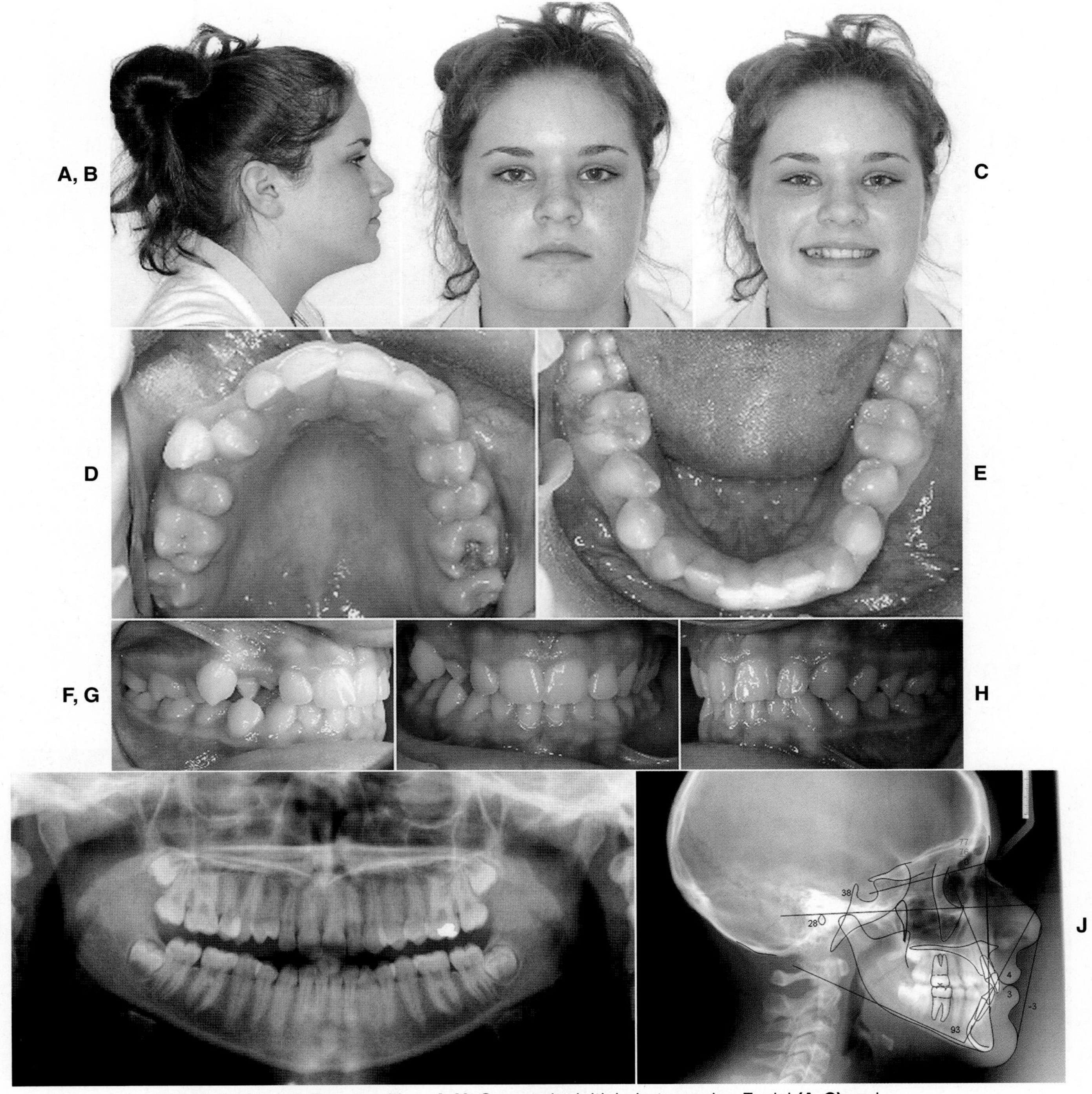

FIG 6-7 Case 7: Transposition. **A-H,** Composite initial photographs. Facial **(A-C)** and intraoral **(D-H)**. **I,** Initial panoramic radiograph. **J,** Initial cephalometric tracing.

Continued

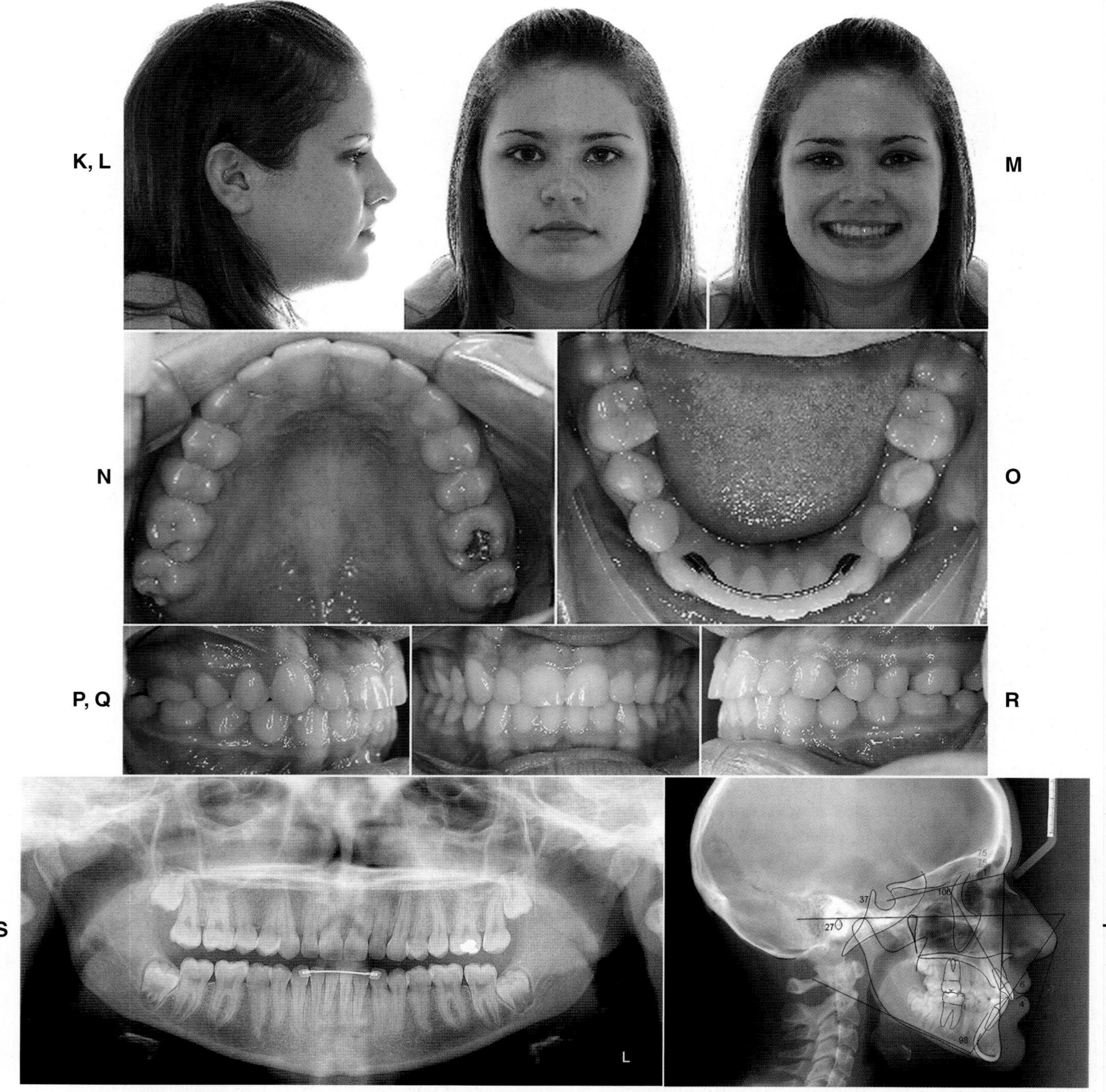

FIG 6-7—cont'd K-R, Composite final photographs. Facial **(K-M)** and intraoral **(N-R)**. **S,** Final panoramic radiograph. **T,** Final cephalometric tracing.

TABLE 6-9 Diagnostic Summary (3D-3T): Case 7—Transposed Teeth (B.H., 13 y 10 m)

	ANTEROPOSTERIOR	TRANSVERSE	VERTICAL
Skeletal	SNA = **77°** SNB = **76°** ANB = **0°**	6-6 Width = **32.8 mm** 6' to 6' Width = **39.5 mm**	SN-GoGn = **38°** FMA = **28°**
Soft Tissue	Profile = **slightly concave** NLA = **normal** E-line = **−3 mm**	Buccal corridors = **normal**	Lips Competent Mesofacial
Dental	Molar: **Class I** OJ = **3 mm** 1 to NA = **4 mm** 1' to NB = **3 mm** 1 to SN = **97°** 1' to GoGn = **93°**	UDML = **1.5 mm to R** LDML = **coincident** U-ALD = **2.5 mm** L-ALD = **4 mm** 3' to 3' Width = **25 mm**	OB = **3.5 mm**
Other Considerations	Mand Arch Form = **Ovoid** DI = **17** Perio/OH = **Good oral hygiene**		

PRIORITIZED TREATMENT OBJECTIVES	TREATMENT PLAN
1. Improve dental & facial esthetics	1. Place RPE arch, expand 1× day for 30 days; bond L7-7
2. Establish ideal OB/OJ with coincident midlines	2. Band and bond U7-7
3. Correct transposition, rotations, and crowding	3. Replace RPE with TPA soldered with retraction hook to retract UR4 palatally, protract UR3
4. Obtain Class I molar & cuspid, with cuspid guidance	4. Level and align
5. Maintain oral hygiene	5. Detail occlusion
6. Establish Class I mutually protected occlusion	6. Retain: Mx Wrap Mn 3-3
	7. Evaluate for perio graft UR3

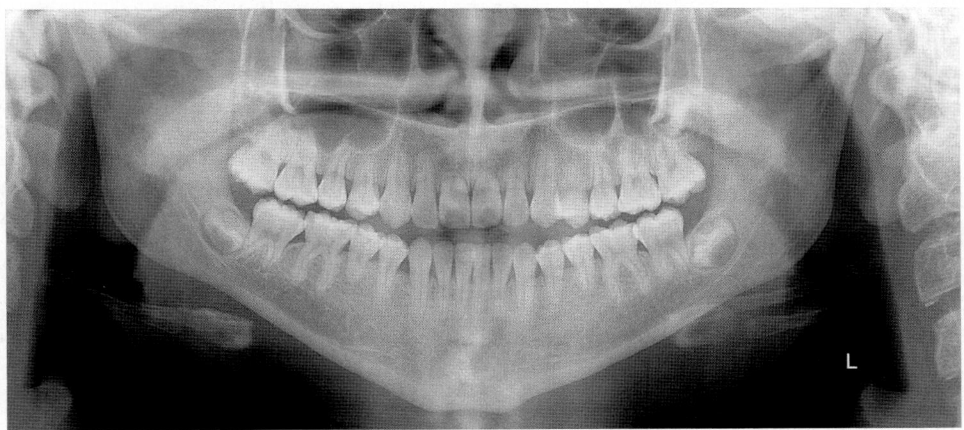

FIG 6-8 Case 8: Root resorption. Root resorption prior to orthodontic treatment on initial panoramic radiograph.

Case 8: Root Resorption

(Fig. 6-8)

22. Which measures should be taken in the orthodontic management of teeth presenting with root resorption or dilacerations?

Resorption of a tooth is the dissolution of the root by osteoclasts in response to caries, trauma, crowding, orthodontic tooth movement, or physiological movement in the transition from primary to permanent dentition.[39-41] It results in blunting of the root apex and internal loss of dentin from the pulpal part of the root, and it may lead to loss of the affected tooth depending on the severity of the process. If root resorption of a permanent tooth is radiographically detected, the area should be observed for clinical symptoms and the crown-root ratio should be closely monitored. However, root resorption resulting from orthodontic treatment has been found to be more common and more severe in initially resorbed teeth, but even in these cases it is usually without significant clinical consequences for the patient (see Figure 6-8). *Dilaceration* is the severe distortion of the root of a tooth, whereas a sharp curve or twist is termed *flexion*. The orthodontist should ascertain that dilacerated roots are not causing resorption to adjacent teeth. In the course of orthodontic alignment of the dilacerated roots within the arch, alteration of the crown shape of the corresponding tooth may be necessary to achieve an aesthetically pleasing result.

REFERENCES

1. Order from Chaos: Linnaeus Disposes. Available at http://huntbot.andrew.cmu.edu/HIBD/Exhibitions/OrderFromChaos/pages/intro.shtml. Accessed on July 25, 2007.
2. Angle EH: *The Treatment of Malocclusion of the Teeth. Angle's System*, edition 6. Philadelphia: The SS White Dental Manufacturing Company, 1907.
3. Magie WF, Carnot S, Clausius R, Kelvin WT: *The Second Law of Thermodynamics; Memoirs by Carnot, Clausius, and Thomson*, New York: Harper & Brothers, 1899.
4. Nanda R: Patterns of vertical growth in the face. *Am J Orthod Dentofacial Orthop* 1988;93:103-116.
5. Pearson LE: Vertical control in fully banded orthodontic treatment. *Angle Orthod* 1986;56:205-224.
6. Sankey WL, Buschang PH, English JD, Owens A: Early treatment of vertical skeletal dysplasia: The hyperdivergent phenotype. *Am J Orthod Dentofacial Orthop* 2000;118(September):317-327.
7. Vaden J: Nonsurgical treatment of the patient with vertical discrepancy. *Am J Orthod Dentofacial Orthop* 1988;113:567-582.
8. Rakosi T, Jonas I, Graber TM: *Color atlas of dental medicine: Orthodontic diagnosis.* New York: Thieme Medical Publishers, 1993.
9. Proffit WR: *Contemporary Orthodontics*, edition 3. St Louis: Mosby, 2001.
10. Graber TM, Vanarsdall RL, Vig K: *Orthodontics: current principles and techniques*, edition 4., St Louis: Elsevier, 2005.
11. Riolo ML, Avery JK: *Essentials for orthodontic practice*, edition 1. Ann Arbor and Grand Haven, MI: EFOP Press, 2003.
12. Nanda R, Ghosh J: Facial soft tissue harmony and growth in orthodontic treatment. *Semin Orthod* 1995;1(2):67-81.
13. Arnett GW, Bergman RT: Facial keys to orthodontic diagnosis and treatment planning. Part I. *Am J Orthod Dentofacial Orthop* 1993;103:299-312.
14. Reyneke JP: *Essentials of Orthognathic Surgery*. Carol Stream, IL: Quintessence Publishing, 2003.
15. Schiffman PH, Tuncay OC: Maxillary expansion: a meta analysis. *Clin Orthod Res* 2001; 4:86-96.
16. Horn A: Facial height index. *Am J Orthod Dentofacial Orthop* 1992;102:180.
17. Cangialosi T, Riolo ML, Owens SE Jr, et al: The ABO discrepancy index: A measure of case complexity. *Am J Orthod Dentofacial Orthop* 2004;125(3):270-278.
18. O'Reilly MT, Nanda SK, Close J: Cervical and oblique headgear: A comparison of treatment effects. *Am J Orthod Dentofacial Orthop* 1993;103(June):504-509.
19. Chua A, Lim J, Lubit E: The effects of extraction versus nonextraction orthodontic treatment on the growth of the lower anterior face height. *Am J Orthod Dentofacial Orthop* 1993;104: 361-368.
20. Bowman J, Johnston LE Jr.: The esthetic impact of extraction and nonextraction treatments on Caucasian patients. *Angle Orthod* 2000;70(February):3-10.
21. Johnson D, Smith R: Smile esthetics after orthodontic treatment with and without extraction of four first premolars. *Am J Orthod Dentofacial Orthop* 1995;108:162-167.
22. Sheridan JJ: Air-rotor stripping. *J Clin Orthod* 1985;19:43-59.
23. Sheridan JJ: Air-rotor stripping update. *J Clin Orthod* 1987;21:781-788.
24. Haas AJ: The treatment of maxillary deficiency by opening the mid-palatal suture. *Angle Orthod* 1965;35:200-217.
25. Haas AJ: Palatal expansion: just the beginning of dentofacial orthopedics. *Angle Orthod* 1970;57:213-255.
26. Haas AJ: Long-term post-treatment evaluation of rapid palatal expansion. *Angle Orthod* 1980;50:189-217.
27. Wertz RA: Skeletal and dental changes accompanying rapid midpalatal suture opening. *Am J Orthod* 1970;58:41-66.
28. McNamara JA Jr.: Early intervention in the transverse dimension: is it worth the effort?. *Am J Orthod Dentofacial Orthop* 2002;121:572-574.
29. Bishara S: Impacted maxillary canines: A review. *Am J Orthod Dentofacial Orthop* 1992;101:159-171.
30. Kokich VG: Surgical and orthodontic management of impacted maxillary canines. *Am J Orthod Dentofacial Orthop* 2004;126(Sept):378-383.
31. Spear FM, Mathews DM, Kokich VG: Interdisciplinary management of single-tooth implants. *Semin Orthod* 1997;3:45-72.
32. Damm N, Bouquot A, editors: Abnormalities of teeth. In *Oral and maxillofacial pathology*, edition 2. Philadelphia: WB Saunders, 2002.
33. Steiner DR: Timing of extraction of ankylosed teeth to maximize ridge development. *J Endod* 1997;23:242-245.
34. Kofod T, Würtz V, Melsen B: Treatment of an ankylosed central incisor by single tooth dento-osseous osteotomy and a simple distraction device. *Am J Orthod Dentofacial Orthop* 2005;127(1):72-80.
35. Peck S, Peck L: Classification of maxillary tooth transpositions. *Am J Orthod Dentofacial Orthop* 1995;107:505-517.
36. Kavadia S: A clinical study of maxillary canine transposition and their orthodontic management. *Euro J Orthod* 2003;25(5):531.
37. Shapira Y, Kuftinec M: Orthodontic management of mandibular canine – incisor transposition. *Am J Orthod Dentofacial Orthop* 1983;83(4):271-276.
38. Shapira Y, Kuftinec M: Intrabony migration of impacted teeth. *Angle Orthod* 2003;73(6):738-744.
39. Sameshima GT, Sinclair PM: Predicting and preventing root resorption: Parts I and II. *Am J Orthod Dentofacial Orthop* 2001;119:505-515.
40. Linge L, Linge BO: Patient characteristics and treatment variables associated with apical root resorption during orthodontic treatment. *Am J Orthod Dentofacial Orthop* 1991;99:35-43.
41. Harris EF, Baker WC: Loss of root length and crestal bone height before and during treatment in adolescent and adult orthodontic patients. *Am J Orthod Dentofacial Orthop* 1990;98:463-469.

Orthodontic Appliances

CHAPTER 7

P. Emile Rossouw

The introduction of fixed appliances to the teeth with bands or brackets set a milestone in the discipline of orthodontics. Orthodontic treatment options increased significantly; moreover, three-dimensional (3D) control of tooth movement became a standard goal of orthodontic treatment. Contemporary fixed appliances now have incorporated first-, second-, and third-order prescriptions. Numerous attachments and/or auxiliary appliances can now be attached to the fixed appliance, hence the term *fixed-removable* for such appliances as the headgear, removable transpalatal arch, and removable lingual arch. Fixed appliances, which encompass the various designs of brackets (directly bonded to enamel or laser welded to bands and cemented to teeth), tubes, buttons and others, with the activated arch wires in place, move teeth into new positions. Orthodontics reached out to industries with requests for "space-age" and biocompatible materials to facilitate and enhance treatment options. It is thus not surprising that the discipline went from the large gold bands and wires of Dr. Angle to the small, esthetic appliances constructed from various materials, including stainless steel, titanium, and ceramic, as well as combinations of the noted materials. In addition, arch wires that exhibit amazing memory and heat-activation characteristics have become the order of the day.

The amazing bracket designs comparable to classic art work and the highly developed arch wires have changed orthodontic treatment from laborious and time consuming to a very refined, efficient, and reliable practice; this is truly a remarkable ingredient in providing quality of life to millions of patients.

The development of the fixed appliance over the last 100 years incorporated sophistication second to none. The purpose of this chapter is to provide insight into these developments and stimulate further study by providing a brief overview of fixed orthodontic appliances.

1. What is a fixed orthodontic appliance?

A fixed orthodontic appliance has the capability of being fixed to teeth. Its design dictates either direct fixation by bonding to the enamel surface with composite cement or cemented via a band around the crown of a tooth. The nature of the appliance prevents removal by the patient, except if it is a fixed-removable appliance such as a headgear. The arch wires are then fixed to the brackets or tubes by clips, steel ligatures, or elastomeric o-rings to form the total fixed appliance and when activated leads to tooth movement.[1]

2. What characteristics should fixed orthodontic brackets or appliances exhibit?[2-4]

Fixed orthodontic appliances or braces, commonly referred to as orthodontic brackets attached to teeth, should exhibit the following properties:

- They should be simple to place and activate, thus should easily pull, push, and rotate teeth
- They should be fixed in a stable position to the teeth in order to accept the applied forces without failure but could be removed by choice without tissue damage
- Tooth movement must occur efficiently (refer to friction requirements) and anchorage provided must negate Newton's third law (for every action there is an equal and opposite reaction)
- Braces should be large enough for effective application, but also delicate enough to avoid tissue trauma; however, they must not cause inflammation and soreness
- Braces must be small and inconspicuous; thus, esthetically acceptable

3. When and by whom was the edgewise appliance introduced to the discipline of orthodontics?

The appliance was introduced by Dr. Edward Hartley Angle in 1928.[2]

4. Which appliance preceded the edgewise appliance?

The Angle System (Fig. 7-1) by Dr. Edward H. Angle (1887) preceded the edgewise appliance. It consisted of adjustable clamp bands closely adapted to the teeth and held in place by friction. The clamp bands had soldered retraction screws to enable closure of space; moreover, prototype bands on incisors and cuspids had soldered tubes into which rotation springs were inserted. Jackscrews crossed the palate for arch expansion. The E arch (expansion arch) replaced jackscrews; the latter

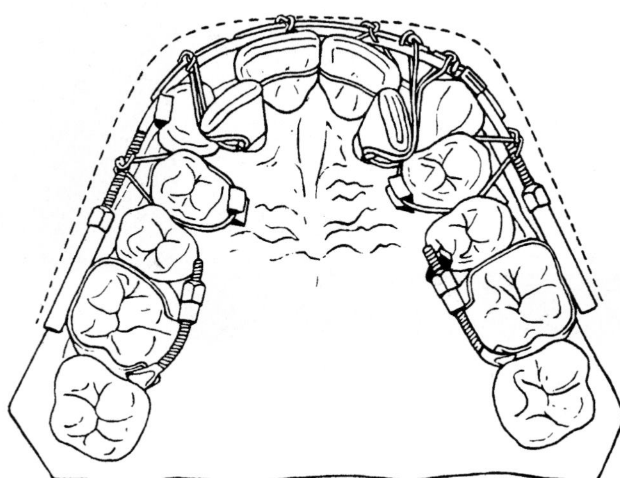

FIG 7-1 The Angle System. (From Angle EH: *Treatment of malocclusion of the teeth*. Philadelphia: SS White Dental Manufacturing, 1907.)

were soldered to the buccal aspects of molar bands. The E arch appliance was used to expand the arches.[2]

5. Why did Angle develop the pin and tube appliance?

Angle realized that the axial inclinations of teeth needed to be corrected. He developed the pin and tube appliance to enable orthodontists to accomplish root movement (Fig. 7-2). The pins had to be expertly soldered to the arch wire, fitted perfectly into the tubes on the bands, removed as the movement progressed, moved along the arch wire, soldered again, and fitted once more into the tubes on the bands. This precise and delicate procedure had to be completed at each patient visit, often with activation every few days, which was a laborious and difficult task and not user friendly.[2]

6. Which appliance did Angle develop in 1915 to replace the cumbersome pin and tube appliance?

The ribbon arch appliance (Fig. 7-3) was a much simpler appliance to construct and activate. The brackets, which were soldered to bands, consisted of a vertical slot (in contrast to contemporary edgewise brackets, which have horizontal slots). Brass pins, inserted from the occlusal aspect of the vertical tube, held the arch wire in place. The teeth could now freely move along the arch wire, similar to a string of beads.[2]

7. Which modern appliance is based on the Ribbon Arch appliance?

The Begg appliance of Dr. Raymond Begg uses the vertical bracket slot principle; however, the bracket is upside down with the arch wire inserted from the gingival aspect and then held in place with a variety of pins. Each pin fulfills a different function (Fig. 7-4). The Begg light wire technique or appliance uses mostly round arch wires with numerous auxiliary springs inserted into the vertical slots to achieve the required tooth movement. The treatment with

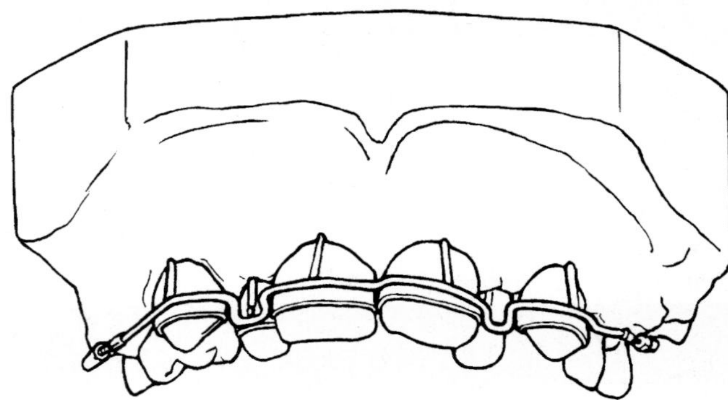

FIG 7-2 Angle pin and tube appliance. Note the wire inserted occlusally. (From Steiner CC: *Angle Orthod* 1933;3[4]:277.)

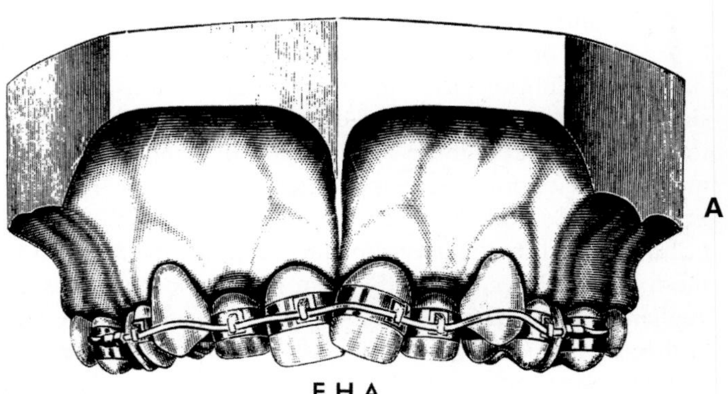

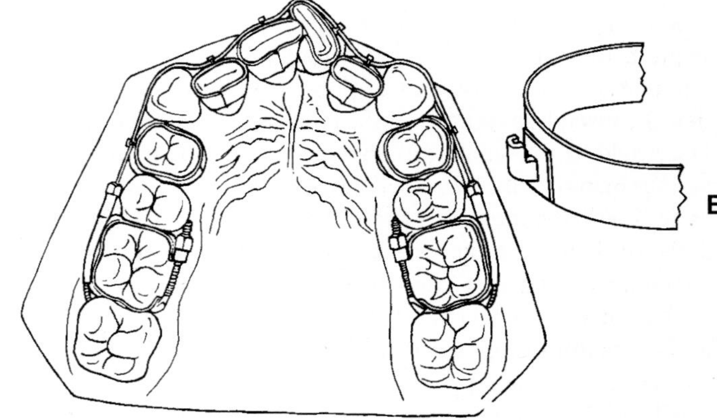

FIG 7-3 **A** and **B,** Angle's ribbon arch appliance. Note the wire inserted occlusally. (From Steiner CC: *Angle Orthod* 1933;3[4]:277.)

this appliance consists of different stages. For example, Stage 1 starts with the initial alignment and bite opening, Stage 2 is mostly space closure, and the final Stage 3 is where all the detail of the occlusion is consolidated.[2,4,5]

8. What is the Tip-Edge bracket?

The Tip-Edge bracket or appliance developed by P.C. Kesling[6] is basically a combination of the Edgewise and Begg bracket. The bracket has been modified to include a specialized slot—in general, an edgewise bracket that had two wedges removed from each side of the slot (Fig. 7-5, *A*) to provide a bracket that would permit free crown tipping (such as with Begg) followed by controlled root uprighting (Begg with auxiliary spring and Edgewise). The initial Tip-Edge bracket had a vertical slot and rotation wings. The Tip-Edge Plus bracket was introduced in 2003 and incorporated the latter as well as a horizontal slot for enhanced tooth movement in the final stages of treatment (Fig. 7-5, *B*).

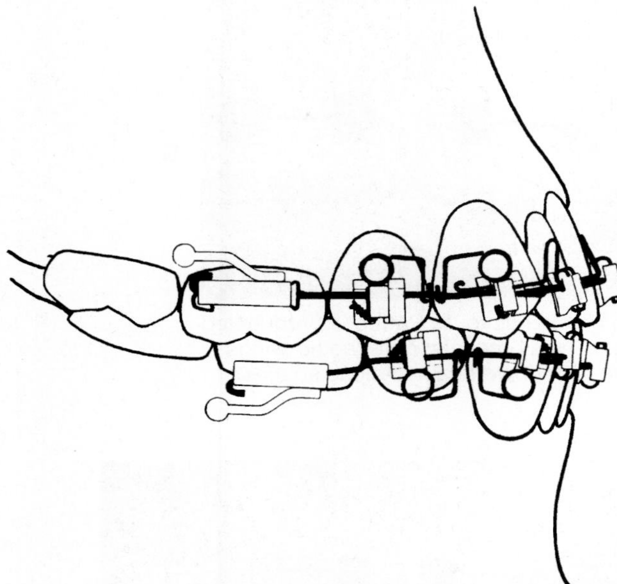

FIG 7-4 The Begg Appliance in Stage 3; this stage uses various springs. The uprighting springs as shown allow for correct tooth inclination. Note that these are inserted in the vertical slot of the bracket and the arch wire is inserted gingivally. (From Begg PR, Kesling PC: *Begg orthodontic theory and technique,* edition 2. Philadelphia: WB Saunders, 1971.)

9. How did the edgewise appliance evolve?

En masse movement of teeth, particularly in an anteroposterior direction, was extremely difficult with the ribbon arch appliance. Dr. Angle changed the bracket format; he placed the slot in the center of the bracket and fitted the bracket slot in a horizontal plane to the band rather than vertically. One could say that the vertical bracket now had its edge in a sidewise position; arch wire insertion accordingly was with the edge on its side, hence the very appropriate term *edgewise appliance.*[2]

10. What made the new edgewise bracket different from the original pin and tube vertical bracket?

The vertical bracket had two walls and a pin held the arch wire in place. The new edgewise bracket, 0.022 × 0.028 inch in dimension with the slot opening horizontally, consisted of a rectangular box with three walls within the bracket. The new design provided a more efficient mechanism with which to torque teeth.[2]

11. Who started the first pure edgewise specialty practice?

A student of Dr. Edward Angle, Dr. Charles H. Tweed, followed Dr. Angle's advice that one could only master the edgewise appliance if the practitioner limited the practice solely to the use of this appliance. Tweed, who received the first specialty certificate in Arizona, devoted 42 years to the advancement of the edgewise appliance. The Tweed philosophy has undergone contemporary changes and is still taught at the Tweed Foundation for Orthodontic Research in Tucson, Arizona, where it has developed the reputation as one of the finest basic edgewise courses.[2]

12. How is the arch wire in the edgewise appliance held in place?

Various methods are used, ranging from the original brass wire ligature to delicate stainless steel wire ligatures; however, elastic o-rings are more often used today (Fig. 7-6, *A* and *B*).

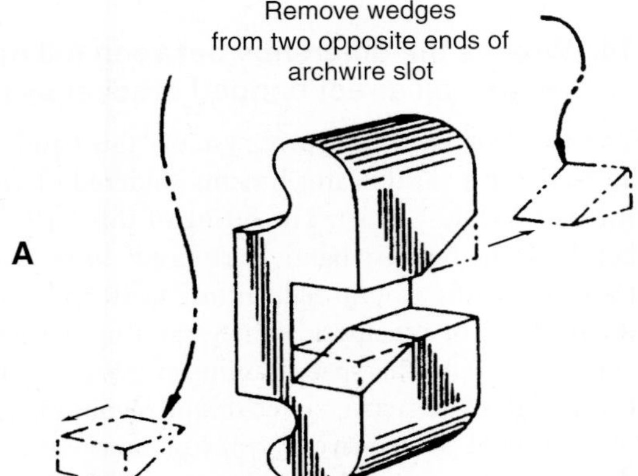

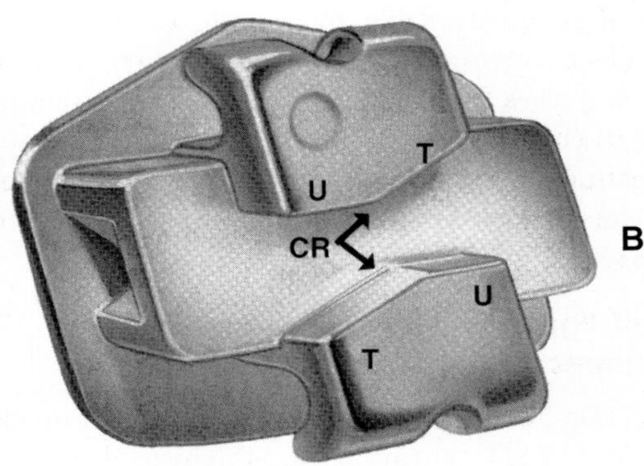

FIG 7-5 A, Removal of diagonally opposed corners of a conventional edgewise bracket arch wire slot to create the basic Tip-Edge bracket. **B,** The addition of a horizontal tunnel intersects the vertical slot, therefore the bracket profile remains low. The tipping surfaces *(T)* limit the degree of initial crown tipping, and the uprighting surfaces *(U)* control final tip and torque angles for a specific tooth. The central ridges *(CR)* provide vertical control during the noted tooth movements. (Reprinted from Kesling PC: Tip-Edge Plus Guide, edition 6. La Porte, IN: TP Orthodontics, Inc., 2006. With permission from Dr. Peter C. Kesling.)

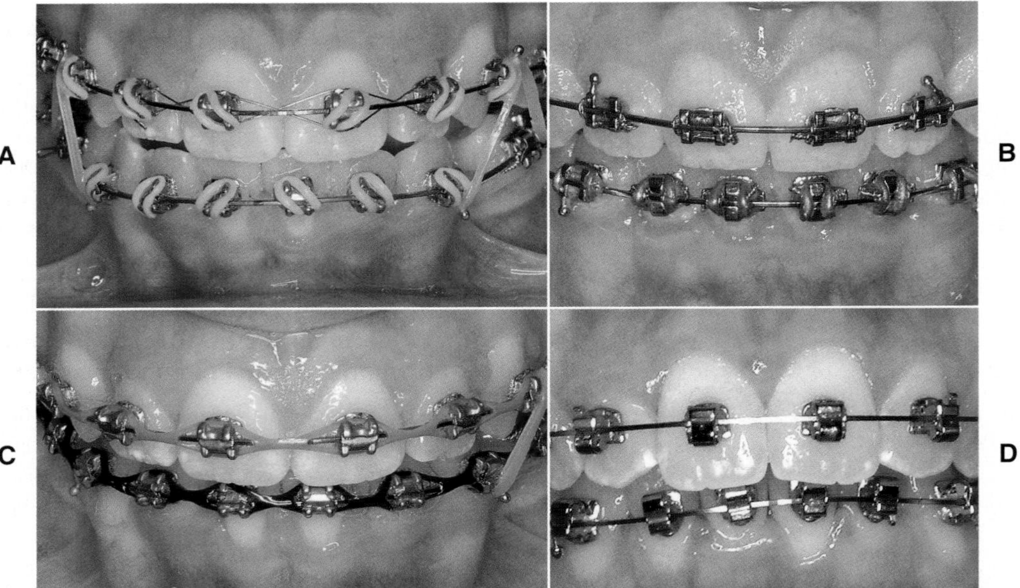

FIG 7-6 Various means of securing arch wires into bracket slots. **A,** Pattern as requested by a patient. **B,** Stainless steel ligatures on Siamese or Twin brackets; note the tie-wings used as retention for the ligatures. **C,** Halloween time with powerchain to close spaces. **D,** Self-ligating bracket.

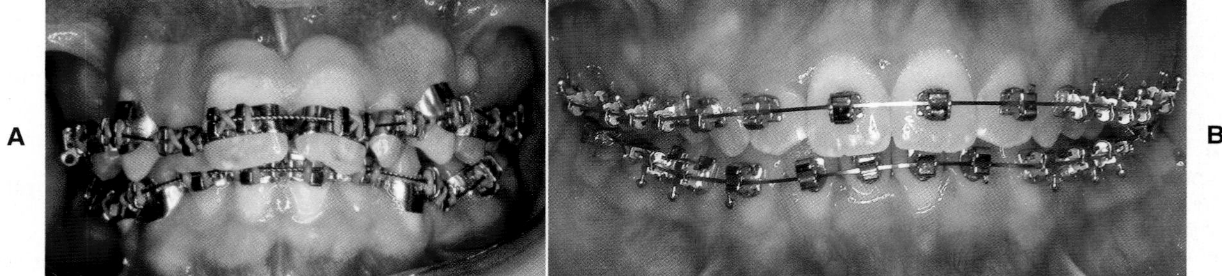

FIG 7-7 **A,** Full bands versus part B which shows direct bonding. **B,** SPEED™ bracket multi-piece construction.

The elastic o-rings are available in various colors, which orthodontic patients often request to provide esthetic themes such as orange and black for Halloween (Fig. 7-6, *C*). A significant milestone in contemporary orthodontics is the development of self-ligating brackets (Fig. 7-6, *D*), which incorporates a spring or gate mechanism as an integral part of the bracket to secure the arch wire in place.[2,3]

13. Do all self-ligating brackets function in the same manner during active treatment?

No. Larger twin (Damon[c]; In-Ovation,[b] and Time[a]) and smaller single brackets (SPEED[d]) are available. Moreover, active clip (SPEED[d] and In-Ovation[b]) and passive clip (Damon[c]) mechanisms exist.[3,4]

[a]American Orthodontics, Sheboygan, Wisconsin; [b]GAC International, Bohemia, New York; [c]Ormco Corporation, Glendora, California; [d]SPEED™ Systems, Strite Industries Ltd, Ontario, Canada

14. What is the difference between full banded versus full direct bonded bracket systems?

The banded fixed appliance systems use bands cemented to all teeth with various attachments soldered or laser welded to the bands (Fig. 7-7, *A*). The fitting of this type of appliance is cumbersome because band space needs to be created in order to fit the bands around tight fitting teeth and even more so in the presence of a malocclusion. Separating elastics, ligatures, or clips are used for this space-gaining exercise. In contrast, the introduction of the acid etch technique revolutionized orthodontic treatment as numerous types of brackets were developed that could be attached directly to enamel by composite/resin or resin-reinforced glass-ionomer cements (Fig. 7-7, *B*). Direct bonded appliances are the choice of the majority of clinicians today as they fulfill all the basic requirements of fixed appliance treatment; that is, an esthetic and stable attachment, which can be efficiently placed with no trauma to the tissues during functioning. Direct bonded attachments can be placed in lingual positions to fulfill the "invisible appliance" requirement or individual attachments on the lingual surfaces facilitate correction of crossbites.[4]

15. What is meant by the bracket prescription or preadjusted appliance?

Tooth movement normally occurs in three dimensions. The dimensions were originally incorporated in the edgewise mechanotherapy by specific adjustments to the arch wires, since the first generation of brackets was known as standard edgewise brackets with no prescription. The arch wire adjustments are called first-, second-, and third-order bends. First-order bends are the so-called in-out bends, which are represented by the distance of the bracket slot to the tooth surface and is a horizontal adjustment. This accommodates for the differences in the buccal tooth anatomy. Second-order bends refer to the vertical adjustments, up and down or tip bends, to provide correct axial inclination and tooth-root alignment in a mesiodistal dimension. The mesial to distal tip of the bracket slot in respect to the long axis of the tooth represents this adjustment of the bracket prescription. Third-order or torque adjustments refer to the bucco-palatal or bucco-lingual position of the roots in respect to the crowns of the teeth. All three orders are built into the bracket by the manufacturer and thus represent the prescription of contemporary brackets and in turn meet the requirements of the straight-wire or preadjusted appliance.[2]

16. How does tooth movement occur with fixed appliances?

Tooth movement occurs when a force is applied to the tooth through the bracket, usually an elastic band, coil spring, or specific types of loops or bends in the arch wire. This initiates the resorption of bone on the pressure side and deposition of bone on the tension side of the tooth: the biologic process of tooth movement. A moment is created as a result of the distance of the force application to the center of resistance of the tooth. The center of resistance coincides with the centroid of the root, which in a single-rooted tooth is the geometric center of the root between the apex and alveolar crest. Depending on the significance of the moment, the tooth will translate, tip, or rotate. The latter movements are obviously influenced by the contact of the arch wire and the bracket; thus, a full-thickness arch wire will allow a different type of movement when compared with a thinner dimension and likely more flexible arch wire. In most instances several stages of tooth movement occur with fixed appliances. Examples of these stages include the initial level and alignment stage using smaller size wires, which could be a flexible nitinol or supercable of 0.016-inch size for a 0.018 × 0.25–inch bracket slot. The wire rigidity and size dimension increase as treatment progresses, and this allows dental arch form control.[2,4]

17. How is a direct bonded bracket constructed?

Construction of brackets is a complex process, which is executed with infinite precision. Brackets are designed for each tooth individually because 3D prescriptions differ for the different teeth. Moreover, bracket base designs have to include adaptation for

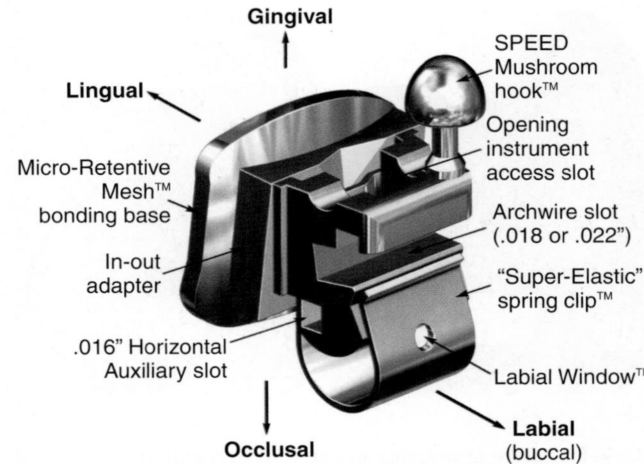

FIG 7-8 The different parts of a modern fixed appliance bracket are seen on the SPEED™ bracket multi-piece construction. (Reproduced by permission of Strite Industries Ltd, Cambridge, Ontario, Canada.)

the various anatomical configurations of the tooth surfaces. The SPEED[d] bracket is an example of a modern bracket constructed through a complex process; however, it is simple to use (Fig. 7-8). Self-ligation is a popular choice today and the SPEED[d] bracket will be described to show the various components of a contemporary self-ligating direct bonded bracket.[3]

18. What are the components of a direct bonded bracket?

The bracket can be a one- or multi-piece bracket. A one-piece bracket is rigid and manufactured usually by injection molding. A multi-piece bracket is usually milled from metal pieces and welded together to form the bracket. Irrespective of construction, there is normally a bracket base, stem with bracket slot, tie-wings to retain the ligatures or o-rings as it secures the arch wire into the slot, and some form of hook used for intramaxillary or intermaxillary attachment of elastics or coils. The very popular self-ligating or self-locked brackets also include a passive or active clip to secure the arch wire.[2-4]

19. What is a self-ligating bracket?

A self-ligating bracket is defined as "a bracket, which utilizes a permanently installed, moveable component to entrap the arch wire." Self-ligating brackets may be classified into two categories: passive and active.[3]

20. What is an active self-ligating bracket?

Active brackets use a flexible component to entrap the arch wire (Fig. 7-9). The active component or flexible clip constrains the arch wire in the arch wire slot and has the ability to store and release energy through elastic deflection. A continuous light force is imparted on the tooth and its supporting structures, resulting in precise and controlled movement. The skilled clinician will choose the appropriate bracket-arch wire combination to allow low or friction-free movement when sliding of the teeth on the arch wire is required but use the

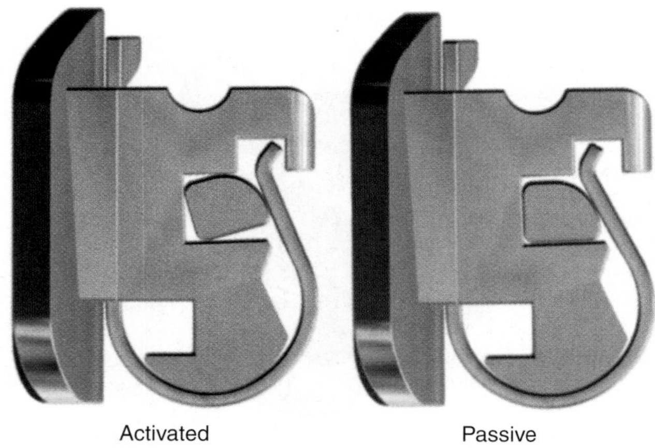

FIG 7-9 Active springclip forces wire into slot. (Reproduced by permission of Strite Industries Ltd, Cambridge, Ontario, Canada.)

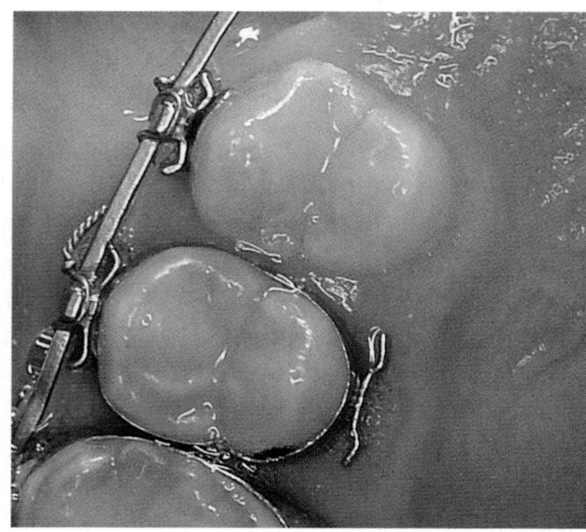

FIG 7-10 The bracket body has wings on each side that rotate teeth when activated. Note the contrast between the band versus the direct bonded bracket and the steel versus the elastic o-ring to secure the wire in position. The steel ligature is often used to enhance the force of activation.

friction provided by the clip pressing on the arch wire when rotational correction is required or when a larger dimension wire is used for 3D control. An example of an active bracket is the SPEED[d] self-ligating bracket, which provides this precise control when required.[3]

21. What is a spring-wing bracket?

A single bracket provides a larger inter bracket distance between teeth and theoretically allows a lighter force to act on the teeth compared with a similar dimension wire in a twin or Siamese bracket. The latter is wider and thus closer together when placed on the teeth. However, rotations are believed to be more difficult to correct with a small and narrow single bracket, hence the additions of rotation arms or wings (Fig. 7-10). These were traditionally named the Steiner wings, Lang antirotation arms, or Lewis spring wings. These wings or arms can be adjusted depending on the rotation and direction of correction required.[2]

22. What is inter-bracket width?

Inter-bracket width refers to the distance between contact points of brackets, also referred to as the distance of arch wire between two neighboring teeth. Siamese or twin brackets generally have less inter-bracket space or width compared with single brackets (see Figures 7-6, *B* and *D*). A small inter-bracket width limits the size of stainless steel wire that will be able to fit in the bracket slots of adjacent teeth. The sooner the clinician is able to engage a full-thickness stainless steel arch wire in the bracket slot, the sooner 3D control of tooth position is initiated. Not all treatment objectives require this procedure; however, if this is part of the treatment plan, then single brackets with larger inter-bracket width obviously have advantages. Clinicians have added multiple loops into arch wires in the past to accommodate more length of wire between brackets in an effort to increase the flexibility of the steel wires. Newer flexible arch wires developed from space-age materials such as nitinol and titanium plus the addition of heat sensitive or heat-activated characteristics have, in the majority of instances, overcome this limitation. Thus, instead of multiple loops between teeth, a straight arch wire is the order of the day. Moreover, all popular contemporary brackets have become smaller; thus inter-bracket width has increased, but single brackets still have the advantage in this area.[2,4]

23. What is a single-, double-, or triple-tube bracket?

These terms most frequently apply to the attachments for the first molar teeth. Depending on the type of mechanotherapy, a clinician may use only one arch wire per treatment stage and thus require only a single slot or tube. Sometimes an auxiliary appliance is used in addition to the base arch wire. Such auxiliaries could be a lip bumper often used in the mandibular arch, utility arch used in both arches (introduced as part of the Bioprogressive system in the late 1970's), and headgears (Fig. 7-11, *A*). If an arch wire and one such auxiliary are used, a double tube is required on the molar bracket and similarly a triple tube where a headgear, base arch wire, and a utility arch are used. Brackets such as the SPEED[d] self-ligating bracket have an auxiliary slot incorporated into the bracket stem and accept an additional wire of up to 0.016 × 0.016 inch dimension to assist with tooth movement where needed (Fig. 7-11, *B*). The latter function is especially effective where a malpositioned tooth is aligned after a full-thickness base arch wire is already in place. An example of the latter is when an impacted tooth, such as a surgically exposed maxillary canine, is brought into an already aligned and stabilized dental arch.[3,4]

24. What is the mechanism to secure a direct bonded appliance to tooth enamel?

The advent of acid etching revolutionized orthodontic fixed appliance therapy. The enamel surface is usually prepared by etching the surface with 37% phosphoric acid for 15 to 30 seconds, then rinsed with water, dried, and sealed with a lightly filled resin. The bracket is then secured or bonded to this prepared surface by

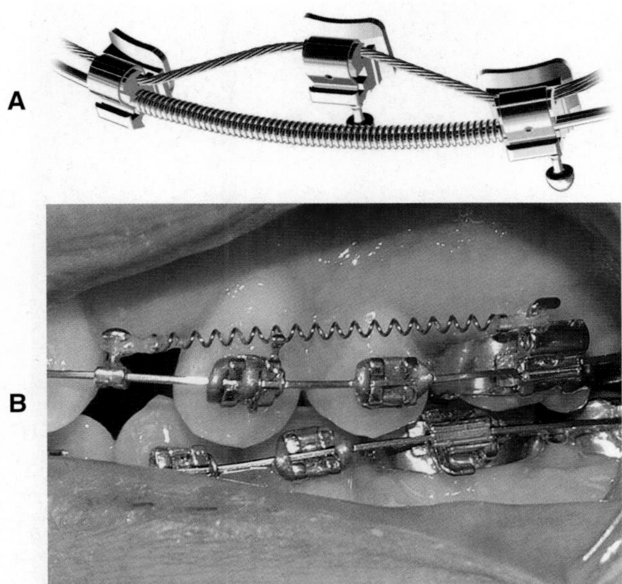

FIG 7-11 **A,** Flexible wire in auxiliary slot while remainder of arch is kept stable with a rigid base arch wire. **B,** Maxillary molar band illustrating a double tube: one for auxiliary such as headgear application and one for arch wire. Mandibular molar illustrates a single tube accommodating only the arch wire. Note the additional hooks on the brackets that are used for retraction coils or elastic traction. (**A,** Reproduced by permission of Strite Industries Ltd, Cambridge, Ontario, Canada.)

a filled or hybrid composite resin adhesive. The latter is available in an auto-polymerizing or self-cured adhesive, which is often referred to as chemical cure; however, light-polymerized adhesives are the most popular composite adhesives. Curing in contemporary clinical practice is accomplished by light-curing using a halogen, argon laser, plasma arc, or light-emitting diode light source. This process of fitting attachments to the enamel has many variants, including using other concentrations of acid, other types of acid, indirect bonding versus direct bonding, moisture-insensitive primers, self-etching primers, acid-resin combinations that are mixed and applied in a single process, and various types of cements that could be resin, glass-ionomer, or a combination resin-reinforced glass ionmer. The bonding process evolved and brackets can be bonded successfully to amalgam, gold, acrylic, or porcelain restorations, provided the surfaces are correctly prepared. Moreover, manufacturers have included another variable in this process: various bonding bases exist (Fig. 7-12). The latter varies from a conventional mesh base (different gauge mesh [e.g., 60-gauge SPEED[d], 80-gauge American master series, 150-gauge SuperMesh SE GAC]) to an integral cast base with undercuts (American Time self-ligating bracket). The metal surfaces can also be sandblasted or micro-etched by the manufacturers, which increases the surface area of the base to enhance bond strength.[3,4,7]

25. What are tie-wings?

Tie-wings are extensions of the conventional bracket (see Figures 7-6, *A-C* and 7-9, *A*). They are used for their undercuts to secure elastic or stainless steel ligatures, which in turn hold the arch wires in place. In addition, tie-wings can be used to secure wire hooks such as Kobayashi tie hooks for elastic traction (Fig. 7-13), if this is required and the bracket design did not provide for this utility.[2-4]

26. What does the bracket slot dimension indicate?

The two most often used dimensions are the 0.018 × 0.025–inch and the 0.022 × 0.028–inch brackets. The main difference is that that the 0.022 slots can accommodate a larger selection of arch wire sizes. No evidence exists to prove that one system is superior to the other; American Board of Orthodontics quality results have been obtained with both. The selection of either is a matter of preference of the clinician. The first number indicates the width of the bracket slot occlusogingivally, and the second number indicates the depth of the slot. Full-thickness arch wires for these two systems are normally 0.017 × 0.025–inch and the 0.021 × 0.028–inch respectively; thus, a rectangular wire of this nature will fill the bracket slot in all dimensions.[2-4]

27. Friction between bracket and arch wire plays an important role during orthodontic tooth movement. How is this factor minimized?

Studies have shown that two absolutely smooth surfaces of similar metals brought into contact and slid over each other can initiate a process called *cold welding,* which literally means that the metals are "fused" together. This obviously increases friction and slows the movement. This also happens between arch wires and bracket slots. Ceramic bracket surfaces have also traditionally provided increased friction values—hence the incorporation of metal slot inserts to decrease sliding friction. It is thus imperative to select appropriate combinations of arch wires and bracket slot dimensions when teeth have to move or slide along an arch wire or when only root or crown movement is required, such as in torquing or third-order movements. When sliding is required, such as during the distal movement of a canine into a space, minimal friction is required. The movement should be accomplished by the use of a smaller diameter wire, which does not bind in the bracket slot. Stainless steel and elastic ligatures increase friction when used to secure arch wires into bracket slots; in addition, the friction is increased when any minor bend in the arch wire comes in contact with the ligature. Self-ligating brackets have basically eliminated this limitation. Most self-ligating brackets are passive (e.g., Damon appliance); there is no action on the wire except when there is wire bracket contact. The active self-ligation brackets have active clip mechanisms to secure the arch wires into the bracket slots. The SPEED[d] bracket clip is unique in that it prevents active contact until full-thickness arch wires are used; this characteristic thus provides low friction during sliding and initial alignment when low friction is required, but it increases the friction when full-dimension arch wires are used for 3D control and when friction free sliding is not a factor.[3,8,9]

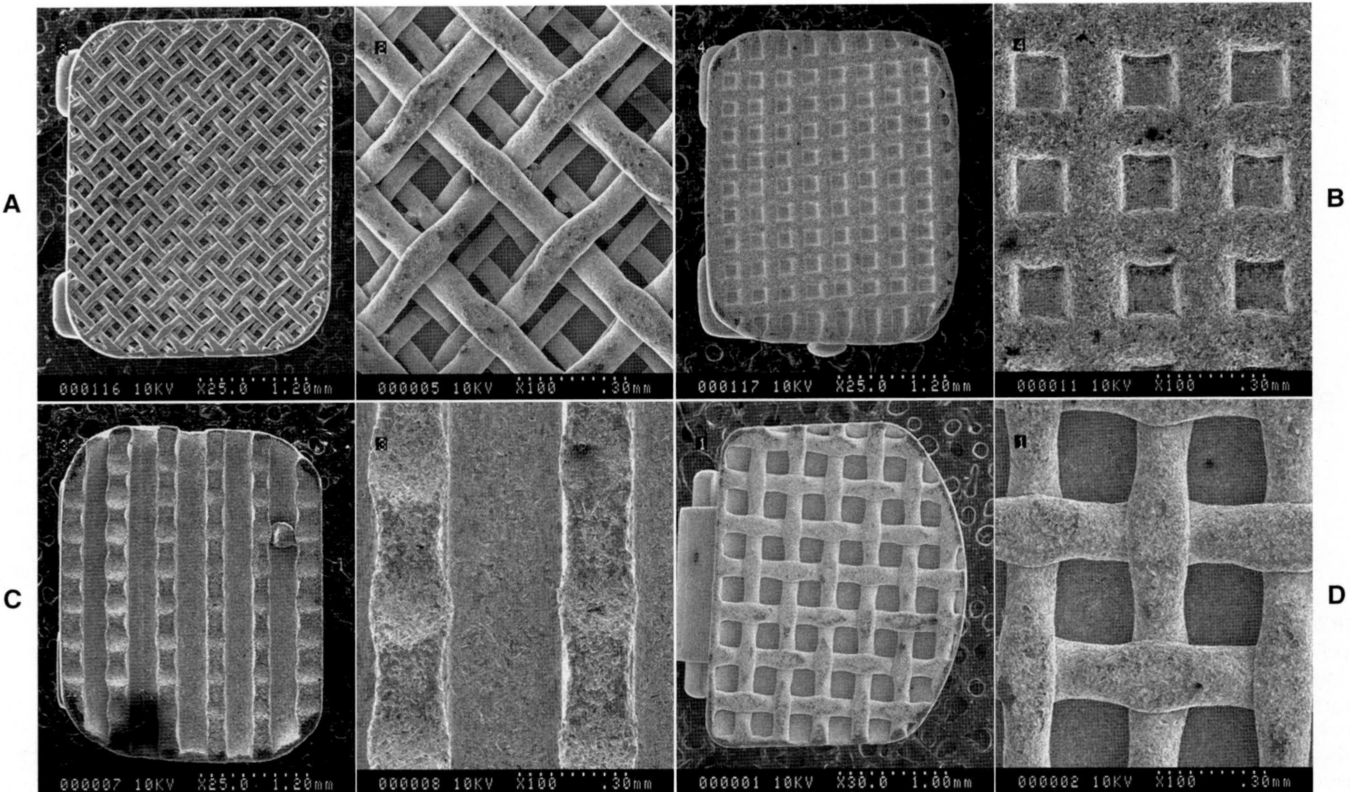

FIG 7-12 SEM images of different bracket base designs. **A,** A 150-gauge SuperMesh. **B** and **C,** Integral cast showing two patterns. **D,** A 60 gauge.

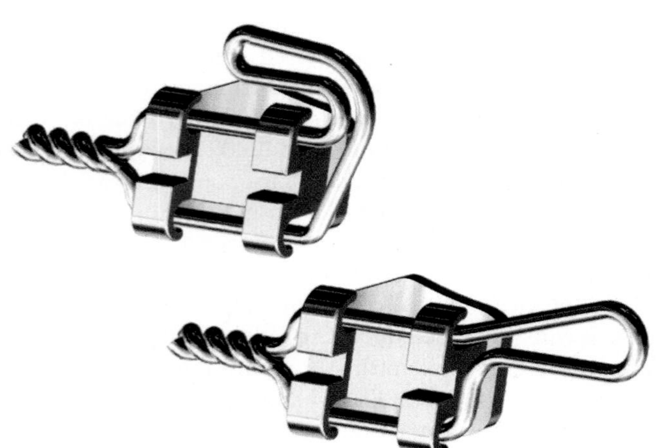

FIG 7-13 Kobayashi tie hooks often used with the conventional edgewise twin bracket. Note that the wire hook can be adjusted to accommodate various directions of elastic traction. (Reproduced by permission of Strite Industries Ltd, Cambridge, Ontario, Canada.)

28. Is a friction-free appliance ideal?

Friction free is only an advantage when the arch wire has to slide. This is most often required during the initial alignment of teeth and when spaces are closed or opened. On the contrary, when corrective movements such as treatment of rotations, movement of severely displaced teeth in only one direction, when teeth are used as anchors, or when torquing movements of teeth are required, then friction is necessary to accomplish the correction. Friction is thus an important factor in attaining successful tooth movements and requires intelligent decision-making.[4,8]

29. How is a bracket constructed?

The two major processes are milling and injection molding. Milling indicates that the bracket is milled out of a piece of metal, sometimes in more than one piece, and then followed by welding together all the pieces to form the bracket for bonding to enamel or welding to a band. Injection molding is a process in which a mold of the bracket is prepared and then filled by a process in which a liquefied metal is poured or injected into the mold; the liquid cools and sets into the bracket form, which is removed and further prepared as a unit for bonding. Brackets are manufactured in stainless steel, titanium, nickel-free alloys, gold plated steel, ceramic, and reinforced polycarbonate materials.[2-4]

30. What is a convertible tube?

In order to provide a tube at the end of the arch wire, mostly for ease of wire insertion, a tube is used for the last tooth in the arch, usually the second molar. However, treatment is often initiated prior to the full eruption of the second molar, and the first molar is then used as the end tooth. A tube is fitted that has a removable plate welded over the slot to provide a slot for ease of placement of the arch wire as noted. Therefore, when the second molar is provided with an attachment, the first molar tube can be converted into a bracket by removing the plate, hence called a *convertible tube/bracket*.[4] The SPEED[d] appliance in contrast uses a bracket on the mesio-buccal cusp of the maxillary molars, and the active clip can be opened to insert the arch wire (see Fig. 7-11, *A*; note that the plate is in place, securing the arch wire in the slot).

31. What is an initial arch wire?

The initial arch wire is usually the first arch wire in a sequence of increasing size and wire stiffness, normally a very flexible wire that exerts a low force to the teeth and that is of a small diameter (Fig. 7-14). It is also required to have super elasticity and shape memory, meaning that lots of flexibility is available to allow the wire to engage all the irregularly positioned teeth without a high force caused by the deflection of the wire. Examples of such wires are 0.012-inch stainless steel, 0.014-inch nitinol, or 0.016-inch Supercable arch wires. Rectangular arch wires of similar characteristics have been introduced recently, and this would be the choice as a starting wire when possible to initiate 3D control from the beginning. The initial arch wire first focuses on tooth rotations and alignment of the marginal ridges, which is followed by vertical and then anteroposterior correction of the malocclusion using more rigid arch wires, sometimes with intermaxillary mechanotherapy added as needed.[2-4]

32. What is sliding mechanics?

Sliding mechanics literally means that the teeth are sliding on the arch wire. A single tooth or en masse movement can be provided. Usually a stainless-steel wire of smaller dimension than the bracket slot is used for this movement in order to prevent friction that will slow movement. There are various ways to activate this movement, including powerchain, conventional rubber/elastic bands, or coil springs such as the Pletcher coil spring, present day nitinol, and titanium closing coils (Fig. 7-15). This type of movement is in contrast to the traditional closing loop arch wire in which the activation of the closing loop allows for the teeth to move and spaces to close where indicated.[2-4]

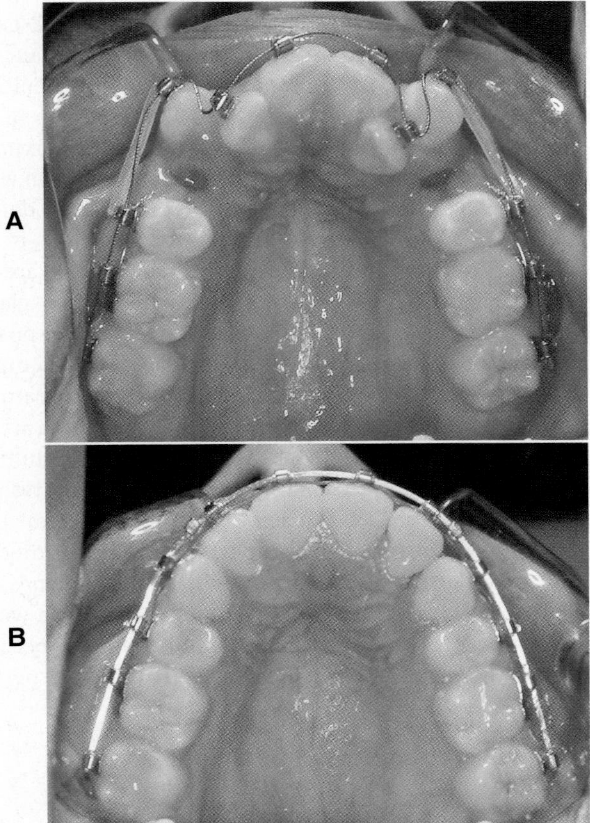

FIG 7-14 Note the flexible initial wire (0.016 supercable) in the crowded dentition **(A)** versus the rigid rectangular stainless steel wire (0.017 × 0.025 SS) in the aligned dentition **(B)** where 3D control is important, such as arch form and crown-root alignment.

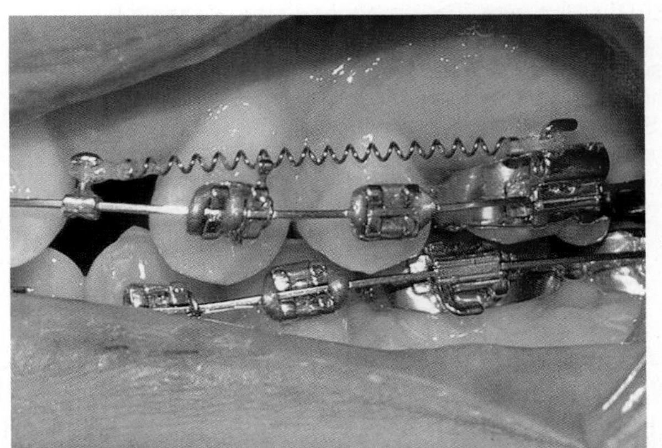

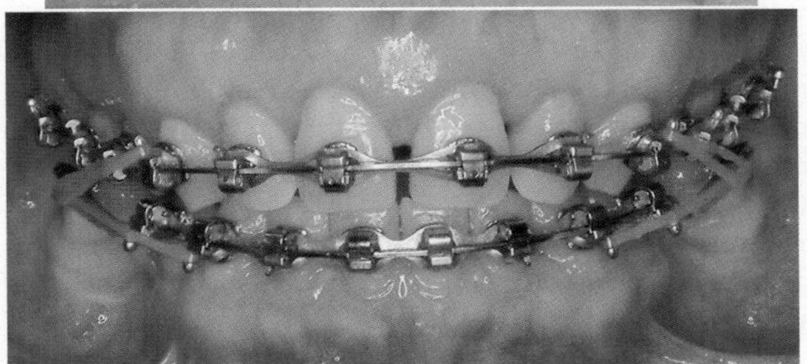

FIG 7-15 **A,** Conventional Edgewise appliance illustrating o-ring ties to secure arch wire in place as well as a nitinol coil spring to retract the anterior teeth into the space. **B,** Powerchain positioned under the arch wire in a self-ligating SPEED™ appliance to enhance space closure in a sliding format. Note also the intramaxillary and intermaxillary elastic traction to facilitate correction of the malocclusion.

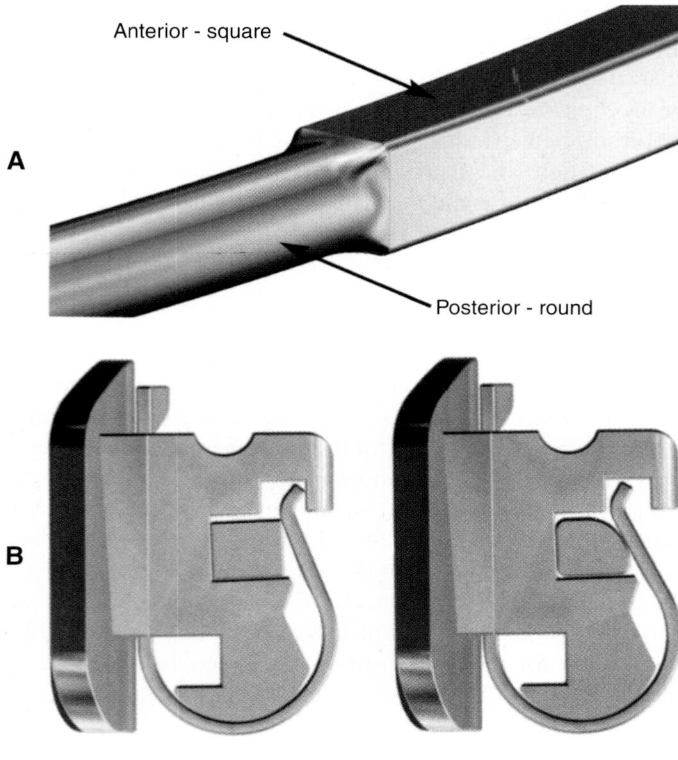

FIG 7-16 **A,** The dual-dimension wire as shown is the SPEED™ Hills wire. The anterior section of the arch wire is square for torque control, and the posterior section is round to facilitate sliding of the wire. **B,** The C-wire is shown in comparison to a rectangular wire in the cross-section of the SPEED™ self-ligating bracket. Note that the C-shape rounding of the edge of the rectangular wire facilitates the active clip to close securely in position. (Reproduced by permission of Strite Industries Ltd, Cambridge, Ontario, Canada.)

33. What is a D-shaped, C-shaped, or dual-dimension arch wire?

These wires are important when self-ligation appliances are used, in particular the SPEED[d] appliance with its active clip mechanism (Fig. 7-16). For effective use of the energy exerted by the active spring on arch wires, it is important that the spring be locked in a secure position. The use of full-thickness arch wires facilitates 3D control; thus, when D- or C-shaped arch wires are used for this purpose, the D or C side of the arch wires allows easy closure of the active clip. The edge of a rectangular or square wire of the same dimension causes difficulty in clip closure; moreover, forceful closure of the clip can damage the clip and negate the energy release for accurate tooth movement.[3]

34. What are the properties of an ideal orthodontic arch wire?

The ideal orthodontic arch wire is one that has a high elastic limit but is not too brittle to break under loading and exhibits a low load-deflection rate. The latter function is determined by the modulus of elasticity (or in simple terms, the rigidity of the wire). Stainless steel, for example, has a modulus of elasticity 1.8 times greater than that of gold. If this example is used for the reactive part of an appliance, which is the part that provides the anchorage against movement, then stainless steel will be 1.8 times more resistant to deflection compared with a reactive component made from gold wire. Moreover, activations made in a steel wire for tooth movement will produce a load-deflection rate almost twice that of a similar activation made in an identical dimension gold wire. In addition, the orthodontic alloy should also be resistant to corrosion when exposed to the oral environment, should not fracture to accidental loading in the mouth or during fabrication of an appliance, should be formed in a soft state and then be heat treated to hard temper, and lastly should allow easy soldering of attachments. Manufacturers provide cross-section stiffness (C_s) and material stiffness (M_s) numbers to wires to allow clinicians to compare arch wires with different dimensions and alloys with one another. Provided the alloy is the same, a 0.014-inch wire will have a significantly smaller C_s compared with a 0.018-inch wire; the first will be able to deflect more when exposed to a force if of the same design.[3,4]

35. What is the difference between nitinol, beta-titanium and stainless steel wires?

Nickel-titanium (nitinol) and beta-titanium (TMA) are shape memory alloys with low-force high-springback capabilities. Nitinol in particular has a tremendous resistance to permanent deformation. The modulus of elasticity of Nitinol is only 0.26 that of stainless steel; thus, a comparison of the M_s shows that a 0.018-inch nitinol wire has the approximate stiffness of a 0.013-inch stainless steel wire. Nitinol arch wires are thus particularly useful when low forces and large deflections are required in relatively straight wires, such as in the initial phases of orthodontic treatment when the teeth are too irregularly aligned to use stainless-steel wires. Super-elastic nitinol wires are also available that are activated by exposure to mouth temperature; they are very flexible at room temperature and become more rigid at higher mouth temperatures. This property allows the wire to be inserted when teeth are severely displaced (see Fig. 7-14). TMA wires have a modulus of elasticity that falls between that of steel and nitinol wires and can be deflected almost twice as much as steel without permanent deformation. Unlike nitinol, TMA can accommodate some adjustments, and auxiliaries such as finger springs can be welded to the wire. TMA can be used as an active working wire; however, it is often used as a finishing wire because small adjustments can be bent into the wire to secure perfect alignment of teeth.[3,4]

36. What is a straight wire appliance and who popularized the concept?

Dr. Larry F. Andrews published his classic article "The Keys of Normal Occlusion" in 1972. He used the six keys to ideal occlusion (Fig. 7-17) to develop and introduce the straight wire appliance to orthodontics, which is basically an appliance with built-in 3D prescription to represent ideal tooth positions.

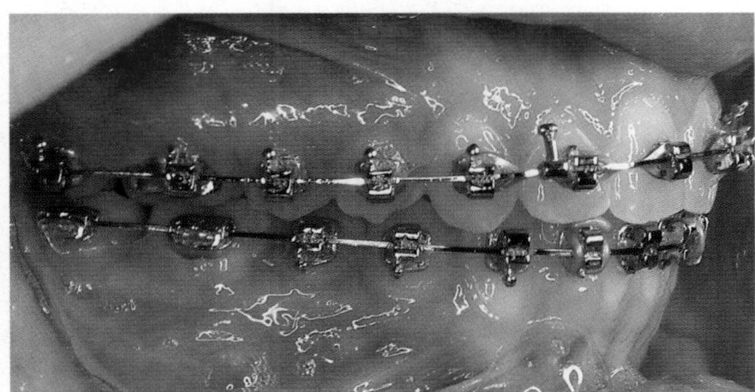

FIG 7-17 The keys to a Class I occlusion in the making. Note that the mesiobuccal cusp of the maxillary first molar is occluding in the buccal groove of the mandibular first molar. This allows all the posterior teeth as shown to occlude in correct Class I relationships.

The slots are all aligned parallel to the occlusal plane when the teeth are in ideal occlusion, provided the brackets are correctly placed on the tooth surface. Andrew's bracket had a base contoured occlusogingivally and mesiodistally; when fitted correctly, it would avoid any arch wire adjustments as reflected in the original no-prescription appliances with the three orders bent into the arch wires; hence, the straight wire appliance.[2,10]

37. Does bracket position on the tooth influence treatment?

With the advent of preadjusted, straight wire or fully programmed appliances, as the plethora of new developments in bracket systems were called, bracket position became very important both occlusogingivally and mesiodistally. The specific heights can be measured using such instruments as an Andersen gauge or Boone gauge. The skilled clinician can position most of the brackets correctively most of time; however, with efficiency and chair time in the modern orthodontic office at a premium, another technique of bracket placement surfaced. This indirect bonding technique differs from the direct placement in the mouth; a preliminary impression is provided and the brackets accurately positioned in the laboratory whereupon a transfer tray allows the brackets to be bonded to the enamel in the conventional manner through acid-etching and resin cements.[3,4]

38. Why is a power arm attached to a bracket?

In order to provide planned tooth movement (i.e., translation versus tipping), the clinician must plan the point of force application on the tooth and the direction of the force in respect to the center of resistance of the tooth (Fig. 7-18). The center of resistance is mostly situated between the root apex and alveolar bone crest. This makes it impossible to apply force to a bracket unless a power arm is attached to the bracket, which allows for the applied force to be closer to the center of resistance. If a force is applied in this way, the clinician has the ability to control the translation or rotation/tipping of a tooth or group of teeth.[2-4,11]

39. What is a ceramic bracket?

Orthodontic materials have developed significantly over the last 20 years, resulting in an increasing number of adult patients seeking orthodontic treatment. These patients requested the use of more esthetic appliances. Direct bonded brackets replaced bands, brackets became smaller, and lingual appliances became popular and ceramic (clear or tooth-colored) brackets were introduced (Fig. 7-19). Ceramic brackets were initially very fragile, but the bonding to the enamel occurred initially through a Silane layer resulting in a chemical bond of very high bond strength. Not only did the brackets fracture during treatment, but more important, enamel fracture occurred during bracket removal. The ceramic was also more resistant to wear compared with enamel, which resulted in enamel wear if an opposing tooth touched the bracket. A new generation of ceramic bracket was introduced with a lower profile and a mechanical retentive bonding base without these flaws. It is recommended to avoid contact of an opposing tooth to a ceramic bracket. High friction between arch wire and the ceramic bracket slot was also evaluated, resulting in ceramic brackets with smoother surfaces as well as stainless steel inserts into the slots reducing friction for sliding and thus aiding tooth movement.[2-4]

40. What is a lingual appliance?

Esthetic requirements differ from person to person. Mostly, it is a decision of obtrusiveness. Clear or ceramic appliances may satisfy some, others prefer a small stainless-steel self-ligating bracket, others prefer the conventional bracket with various colored o-rings to secure wires, and then there is an option of lingual braces. Lingual braces are secured to the lingual surfaces of the teeth (Fig. 7-20). Surprisingly, the problem with lingual braces is not the retention of the attachments on the enamel surfaces, but rather that some pronunciation difficulties occur after insertion. Furthermore, the technique is difficult and time consuming, and the working position is awkward. The interbracket distance is also reduced on the lingual surfaces, which limits adjustments. To facilitate treatment, customized brackets are presently produced with accompanying custom arch wires using scanning and computerized robotics.[3]

41. What does Hooke's Law define in respect to orthodontic arch wires?

Hooke's law refers to load and deflection of wires (Fig. 7-21). If a linear relationship exists between loading and deflection, when the force exerted on the wire increases, the deflection will increase. This proportionality is referred to as Hooke's law. Load-deflection diagrams differ for different wires. Activation and deactivation curves also provide relevant information as to the load and deflection properties of wires.[3]

42. How does contamination of the bracket base affect the bonding to enamel?

Contamination of the bracket base with substances such as talc powder, skin oil, laboratory wax, and others significantly reduces the bond strength of the bracket to the enamel surface

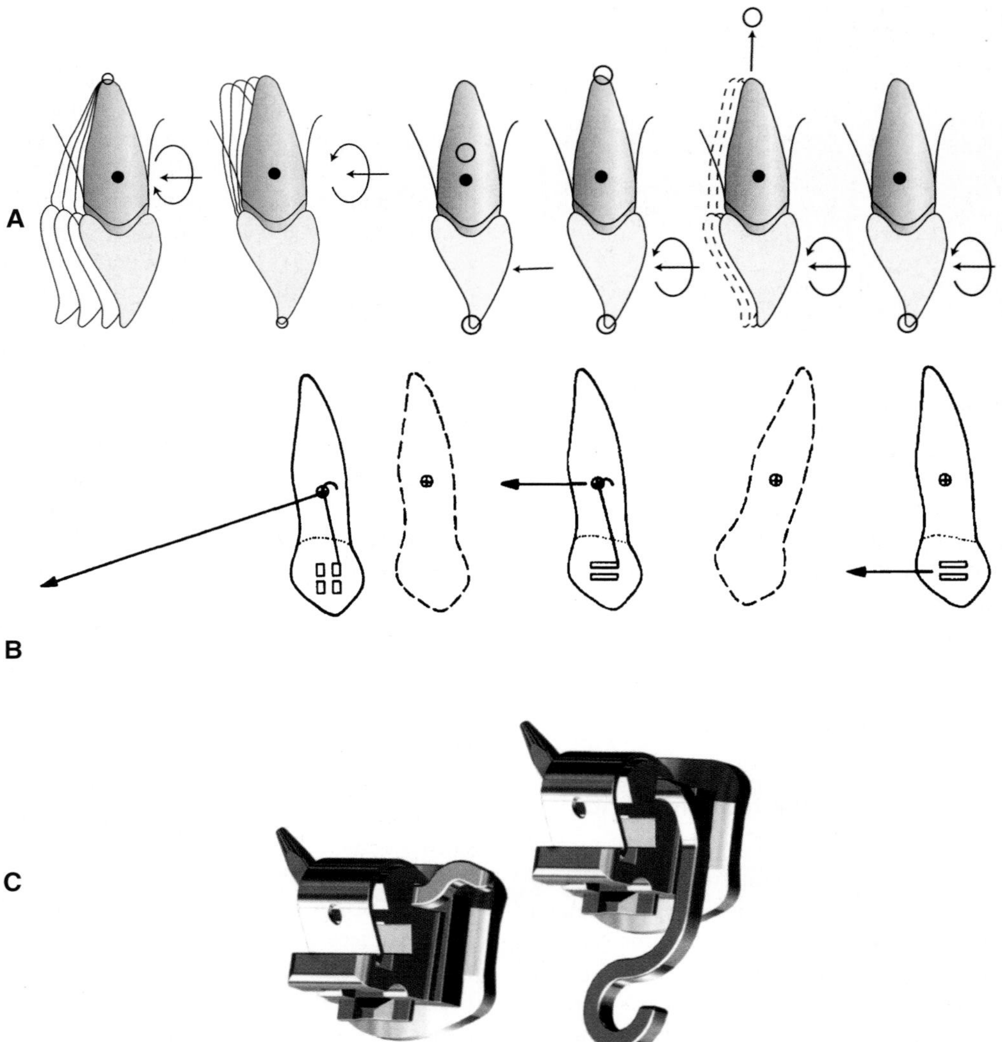

Performed SPEED hooks installed in SPEED brackets

FIG 7-18 A, The center of resistance (black dot in middle of root) and the center of rotation (circle root apex and crown tip) are illustrated. The horizontal arrow indicates the force vector; two moments are shown: (1) the moment where the center of rotation is at the root apex and the resultant movement is tipping of the crown; the force application is at the bracket on the crown and the arch wire could be a round wire, and (2) the moment where root torque is accomplished with the center of rotation at the crown tip; a rectangular wire could be inserted and the torque prescription is causing the root tip. **B,** Power arms can be inserted as shown with the SPEED™ hooks. Bodily movement is encouraged with the power arm, allowing the force vector through the center of resistance. **C,** Power arms can be inserted into an auxiliary slot (0.016 × 0.016 inch) as shown with the SPEED™ hooks. (**A** from Graber TM, Vanarsdall RL Jr, Vig KWL: *Orthodontics: current principles and techniques,* edition 4. St Louis: Mosby, 2005. **B** from Smith RJ, Burstone CJ: *Am J Orthod* 1984;85[4]:294-307. **C** Reproduced by permission of Strite Industries Ltd, Cambridge, Ontario, Canada.)

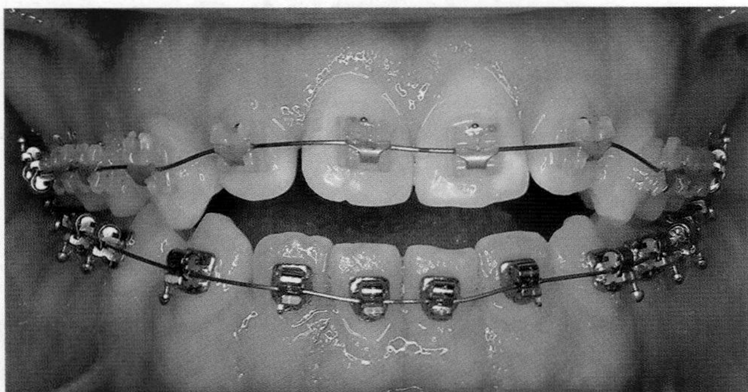

FIG 7-19 Two self-ligating brackets: ceramic In-Ovation in the maxillary arch and stainless steel SPEED™ in the mandibular arch being used to close an anterior open bite.

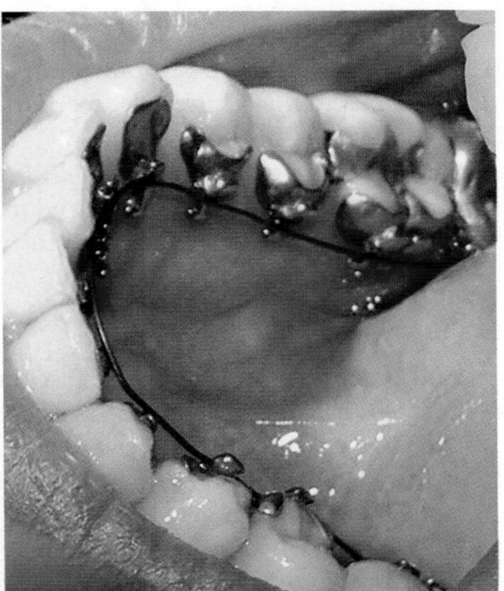

FIG 7-20 Lingual appliances fitted by indirect bonding actively aligning the lower teeth.

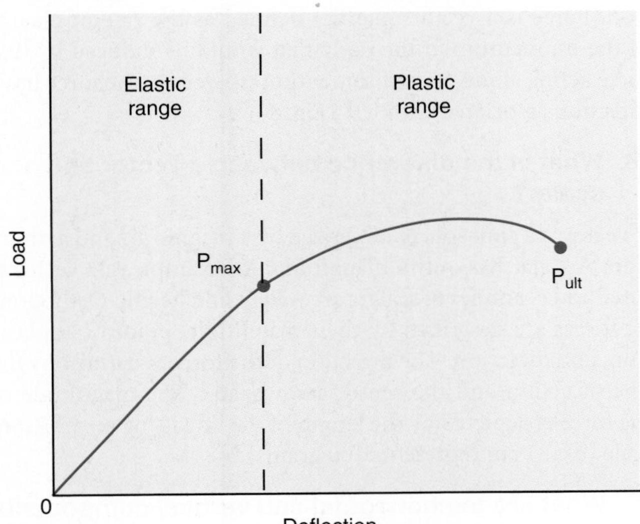

FIG 7-21 The linear display of the graph from 0 to P_{max} represents Hooke's law. (From Graber TM, Vanarsdall RL Jr, Vig KWL. *Orthodontics: current principles and techniques,* edition 4. St Louis: Mosby, 2005.)

and subsequently leads to premature bracket bond failure. It is imperative to follow a meticulous protocol for bonding fixed appliances to the teeth for successful orthodontic treatment.[12]

REFERENCES

1. Daskalogiannakis J: *Glossary of orthodontic terms*. Berlin: Quintessence Publishing, 2000.
2. Vaden JL, Dale JG, Klontz HA: The Tweed-Merrifield Edgewise appliance: philosophy, diagnosis, and treatment. In Graber TM, Vanarsdall RL, Vig WL: *Orthodontics: current principles and techniques*, edition 2. St Louis: Mosby, 2000, pp 627-684.
3. Woodside DG, Berger JL, Hanson GH: Self-ligation orthodontics with the speed appliance. In Graber TM, Vanarsdall RL, Vig WL: *Orthodontics: current principles and techniques*, edition 2. St Louis: Mosby, 2005, pp 717-752.
4. Proffit WR, Fields HW: *Contemporary orthodontics*, edition 2. St Louis: Mosby, 2000, pp 326-361, 385–416.
5. Begg PR, Kesling PC: *Begg orthodontic theory and technique*. edition 2. Philadelphia: WB Saunders, 1971.
6. Kesling PC: *Tip-Edge Plus Guide,* edition 6. La Porte, Ind: TP Orthodontics, 2006.
7. Sharma-Sayal, Rossouw PE, Kulkarni GV, Titley KC: The influence of orthodontic bracket base design on shear bond strength. *Am J Orthod Dentofac Orthop* 2003;124(1):74-82.
8. Rossouw PE: Friction—an overview. *Semin Orthod* 2003; 9(4):218-222.
9. Rossouw PE, Kamelchuk LS, Kusy RP: A fundamental review of variables associated with low velocity frictional dynamics. *Semin Orthod* 2003;9(4):223-235.
10. Andrews LF: The keys of normal occlusion. *Am J Orthod* 1972;63:296.
11. Smith RJ, Burstone CJ: Mechanics of tooth movement. *Am J Orthod* 1985;85(4):294-307.
12. Rossouw PE, Penuvchev AV, Kulkarni K: The influence of various contaminants on the bonding of orthodontic attachments. *Ont Dentist* 1996;sept:15-22.

CHAPTER 8

Biomechanics in Orthodontics

André Haerian • Sunil Kapila

In general terms, mechanical principles that govern the behavior of devices that interface with biological tissues are collectively termed *biomechanics*. At the core of all orthodontic treatment are the devices or appliances that deliver controlled forces to the teeth and jaws. Therefore, the mechanics of force delivery is an integral part of orthodontics. The principles of biomechanics therefore are a common thread in all orthodontic curricula.[1] This chapter addresses some of the basic biomechanical principles that are critical in clinical orthodontics. An understanding of these principles and their appropriate application provides the clinician the ability to achieve consistent and controlled tooth movement.[1]

Orthodontic appliances—simple or complicated, fixed or removable—are all subject to laws of physics.[1] Therefore, the discussion in biomechanics often begins with an introduction to Newtonian mechanics.

1. What is biomechanics?

Biomechanics is the research and analysis of the mechanical properties of living tissues and non-living objects that affect those living tissues. In orthodontics, this analysis of biomechanical properties is used to determine the effect of orthodontic appliances on oral tissues, particularly teeth and bone. The analysis of the non-living component simply follows Newtonian mechanical principles. In contrast, the biomechanical properties of living tissue are more complicated and often not thoroughly understood.[2,3]

2. What is Newtonian mechanics?

Newton's three Laws of Motion describe the relationship between the external forces acting on an object and the motion of that object, which form the basis for classical mechanics. Mechanics is the branch of physics concerned with the behavior of objects when subjected to forces or displacements. These laws were first formulated by Sir Isaac Newton and published in his work *Philosophiae Naturalis Principia Mathematica* (1687).[4,5]

3. What are Newton's three laws of motion?

- **First Law:** A body at rest remains at rest, and a body in motion continues to move in a straight line with a constant speed unless and until an external unbalanced force acts upon it.[4,5]
- **Second Law:** The rate of change of momentum of a body is directly proportional to the impressed force and takes place in the direction in which the force acts.[4,5]
- **Third Law:** Whenever *A* exerts a force on *B*, *B* simultaneously exerts a force of the same magnitude and in the opposite direction on *A*. This can be stated simply as: "For every action, there is an equal and opposite reaction."[4,5]

4. What is force in physics?

In physics, force is an influence that may cause an object to change its velocity (accelerate). It may be experienced as a lift, a push, or a pull, and it has a magnitude and a direction and hence is mathematically represented by a vector. The actual acceleration of the body is determined by the vector sum of all forces acting on it. Forces can also cause deformation or rotations of an object.[6,7]

5. What is a vector in physics?

A vector is a concept characterized by a magnitude and a direction. Force is a vector quantity defined as the rate of change of the momentum of the body that would be induced by that force acting alone. Since momentum is a vector, the force has a direction associated with it[6,7] (Fig. 8-1).

6. What is the difference between a vector and a scalar?

A vector is a concept characterized by a magnitude and a direction. A scalar has only a magnitude. An example of a vector is force and examples of scalars are weight and height. Orthodontic forces are described by their magnitude, point of application, and direction. The direction of the force is defined by the line of action and the sense (arrowhead). The magnitude of the force is depicted by the length of the line using an arbitrary scale (e.g., 1 cm represents 100 grams).[6,7]

7. What are the horizontal and vertical components of an orthodontic force?

Any force applied to a tooth can be broken up into its vertical and horizontal components using the occlusal plane as the horizontal reference of an orthogonal coordinate system. The

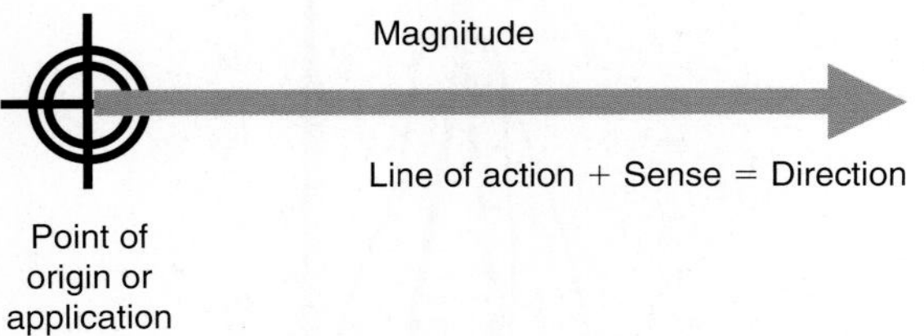

FIG 8-1 Force vector.

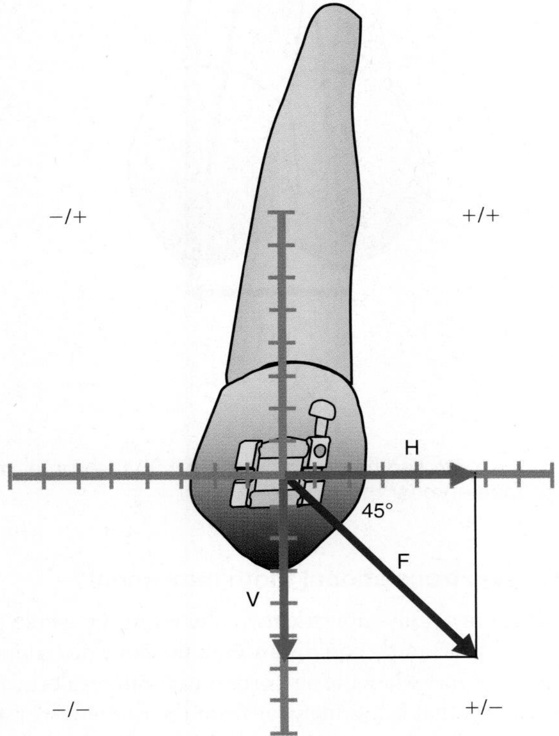

FIG 8-2 Horizontal and vertical components of a force F applied to a tooth.

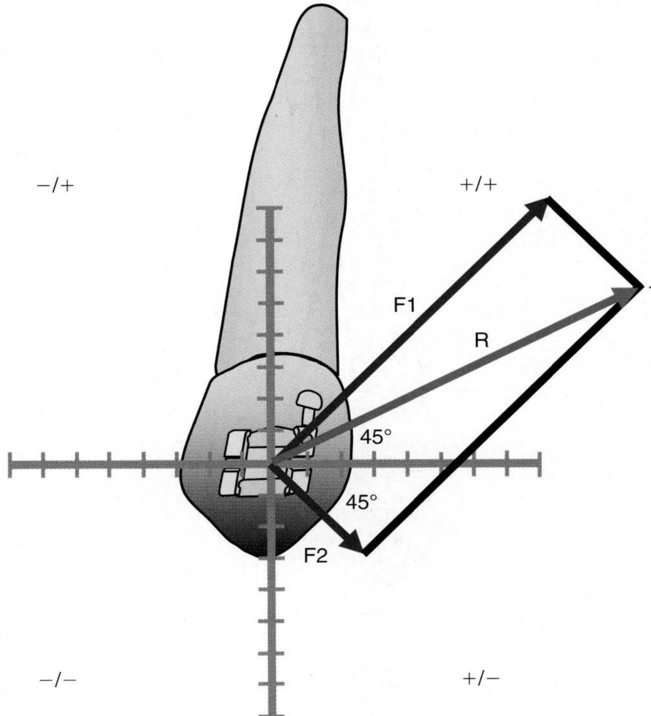

FIG 8-3 The resultant *(R)* for two concurrent forces F1 and F2 acting on a tooth.

calculations of magnitude and direction of the components can be carried out geometrically as in Fig. 8-2 or by using trigonometric methods.[8]

8. What is an orthodontic force system?

Delivery of physical force to the dentition is achieved by using a combination of force delivery methods. These include orthodontic wires, springs, elastic chains, and headgears. The force system describes all the forces involved and allows for analysis and calculation of resultant forces on a tooth or a group of teeth.[2]

9. What are two methods to calculate the resultant of two concurrent forces?

Concurrent forces depicted as vectors can be added together to calculate the resultant by using the parallelogram method or by addition of their components in a reference system. For the latter method, the horizontal and vertical components of each of the two forces can be added to calculate the resultant as follows: If $F_1 = h_1+v_1$ and $F_2 = h_2+v_2$, then $R = F_1+F_2 = (h_1+h_2) + (v_1+v_2)$.

The parallelogram method used to derive resultant forces entails drawing the two concurrent forces (F1 and F2 in Fig. 8-3) to scale at appropriate angulations. The ends of these lines are joined together with a parallelogram. The diagonal of this parallelogram from the point of force application, when measured and converted using the specified scale, gives the magnitude of the resultant (R). The direction of the resultant relative to any plane (e.g., the occlusal plane) can be determined using a protractor.[6,7]

10. What is the center of resistance (centroid)?

The center of resistance is analogous to the center of mass of a free body or its balance point. In physics, the center of mass of a system of particles is a specific point at which the system's mass behaves as if it were concentrated. This center of resistance or centroid of the physical object coincides with its center of mass if the object has uniform density, or if the object's shape and density are symmetric. In orthodontics this centroid or center of resistance of a tooth is a point in the tooth at which a force application results in translational movement. The center of resistance remains constant and is located about one third to one fourth of the root length from the cemento-enamel junction.[3,8]

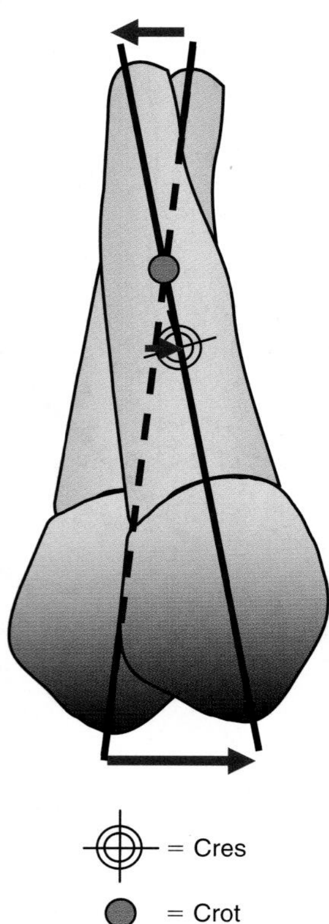

FIG 8-4 Uncontrolled tipping movement showing the location of the center of rotation *(Crot)* relative to the center of resistance *(Cres)*.

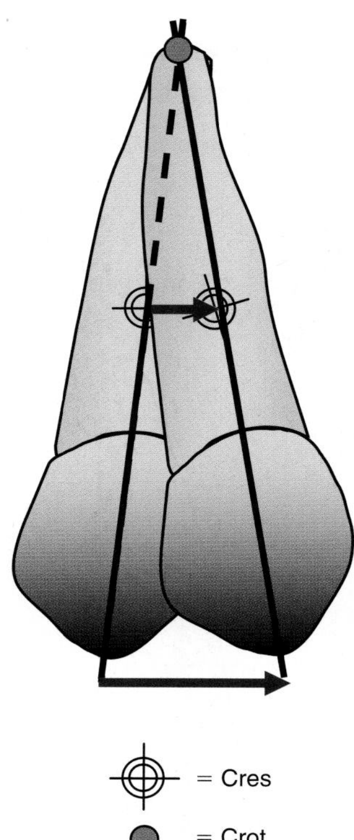

FIG 8-5 Controlled tipping movement with the center of rotation located near the root apex.

11. What is the center of rotation?

The center of rotation of a tooth is the point around which the tooth rotates. A very small rotational tooth movement can be considered as part of a circle (arc), the center of which is called the *center of rotation* for that movement. The location of the center of rotation is not constant and is determined by the type of movement that the tooth is undergoing. For example, in translational tooth movement, the center of rotation is located at an infinite distance from the center of resistance.[9,10]

12. What is uncontrolled tipping?

Uncontrolled tipping movement results when the tooth crown and root move in opposite directions. It occurs when the net force on a tooth results in a center of rotation that is near the center of resistance of that tooth. Removable appliances usually produce this type of tooth movements (Fig. 8-4).[11]

13. What is controlled tipping?

Controlled tipping movement occurs when the net force on a tooth results in a center of rotation that is near the apex of that tooth. This results in the crown moving in the direction of the force, but the root tip moving minimally. Orthodontic treatment requires this type of tooth movement in many instances (Fig. 8-5).[11]

14. What is translational tooth movement?

Translation or bodily movement results when the whole tooth (crown and root) move equidistances in the same direction. The movement occurs when the net force on a tooth results in a center of rotation that is infinitely far from the center of resistance of that tooth. Tooth translation is essential in major correction during orthodontic treatment. This type of tooth movement is achieved by using a force system that has an equivalent force applied to the center of resistance (Fig. 8-6).[11]

15. What is root torque?

Root torque is produced when the root and crown move in the same direction, with the root moving a greater distance than the crown. This type of movement occurs when the net or equivalent force on tooth results in a center of rotation at the incisal tip of that tooth (Fig. 8-7).[11]

16. What is the moment of force?

In classical mechanics, the moment of force is a quantity that represents the magnitude of a given force applied to a rotational system at a distance from the axis of rotation. The SI unit for moment is the Newton meter (Nm). The moment of the force (Mf) has both magnitude and direction (clockwise or counterclockwise) and is therefore a vector.[12,13]

$$\text{Moment of the force} = \text{Magnitude of Force} \times \text{Perpendicular distance to the center of resistance of the tooth}$$

Or

$$Mf = F \times D$$

17. What is the unit of moment of the force?

The unit of moment of a force is the unit of force (Newtons) and distance (meter), which is designated Nm. Given the distance (D) and force (F), calculate the moment of force placed on a tooth in three planes of space in Fig. 8-8.[12,13]

18. What is a couple?

A couple is composed of two equal but opposite non-coplanar forces acting on an object (Fig. 8-9).[11]

19. What is the moment of the couple?

Moment of the couple is the sum total of the moments created by individual force components of a couple. The magnitude of moment of a couple (Mc) is equivalent to the magnitude of the component forces multiplied by the distance between the two component forces at the point of application. The moment of the couple in full-fixed appliance orthodontic treatment results from the deflection of the orthodontic wire against the bracket that produces the couple (f) on the bracket and the tooth (Fig. 8-10).[12,13]

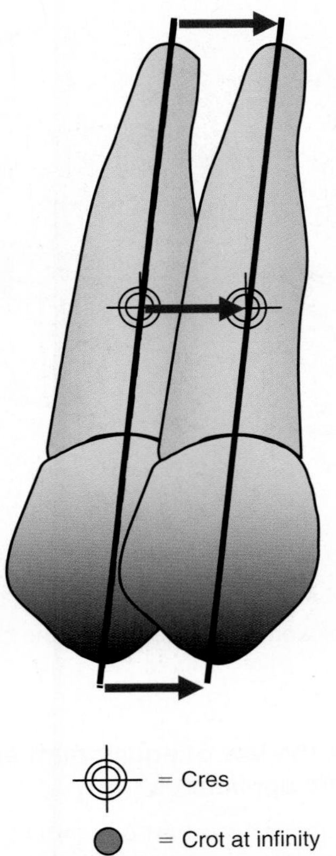

FIG 8-6 Translational tooth movement in which all points on the tooth have moved equally in the same direction and the center of rotation is located at infinity.

20. How is moment of couple instrumental in creating translational movement?

When a force F is applied to a tooth, it produces a moment of the force (Mf), which tends to rotate the tooth in a counterclockwise direction. The tipping of the tooth and bracket tip relative to the wire deflects the wire, creating a couple whose moment (Mc) equals $f \times d$ (where d is the mesiodistal dimension of the bracket) in a clockwise direction. As the tip of the bracket relative to the wire increases, the Mc progressively increases and can eventually become of equal magnitude, but opposite in direction to the moment of the force. The Mf and Mc cancel each other out, resulting in a net effective moment of zero. This places the equivalent of the force F through the center of resistance, producing translational tooth movement (Fig. 8-11).[13,14]

21. When retracting a cuspid on an archwire, what determines the moment of the couple?

The moment of the couple is determined by the magnitude of its component force times the distance between the opposing force's point of action. In the previous example, the distance between acting component forces is fixed (bracket width), but the magnitude of the component force varies based on the wire bracket interaction. Therefore, it is the amount of force delivered by the wire that determines the moment of the couple, and in turn the force delivered by the wire results from the wire's compositions, its geometry, and amount of deflection.[13,14]

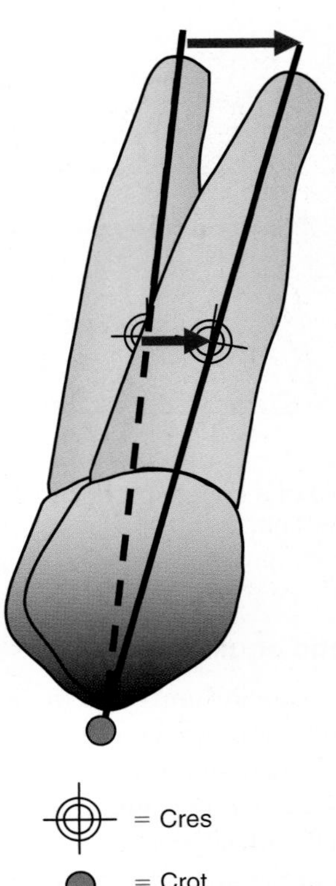

FIG 8-7 Root torque is represented by movement in which the root apex moves more than the incisal edge and the center of rotation is located close to the incisal edge of the tooth.

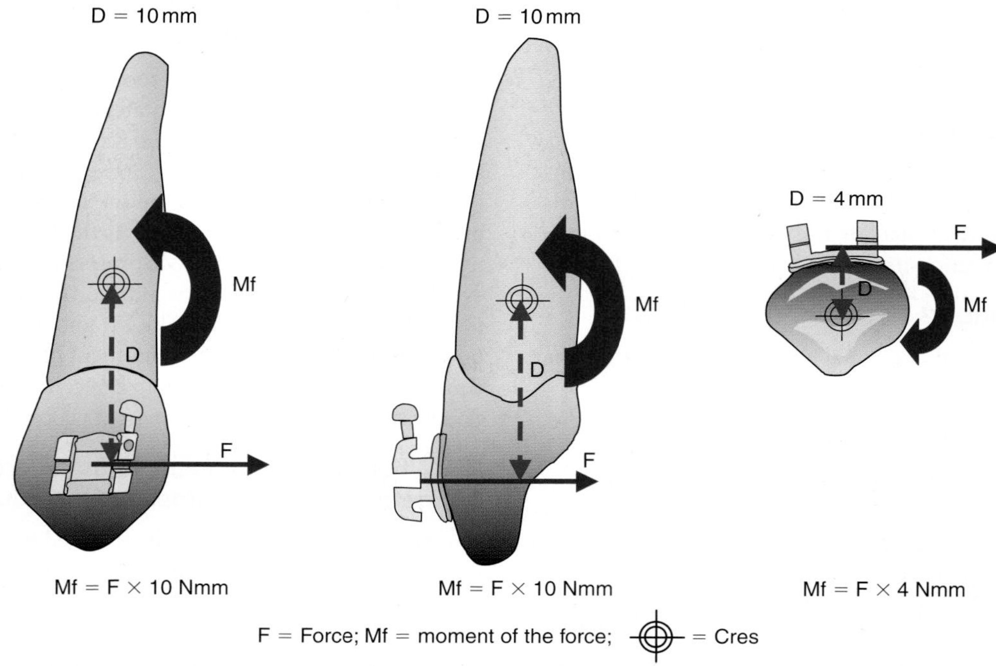

FIG 8-8 Depiction of the moment of force (Mf) in three planes of space that results from the application of the force F on the tooth crown.

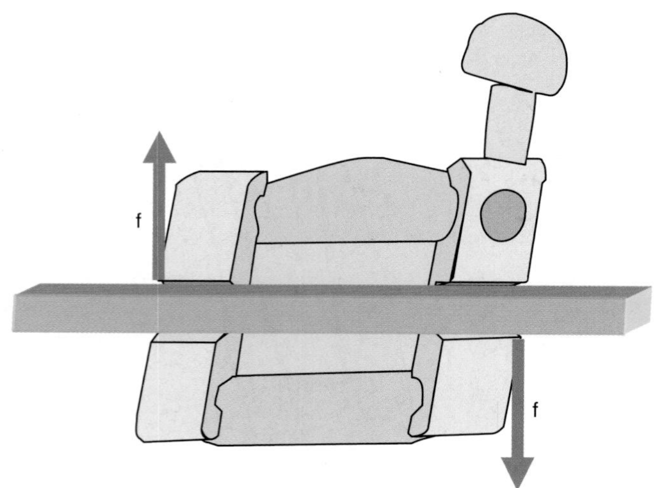

FIG 8-9 Example of a couple produced as a result of bracket wire interaction.

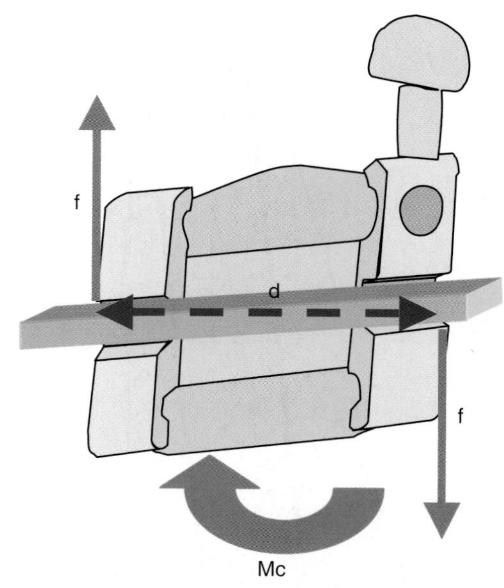

FIG 8-10 Depiction of the moment of the couple: $Mc = f \times d$.

22. What is static equilibrium?

A rigid body is in equilibrium when the external forces acting on it form a system of forces and moments whose sum is equivalent to zero. Therefore, the requirements for system to be in equilibrium are that the sum of all of horizontal forces = 0, the sum of all vertical forces = 0, the sum of all transverse forces = 0, and the sum of all moments = 0. An object in mechanical equilibrium is neither undergoing linear nor rotational acceleration; however, it could be translating or rotating at a constant velocity.[8,12]

23. How does the law of equilibrium apply to orthodontic appliances?

Application of force on one part of a system leads to an equal and opposite force on another part of the system. For example, extraoral appliances deliver active forces intraorally, while the reactive forces are extraoral. Another example is the intermaxillary elastics where the active and reactive forces are

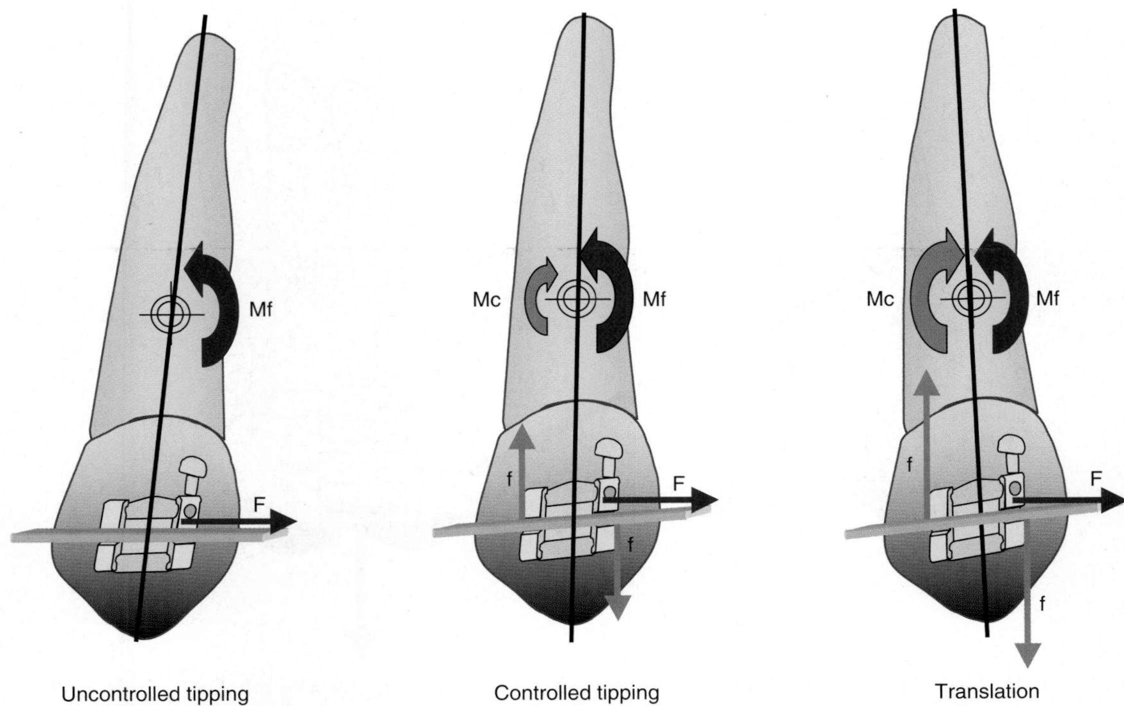

FIG 8-11 Depiction of changes in the types of tooth movement as the moment of the couple increases because of wire deflection or increasing wire stiffness from left to right.

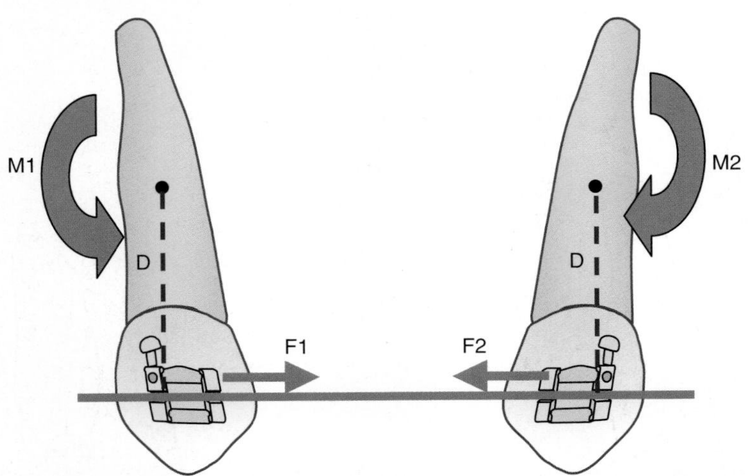

FIG 8-12 Static equilibrium in a simple orthodontic force system.

in the opposite arches. Similarly, the consolidation of spaces in intra-arch mechanics results in static equilibrium.[8,12]

24. Give an example of equilibrium in an orthodontic appliance system.

In the previous example, the forces F1 and F2 produced by an elastic chain are equal and opposite such that their sum is zero. The moment created by F1 is $F1 \times D = M1$ in a counterclockwise direction, whereas that from F2 is $F2 \times D$ in a clockwise direction. Since F1 equals F2 and the distances D are equal, M1 equals M2 but in opposite directions. Therefore, the sum of M1 and M2 is also zero. Because the sum of all forces is zero, and the sum of all moments is also zero, this orthodontic appliance system is in equilibrium (Fig. 8-12).[11,15]

25. What is a one-couple orthodontic force system?

A one-couple orthodontic force system results with an orthodontic appliance that has two points of action in the system, each with the capability to deliver a force but only one of which generates a couple. An example of a one-couple orthodontic force system is an intrusion arch that applies a point force on an anterior tooth or segment of teeth and is engaged in the molar bracket, as depicted in Fig. 8-13. This arrangement results in the single moment of the couple on the molar and intrusive and extrusive forces on the canine and molar,

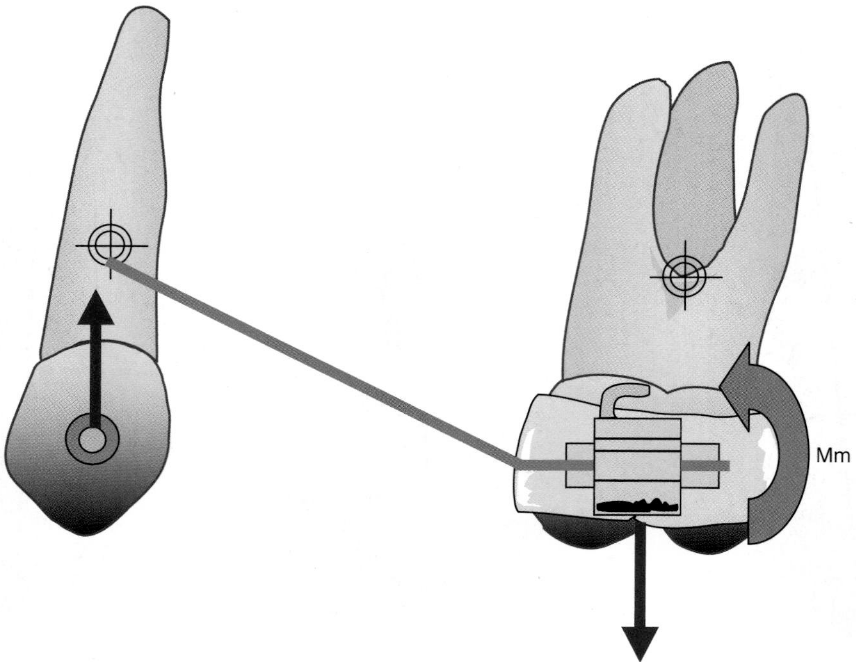

FIG 8-13 Example of a one-couple orthodontic force system. The wire bracket interaction produces a couple at only one end of the system, in this case on the molar. *Mm*, moment on molar.

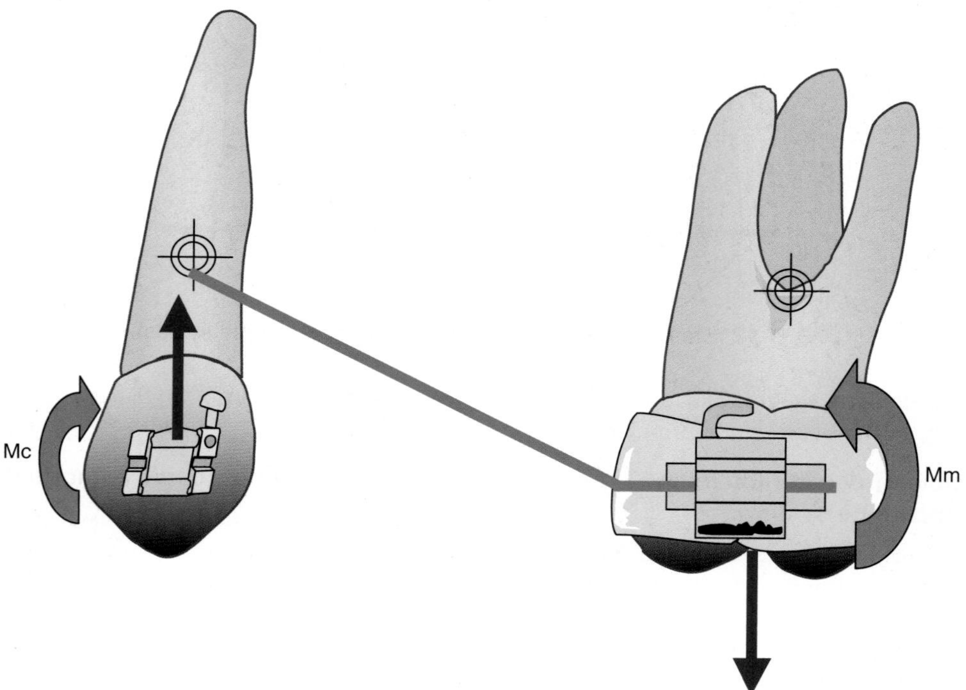

FIG 8-14 An example of a two-couple orthodontic force system. The wire bracket interaction produces two couples, one at each end of the system, namely on the canine and on the molar in this case. *Mc*, moment on canine; *Mm*, moment on molar.

respectively. The couple on the molar will result in a counterclockwise rotation of this tooth. Because the molar extrudes and the incisors intrude, the whole system can be thought to have a clockwise rotation (Fig. 8-13).[11,16-18]

26. What is a two-couple orthodontic force system?

An orthodontic appliance that has two points of action in the system with capability to deliver force at both points that result in separate couples at each of these sites is a two-couple orthodontic force system. An example of a two-couple orthodontic force system is an intrusion arch that engages brackets both in the anterior and posterior teeth, or a canine bracket intrusion arch in which the wire engages the brackets at both the canine and molar, as shown in Fig. 8-14.[11,16-18]

REFERENCES

1. Burstone C: Orthodontics as a science: The role of biomechanics. *Am J Orthod Dentofacial Orthoped* 2000;117(5):598-600.
2. Burstone CJ, Koenig HA: Force systems from an ideal arch. *Am J Orthod* 1974;65(3):270-289.
3. Hocevar RA: Understanding, planning, and managing tooth movement: orthodontic force system theory. *Am J Orthod* 1981;80(5):457-477.
4. Cohen IB, Smith GE: *The Cambridge companion to Newton*. Cambridge, UK; New York: Cambridge University Press, 2002.
5. Tait PG: *Newton's laws of motion*. London: A. & C. Black, 1899.
6. Abraham R, Marsden JE: *Foundations of mechanics; a mathematical exposition of classical mechanics with an introduction to the qualitative theory of dynamical systems and applications to the three-body problem*. New York: W. A. Benjamin, 1967.
7. Becker RA: *Introduction to theoretical mechanics*. New York: McGraw-Hill, 1954.
8. Smith RJ, Burstone CJ: Mechanics of tooth movement. *Am J Orthod* 1984;85(4):294-307.
9. Burstone CJ, Pryputniewicz RJ: Holographic determination of centers of rotation produced by orthodontic forces. *Am J Orthod* 1980;77(4):396-409.
10. Christiansen RL, Burstone CJ: Centers of rotation within the periodontal space. *Am J Orthod* 1969;55(4):353-369.
11. Nanda R: *Biomechanics in clinical orthodontics*. Philadelphia: Saunders, 1997.
12. Shellhart WC: Equilibrium clarified. *Am J Orthod Dentofacial Orthop* 1995;108(4):394-401.
13. Tanne K, Koenig HA, Burstone CJ: Moment to force ratios and the center of rotation. *Am J Orthod Dentofacial Orthop* 1988;94(5):426-431.
14. Gjessing P: Controlled retraction of maxillary incisors. *Am J Orthod Dentofacial Orthop* 1992;101(2):120-131.
15. Mulligan TF: Common sense mechanics. 3. *J Clin Orthod* 1979;13(11):762-766.
16. Nikolai RJ: Rigid-body kinematics and single-tooth displacements. *Am J Orthod Dentofacial Orthop* 1996;110(1):88-92.
17. Isaacson RJ, Lindauer SJ, Rubenstein LK: Activating a 2×4 appliance. *Angle Orthod* 1993;63(1):17-24.
18. Demange C: Equilibrium situations in bend force systems. *Am J Orthod Dentofacial Orthop* 1990;98(4):333-339.

CHAPTER

9 Treatment Planning

James L. Vaden • Cheryl A. DeWood

Treatment planning is the critical first step in orthodontic treatment. Without an adequate treatment plan, proper treatment cannot be rendered. Indeed, the patient's destiny is determined by the treatment plan that is arrived at by the treating clinician. This chapter delves into some of the common areas that should be considered during the treatment planning process. The chapter is divided into a discussion of the dimension of the dentition concept, and subsequent illustrations discuss the facial, skeletal, and dental components of a malocclusion. It is hoped that the person who reads the chapter will have a deeper understanding of the treatment planning process.

1. When a treatment plan for a patient is being developed, what should be the goal?

The goal that should be inherent in any and all treatment plans should be to make the decisions that will allow the orthodontist to:

- Prioritize objectives—both the patient's and the orthodontist's[1]
- Make decisions that will allow the orthodontist to treat the patient so that the greatest number of attainable objectives is reached

For most patients, the objectives are esthetics, health and function, and stability. If a growing child is being treated, an additional objective should be to use forces that are in harmony with growth and development.[2,3]

2. Is there "room for error" during the treatment planning process?

Absolutely not. The orthodontic clinician must use a systematic approach to each and every treatment plan. This systematic approach must be based on sound fundamental principles that have been scientifically validated.[1,4-6] Treatment plans should not be formulated with the use of anecdotal evidence that is contraindicated by scientific data.[7]

3. Should patient/parent desires be considered when a treatment plan is developed?

Absolutely, but only if the patient/parent desires are[1,7-9]:

- In harmony with the scientific body of evidence
- Consistent with what can reasonably be delivered by the competent and caring orthodontic specialist

DESIRES THAT ARE CONSISTENT WITH THE SCIENTIFIC BODY OF EVIDENCE

A patient who presents with minor mandibular crowding and a reasonably steep mandibular plane angle wants a "movie star" smile and a great occlusion—BUT NO EXTRACTIONS! Fig. 9-1, *A-C* shows the facial photographs of such a patient. Fig. 9-1, *D* and *E* illustrates the pretreatment casts. Note the crowding; it is not severe. Figure 9-1, *F* and *G* shows the cephalogram—its tracing and the cephalometric values. The patient was treated—according to the patient's wishes and the general dentist's wishes—with no extractions. Fig. 9-1, *H-M* exhibits a comparison of the pretreatment/"progress" photographs. Is the face better or worse? Fig. 9-1, *N* and *O*, the pretreatment/"progress" cephalograms and their tracings (Fig. 9-1, *P* and *Q*) confirm the fact that the teeth were not "retracted" as the patient/parent desired. The facial esthetics was significantly compromised as is evidenced in Figures 9-1, *H-M*. What happened? The answer is quite simple. Parent desires were not consistent with the scientific evidence in orthodontics—evidence that speaks to expansion orthodontic treatment and facial esthetics. The fact that mandibular incisors must be uprighted in certain skeletal patterns in order to improve facial esthetics was forgotten during formulation of the treatment plan. Simply stated, the patient's treatment plan and her desires were not consistent with the body of knowledge in orthodontics. It is the clinician's duty to explain all of these things to a family when the treatment plan is presented. Not to do so can be disastrous. The patient/parent must be made to understand that desires, at times, cannot be achieved unless preferences or wishes—in this case, no extractions—are modified.

RESULTS THAT CAN REASONABLY BE DELIVERED

The patient and the parent requested "retreatment." Four premolars were extracted. Fig. 9-2, *A-D* shows the pretreatment/posttreatment dentition. Fig. 9-2, *E-M* illustrates the pretreatment, "progress," and posttreatment facial esthetics. The cephalometric tracings (Fig. 9-2, *N-P*) reflect the tooth movement. Fig. 9-2, *Q-S* confirms that the patient has a very nice and pleasing smile at the cessation of

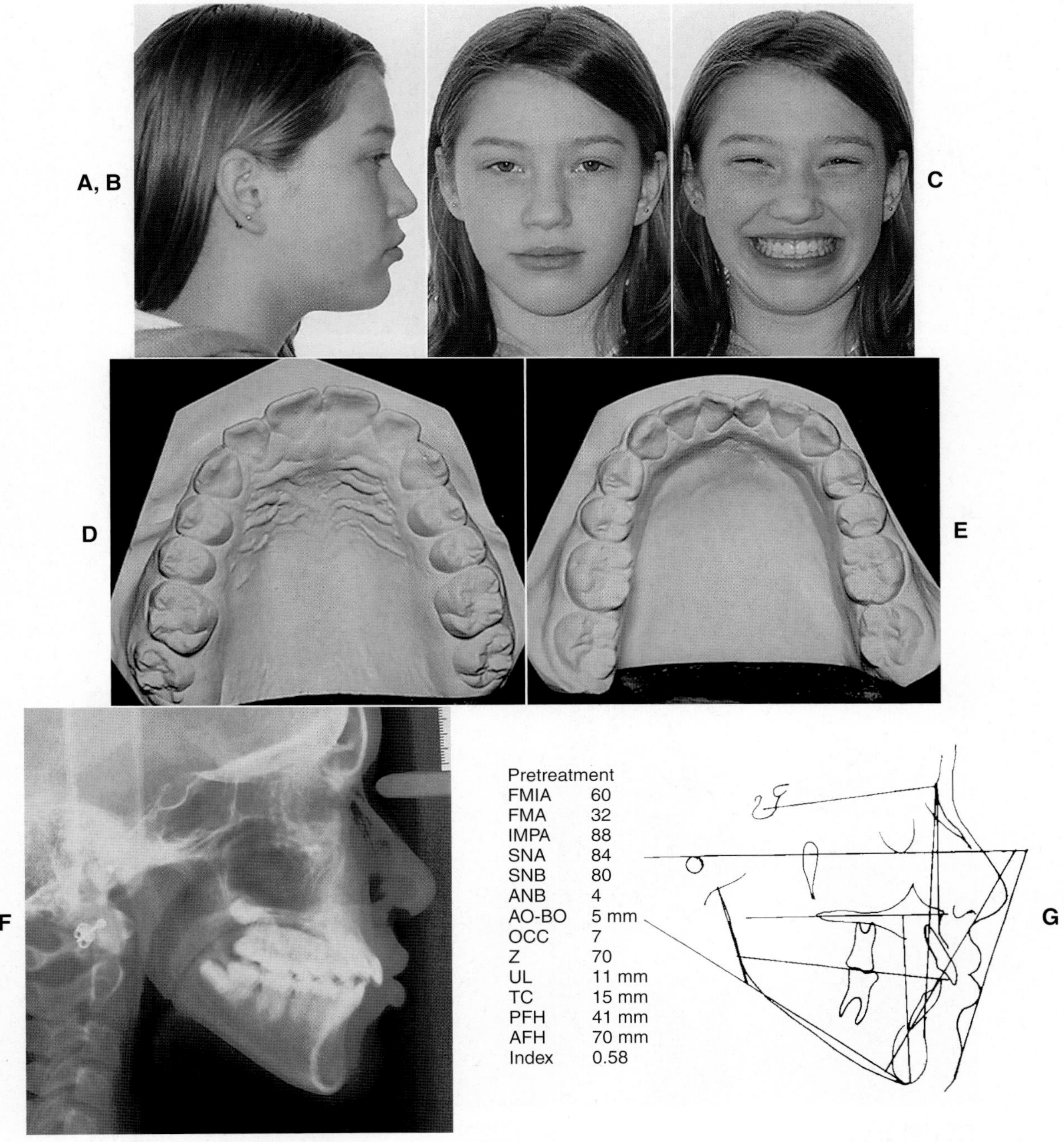

A, B
C
D
E
F
Pretreatment
FMIA 60
FMA 32
IMPA 88
SNA 84
SNB 80
ANB 4
AO-BO 5 mm
OCC 7
Z 70
UL 11 mm
TC 15 mm
PFH 41 mm
AFH 70 mm
Index 0.58
G

FIG 9-1 Patient with minor mandibular crowding and a reasonably steep mandibular plane angle. **A-C,** Facial photographs. **D** and **E,** Cast occlusals. **F,** Cep halogram. **G,** Tracing and numbers.

Continued

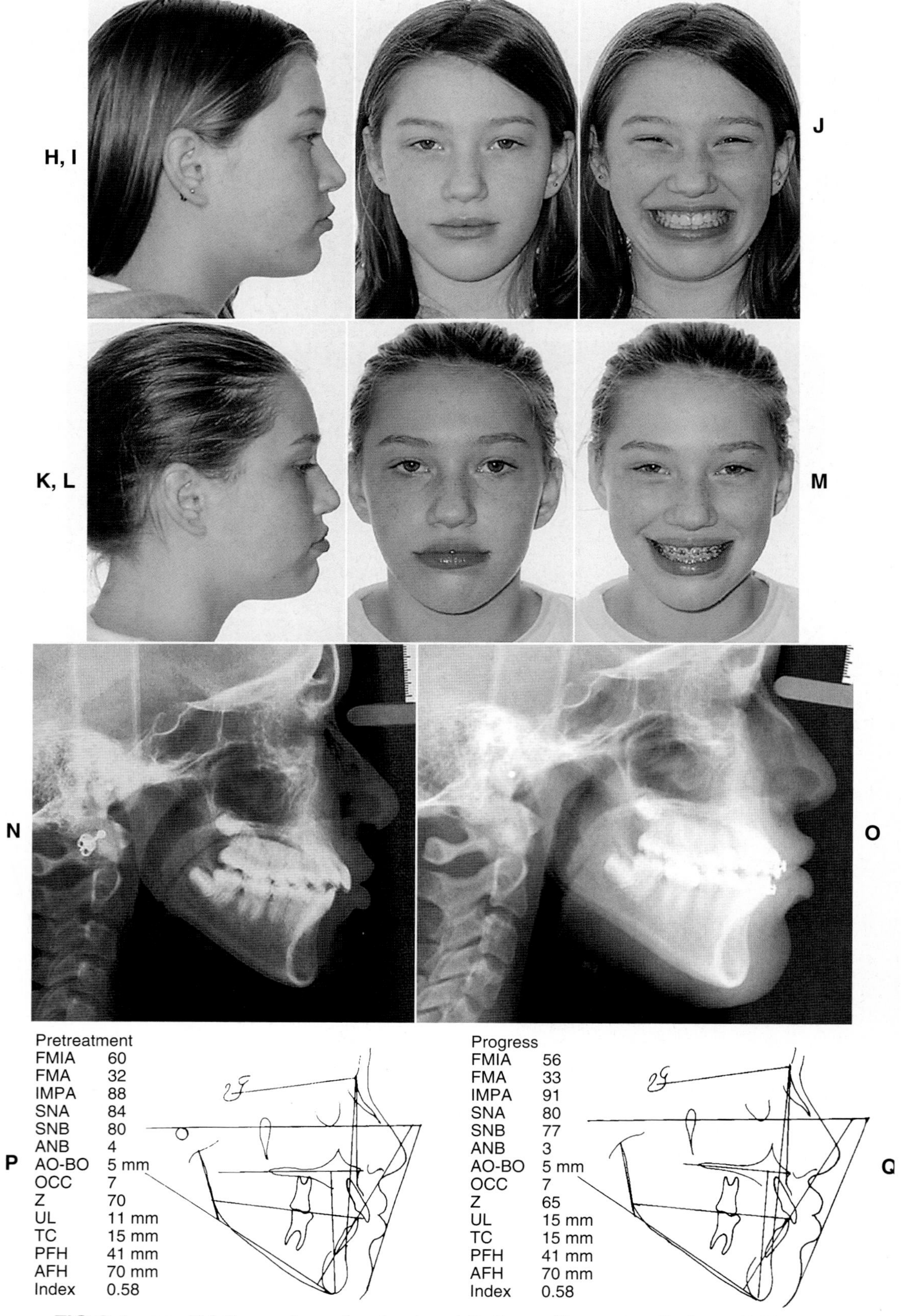

FIG 9-1—cont'd Comparison of pretreatment findings with progress findings. **H-M,** Pretreatment **(H-J)** and treatment progress **(K-M)** photos. **N,** Pretreatment cephalogram. **O,** Progress cephalogram. **P,** Pretreatment tracing and numbers. **Q,** Progress tracing and numbers.

treatment. These results were "reasonable."[10-12] The altered treatment plan and the patient's altered expectations became harmonious with the scientific evidence. This patient wanted "straight" teeth and a nice smile that a flawed treatment plan could not deliver, so a scientifically sound plan was initiated.

4. Is there an underlying concept that should be considered when a treatment plan is developed? If so, how can the concept be simply and succinctly explained?

A fundamental treatment planning concept that should be considered when every treatment plan is developed is that there is a finite dimension of the dentition.[13] This concept has been expressed in various ways. Merrifield[14] expressed it best when he stated that the dimension of the dentition concept has four premises *provided the musculature is normal.*

PREMISE #1—ANTERIOR LIMIT OF THE DENTITION

An anterior limit of the dentition exists (Fig. 9-3, *A*). The teeth must not be placed forward, off basal bone. If the teeth are too far forward, all objectives of treatment are compromised. The photographs (Fig. 9-3, *B-G*) of this patient provide illustration of this important concept. The pretreatment photographs reflect a mildly protruded facial profile. There was a need for some lip retraction. Instead, the patient was treated without extractions, even though there was mandibular anterior crowding. Teeth were pushed forward. The anterior limit of the dentition was violated.[13-15] The lip procumbency is much worse. Facial esthetics was compromised because the anterior limit of the dentition was violated even more.

PREMISE #2—POSTERIOR LIMIT OF THE DENTITION

A posterior limit of the dentition exists (Fig. 9-4, A). Teeth can be positioned and/or impacted into the area behind the mandibular first molar in the mandibular arch even as they can be moved too far forward off basal bone. Easier than posterior movement of mandibular teeth is posterior movement of maxillary teeth. Maxillary posterior expansion is easy to accomplish but equally disastrous. In many instances posterior expansion leads to impaction of the second molars and, more often than not, vertical expansion because posterior teeth, when pushed distally into a smaller part of a "wedge," unfavorably impact the posterior vertical dimension.[13] The pretreatment/6-month cephalograms of a patient (Fig. 9-4, *B* and *C*) exhibit the most common problem: hopeless impaction of the second molars. The patient was subsequently treated with premolar extraction. The pretreatment/posttreatment cephalograms (Fig. 9-4, *D* and *E*) and the pretreatment/posttreatment facial photographs (Fig. 9-4, *F-I*) illustrate the resolution of a posterior discrepancy problem along with maintenance of facial balance and harmony.

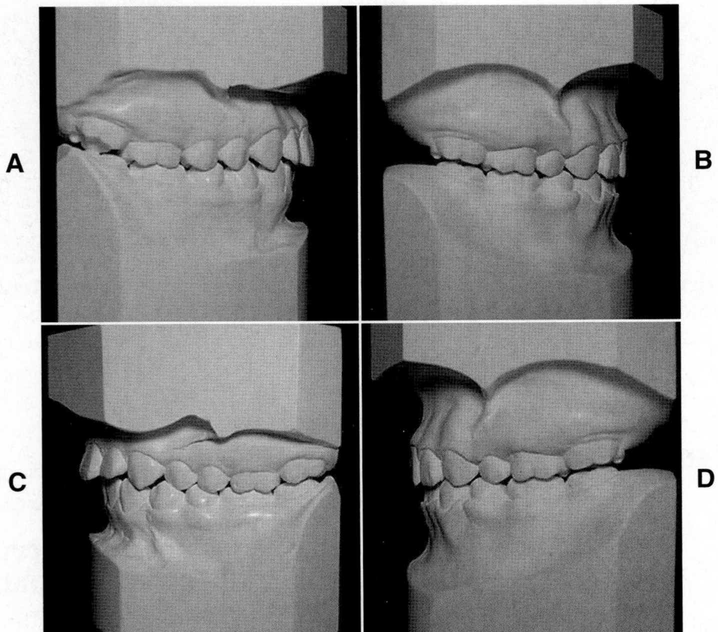

FIG 9-2 "Retreatment" of patient seen in Fig. 9-1. **A** and **B,** Pretreatment casts. **C** and **D,** Posttreatment casts.

Continued

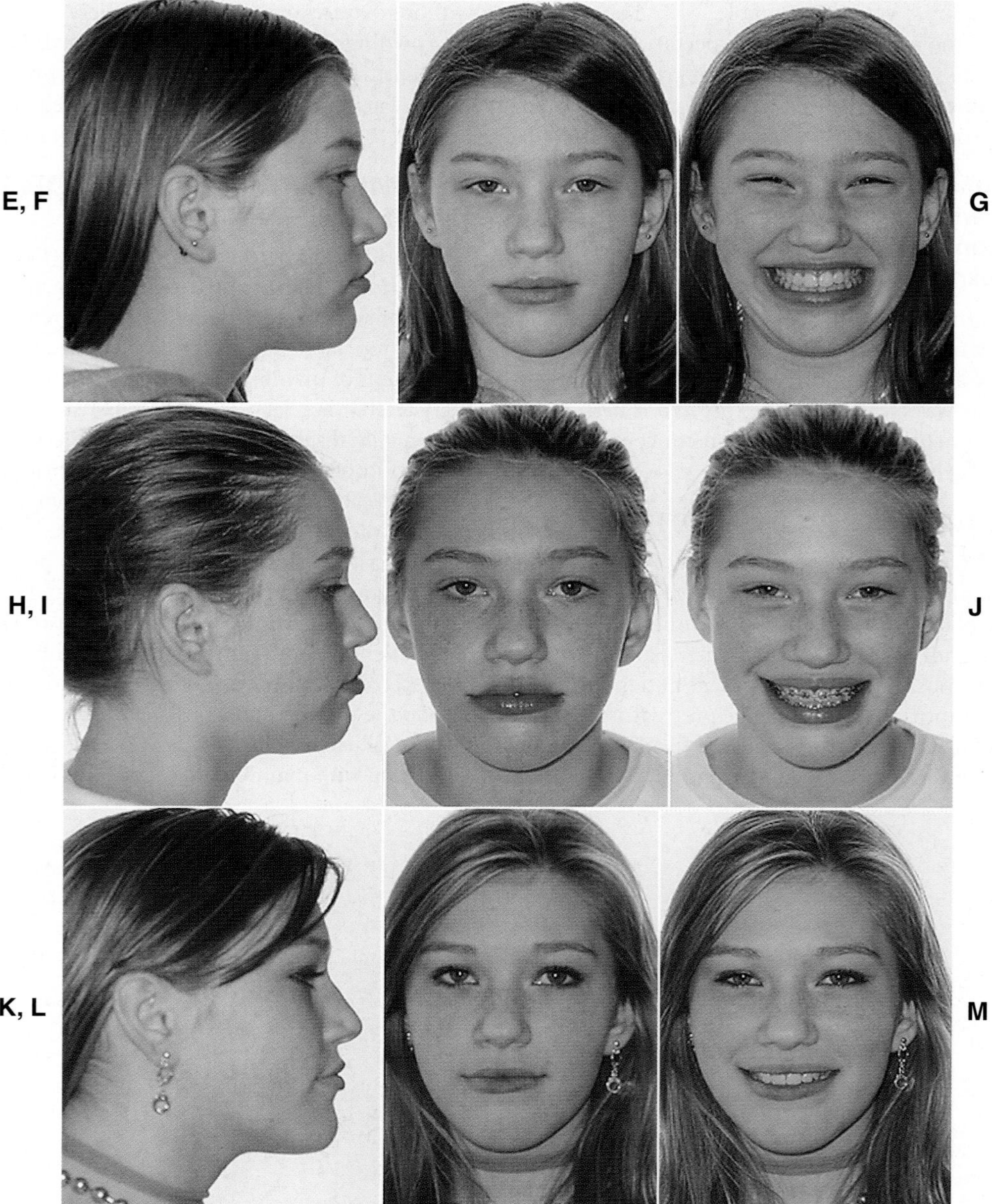

FIG 9-2—cont'd Comparison of facial esthetics. **E-G,** Pretreatment photographs. **H-J,** Progress photographs. **K-M,** Posttreatment photographs.

PREMISE #3—LATERAL LIMIT OF THE DENTITION

A lateral limit of the dentition exists (Fig. 9-5, *A*). If the teeth are moved buccally into the masseter and buccinator muscles, relapse is likely to result over the long term. This fact has been repeatedly reported in the scientific literature.[16] Most unstable of all lateral expansion is mandibular canine expansion. The mandibular casts (Fig. 9-5, *B-C*) of a patient who was treated as a teenager with extraction—but with mandibular canine expansion—graphically illustrate this concept of the lateral limit of the dentition. The relapse shown in Fig. 9-5, *D*, is to be expected if mandibular canines are expanded.

PREMISE #4—VERTICAL LIMIT OF THE DENTITION

A vertical limit of the dentition exists (Fig. 9-6, *A*). Vertical expansion is harmful to facial balance and harmony in the sagittal plane except in deep bite situations.[17] To allow the maxillary and mandibular molars to extrude during treatment—in the moderate to high mandibular plane

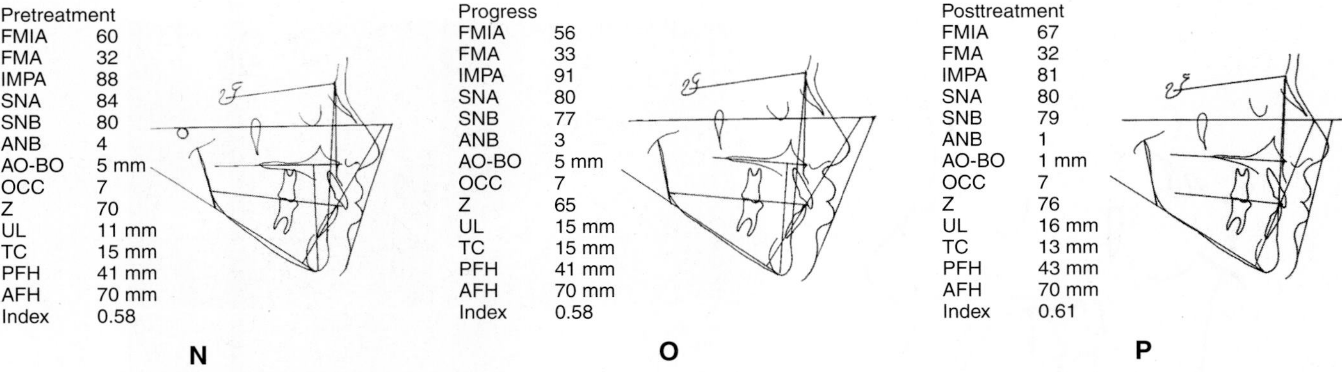

Pretreatment
FMIA 60
FMA 32
IMPA 88
SNA 84
SNB 80
ANB 4
AO-BO 5 mm
OCC 7
Z 70
UL 11 mm
TC 15 mm
PFH 41 mm
AFH 70 mm
Index 0.58
N
Progress
FMIA 56
FMA 33
IMPA 91
SNA 80
SNB 77
ANB 3
AO-BO 5 mm
OCC 7
Z 65
UL 15 mm
TC 15 mm
PFH 41 mm
AFH 70 mm
Index 0.58
O
Posttreatment
FMIA 67
FMA 32
IMPA 81
SNA 80
SNB 79
ANB 1
AO-BO 1 mm
OCC 7
Z 76
UL 16 mm
TC 13 mm
PFH 43 mm
AFH 70 mm
Index 0.61
P

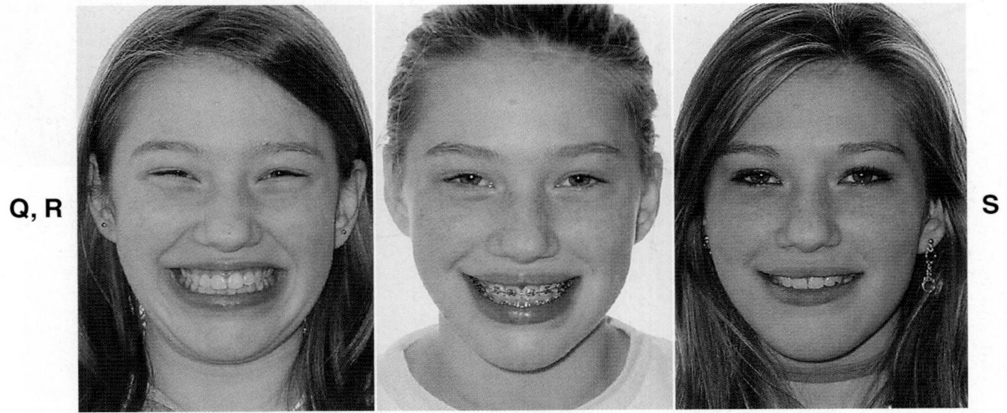

FIG 9-2—cont'd Comparison of tracing and numbers: pretreatment **(N)**, progress **(O)**, and posttreatment **(P)**. **Q-S,** Smiling photographs: pretreatment **(Q)**, progress **(R)**, and posttreatment **(S)**.

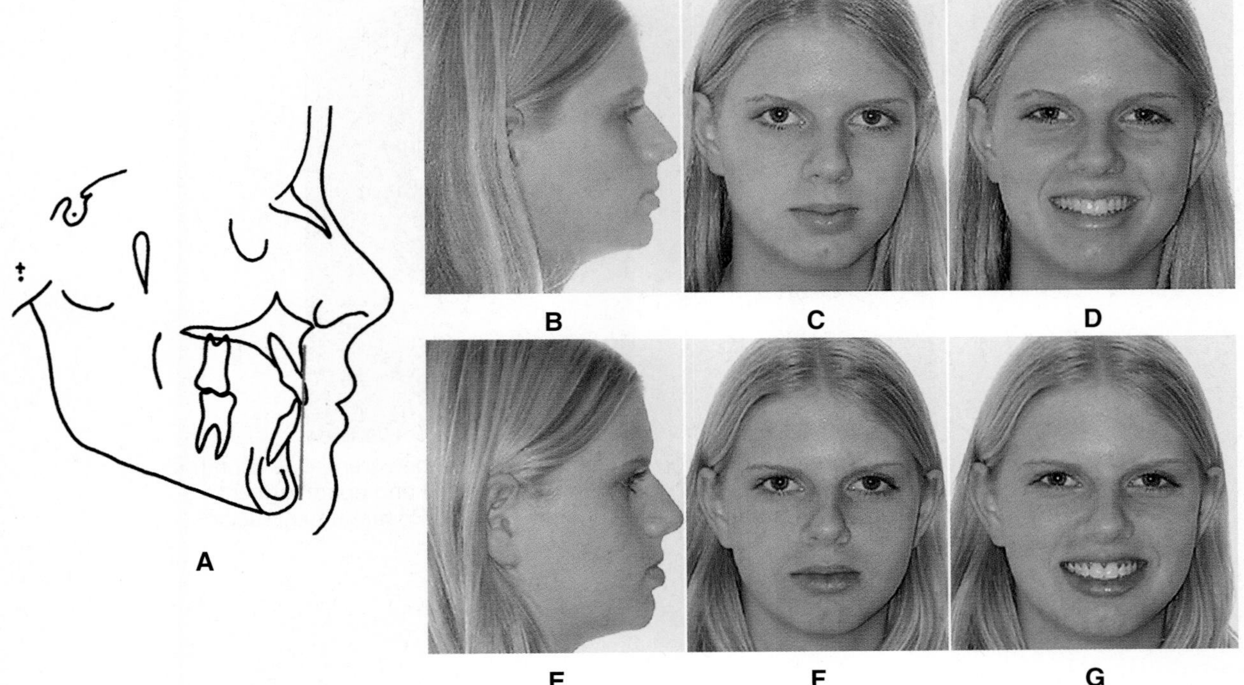

FIG 9-3 A, Anterior limit of the dentition. **B-D,** Pretreatment photos. **E-G,** Posttreatment photos.

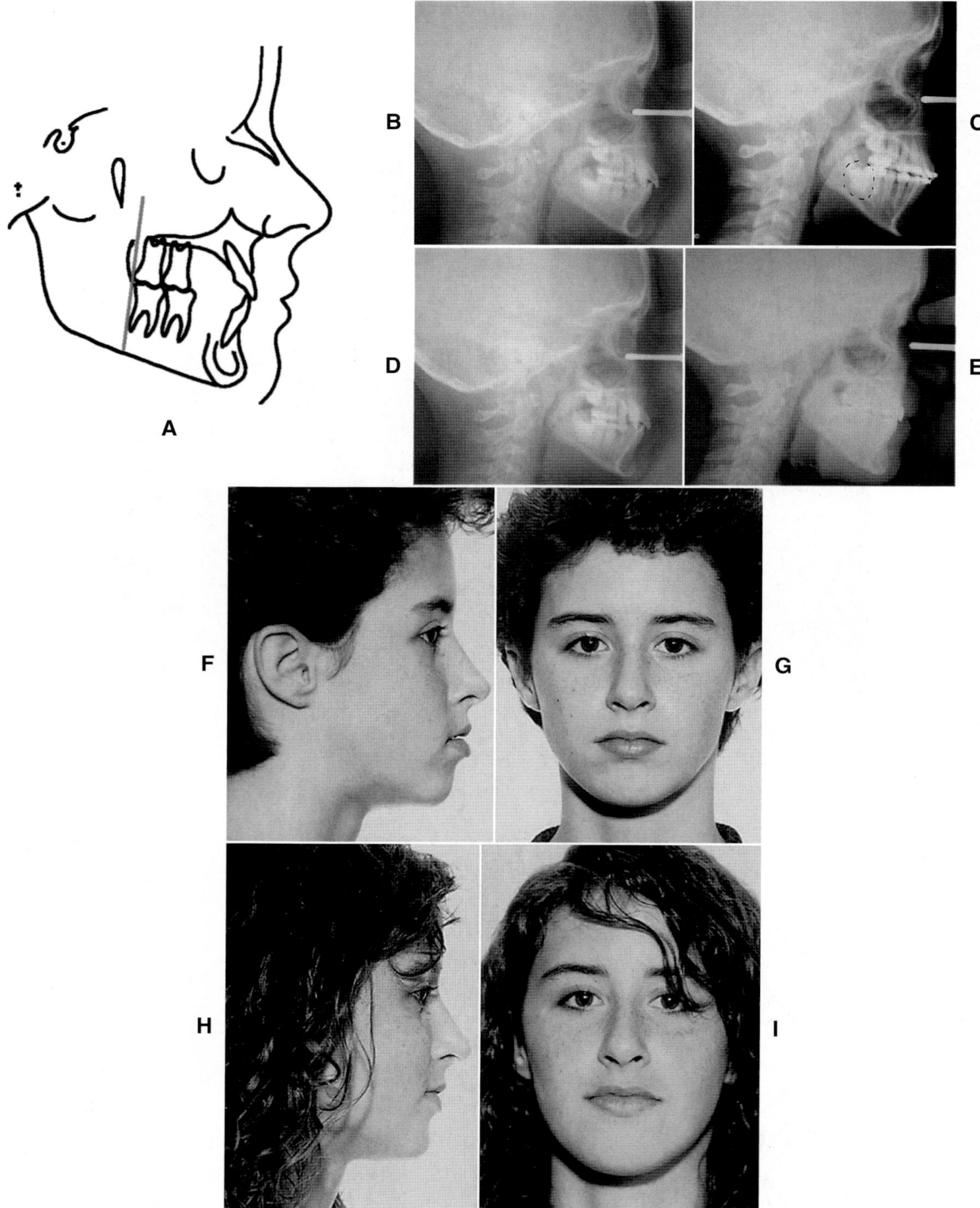

FIG 9-4 **A,** Posterior limit of the dentition. **B,** Pretreatment cephalogram. **C,** 6-month progress cephalogram. **D** and **E,** Comparison of pretreatment **(D)** and posttreatment **(E)** cephalograms. **F** and **G,** Pretreatment facial photos. **H** and **I,** Posttreatment facial photographs.

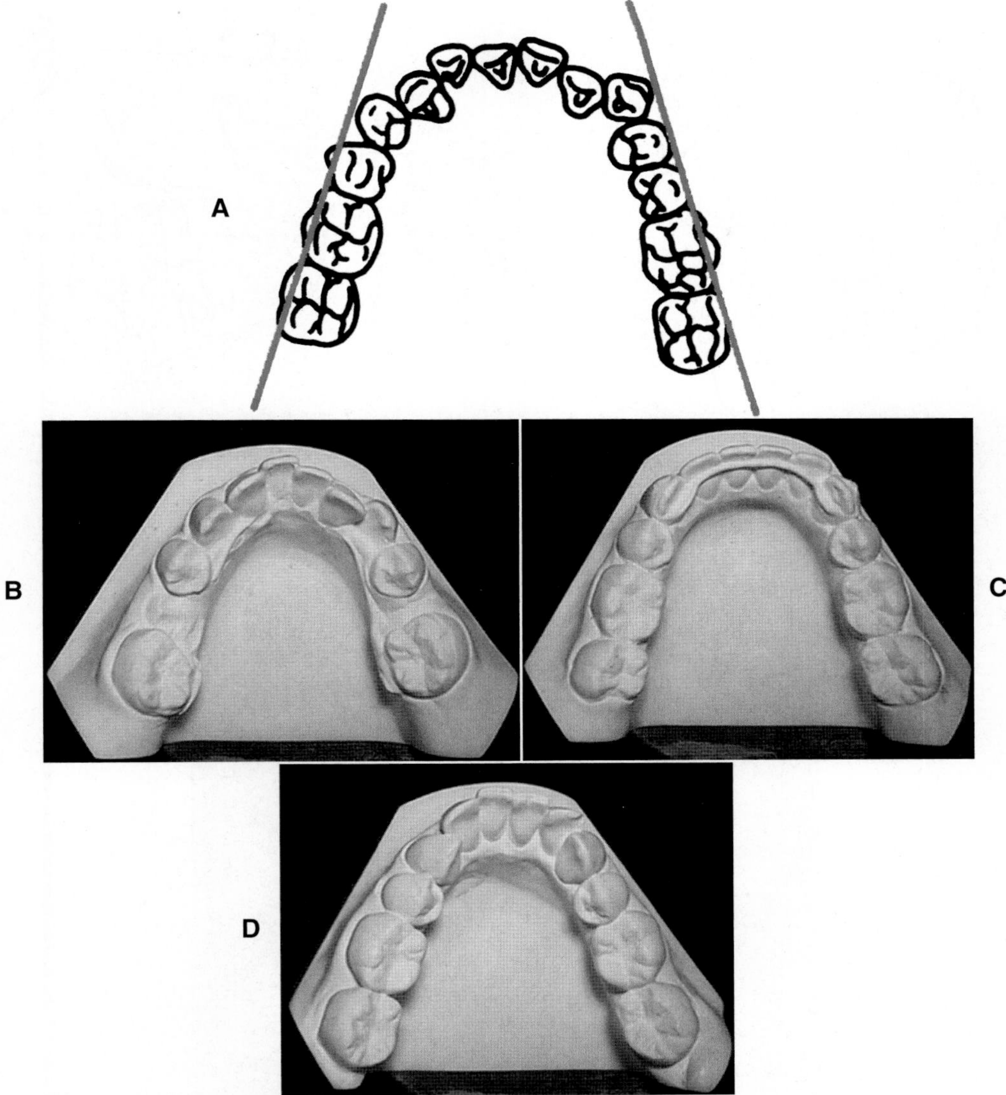

FIG 9-5 **A,** Lateral limit of the dentition. **B,** Pretreatment cast. **C,** Posttreatment cast. **D,** "Relapse" cast.

angle skeletal pattern—can lead to a "stretched" unaesthetic face. The pretreatment/posttreatment superimpositions of a patient (Fig. 9-6, *B*) and the patient's pretreatment/posttreatment facial photographs (Fig. 9-6, *C-F*) illustrate the point.

SUMMARY

In summary, orthodontists must recognize the limitations of the dental environment and plan treatment to conform to these dimensions *when normal muscle balance exists.*

5. Is there a way to "simplify" the treatment planning process by analyzing the malocclusion in "components"?

One way to analyze the malocclusion in a systematic manner is to examine a patient's problem by studying:

- The face
- The skeletal pattern
- The teeth

By looking at each of these three separate yet related entities, the clinician can compile information that will be invaluable to the formation of a treatment plan.[14,18]

THE FACIAL COMPONENT

6. What should be considered when a face is evaluated?

This answer requires books! The orthodontic literature abounds with articles about "the face." Many authors and investigators have studied the face. For the purposes of this treatment planning chapter, the answer will be as succinct as possible. To answer this question requires more questions, the answers to which should guide the practitioner to a consideration of what role the face plays in the formulation of a treatment plan. The following questions, and the answers to these questions, should guide the clinician to make reasonable treatment planning decisions that

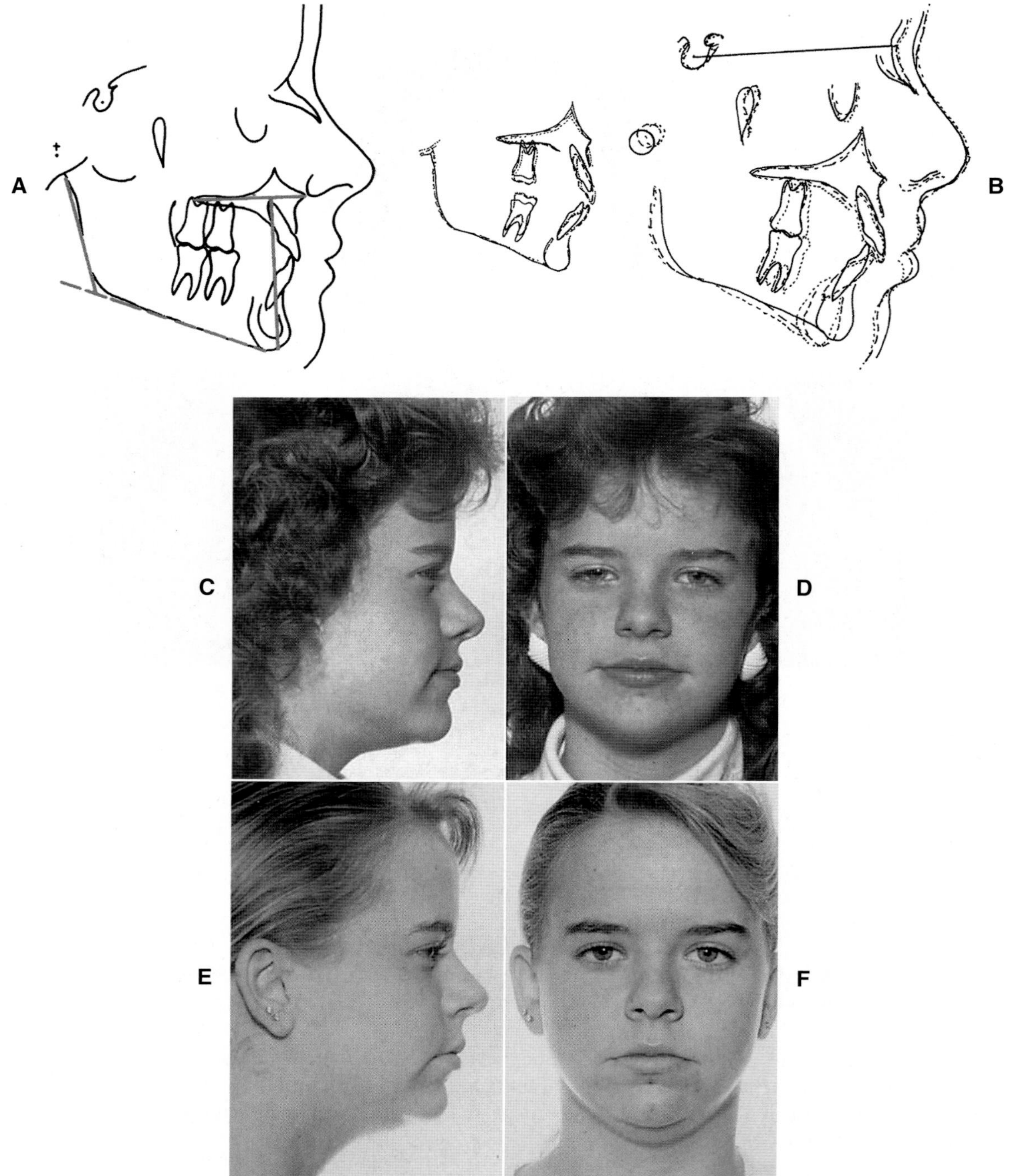

FIG 9-6 A, Vertical limit of the dentition. **B,** Superimposition tracing. **C** and **D,** Pretreatment facial photographs. **E** and **F,** Posttreatment facial photographs.

will maintain a "good" face and, when possible, improve a "poor" face.[19-21]

7. What are the prerequisites for a "good face"?

Prerequisites for a good face are[22-26]:

- **The soft tissue chin is nicely positioned in the facial profile.** A patient who has a weak chin (i.e., a retrognathic mandible) cannot have a face with significant chin projection unless surgery is used. Conversely, a patient who has a Class II malocclusion but who has a fairly "strong" chin can have a more balanced face after orthodontic treatment (Fig. 9-7).
- **No serious skeletal convexity problem exists.** This problem is directly related to the "nicely positioned chin" which has been explained.[27-31]A serious skeletal convexity will generally predispose a patient to a recessive chin after orthodontic

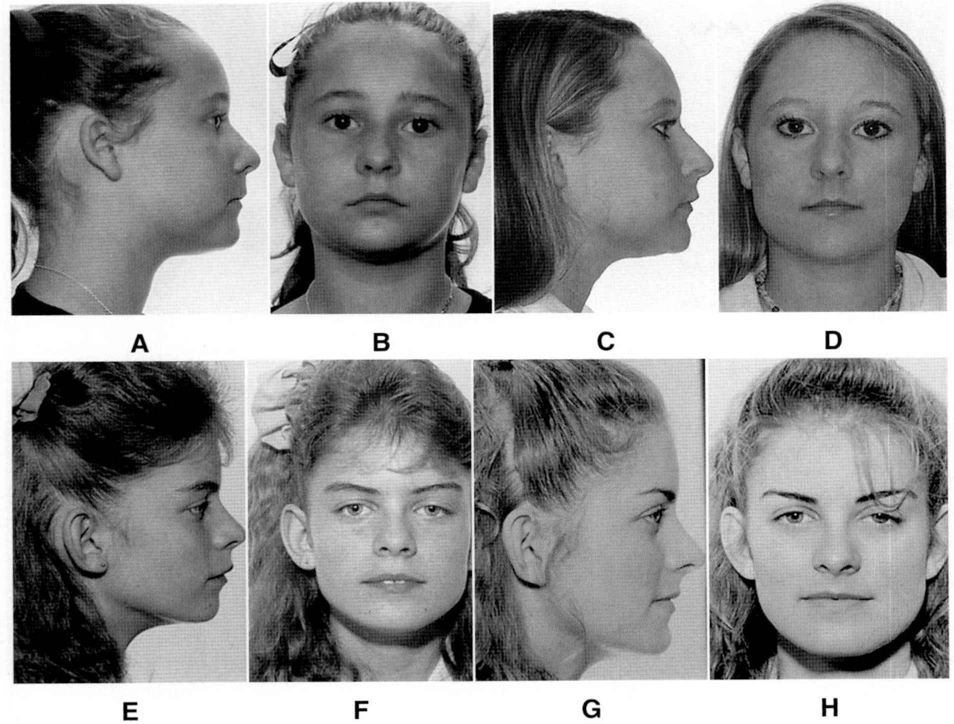

FIG 9-7 Patients who have Class II malocclusion but a fairly "strong" chin can achieve a more balanced face. Patient 1: **A** and **B,** Pretreatment photographs; **C** and **D,** Posttreatment photographs. Patient 2: **E** and **F,** Pretreatment photographs. **G** and **H,** Posttreatment photographs.

treatment. A patient who has a significant malocclusion but who has no serious skeletal convexity should have a very orthognathic profile after proper treatment (Fig. 9-8).

- **Adequate lip fullness—the lower lip should lie on the profile line**. A lower lip that is severely retruded or very "weak" lips will predispose a patient to poor facial esthetics. There is nothing an orthodontist can do about this problem because the patient has inherently poor lip structure.[32] On the other hand, a patient with more lip fullness will always have a more pleasing face if treated properly (Fig. 9-9).
- There should be a definite curl to the upper lip, which measures 3 to 5 mm in depth. Lower lip form and curl must be in harmony with upper lip form and curl (Fig. 9-10).[33]

8. What measurements allow the clinician to quantify or measure, a "good" face?

There are several ways to quantify a pleasing face. A very simple way is to draw a profile line on the face. The profile line is drawn from soft tissue chin and touches the most prominent lip (Fig. 9-11, *A* and *B*). If the profile line lies outside the nose, the patient has a protrusion. If the profile line is inside the tip of the nose, the patient generally has pleasing facial balance. Merrifield[34] used the profile line and suggested that the angle the profile line makes with Frankfort horizontal, called the Z angle, is an excellent way of quantifying facial balance.[35,36] A normal Z angle for a pleasing face is 72 to 78 degrees (Fig. 9-11, *C* and *D*). Reed Holdway[37] developed the Holdway angle, which he used to quantify facial balance. Steiner[38] developed a series of angles, which he also used to quantify facial balance (Fig. 9-12). Ricketts[39] used the facial esthetic line. He felt that a patient who had facial balance had lips that were approximately 4 mm inside a line drawn from soft tissue chin to the tip of the nose (Fig. 9-13).

9. What factors affect facial balance/facial harmony?

There are essentially three factors that influence facial balance or the lack thereof [14,40-43]:

1. The position of the teeth
2. The skeletal pattern
3. The soft tissue overlay

10. How do teeth affect facial balance?

Facial balance is affected by marked protrusion and/or crowding of the teeth or, conversely, by retrusion of the teeth. The upper lip rests on the upper two thirds of the labial surface of the maxillary incisors, and the lower lip is supported by the lower one third of the labial surface of the maxillary incisors; thus, lip protrusion or retrusion is a reflection of the position of maxillary incisors. Maxillary incisor position is, of course, directly related to the position of the mandibular incisors. Protruded teeth cause facial imbalance. Reduction of a protrusion improves facial balance (Fig. 9-14).[44-49]

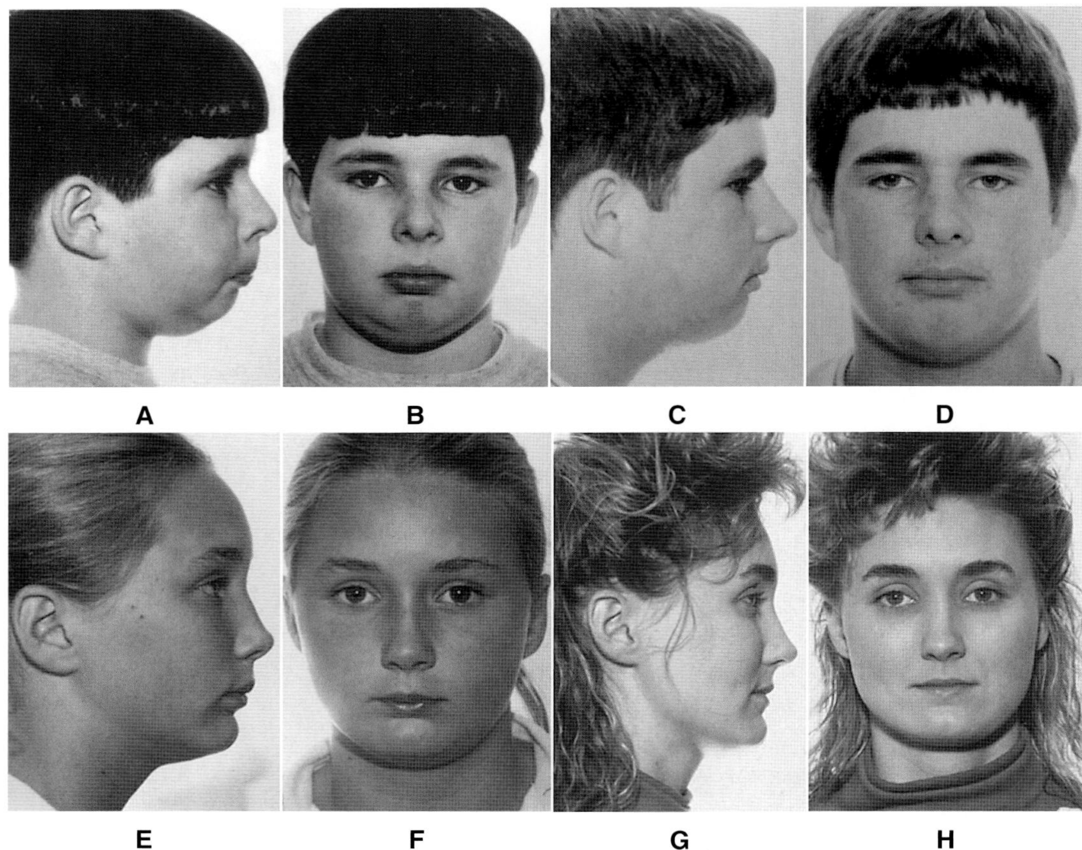

FIG 9-8 Patients who have a significant malocclusion but no serious skeletal convexity can achieve a very orthognathic profile. Patient 1: **A** and **B,** Pretreatment photographs; **C** and **D,** Posttreatment photographs. Patient 2: **E** and **F,** Pretreatment photographs; **G** and **H,** Posttreatment photographs.

11. What does a skeletal pattern have to do with facial balance?

The underlying theme that surfaces from all artists and orthodontic investigators is the concept that there cannot be good balance and harmony in the lower face unless the vertical dimension is within normal limits. The most important prerequisite for facial balance is normal vertical dimension of the lower face. Poulton[50] conducted a study on cervical traction and found that large lower anterior facial heights were most often associated with a displeasing face. In their article on soft-tissue profile preference, DeSmit and Dermaut[51] created three different series of nine profile photographs so that a total of more than 200 profiles could be ranked by graduate dental students. They found that differences in gender and orthodontic knowledge of the students seemed to have no significant influence on their esthetic preference. The results of their study confirmed the importance of anteroposterior deviations but suggest that unaesthetic facial profiles that were a result of anteroposterior deviations were completely overshadowed by long-face features—the long-face feature being more unaesthetic.

Before discussing the abnormal, it is prudent to understand the normal. The "ideal" face is vertically divided onto equal thirds by horizontal lines that approximate the hairline, the bridge of the nose, the ala of the nose, and menton (Fig. 9-15). These divisions of the face can be used by the clinician to help diagnose vertical dimension problems. For example, does a patient have a disproportionately long lower facial height because of vertical maxillary excess or because of excessive chin height?[52-57] Conversely, is a short facial height caused by vertical maxillary deficiency or by short chin height? By using these accepted proportions as a guide, the patient shown in Fig. 9-16, *A*, has an excessive lower anterior facial height, whereas the patient shown in Fig. 9-16, *B*, has diminished lower anterior facial height. A careful determination of the vertical proportions of the face is the first step in the diagnosis of a vertical dimension problem.

12. What part does soft tissue overlay or a maldistribution of soft tissue have on facial balance?

Facial disharmonies that are *not* the result of skeletal or dental distortion are generally the result of poor soft tissue distribution.[33,58] This problem needs to be identified during differential diagnosis and treatment planning so that needed dental compensations can be planned. The millimetric measurements of total chin thickness and upper lip thickness are essential components in any study of

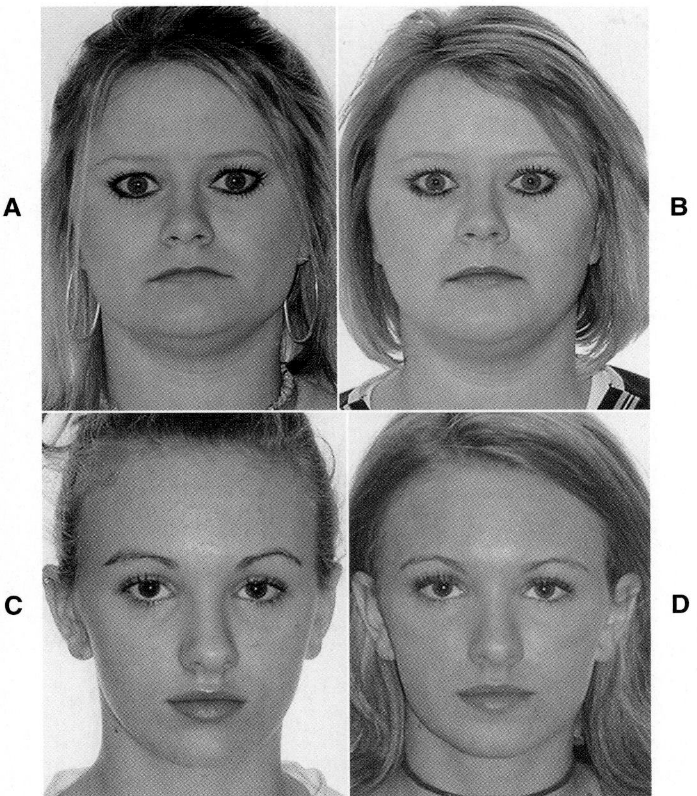

FIG 9-9 Patients with more lip fullness will achieve a more pleasing face. Patient 1: **A,** Pretreatment photograph. **B,** Posttreatment photograph. Patient 2: **C,** Pretreatment photograph. **D,** Posttreatment photograph.

facial balance. Upper lip thickness is measured from the greatest curvature of the labial surface of the maxillary central incisor to the vermilion border of the upper lip. The total chin thickness is measured horizontally from the NB (Nasion Pt. B) line extended to the soft tissue pogonion (Fig. 9-17). Total chin thickness should equal upper lip thickness. If it is less that upper lip thickness, the anterior teeth must be uprighted further to facilitate a more balanced facial profile because lip retraction follows tooth retraction.

THE SKELETAL COMPONENT

13. How does one begin to analyze the skeletal problem and its impact on a malocclusion?

For simplicity, the skeletal pattern analysis can be subdivided into three components: vertical, anteroposterior, and transverse. The skeletal patterns with which the clinician must deal are not only varied, they are multifactorial.

Like the discussion of the "face," it is prudent to discuss the skeletal component of the treatment planning process in categories. Again, books have been written about the subject. Many combinations of skeletal aberrations can exist.[59-61] These may include, but are not limited to, the following:

- **Maxilla:** maxillary posterior alveolar excess and inferiorly or superiorly positioned maxilla

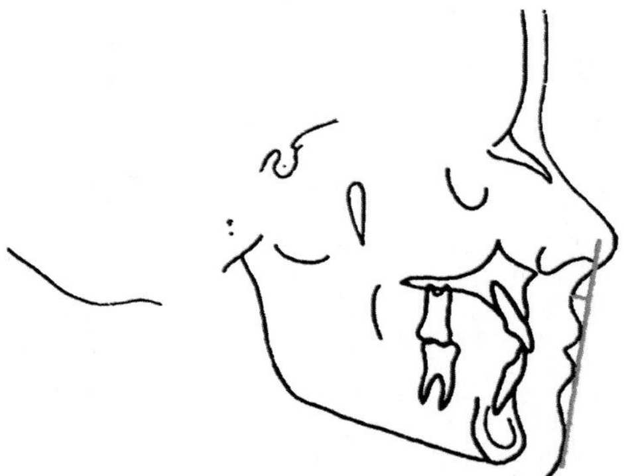

FIG 9-10 Upper lip thickness.

- **Mandible:** mandibular posterior alveolar excess and short/long mandibular rami

Other abnormalities may include superiorly positioned condylar fossa, obtuse cranial base angle, and condylar resorption.

Any of these conditions, with or without aberrant mandibular growth rotation, can be a causative factor in the skeletal discrepancy. It must also be understood that any malocclusion may present with a combination of skeletal problems. For example, a patient with a significantly increased or decreased anterior facial height may have an anteroposterior problem and/or a transverse problem.

THE VERTICAL COMPONENT OF THE SKELETAL PATTERN PUZZLE

14. What factors influence a skeletal pattern in the vertical plane?

There are several factors, but the two most significant ones seem to be condylar growth and dentoalveolar development.[62-67] The role of "environmental factors" like swallowing and tongue posture continue to be debated.

15. What does condylar growth have to do with the skeletal pattern and, ultimately, with treatment planning?

Mandibular growth and growth rotation can unfavorably impact dentoalveolar development in both the maxilla and mandible.[68] Bjork and Skieller[69] have performed numerous studies that have shown that the most common direction of condylar growth is vertical, with some anterior component. Patients with a pronounced short lower anterior facial height (Fig. 9-18, *A-C*) generally exhibit upward and forward condylar growth. These individuals generally have a deep vertical overbite with a deep mentolabial sulcus and a strong overclosed appearance. In contrast, patients with long-face syndrome (Fig. 9-18, *D-F*) have a more posteriorly directed growth pattern of the mandibular condyle. These backward growth rotators have increased anterior facial height, a more posterior position of the chin, and, in extreme cases, an anterior open bite may exist.[70]

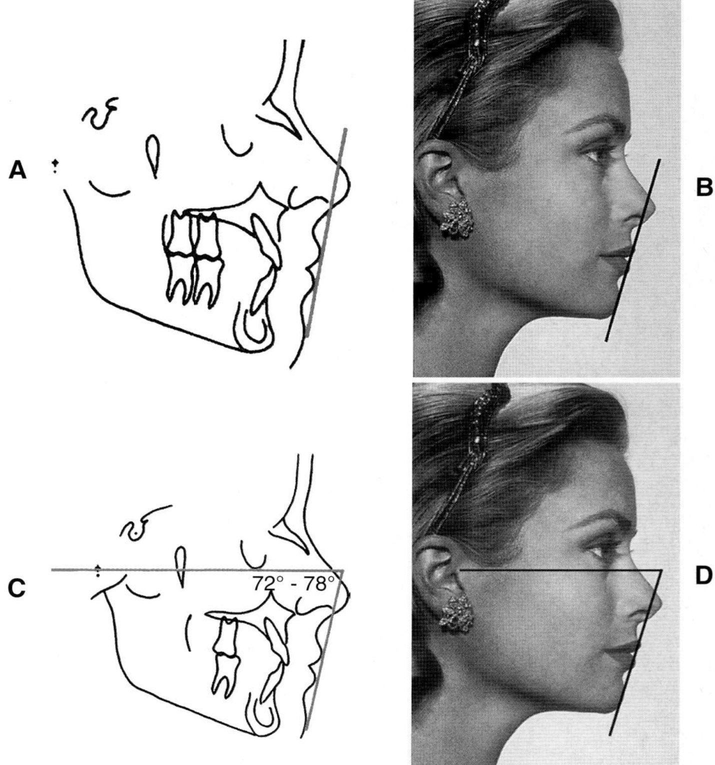

FIG 9-11 Profile line to nose, drawing **(A)** and photo **(B)**. Z angle, drawing **(C)** and photo **(D)**.

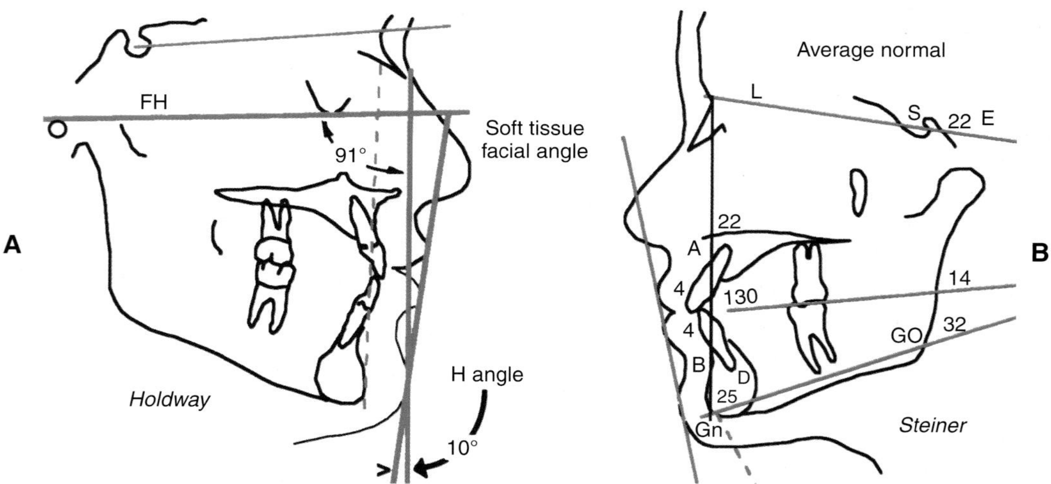

FIG 9-12 **A,** Holdway analysis. **B,** Steiner analysis.

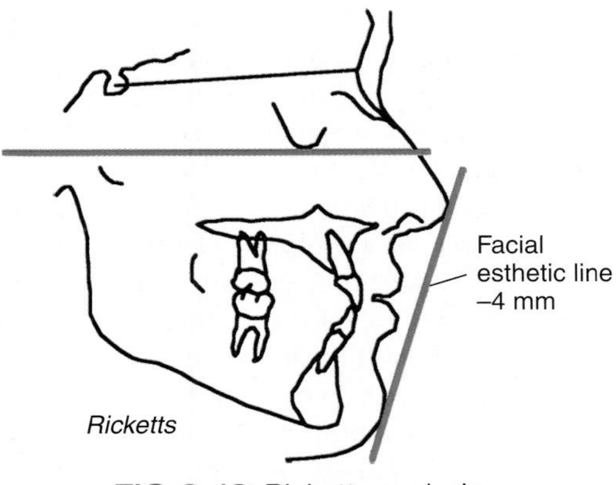

FIG 9-13 Ricketts analysis.

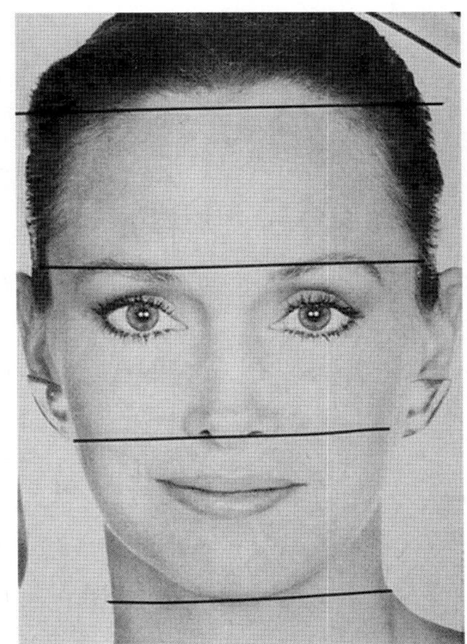

FIG 9-15 Divisions of the face.

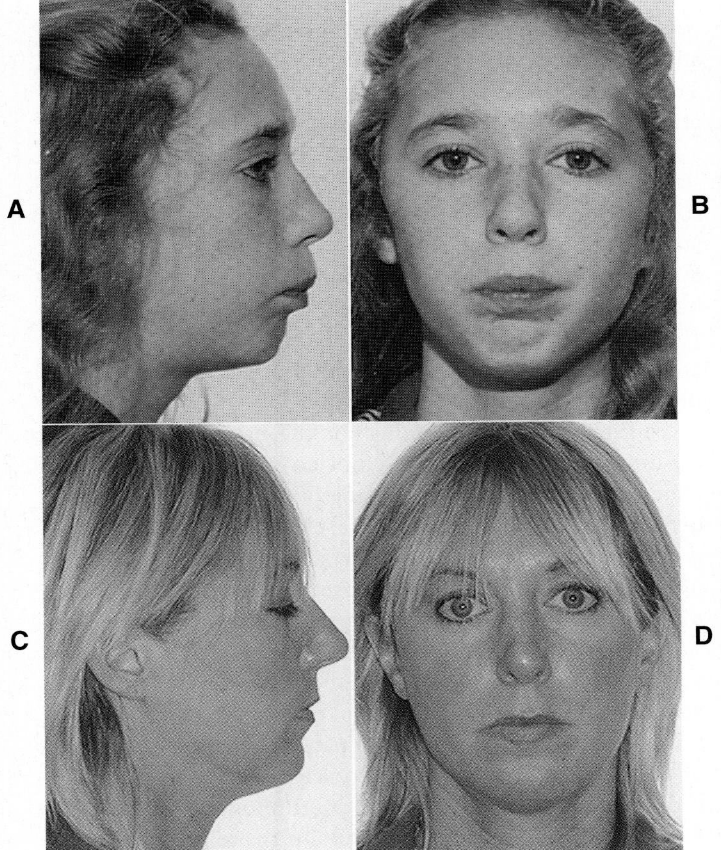

FIG 9-14 Reduction of a protrusion to improve facial balance. **A** and **B,** Pretreatment photos. **C** and **D,** Posttreatment photos.

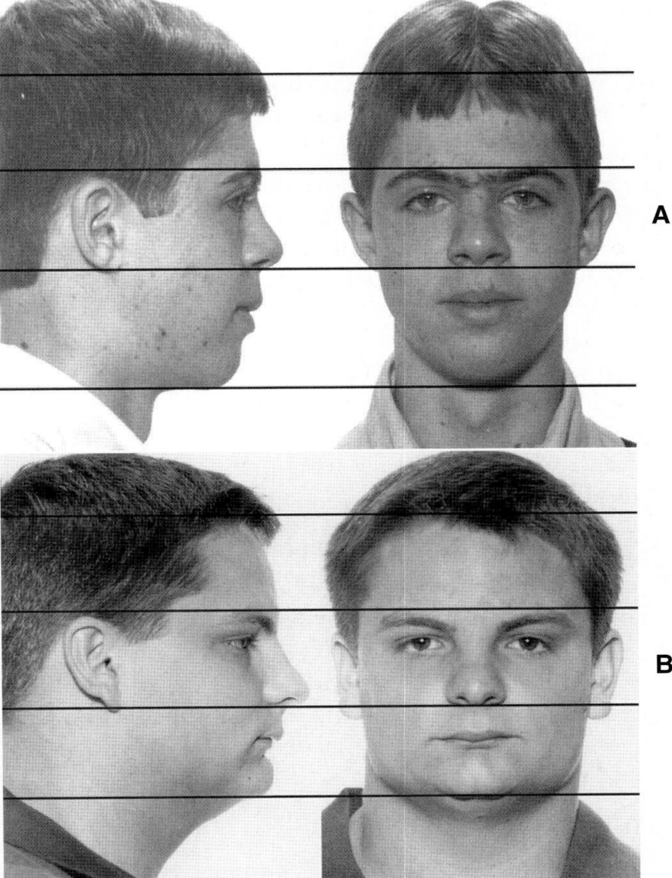

FIG 9-16 **A,** Excessive lower anterior facial height. **B,** Diminished lower anterior facial height.

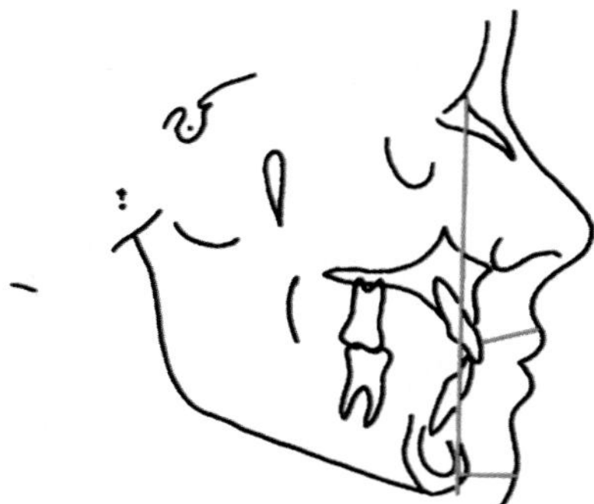

FIG 9-17 Soft-tissue thickness.

Isaacson et al.[71,72] and Schudy,[73] following Bjork's reports, studied jaw rotation caused by vertical condylar growth. A succinct summary of the findings of these investigators is that forward mandibular rotation occurs when vertical condylar growth exceeds the sum of the vertical growth of the maxillary sutures and the maxillary/mandibular alveolar processes. A backward rotation occurs, and the face becomes longer, when alveolar process growth exceeds condylar growth. An understanding of the effect of condylar growth on mandibular position is fundamental if the clinician is to adequately and appropriately diagnose a vertical dimension abnormality.

16. What role does dentoalveolar development have in the skeletal pattern scenario?

Isaacson et al.[72] studied dentoalveolar development in three groups of subjects: (1) those with short anterior facial height, (2) those with average anterior facial height, and (3) those with excessive anterior facial height. In patients with long anterior facial height, the mean distance from the occlusal plane to the inferior edge of the palate was 22.50 mm. This distance decreased to 19.6 mm for the average group and 17.1 mm for the group with short anterior facial height (low MP-SN angles). This difference of 5.1 mm of dentoalveolar development between the high-angle and low-angle groups is of no small significance when the vertically compromised skeletal pattern is studied.

17. As one considers the skeletal problems during the treatment planning process, is the role of environmental factors clear? How should these factors be assessed?

The role of tongue posture, swallowing, and breathing is a subject of debate, argument, and study in orthodontics. Their respective impact on the vertical dimension is in need of continued study and research.

MOUTH BREATHING

The relationship between mouth-breathing, altered mandibular posture, and the development of malocclusion is not as clear cut as the theoretical outcome of shifting to oral respiration might appear at first glance. Airway problems, such as large adenoids, tonsils, or blocked airways caused by septum deviations, large conchae, or allergies, are frequently observed in high-angle patients and may affect mandibular posture, allowing more freedom for posterior eruption. This hypothesis is supported by Linder-Aronson,[74] who showed closing of the mandibular plane angle and reduction in the anterior face height after removal of adenoids and tonsillectomy. Recent experimental studies have only partially clarified the situation. Current experimental data for the relationship between malocclusion and mouth-breathing are derived from studies of the nasal/oral ratio in normal versus long-face children. The data from the study show that both normal and long-face children are likely to be predominantly nasal breathers *under laboratory conditions*.[75,76]

In conclusion, it appears that mouth-breathing may contribute to the development of orthodontic problems but is difficult to indict as a primary etiologic agent. Clinically, most orthodontists refer mouth-breathers to an otolaryngologist for an evaluation. This problem should be evaluated carefully during the diagnosis of a patient with excess vertical dimension.

SWALLOWING AND TONGUE POSTURE

Many clinicians believe that if a patient has a forward resting posture of the tongue, the duration of this pressure, even if very light, could affect tooth position vertically or horizontally. Tongue-tip protrusion during swallowing is sometimes associated with a forward tongue posture.[77]

Others argue that tongue thrust swallowing simply has too short a duration to have an impact on tooth position. Pressure by the tongue against the teeth during a typical swallow lasts for approximately 1 second. A typical individual swallows 800 times per day while awake but has only a few swallows per hour while asleep. The total per day, therefore, is usually under 1000. One thousand seconds of pressure, of course, totals only a few minutes—not nearly enough time, it is argued, to affect the equilibrium.

During treatment planning for the patient with a vertical dimension problem, the clinician must understand that condylar growth, sutural lowering of the maxillary complex, dentoalveolar development, dental eruption, and the patient's oral environment/habits are interrelated. There is generally not a single causative factor that predisposes the patient to too much or too little vertical development of lower facial height. To simplify, one might conclude as a general rule that when vertical condylar growth exceeds tooth eruption (alveolar development), forward mandibular rotation occurs. The result is increased posterior facial height and an increase in the ratio of posterior facial height to anterior facial height. Conversely, if dentoalveolar growth and tooth eruption are greater than vertical condylar growth, the resultant mandibular change is backward rotation. The anterior facial height/posterior facial height ratio decreases. Environmental factors can play a role, but the role is, at times, difficult to assess and varies from patient to patient.

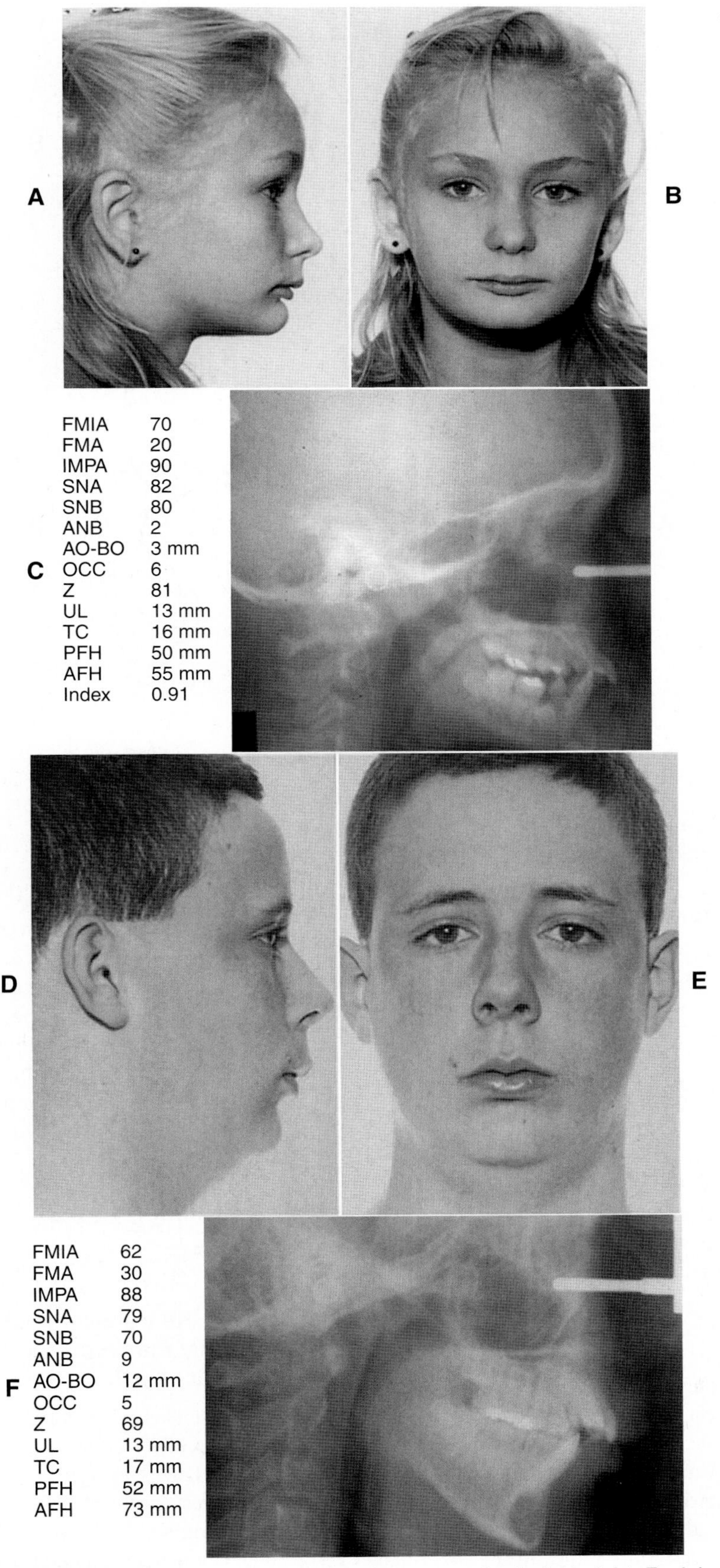

A
B
C
FMIA 70
FMA 20
IMPA 90
SNA 82
SNB 80
ANB 2
AO-BO 3 mm
OCC 6
Z 81
UL 13 mm
TC 16 mm
PFH 50 mm
AFH 55 mm
Index 0.91
D
E
F
FMIA 62
FMA 30
IMPA 88
SNA 79
SNB 70
ANB 9
AO-BO 12 mm
OCC 5
Z 69
UL 13 mm
TC 17 mm
PFH 52 mm
AFH 73 mm

FIG 9-18 **A-C,** Patient with pronounced short lower anterior facial height. Facial photos **(A** and **B)** and cephalogram and numbers **(C)**. **D-F,** Patient with long-face syndrome. Facial photos **(D** and **E)** and cephalogram and numbers **(F)**.

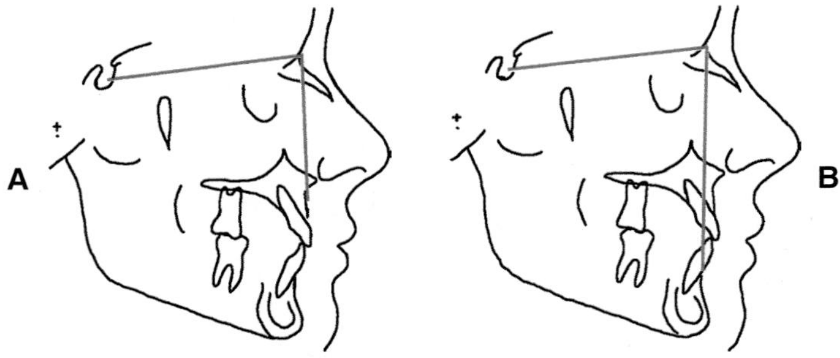

FIG 9-19 **A,** SNA. **B,** SNB.

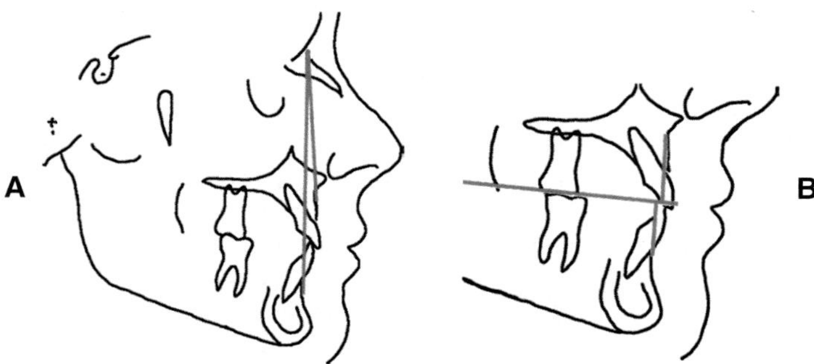

FIG 9-20 **A,** ANB. **B,** AO-BO.

THE ANTEROPOSTERIOR COMPONENT OF THE SKELETAL PATTERN

18. How can anteroposterior skeletal problems be assessed?

Several cephalometric values can be used. The most common follow:

SNA—This angular value gives guidance in determining the relative horizontal position of the maxilla to cranial base. A range of 80 to 84 degrees is normal at the end of growth and development.[78]

SNB—This value expresses the horizontal relationship of the mandible to the cranial base, and a range of 78 to 82 degrees indicates normal horizontal mandibular position.[78] If the value is below 74 degrees, it might indicate that orthognathic surgery would be a valuable adjunct to treatment. The same concern should be accorded a value of over 84 degrees (Fig. 9-19).

ANB—The normal range is 1 to 5 degrees. This significant value expresses a direct horizontal relationship of the maxilla to the mandible.[79] As the Class II malocclusion becomes proportionally more difficult, the higher the ANB. An ANB above 10 degrees usually indicates that surgery should be a possible adjunct to treatment. A negative ANB value is perhaps even more indicative of horizontal facial disproportion. For example, an ANB of –3 degrees or more, if the mandible is in its true position, should indicate careful monitoring with the possibility of surgical assistance for Class III correction.[78,79]

AO/BO—The relationship will verify the horizontal relationship of the maxilla to the mandible. It is perhaps more sensitive to malrelationships than ANB because it is measured along the occlusal plane.[80-82] Treatment becomes more difficult if the value is outside the normal range of 0 to 4 mm. AO/BO is affected by the steepness or flatness of the occlusal plane, since the measurement is made from a perpendicular to occlusal plane from Point A and Point B (Fig. 9-20).

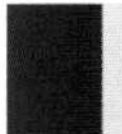

THE TRANSVERSE COMPONENT OF THE SKELETAL PATTERN

19. How is the transverse skeletal problem generally manifest—or more simply stated, how is it seen?

The transverse skeletal problem is most often seen when the dentition is carefully examined. A patient who has a very high mandibular plane angle (i.e., a hyperdivergent skeletal pattern) will, if a transverse problem exists, exhibit posterior crossbites (Fig. 9-21, *A-C*). Conversely, a patient who has a very low mandibular plane angle—the hypodivergent patient—will have a bypass bite, commonly referred to as a "Brodie bite" (Fig. 9-21, *D-F*).

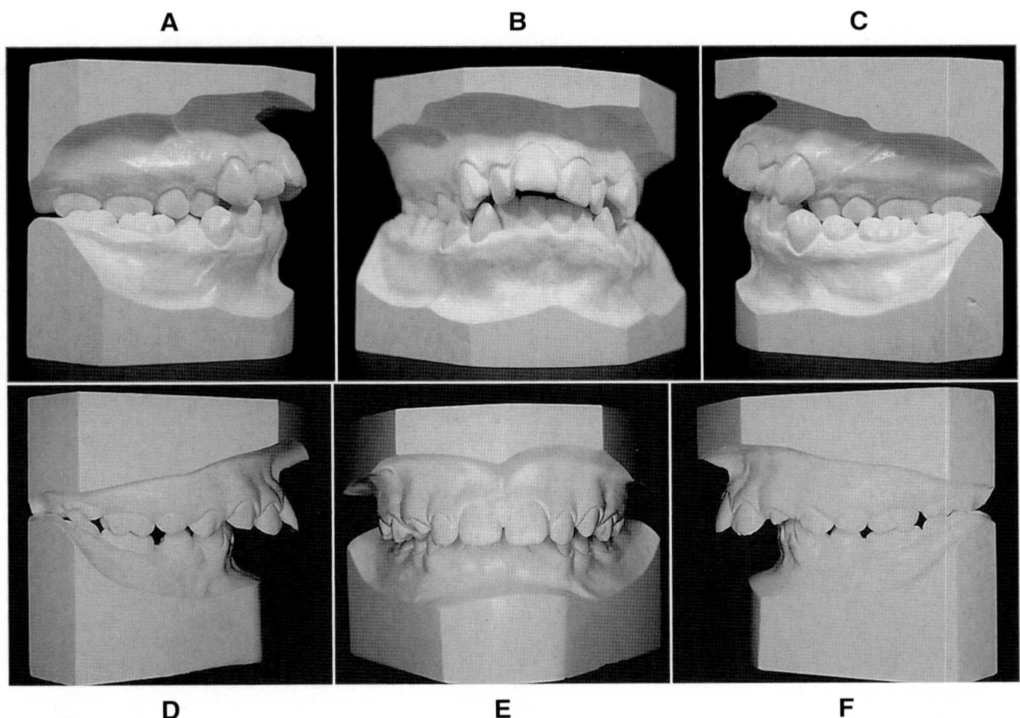

FIG 9-21 **A-C,** Posterior crossbites are seen on these pretreatment casts. **D-F,** A "Brodie bite" is seen on these pretreatment casts.

THE DENTITION

20. How can the dentition and space for the teeth or lack thereof be evaluated carefully?

For most patients, a dental disharmony is manageable. To correctly diagnose the dental problem, a careful dentition space analysis and a study of the occlusal relationships is essential. The dentition is divided into three areas: anterior, midarch, and posterior. This division is made for two reasons: simplicity in identifying the area of space deficit or space surplus, and the possibility of arriving at a more accurate differential diagnosis.[14,83]

ANTERIOR SPACE ANALYSIS

The anterior space analysis includes the difference in millimeters between the space available in the mandibular arch from the distal of the contralateral canines and the mesiodistal widths of all the six anterior teeth. Essentially, the space available is measured (Fig. 9-22, *A-C*). Space required is measured (Fig. 9-22, *D-I*). The difference between these measured values is referred to as a *surplus* or a *deficit.*

A head-film discrepancy, or a calculation of how much space is necessary for mandibular incisor uprighting, must be added to the anterior space surplus or deficit. *Cephalometric discrepancy* is a term that originated with Charles Tweed.[84] He studied the cephalograms of 37 consecutively treated patients and integrated his findings with those of Brodie, Downs, and B. Holly Broadbent. He found that the patients who exhibited pleasing facial esthetics had an Frankfort mandibular incisor angle (FMIA) between 62 and 70 degrees, no matter what their Frankfort mandibular plan angle (FMA). This led Tweed to propose his formula for cephalometric correction (mandibular incisor uprighting) to arrive at a favorable FMIA for each patient. Tweed's formula is as follows:

FMA 21 to 29 degrees: FMIA should be 68 degrees
FMA 30 degrees or greater: FMIA should be 65 degrees
FMA 20 degrees or less: IMPA should not exceed 92 degrees

Tweed measured his cephalometric correction on an x-ray by doing the following:

> A lateral head plate is made of the patient and the triangle is drawn on the head plate with white ink. A dotted line starting at the apex of the mandibular incisor is drawn upward to intercept the Frankfort plane at an angle of 65° The distance between the solid line, which is the existing inclination of the mandibular incisor, and the dotted line, which is the desired incisal inclination (measured at the incisal edge of the mandibular incisor), is the distance in millimeters that the mandibular incisors must be tipped lingually to satisfy the minimum requirement for an FMIA of 65°.

The number of millimeters from the desired position of the mandibular incisor edge to the actual position of the mandibular incisor edge is multiplied by 2 because both sides of the arch have to be considered (Fig. 9-23).

The sum of the anterior tooth arch surplus or deficit and the cephalometric discrepancy is referred to as the *anterior discrepancy.*

MIDARCH SPACE ANALYSIS

The midarch area includes the mandibular first molars, the second premolars, and the first premolars. Careful analysis of this area can show mesially inclined first molars, rotations,

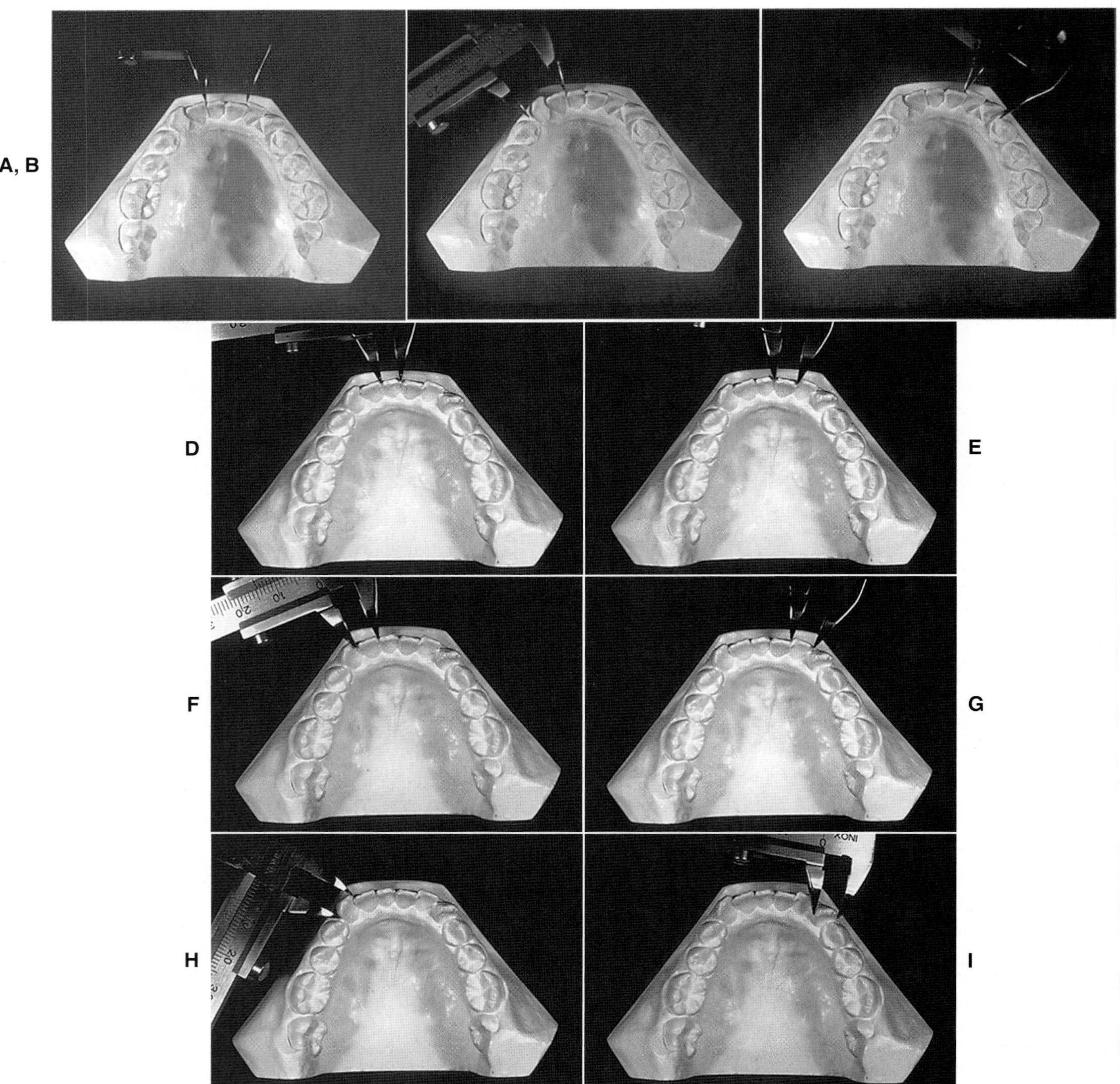

FIG 9-22 Anterior space analysis. **A-C,** Measurement of anterior space available. **D-I,** Measurement of space required.

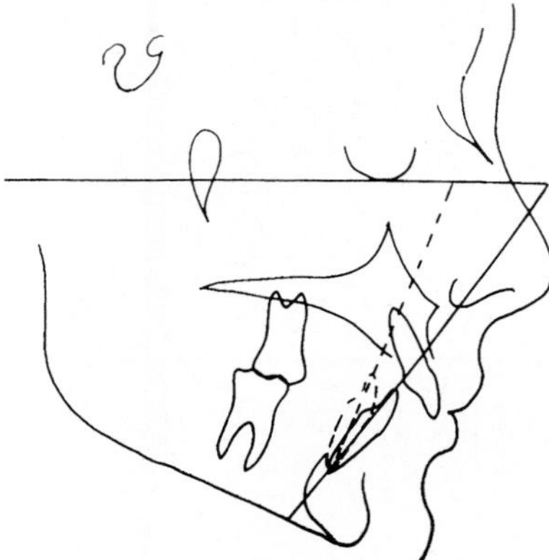

FIG 9-23 Calculation of cephalometric discrepancy.

spaces, a deep curve of Spee, cross bites, missing teeth, habit abnormality, blocked-out teeth, and occlusal disharmonies. This is an extremely important area of the dentition because it allows for space management for posterior malocclusion correction. A careful measurement of the space from the distal of the canine to the distal of the first molars should be recorded as available midarch space (Fig. 9-24, *A* and *B*). An equally accurate measurement of the mesiodistal widths of the first premolar, the second premolar, and the first molar should also be recorded (Fig. 9-24, *C-H*). The lesser value is subtracted from the greater value. To the space surplus or deficit is added space required to level the curve of Spee. To calculate the amount of space required to level the curve of Spee, the greatest depth of the curve is measured on both sides (Fig. 9-24, *I*), the values are summed, and then the sum is divided by two.[85] From these space analysis and curve of spree measurements, one can determine the total space deficit or surplus in the midarch area.

Although not a part of the actual midarch space analysis, occlusal disharmony, a Class II or Class III buccal segment relationship, must be measured because an occlusal disharmony adds a great deal to the difficulty of correction of any malocclusion and requires a careful treatment strategy.

Occlusal disharmony is measured by articulating the casts and using the maxillary first premolar cusp as a reference.[86] The clinician should measure mesially or distally from the maxillary first premolar buccal cusp to the embrasure between the mandibular first and second premolars. This measurement is made on both sides and is then averaged to determine the occlusal disharmony (Fig. 9-25). During the treatment planning process, it must be remembered that movement of the posterior teeth requires space management.

POSTERIOR SPACE ANALYSIS

This area of the dentition has great importance. Before any measurement of posterior space can be made, it must be understood that there is a posterior limit of the dentition. Rarely are healthy functioning mandibular teeth located posterior to the anterior border of the ramus. Regardless of age, the anterior border of the ramus appears to be the posterior limit of the dentition.

The required space is the sum of the mesiodistal widths of the mandibular second molars and third molars (Fig. 9-26, *A-C*). The available space is more difficult to ascertain on the immature patient. It is:

- A measurement in millimeters of the space distal to the mandibular first molar, along the occlusal plane, to the anterior border of the ramus (Fig. 9-26, *D*)
- An estimate of posterior arch length increase based on both age and sex

A literature study suggests that 3 mm of increase occurs per year until age 14 for girls and until age 16 for boys.[87-89] This would be 1.5 mm of increase on each side each year after the full eruption on the mandibular first molars. In mature patients, girls over 14 years old and boys over 16 years old, one can measure from the distal of the first molar to the anterior border of the ramus at the level of the occlusal plane and have an accurate determination of the space available in the posterior area. It is of extreme importance in diagnosis and treatment planning to know whether there is a space surplus or deficit in this area. The orthodontist should not create severe posterior discrepancies while making adjustments in the midarch and anterior arch deficits.

21. How can information assembled by a careful study of the facial, skeletal, and dental components of a malocclusion be "assimilated" so that it can be used during the treatment planning process?

The answer is simple and yet very complex. First, analyze the face. Does the face need to be changed? If so, why? Is the problem skeletal, dental, or both? If it is skeletal, can orthodontics alone change it? Probably not. To change it will require a surgical procedure. Is there a dental protrusion? If the face is protruded, but the skeletal pattern is normal and the teeth are crooked and protruded, one can favorably change the face by extracting teeth. Is there dental retrusion? If the skeletal pattern is hypodivergent and the face is "flat," facial change will be much more difficult. Suffice it to say that as a general rule, a rule to which there are always exceptions, the following concepts are very applicable to treatment planning:

- The more hyperdivergent the face and the skeletal pattern, the more mandibular incisors need to be upright in order to achieve facial balance. If there is any crowding at all, teeth must be extracted if a facial change is desired. The teeth that are extracted must be determined by the amount of crowding, the status of the dentition, the soft tissue overlay, and the amount of anteroposterior problem that exists.
- The more hypodivergent the skeletal pattern and the face, the more mandibular incisors need to remain in their pretreatment positions. Mandibular incisor uprighting will generally harm the facial esthetics of these patients. However, these patients, if severe crowding is present, must not be treatment planned so that the mandibular teeth are proclined from their original positions. Proclination of the teeth has deleterious effects on both the face and the stability of the teeth.[90-93]

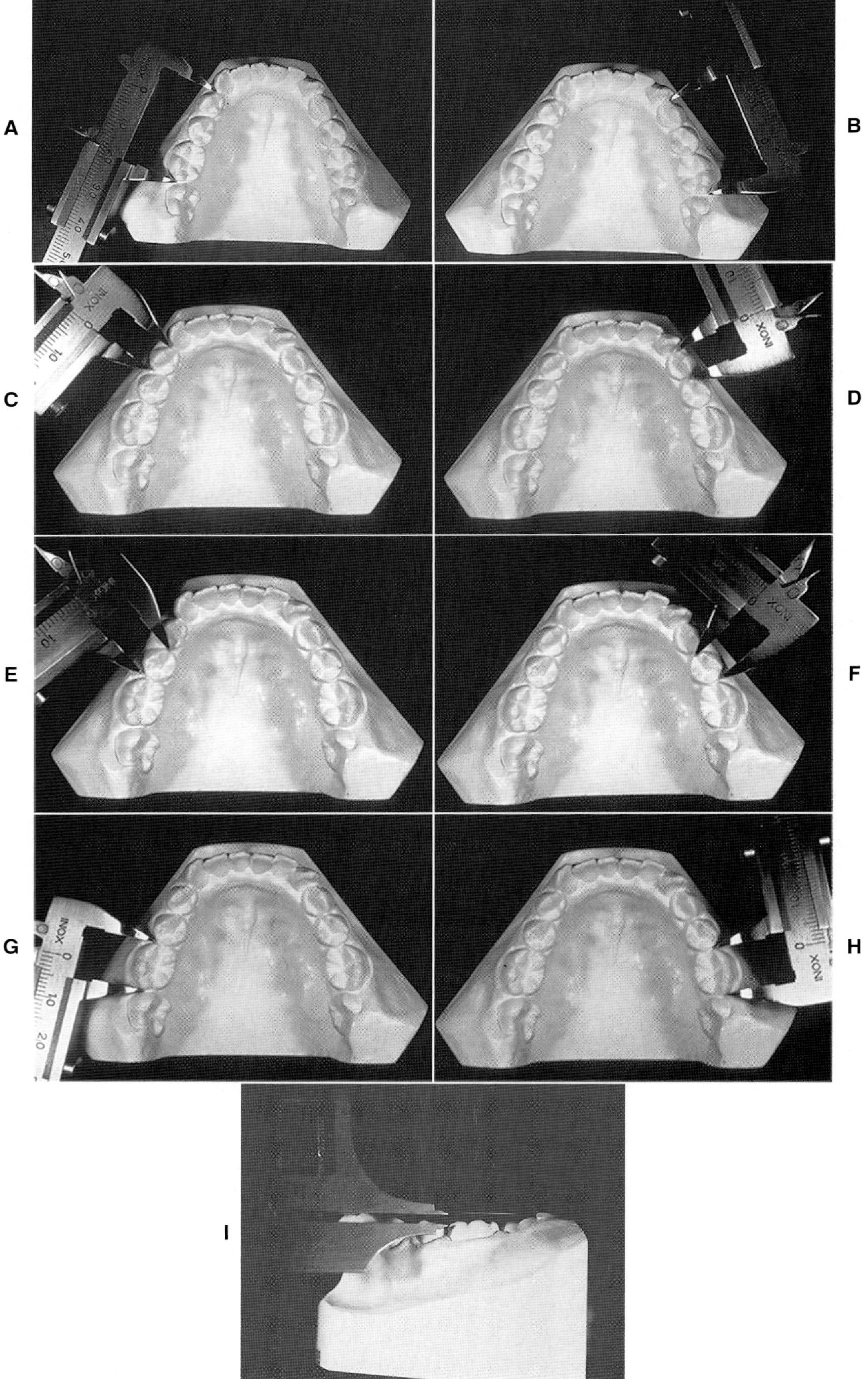

FIG 9-24 Midarch space analysis. **A** and **B,** Midarch space available. **C-H,** Midarch space required. **I,** Measurement of depth of curve of Spee.

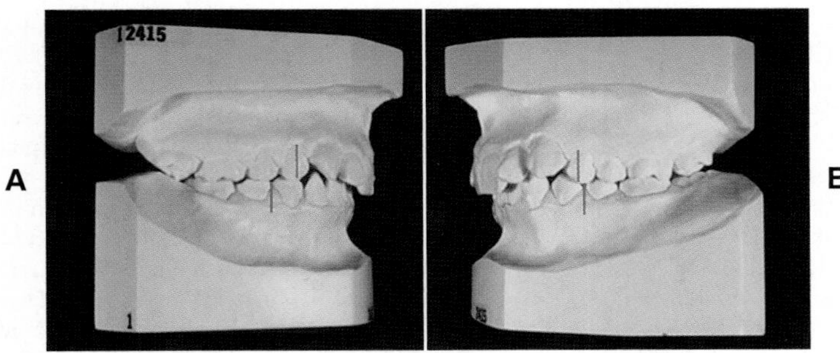

FIG 9-25 **A** and **B,** Class II measurement.

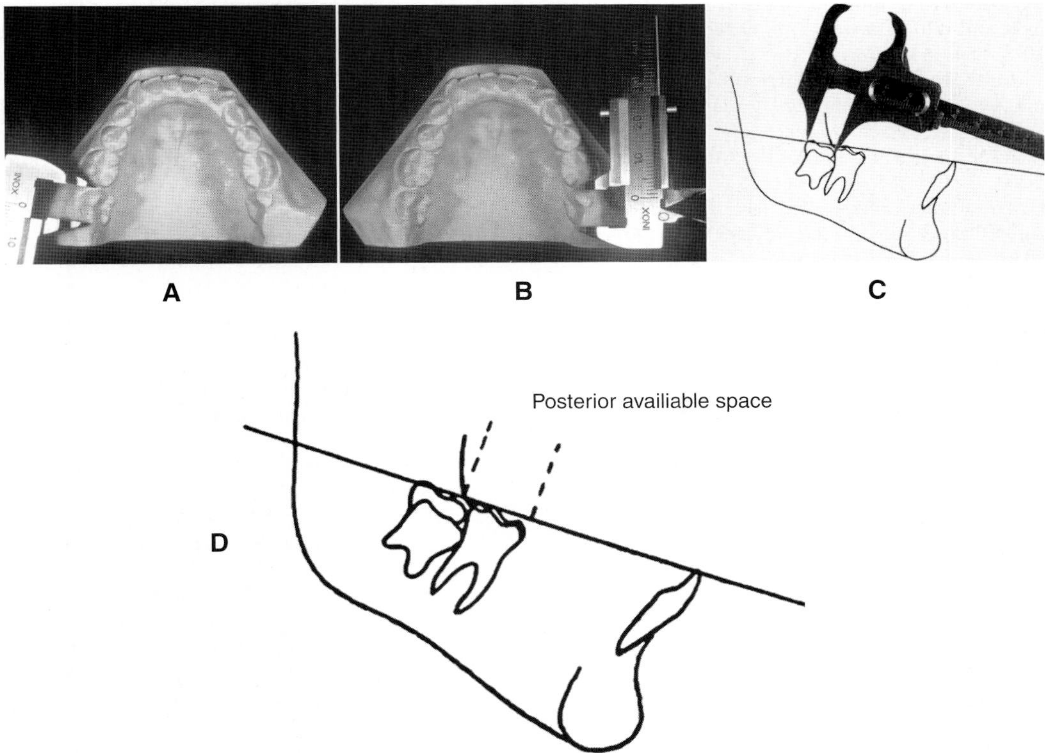

FIG 9-26 Posterior space analysis. **A-C,** Posterior dentition required space. **D,** Posterior space available.

Treatment planning is a very complex process. A multiplicity of factors must be considered. For this reason, it is essential to organize the process by studying the face, the skeletal pattern, and finally the teeth. The interrelationship of all these must be understood in order for a viable treatment plan to be developed.[94-98]

REFERENCES

1. Gianelly A: Evidence-based therapy: an orthodontic dilemma. *Am J Orthod Dentofacial Orthop* 2006;129(5):596-598.
2. Johnston LE Jr: The value of information and the cost of uncertainty: who pays the bill?. *Angle Orthod* 1998;68(2)(99):101-102.
3. Lee R, MacFarlane T, O'Brien K: Consistency of orthodontic treatment planning decisions. *Clin Orthod Res* 1999;2(2):79-84.
4. Curtis DA, Lacy A, Chu R, et al: Treatment planning in the 21st century: what's new?. *Calif Dent Assoc* 2002;30(7):503-510.
5. Huang GJ: Making the case for evidence-based orthodontics. *Am J Orthod Dentofacial Orthop* 2004;125(4):405-406.
6. Sagehorn EG: Competency—that elusive quality. *Am J Orthod* 1980;78(3):341-345.
7. Ackerman M: Evidence based orthodontics for the 21st century. *J Am Dent Assoc* 2004;135(2):162-167.
8. Bass NM: From treatment planning to treatment results: the luck of the draw? *Am J Orthod Dentofacial Orthop* 2000;118(2):142-149.
9. Graber TM: Pride in orthodontics. *Am J Orthod Dentofacial Orthop* 2000;117(5):618-620.

10. Labarrere H: To extract or not to extract: is that the right question? *J Clin Orthod* 2004;38(2):63-78.
11. Roberts-Harry D, Sandy J: Orthodontics. Part 4: Treatment planning. *Br Dent J* 2003;195(12):683-685.
12. Vaden JL, Kiser HE: Straight talk about extraction and non-extraction: a differential diagnostic decision. *Am J Orthod Dentofacial Orthop* 1996;109(4):445-452.
13. Merrifield LL: The dimensions of the denture: back to basics. *Am J Orthod Dentofacial Orthop* 1994;106(11):535-542.
14. Merrifield LL: Differential diagnosis. *Semin Orthod* 1996;2(4):241-253.
15. Merrifield LL, Cross JJ: Directional force. *Am J Orthod* 1970;57(5):435-464.
16. Joondeph DR: Retention and relapse. In: Graber TM, Vanarsda RL, Vig KWL, eds. *Orthodontics: current principles & techniques*, edition 4. St Louis: Elsevier; 2005.
17. Merrifield LL, Gebeck TR: Orthodontic diagnosis and treatment analysis: concepts and values, part II. *Am J Orthod Dentofacial Orthop* 1995;107(5):541-547.
18. Merrifield LL, Klontz HA, Vaden JL: Differential diagnostic analysis systems. *Am J Orthod Dentofacial Orthop* 1994;106(12): 641-648.
19. Bowman SJ: Facial aesthetics in orthodontics. *Aust Orthod J* 2001;17(3):17-26.
20. Peck S, Peck H: The aesthetically pleasing face: an orthodontic myth. *Trans Europ Orthod Soc* 1971;47:175-185.
21. Riggio RF, Widamann KF, Tucker JS, Salinas C: Beauty is more than skin deep: components of attractiveness. *Basic Appl Soc Psychol* 1991;12(1):423-439.
22. Angle EH: *The treatment of malocclusion of the teeth*, edition 7. Philadelphia: SS White; 1907.
23. Langlois JH, Roggman LA, Musselman L: What is average and what is not average about attractive faces. *Psychol Sci* 1994;5: 214-220.
24. McNamara JA Jr, Brust EW, Riolo ML: Soft tissue evaluation of individuals with an ideal occlusion and a well-balanced face. In: McNamara JA Jr, ed. *Esthetics and the treatment of facial form, vol 28, Craniofacial Growth Series*, Ann Arbor: Center for Human Growth and Development, University of Michigan; 1993.
25. Olds C: Facial beauty in Western art. In: McNamara JA Jr, ed. *Esthetics and the treatment of facial form, vol 28, Craniofacial Growth Series*, Ann Arbor: Center for Human Growth and Development, University of Michigan; 1993.
26. Peck H, Peck S: A concept of facial esthetics. *Angle Orthod* 1970;40:284-317.
27. Klontz HA: Facial balance and harmony: an attainable objective for the patient with a high mandibular plane angle. *Am J Orthod Dentofacial Orthop* 1998;114:176-188.
28. Pearson LE: The management of vertical dimension problems in growing patients, the enigma of the vertical dimension. In: McNamara JA Jr, ed. *Craniofacial Growth Series 36*, Ann Arbor: Center for Human Growth and Development, University of Michigan; 2000.
29. Tweed CH: Indications for the extraction of teeth in orthodontic procedure. *Am J Orthod* 1994;30:405-428.
30. Vaden JL: Alternative nonsurgical strategies to treat complex orthodontic problems. *Semin Orthod* 1996;2:90-113.
31. Wylie WL, Johnson EL: Rapid evaluation of facial dysplasia in the vertical plane. *Angle Orthod* 1952;22(3):165-182.
32. Satravaha S, Schlegel KD: The significance of the integumentary profile. *Am J Orthod Dentofacial Orthop* 1987;92:422-426.
33. Burstone CJ: Lip posture and its significance in treatment planning. *Am J Orthod* 1967;53:262-284.
34. Merrifield LL: The profile line as an aid in critically evaluating facial esthetics. *Am J Orthod* 1966;52:804-821.
35. Jacobs JD: Vertical lip changes from maxillary incisor retraction. *Am J Orthod* 1978;74:396-404.
36. Hulsey CM: An esthetic evaluation of lip-teeth relationships present in the smile. *Am J Orthod* 1970;57:132-144.
37. Holdway RA: A soft tissue analysis and its use in orthodontic treatment planning: Part I. *Am J Orthod* 1983;84:1-28.
38. Steiner C: Cephalometrics in clinical practice. *Angle Orthod* 1959;29(1):8-29.
39. Ricketts RM: Perspectives in the clinical application of cephalometrics. *Angle Orthod* 1981;51(2):115-150.
40. Czarnecki ST, Nanda R, Currier F: Perceptions of a balanced facial profile. *Am J Orthod Dentofacial Orthop* 1993;104:180-187.
41. Herzberg BL: Facial esthetics in relation to orthodontic treatment. *Angle Orthod* 1952;22(1):3-22.
42. Ricketts RM: Divine proportions in facial esthetics. *Clin Plastic Surg* 1982;9:401-422.
43. Steiner CC: Cephalometrics for you and me. *Am J Orthod* 1953;39:729-755.
44. Angle EH: *The treatment of malocclusion of the teeth and fractures of the maxillae*, edition 6. Philadelphia: SS White; 1900.
45. Vaden JL, Dale JG, Klontz HK: The Tweed Merrifield Edgewise Appliance: philosophy, diagnosis and treatment. In: Graber TM, Vanarsda RL, Vig KWL, eds. *Orthodontics: current principles & techniques*, edition 4. St Louis: Elsevier; 2005.
46. Tweed CH: A philosophy of orthodontic treatment. *Am J Orthod Oral Surg* 1945;31(2):74-103.
47. Tweed CH: *Clinical orthodontics, vols. 1 and 2*, St Louis: Mosby; 1966.
48. Tweed CH: The application of the principles of the edgewise arch in the treatment of Class II, Division 1, Part II. *Angle Orthod* 1936;6(4):255-257.
49. Tweed CH: The Frankfort mandibular incisor angle (FMIA) in orthodontic diagnosis, treatment planning and prognosis. *Am J Orthod Oral Surg* 1954;24:121-169.
50. Poulton DR: The influence of extraoral traction. *Am J Orthod* 1967;53:8-18.
51. DeSmit A, Dermaut L: Soft-tissue profile preference. *Am J Orthod* 1984;86:67-73.
52. Fields HW, Proffitt WR, Nixon WL, et al: Facial pattern differences in long face children and adults. *Am J Orthod* 1984;85: 217-223.
53. Isaacson JR, Isaacson RJ, Speidel TM, et al: Extreme variation in vertical facial growth and associated variation in skeletal and dental relations. *Angle Orthod* 1971;41:219-229.
54. Pearson LE: Vertical control in treatment or patients having backward rotational growth tendencies. *Angle Orthod* 1978;43:132.
55. Pearson LE: Vertical control. In fully-banded orthodontic treatment. *Angle Orthod* 1986;56:205.
56. Peck S, Peck L, Kataja M: The gingival smile line. *Angle Orthod* 1992;62:91-100.
57. Schendel SA, Eisenfeld J, Bell WH, et al: The long face syndrome: vertical maxillary excess. *Am J Orthod* 1976;70:398-408.
58. Burstone CJ: The integumental contour and extension patterns. *Angle Orthod* 1950;29:93.
59. Bjork A: Facial growth in man, studied with the aid of metallic implants. *Acta Odontol Scand* 1955;13:9-34.
60. Bjork A: Variations in the growth pattern of the human mandible: longitudinal cephalometric study by the implant method. *J Dent Res* 1963;400-411.
61. Sarver D, Proffit W, Ackerman J: Diagnosis and treatment planning in orthodontics. In: Graber TM, Vanarsdall RL, eds. *Current principles and techniques*, edition 3. St Louis: Mosby; 2000.
62. Bjork A: Sutural growth of the upper face studied by the implant method. *Acta Odontol Scand* 1966;24:109-129.
63. Bjork A: The use of metallic implants in the study of facial growth in children, method and application. *Am J Phys Anthropol* 1968;29:243-254.

64. Neilsen IL: Vertical malocclusions: etiology, development, diagnosis and some aspects of treatment. *Angle Orthod* 1978;48: 130-140.
65. Schudy FF: Vertical growth vs. anteroposterior growth as related to function and treatment. *Angle Orthod* 1964;24:75-93.
66. Skieller V: Cephalometric analysis in the treatment of overbite. *Rep Congr Eur Orthod Soc* 1967;147-157.
67. Vaden JL, Pearson LE: Diagnosis of the vertical dimension. *Semin Orthod* 2002;8(9):120-129.
68. Bjork A: Prediction of mandibular growth rotation. *Am J Orthod* 1969;55:585-599.
69. Bjork A, Skieller V: Normal and abnormal growth of the mandible: a synthesis of longitudinal cephalometric implant studies over a period of 25 years. *Eur J Orthod* 1983;5:1-46.
70. Proffit WM: The development of orthodontic problems. In: Proffit WM, Fields HW, eds. *Contemporary orthodontics*, St Louis: Mosby; 2000.
71. Isaacson RJ: The geometry of facial growth and its effects on the dental occlusion and facial form. *J Charles H Tweed Int Found* 1981;9:21-38.
72. Isaacson JR, Isaacson RJ, Speidel TM, et al: Extreme variation in vertical facial growth and associated variation in skeletal and dental relationships. *Angle Orthod* 1971;41:219-228.
73. Schudy FF: The rotation of the mandible resulting from growth: Its implications in orthodontic treatment. *Angle Orthod* 1965;35:36-50.
74. Linder-Aronson S: Effects of adenoidectomy on the dentition and facial skeleton over a period of five years. In: Cook JT, ed. *Transactions of the Third International Orthodontic Congress*, St Louis: Mosby; 1975.
75. Vig KWL: Nasal obstruction and facial growth: The strength of evidence for clinical assumptions. *Am J Orthod Dentofacial Orthop* 1998;113:603-611.
76. Fields HW, Warren DW, Black K, et al: Relationship between dentofacial morphology and respiration in adolescents. *Am J Orthod Dentofacial Orthop* 1991;99:147-154.
77. Ingervall B, Thilander B: Relationship between facial morphology and activity of the masticatory muscles. *J Oral Rehab* 1974;1: 131-147.
78. Reidel RA: The relation of maxillary structures to cranium in malocclusions and in normal occlusion. *Angle Orthop* 1952;22: 140-145.
79. Riolo ML, Moyers RE, McNamara JA, Hunter WS: *An atlas of craniofacial growth*, volume 2. Ann Arbor: 1974.
80. Jacobson A: Update on the "wits" appraisal. *Angle Orthod* 1988;58:205-219.
81. Jacobson A: The 'wits' appraisal of jaw disharmony. *Am J Orthod Dentofacial Orthop* 1975;67:125-138.
82. Gramling JF: The probability index. *Am J Orthod Dentofacial Orthop* 1995;107:165-171.
83. Merrifield LL: Differential diagnosis with total space analysis. *J Charles H Tweed Int Found* 1978;6:10-15.
84. Tweed CH: *Clinical orthodontics, volume 1*, pp 252–265 St Louis: Mosby; 1967.
85. Baldridge D: *Leveling the Curve of Spee: Its Effect on Mandibular Arch Length, unpublished master's thesis*, Memphis: The University of Tennessee; June 1960.
86. Katz MI: Angle Classification revisited 2: A modified Angle Classification. *AM J Orthod Dentofacial Orthop* 1995;102(9): 277-284.
87. Richardson ME: Late lower arch crowding: the role of the transverse dimension. *Am J Orthod Dentofacial Orthop* 1995;107:613-617.
88. Richardson ME: The effect of mandibular first premolar extraction on third molar space. *Angle Orthod* 1989;59(4): 291-294.
89. Ledyard BC: A study of the mandibular third molar area. *Am J Orthod* 1953;39:366-373.
90. Glenn G, Sinclair PM, Alexander RG: Nonextraction orthodontic therapy: Posttreatment dental and skeletal stability. *Am J Orthod Dentofacial Orthop* 1987;92:321-328.
91. Haruki T, Little RM: Early vs. late treatment in crowded extraction cases: A postretention evaluation of stability and relapse. *Angle Orthod* 1998;68:61-68.
92. Little RM, Reidel RA, Artun J: An evaluation of changes in mandibular anterior alignment from 10 to 20 years postretention. *Am J Orthod Dentofacial Orthop* 1988;93: 423-428.
93. Little RM, Reidel RA, Engst ED: Serial extraction of first premolars: Postretention evaluation of stability and relapse. *Angle Orthod* 1990;60:255-262.
94. Little RM, Wallen TR, Reidel RA: Stability and relapse of mandibular anterior alignment–first premolar extraction cases treated by traditional edgewise orthodontics. *Am J Orthod* 1981;80:349-365.
95. Little RM: Stability and relapse of mandibular anterior alignment: University of Washington studies. *Semin Orthod* 1999;5:191-204.
96. Nance H: The limitations of orthodontic treatment. *Am J Orthod* 1947;33:253-300.
97. Paquette DE, Beattie JR, Johnston LE: A long-term comparison of non-extraction and premolar extraction edgewise therapy in "borderline" class II patients. *Am J Orthod Dentofacial Orthop* 1992;102:1-14.
98. Vaden JL, Harris EF, Zeigler Gardner RL: Relapse revisited. *Am J Orthod Dentofacial Orthop* 1997;111:543-553.

CHAPTER 10

Treatment Tactics for Problems Related to Dentofacial Discrepancies in Three Planes of Space

Burcu Bayirli • Christopher S. Riolo • Michelle Thornberg • Michael L. Riolo

All orthodontic appliances produce both desired and undesired tooth movements. The science and art of orthodontics is to balance forces in order to maximize the desired movement and minimize the undesired movement. This balance is achieved through proper decision making in three areas: (1) appliance selection, (2) appliance utilization, and (3) timing of appliance therapy.

Appliance selection is critical for successful treatment outcomes. For instance, when selecting a functional appliance, one has to consider that certain functional appliances may lead to undesirably procumbent lower incisors. Proper appliance utilization is critical for minimizing undesired tooth movements, such as flaring of the lower incisors. If lower incisor flaring is a concern, a tissue-borne functional appliance or a tooth-born appliance such as a MARA used in conjunction with fixed appliances using a full-size lower archwire can minimize lower incisor flaring. In addition, the use of Class II elastics without establishing proper anchorage may lead to extrusion of posterior teeth, anterior open bite, and excessive tipping of the occlusal plane.

Although proper appliance selection and utilization are two critical issues in effective orthodontic treatment, successful treatment outcomes may not be achieved without appropriate timing of appliance therapy. Using an orthodontic appliance at an inappropriate time may lead to ineffective treatment and result in undesired tooth movements. For example, the use of a rapid palatal expander (RPE) in a skeletally mature patient may cause excessive tipping of posterior teeth, lingual cusp interferences, anterior open bite, adverse periodontal consequences, and high potential for orthodontic relapse after treatment. Timing of appliance therapy also relates to the sequence of treatment events. Attempting space closure and anterior tooth retraction without proper anchorage preparation may lead to undesired tooth movements that cannot be reversed. Consequently, selection, utilization, and timing of appliance therapy are intertwined and involve a comprehension of tooth movement in the transverse, vertical, and anterior-posterior dimensions.

TRANSVERSE DISCREPANCIES

1. Under what circumstances should a maxillary expansion appliance be used?

- Correction of dental and/or skeletal posterior crossbites that are either unilateral or bilateral.[1-3]
- Correction of anterior crossbites associated with a functional shift or traumatic occlusion. Early expansion sometimes used in conjunction with a protraction facemask or upper fixed appliances on the lateral and central incisors can result in anterior movement of the dental alveolar complex through both dental and skeletal movement.[2]
- Elimination of crowding through an increase in arch length.
- Correction of axial inclinations of posterior teeth.
- Mobilization of circummaxillary sutures to make skeletal protraction possible during facemask treatment.

2. What are the different types of expansion appliances?

BANDED EXPANDERS

Hyrax Expander

The Hyrax expander consists of two bands on the upper first molars and usually two bands on the upper first bicuspids (Fig. 10-1, A). The Hyrax expansion screw located near the midpalate is soldered to the lingual surface of the bands. The expansion screw is usually activated one turn (approximately 0.25 mm) each day. If substantial expansion is required, the expander design should incorporate as many teeth as possible to minimize buccal crown torque (tipping rather than translation) and "hanging" lingual cusps. Excessive buccal crown torque should be avoided, since it can result in adverse periodontal sequelae, relapse of the maxillary constriction, and lingual interferences.

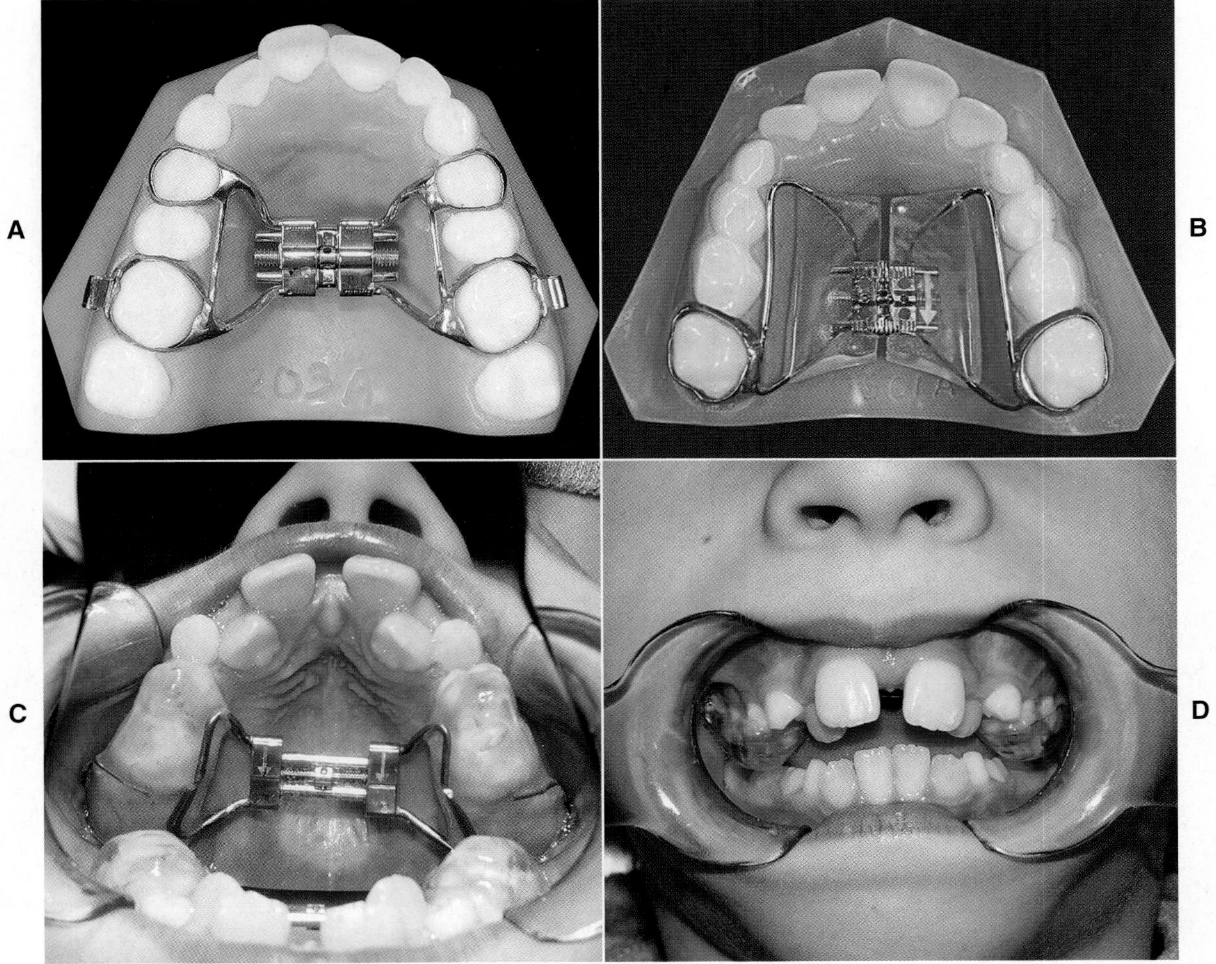

FIG 10-1 A, The Hyrax maxillary expander. **B,** The Haas maxillary expander. **C** and **D,** The bonded rapid palatal expander: palatal view **(C)** and frontal view **(D)**.

Continued

Haas Expander

The Haas expander is a fixed maxillary expander that uses acrylic pads and heavy lingual wires to apply pressure to both the teeth and the palatal tissue during expansion. This expander is thought to result in less tipping of the buccal tooth segments (Fig. 10-1, *B*). The lingual wires are soldered to bands on the first bicuspids and the first molars and extend onto the palate where they are embedded in the acrylic pads. The Haas expander as well as the Hyrax expander moves the palate transversely and increases arch perimeter 0.7 mm for each millimeter of transverse expansion. Most feel that an RPE will move the maxilla inferiorly and anteriorly as well as transversely.

BONDED RAPID PALATAL EXPANDER

Bonded RPE is an alternative to the banded design. It is a fixed appliance that uses posterior acrylic coverage and is directly bonded to the teeth (Fig. 10-1, *C* and *D*). The posterior bite blocks remove cuspal interferences. Headgear tubes, arch wire tubes, and reverse pull hooks for a protraction face mask can all be added as desired. This appliance is typically used when a more rigid appliance is desired to minimize tipping of the buccal segments. It is preferred in mixed dentition patients who do not yet have their upper first bicuspids, but primary molars are present. In addition, it may be used for its bite block effect in patients with an open bite tendency.

LOWER SCHWARTZ APPLIANCE (REMOVABLE)

Lower Schwarz appliance (Fig. 10-1, *E*) is used for minimal arch expansion in the mandible.[4] This appliance is only activated once a week, unlike the RPEs described previously.

FIXED MANDIBULAR EXPANDER

Fixed mandibular expander is used as an alternative to the removable Schwarz appliance. This fixed metal expander provides lateral expansion in the mandibular arch (Fig. 10-1, *F*). The lower fixed expander can be a good option when patient cooperation is an issue.

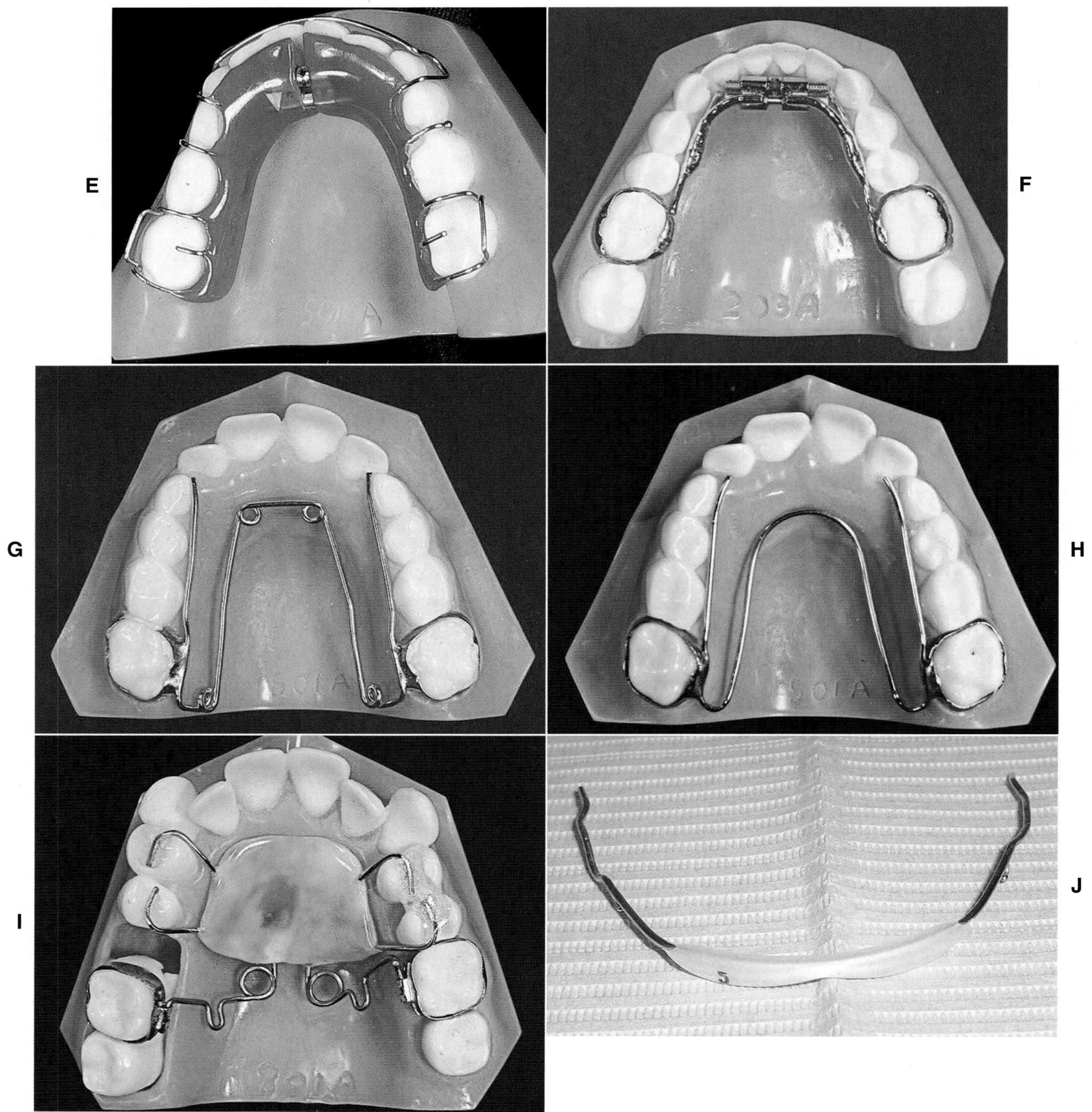

FIG 10-1—cont'd E, Removable Schwartz appliance. **F,** Fixed mandibular expander. **G,** Quadhelix. **H,** W arch. **I,** Pendex appliance. **J,** Lip bumper appliance. (**A, B, E-I,** courtesy AOA Orthodontic Appliances, Sturtevant, Wisc.)

QUADHELIX

This fixed metal expander is capable of applying forces in numerous directions depending upon how it is activated by the orthodontist (Fig. 10-1, *G*). The four helical loops (two in the first bicuspid region and two in the first molar region) can be activated in unison or individually to achieve the desired results. The appliance is soldered to bands on the first molars, and lingual arms run from the bands forward to the cuspids or first bicuspids as desired. In general, quadhelix is used if dental expansion is primarily desired.

W ARCH

W arch is similar to the quadhelix without the four helical loops (Fig. 10-1, *H*). This appliance will lead to more dental expansion as opposed to skeletal expansion than a Hyrax or Haas maxillary expander.

PENDEX

Pendex is a fixed expansion appliance that is also used to distalize and derotate one or both upper first molars (Fig. 10-1, *I*). The Pendex appliance eliminates patient compliance concerns from the distalization treatment objective. A Haas expansion screw is usually incorporated into acrylic pads. This appliance can be designed with bands on the bicuspids and is frequently used in conjunction with wire rests that are bonded to the occlusal surface of bicuspids or primary molars to provide additional anchorage.

LIP BUMPER

A lip bumper (Fig. 10-1, *J*) is a large-diameter round wire that extends from first molar to first molar and rests in the buccal sulcus. It also has an acrylic pad in the anterior region. It can be used in either arch to distalize the first molars and promote transverse development of the arch by removing the pressure of the buccal tissues on the teeth and supporting structures.

CONVENTIONAL FIXED APPLIANCES

Arch wires can be expanded transversely to achieve dental expansion in either the maxilla or mandible.

3. Which expansion appliance should I use?

Factors that influence the selection of an expansion appliance include, but are not limited to, patient's age or skeletal maturity, the clinician's desire for dental versus skeletal expansion, the number of teeth available for anchorage, the expectation for patient compliance, and whether the expander will be used in conjunction with fixed appliances or other appliances, such as a facemask.[5] In general, the more skeletally mature the patient, the number of teeth required for adequate anchorage to minimize dental movement increases. In addition, more rigid expansion appliances are generally required in more mature patients to minimize dental tipping of the buccal segments.

4. When should expansion be initiated?

Treatment of crossbite with a functional shift should be initiated as soon as it is diagnosed. If not treated, these crossbites may adversely affect growth. If the mandible shifts to one side, growth will be asymmetric and the chin will deviate to that side. Also, very narrow upper arches should be treated as early as possible. As the patient matures, it is hard to get skeletal expansion. These narrow upper arches are usually associated with significant crowding and are best corrected when the patient is skeletally immature. Expansion in skeletally mature patients may result in undesired dental movement; therefore, the best time to correct these constricted arches is usually in the mixed dentition.

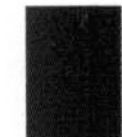

ANTEROPOSTERIOR AND VERTICAL DISCREPANCIES

5. How is Class II malocclusion corrected using fixed appliances?

Correction of a Class II malocclusion using nonextraction orthodontic treatment with fixed appliances requires the distalization of the maxillary teeth and/or anterior movement of the mandibular teeth. Maxillary teeth can be distalized using extra-oral forces (e.g., J-hook headgear or facebow) or intra-oral forces (e.g., Class II elastics or appliances such as the Distal Jet or Pendulum appliance) using the lower arch as anchorage.

6. What type of headgear or facebow should I use?

Extra-oral traction can be used to achieve both tooth movement and modification of bone growth. The type of headgear used depends on the patient's skeletal pattern. The direction of the pull may be adjusted accordingly so that a desirable skeletal and/or dental effect may be achieved and any undesirable effects may be avoided. For instance, a cervical pull headgear should not be used in a patient with hyperdivergent vertical growth tendency, but it is an excellent choice in a hypodivergent patient. A hyperdivergent pattern is best treated with an occipital or high-pull headgear. Also, one must decide if tipping or bodily movement of teeth is preferred. Forces may be arranged to go through the center of resistance of a molar for bodily movement. For distal tipping, the force vector should be below the center of resistance of a molar.

7. When should extra-oral traction therapy be initiated?

Extra-oral traction may be initiated in the mixed dentition, especially if a skeletal effect is desired. It may also be used in patients who are not growing if only tooth movement or anchorage is the goal.

8. What are the indications and contraindications for Class II elastics?

INDICATIONS

- Class II molar or canine dental relationship
- Finishing orthodontic cases to achieve anterior coupling
- Excessive overbite (deep bite)
- Orthognathic facial profile

CONTRAINDICATIONS

- Class III skeletal discrepancy
- Dental open bite or skeletal open bite tendency
- Severe mandibular retrognathia

- Insufficient wire dimension to resist extrusion of teeth associated with the use of Class II elastics
- Excess lower anterior facial height

9. Under what circumstances should orthodontic extractions be considered?

Orthodontic extractions should be considered if there is excessive tooth material for the available arch length. Also, extractions will facilitate the anteroposterior tooth movements needed to attain a Class I canine and molar relationship. In addition, patients with anterior dentoalveolar protrusion as well as patients with a skeletal open bite tendency may benefit from orthodontic extractions. Finally, extractions should be considered in noncompliant patients who refuse to wear headgear or elastics.

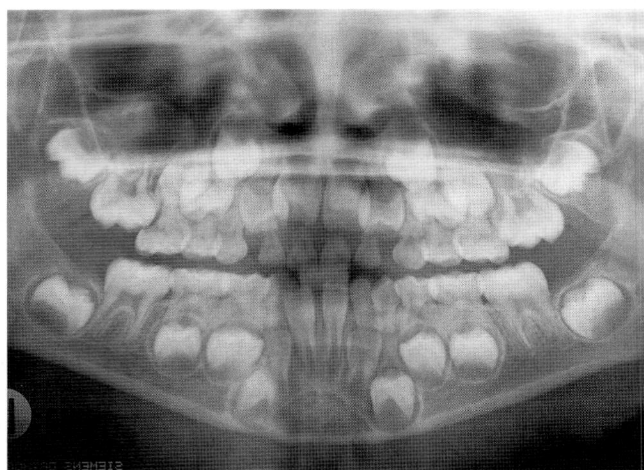

FIG 10-2 Panoramic radiograph depicting ectopic maxillary first permanent molars and early resorption of the roots of the maxillary second deciduous molars.

10. What are the treatment options to correct crowding problems?

There are three basic ways to correct crowding problems:

1. Expansion of the dental arches, including distalization of the posterior segments of the dental arch
2. Extraction of permanent tooth mass
3. Reapproximation to reduce the mesial-distal width of selected teeth

Expansion of the dental arches can be achieved with a variety of appliances. There are a number of factors that should be considered when selecting an expansion treatment tactic. For example, is the crowding problem caused by space loss in the dental arch? Or are one or more of the dental arches constricted? If the arches are constricted, is the constriction primarily dental or skeletal? Crowding as a result of space loss is usually due to either ectopic eruption of the first molars or early loss of primary teeth. If space is not maintained after the early loss of one or more primary teeth, arch length loss can occur. If there is loss of arch length, the clinician must decide to either regain the lost space or maintain the remaining space. Another option is to defer treatment in anticipation of extracting permanent teeth. If the decision is made to regain the space, it is usually best to proceed with treatment as soon as practical. Regaining space caused by the mesial migration of posterior teeth (primarily the first permanent molars) is more easily accomplished before the eruption of the second permanent molars. Space loss caused by ectopic eruption most commonly involves the maxillary first molars (Fig. 10-2). Ectopic mesial eruption may necessitate the early removal of the second deciduous molars in order to allow full eruption of the permanent first molars before regaining the lost arch perimeter.

Fig. 10-2 depicts a panoramic radiograph of ectopic maxillary first permanent molars and early resorption of the roots of the second deciduous molars.

The extraction of permanent teeth can be used to correct tooth size/arch length discrepancies. In deciding which permanent teeth to extract, the practitioner needs to consider both anteroposterior and vertical discrepancies. After the crowding problem is resolved, how will an anteroposterior problem be addressed? Is there a facial asymmetry? If so, can an asymmetric extraction pattern facilitate the orthodontic mechanics? Is there an open bite tendency? If so, will extracting teeth more posteriorly help minimize the mandibular plane angle? Usually, the easiest part of the orthodontic treatment is aligning the teeth. It is very important that the orthodontist think ahead about how a functional and stable canine Class I occlusion will be achieved and how the extraction pattern will either facilitate or impede the orthodontic mechanics.

Reapproximation is the removal of tooth structure or restorative material from the mesial and distal surfaces of the teeth using abrasive strips or a high-speed handpiece.[6] It can be used to gain space to mitigate slight or moderate crowding in the dental arch without increasing the procumbency of the anterior teeth. When reapproximation is carried out, care should be taken to maintain the interproximal contour of the teeth in order to avoid flat broad contacts.

11. When should serial extractions be considered?

Serial extraction is the selected removal of both deciduous and permanent teeth (usually the first premolars) in order to allow severely crowded teeth to erupt into more desirable positions. This sequential removal of primary teeth and permanent teeth is typically followed by comprehensive orthodontic treatment after eruption of permanent teeth has brought about as much improvement as it can on its own.

INDICATIONS FOR SERIAL EXTRACTIONS

- Minimum 7.0 mm of crowding in the anterior areas per arch
- Coincident upper and lower midlines
- Bilateral Class I molar relationship
- Balanced skeletal pattern in all three planes of space

COMPLICATING FACTORS FOR SERIAL EXTRACTIONS

- Class III molar relationships
- Class II molar relationships
- Unbalanced skeletal patterns of any kind (transverse, anteroposterior, or vertical)
- Unequal crowding in the maxillary and mandibular arches
- Unequal crowding bilaterally in either arch
- Midline discrepancies (>2 mm)
- Open bites or impinging deep bites

12. Under what circumstances should orthodontic extractions *not* be considered?

In general, orthodontic tooth extraction should not be considered in Class II division 2 patients for the purpose of anteroposterior correction. An exception can be made in the case of severe crowding. In addition, space closure subsequent to orthodontic extractions can be a problem in patients with an obtuse nasolabial angle. Retraction of upper anterior teeth will increase the nasolabial angle even more and may result in an unpleasant profile in these cases. Moreover, caution should be taken with patients who are more susceptible to having adverse sequelae caused by orthodontic tooth movement. These patients include the following:

- Patients who are periodontally compromised
- Patients who have external root resorption from previous orthodontic treatment
- Patients with short blunted root morphology
- Patients with thin alveolar ridges

Poor oral hygiene is also a problem, especially if oral hygiene deteriorates during treatment and decalcification becomes a serious issue. It is problematic to discontinue treatment until the extraction spaces are closed. Frequently, these spaces are difficult to close because of a generalized lack of cooperation in these patients.

13. Which teeth should be removed in order to facilitate orthodontic tooth movement for the correction of a Class II discrepancy?

This question is very complex; therefore only general guidelines will be presented. Permanent teeth may be extracted in order to use anchorage to protract and retract key tooth segments in order to establish a Class I canine and molar relationship.[7,8] There are a number of important considerations when contemplating permanent tooth extraction. These considerations include:

- The degree of crowding in the dental arches
- The proclination of the anterior teeth, periodontal support, and presence of lip competence
- The interincisal angle and the palatal morphology immediately lingual to the incisors
- The facial profile (orthognathic, retrognathic, prognathic, or excess lower anterior facial height)
- Presence of skeletal or dental open bite or an open bite tendency
- Thickness of the perioral soft tissue
- Molar and canine relationship
- Presence of maxillary and mandibular midline discrepancy—may require an asymmetric extraction pattern
- Missing teeth
- Periodontal condition, or history of periodontal disease
- History of external root resorption, or short thin tapered root morphology
- Anticipated level of patient cooperation

When considering extractions as part of the orthodontic treatment plan and deciding which permanent teeth to extract, the orthodontist must consider whether or not each of the factors just listed will influence the treatment result if specific teeth are extracted.

Most of the orthodontic extractions for the correction of Class II malocclusions involve premolars. Most commonly, maxillary and mandibular first premolars are chosen for extraction; however, in many Class II patients, it is worth considering the extraction of maxillary first premolars and mandibular second premolars so that the correction of the Class II molar relationship may be facilitated. In patients with a Class II molar relationship and minimal mandibular crowding, sometimes only maxillary premolars are selected for extraction. This treatment plan results in final Class II molar and Class I canine occlusal relationship.

Moreover, if the Class II malocclusion is characterized by excessive lower anterior facial height and open bite or an open bite tendency, maxillary and mandibular second premolars are often considered for extractions.[9] Also, asymmetric extraction patterns involving first premolars on one side and second premolars on the other side or unilateral premolar extraction are commonly used to maximize mechanical advantage in the correction of asymmetric Class II malocclusions.

14. What types of functional appliances are available?

Class II correction using functional appliances is achieved by changing the neuromuscular environment of the dentition to promote mandibular growth and guide both the eruption of the permanent teeth and development of the alveolus.[10]

There are many different designs, but all functional appliances have two characteristics in common: they disarticulate the teeth and position the mandible forward. Functional appliances can be categorized into two different broad groups with respect to design: tissue- and tooth-borne appliances. In general, tissue-borne appliances (e.g., a Fränkel appliance) (Fig. 10-3, *A*) produce less dental compensation than tooth-borne appliances. Tooth-borne appliances (Fig. 10-3, *B* and *C*) can be further categorized into two classes: removable and fixed. Figures 10-3, *A* and *B*, show a MARA and a Herbst appliance, respectively, which are examples of fixed tooth-borne functional appliances. Fig. 10-3, *D*, depicts a Bionator, which is a type of removable tooth-borne functional appliance.

15. Which functional appliance should I use?

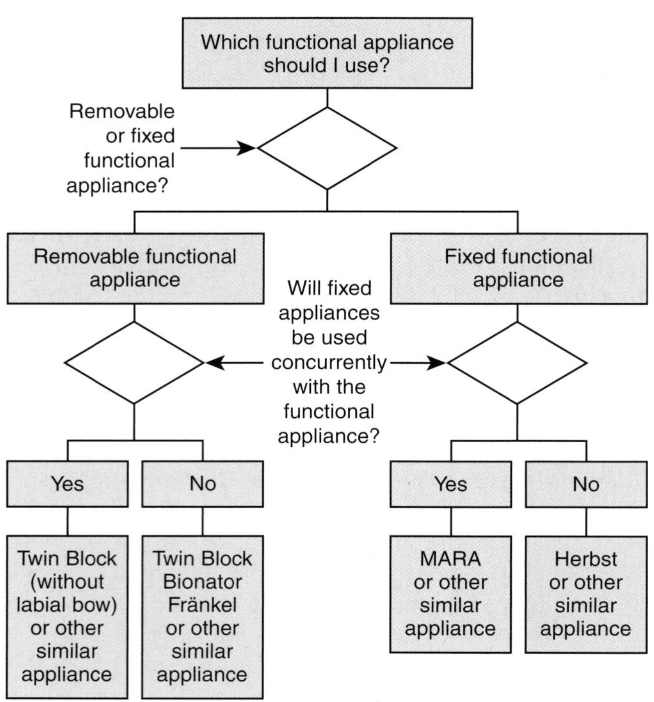

16. When should functional appliance therapy be initiated?

The timing of an early phase of treatment using a functional appliance is a critical decision for the success of a two-phase treatment plan. It is important that the functional appliance therapy be initiated while substantial growth is remaining. A hand-wrist x-ray may be helpful in assessing whether the patient has substantial growth remaining.[11] In addition, removable functional appliances require a high degree of patient compliance. Therefore, the maturity of the patient should be considered before initiating an early phase of treatment using a removable functional appliance. Before the functional appliance can be delivered, the upper anterior teeth may need to be decompensated using fixed appliances on the lateral and central incisors so that the lower arch can be positioned into a Class I molar relationship without anterior occlusal interferences. In addition, the upper arch may require expansion in order to accommodate the lower arch in a Class I molar relationship.

17. When should protraction facemask therapy be initiated?

A protraction facemask is best used for a Class III malocclusion with a low to average mandibular plane angle. Young patients from 6 to 9 years of age demonstrate a greater skeletal response, whereas adolescents show a more dental response to protraction facemask wear.

18. Under what circumstances should orthodontic extractions be used for the correction of a Class III anteroposterior discrepancy?

- Bimaxillary protrusion (in the absence of generalized spacing)
- Anterior open bite or anterior open bite tendency
- Either growth is nearing completion or the orthodontist is confident that the treatment plan has a high probability of success

19. Which teeth should be removed in order to facilitate orthodontic tooth movement for the correction of a Class III discrepancy?

Correction of Class III malocclusions can be achieved by the extraction of permanent teeth.[8,12] The space provided by the extraction of permanent teeth is used to differentially protract and retract posterior and anterior teeth in the maxillary and mandibular arches to achieve a Class I molar and canine relationship.

Asymmetric extraction patterns can be used when correcting unilateral Class III malocclusions. Care should be taken if extracting primary teeth in place of missing succedaneous teeth, because closing the space resulting from agenesis of permanent teeth can be very difficult. Space closure by attempting to protract posterior teeth in the absence of substantial crowding can be particularly problematic.

Bicuspid extraction allows for maximum correction of the Class III molar and canine relationship. Lower first and upper second bicuspid extraction provides substantial mechanical advantage when the treatment plan calls for correction of both the molar and canine Class III relationships. The extraction of the upper and lower first bicuspids is most desirable when the Class III malocclusion is characterized by a bimaxillary protrusion. Typically, differential anchorage is used to correct the molar and canine Class III relationship while uprighting the upper and lower anterior teeth. Four second bicuspid extractions are sometimes used when the Class III malocclusion is accompanied by a skeletal or dental open bite or a skeletal open bite tendency. In this case, differential anchorage is used to correct the molar and canine Class III relationship. The extraction of second bicuspids encourages protraction of posterior teeth and minimizes the tendency for the mandibular plane angle to increase.

Lower first bicuspid extraction alone inevitably leads to a compromised treatment result that should be discussed with the patient before this treatment plan is implemented. As a result of this extraction pattern, a molar Class III and canine Class I relationship, usually characterized by a poor posterior occlusion, is achieved. This result may be an acceptable compromise when a surgical treatment plan is not feasible.

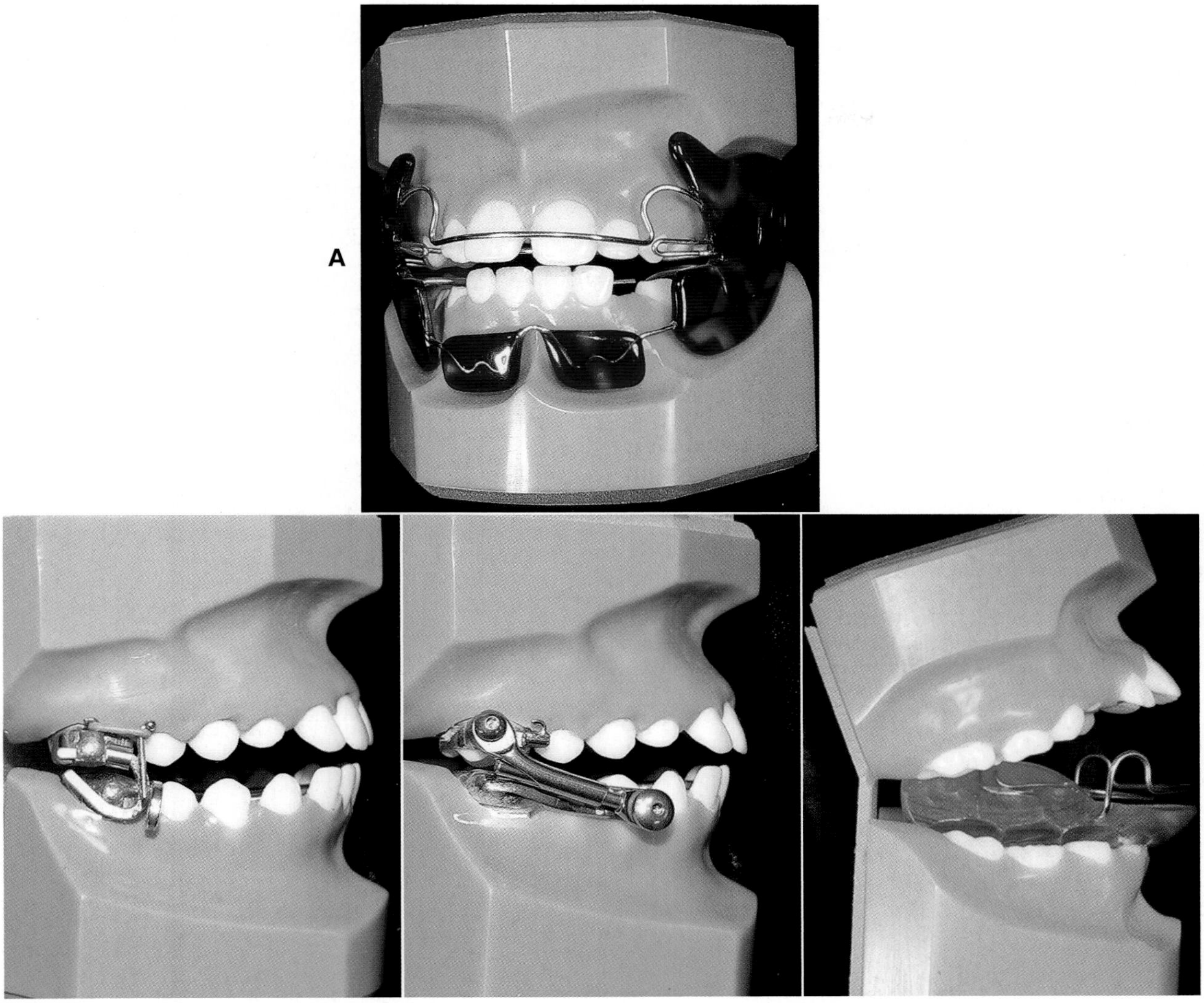

FIG 10-3 **A,** Fränkel appliance. **B,** MARA appliance. **C,** Herbst appliance. **D,** Bionator appliance. (Courtesy AOA Orthodontic Appliances, Sturtevant, Wisc.)

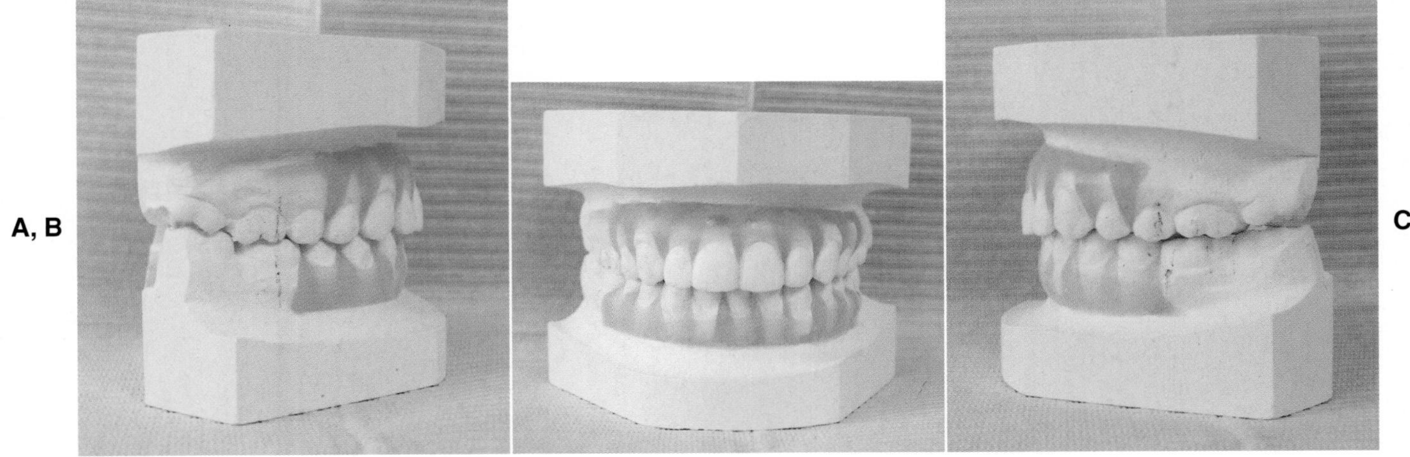

FIG 10-4 **A,** Diagnostic setup—right. **B,** Diagnostic setup—frontal. **C,** Diagnostic setup—left.

A lower incisor extraction can be a good alternative to four bicuspid extraction[13,14] especially in cases where:

- It is desirable to leave the buccal occlusion intact
- A treatment objective is to establish excess overjet for restorative purposes
- It is a high priority to minimize treatment time (9–12 mos)
- A Bolton discrepancy exists

A diagnostic setup (Fig. 10-4) is always a good idea when contemplating a lower extraction treatment plan.

REFERENCES

1. Hayes JL: Rapid maxillary expansion. *Am J Orthod Dentofacial Orthop* 2006;130(4):432-433.
2. Pangrazio-Kulbersh V, Berger JL, Janisse FN, Bayirli BM: Long-term stability of class III treatment: rapid palatal expansion and protraction facemask vs Lefort I maxillary advancement osteotomy. *Am J Orthod Dentofacial Orthop* 2007;131(7):709-719.
3. Salemi G. A photogrammetric technique for the analysis of palatal three-dimensional changes during rapid maxillary expansion. *Eur J Orthod* 2007;29(1):26-30.
4. O'Grady PW, McNamara JA Jr, Baccetti T, Franchi L: A long-term evaluation of the mandibular Schwartz appliance and the acrylic splint expander in the early mixed dentition patients. *Am J Orthod Dentofacial Orthop* 2006;130(2):202-213.
5. Gottlieb LE, Brazones MM, Malerman A, et al: Early orthodontic treatment. 2. *J Clin Orthod* 2004;38(3):135-154.
6. Riolo ML, Avery JK: *Essentials for orthodontic practice.* Ann Arbor and Grand Haven, Michigan: EFOP Press. 2003.
7. Battagel JM: Profile changes in class II, division 1 malocclusions: a comparison of the effects of Edgewise and Frankel appliance therapy. *Eur J Orthod* 1989;11(3):243-253.
8. Russell DM: Extractions in support of orthodontic treatment. *NDA J* 1994;45(2):15-19.
9. Ngan P, Fields HW: Open bite: a review of etiology and management. *Pediatr Dent* 1997;19(2):91-98.
10. Fränkel R: The theoretical concept underlying the treatment with functional correctors. *Rep Congr Eur Orthod Soc* 1966;42: 233-254.
11. Uysal T, Ramoglu SI, Basciftci FA, Sari Z: Chronologic age and skeletal maturation of the cervical vertebrae and hand-wrist: Is there a relationship? *Am J Orthod Dentofacial Orthop* 2006;130(5):622-628.
12. Battagel JM, Orton HS: Class III malocclusion: a comparison of extraction and non-extraction techniques. *Eur J Orthod* 1991;13(3):212-222.
13. Bahreman AA: Lower incisor extraction in orthodontic treatment. *Am J Orthod* 1977;72(5):560-567.
14. Kokich VG, Shapiro PA: Lower incisor extraction in orthodontic treatment. Four clinical reports. *Angle Orthod* 1984;54:139-153.

Phase I: Early Treatment

CHAPTER

11

James A. McNamara, Jr. • Laurie McNamara

Early treatment, also known as *"Phase I treatment,"* represents orthodontic and/or orthopedic therapy that is rendered in the mixed dentition, typically with the expectation of a second phase of orthodontic intervention *("Phase II")* after the eruption of the permanent teeth.[1] The goal of early treatment is to correct existing or developing skeletal, dentoalveolar, and/or muscular imbalances, thereby improving the overall oral environment before the eruption of the permanent dentition is complete. By initiating orthodontic and orthopedic therapy at a younger age, it is anticipated that many future abnormalities in the occlusion (e.g., crowding, excessive overjet, underbite) will be resolved with a relatively straightforward second phase of full fixed appliances in most instances. Thus, the frequency of complex orthodontic treatment involving permanent tooth extraction and/or corrective jaw surgery presumably is reduced.

During the last two decades, there has been increasing interest in early treatment, both within the orthodontic community and among the lay population, with articles on this topic appearing in such prominent lay publications as the *New York Times, The Wall Street Journal,* and *US News and World Report.* Within the dental community there has been an increased attention to intercepting or modifying abnormal orofacial conditions that are recognized early. This growing interest has coincided with a general rise in the level of consciousness concerning preventive dentistry and medicine; parents often seek treatment for their children at a young age, based in part on an esthetics-driven society.

1. What are the contraindications to early treatment?

Early orthodontic treatment is not always necessary or appropriate. Certainly not all orthodontic therapy delivered under the guise of "early treatment" is good treatment, as for example in instances of young patients being treated for extended periods of time with regimens that have ill-defined goals and unpredictable outcomes. In such situations, early treatment may serve only to increase treatment duration and cost; such intervention may result in patient and parental "burnout." Early treatment is not indicated in those instances in which early intervention does not change the environment appreciably for dentofacial development and permanent tooth eruption.

2. Which problems can be treated effectively and efficiently during the mixed dentition?

We are moving toward a better understanding as to the appropriate timing of orthodontic and orthopedic intervention depending on the clinical condition. With the increasing emphasis on "evidence-based" treatments in both medicine and dentistry, we now are gaining an appreciation concerning the nature of the effects produced by specific protocols in patients of varying maturational levels. The orthodontist has many treatment options available, all of which have specific indications. The possibilities range from simple space maintenance to a variety of active orthodontic and orthopedic therapies.

3. What is the purpose of space maintenance?

One of the most basic concepts for both general dentists and specialists to comprehend is the importance of maintaining the so-called "leeway space," or the space that becomes available during the transition from the second deciduous molars to the second premolars. In many borderline crowding cases, the maintenance of the leeway space may mean the difference between treating a patient with or without the removal of permanent teeth.

On average, 2 mm of space per side can be gained in the maxillary arch and 2.5 mm of space per side can be gained in the mandibular arch, because of the differences in the sizes of the second deciduous molars and the succeeding second premolars.[2] To preserve such space, lingual wires attached to bands on the first molars may be placed at the time that the second deciduous molars have become mobile or have significant root resorption as seen in the panoramic radiograph. The major role of these wires in the late mixed dentition is to prevent the mesial migration of the first molars during the transition from the second deciduous molars to the second premolars.

In the maxilla, a transpalatal arch (TPA; Fig. 11-1, *A*) extends from one maxillary first molar along the contour of the palate to the first molar on the opposite side. This appliance is capable of producing molar rotation and changes in root torque and angulation; the TPA may remain in place until the completion of the final comprehensive phase of orthodontic therapy.[1] In the mandible, a lingual arch (Fig. 11-1, *B*) that extends along the lingual contour of the mandibular dentition from first molar to first molar may be used. The lower lingual arch is used less frequently than the transpalatal arch because many patients undergoing early orthodontic treatment do not require the maintenance of the space in the mandibular second premolar region. Thus, the lower lingual arch is used only in patients in whom maximum anchorage is to be maintained. In contrast to the transpalatal arch, the lower lingual arch is usually removed as soon as the mandibular second premolars erupt fully into occlusion.

4. How do you treat patients with crowded teeth?

Patients with developing moderate to severe tooth-size/arch-size discrepancy problems are often treated effectively and efficiently when a patient is 8 or 9 years of age. Normally, this treatment is started after the permanent lower four incisors and the permanent upper central incisors have erupted. In many instances, there is insufficient space to allow for the unimpeded eruption of the maxillary lateral incisors. Depending on the size of the permanent teeth, either a serial extraction or an orthopedic expansion protocol can be used.

5. What is "serial extraction?"

Serial extraction refers to the sequential removal of deciduous teeth to facilitate the unimpeded eruption of the permanent teeth. Such a procedure often, but not always, results in the extraction of four first premolars. The typical serial extraction protocol is initiated about the time of the appearance of the permanent lateral incisors, which erupt in rotated positions or are initially prevented from eruption by the deciduous canines (Fig. 11-2).

In the most commonly used protocol, the first teeth to be removed are the deciduous canines. The removal of these teeth allows for the eruption, posterior movement, and spontaneous improvement in the alignment of the permanent lateral incisors. In about 6 to 12 months, the removal of the four deciduous first molars is undertaken, followed later by the extraction of the first premolars. It is common to observe that the adjacent teeth erupt toward the extraction sites, with the lower incisors often uprighting as well (sometimes too much so). As soon as the second molars near emergence, fixed appliances can be used to align and detail the dentition.

6. When is serial extraction indicated?

According to Graber,[3] serial extraction may be indicated when it is determined "with a fair degree of certainty that there will not be enough space in the jaws to accommodate all the permanent teeth in their proper alignment." A predicted tooth-size/arch-size discrepancy of 7 to 10 mm (or greater) is an indication for serial extraction.[4,5]

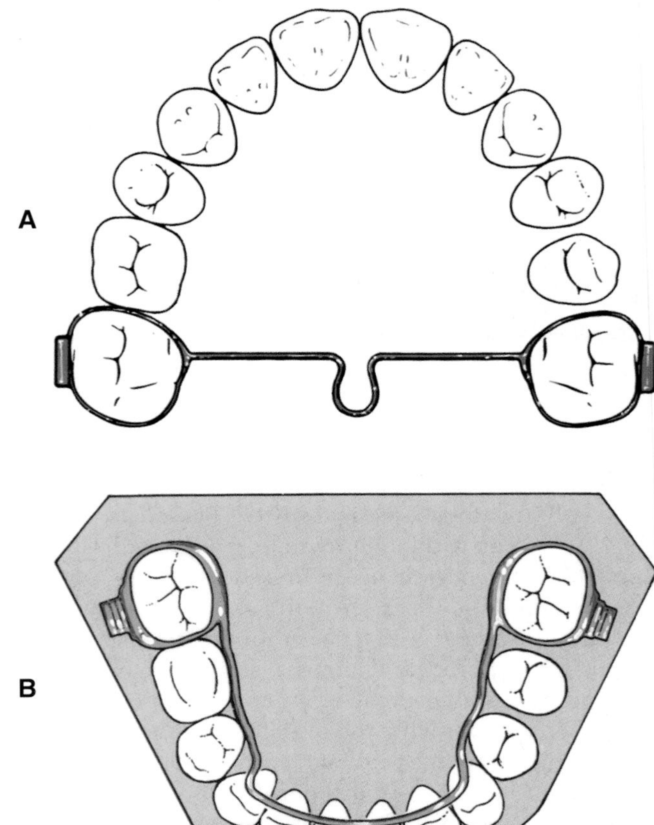

FIG 11-1 A, The transpalatal arch is used to maintain the leeway space during the transition from the mixed to the permanent dentition. It can also be used to rotate the maxillary first molars and to produce buccal root torque as necessary. **B,** The fixed lower lingual arch is used to maintain the lower leeway space during the transition of the dentition. It can also be used to widen the lower posterior dental arch following rapid expansion of the maxilla.

A primary factor to be evaluated when making a treatment decision concerning serial extraction is the *size of the individual teeth*. In instances in which tooth sizes are abnormally large, as indicated, for example, by the width of the erupted maxillary central incisors, serial extraction protocols may be appropriate. A central incisor with a mesiodistal width of 10 mm or greater indicates that the patient may have larger than average teeth.[2]

The presence of gingival recession and alveolar destruction on the labial surface of one or both mandibular central incisors can also indicate the need for this type of treatment regimen.[3] An additional indication is the early loss of one or both mandibular canines and a resultant asymmetrical midline shift.

7. What are the contraindications for serial extraction?

It is well known that serial extraction is not a panacea in all instances of tooth-size/arch-size discrepancy problems, and in fact this protocol is used relatively infrequently in our practice.

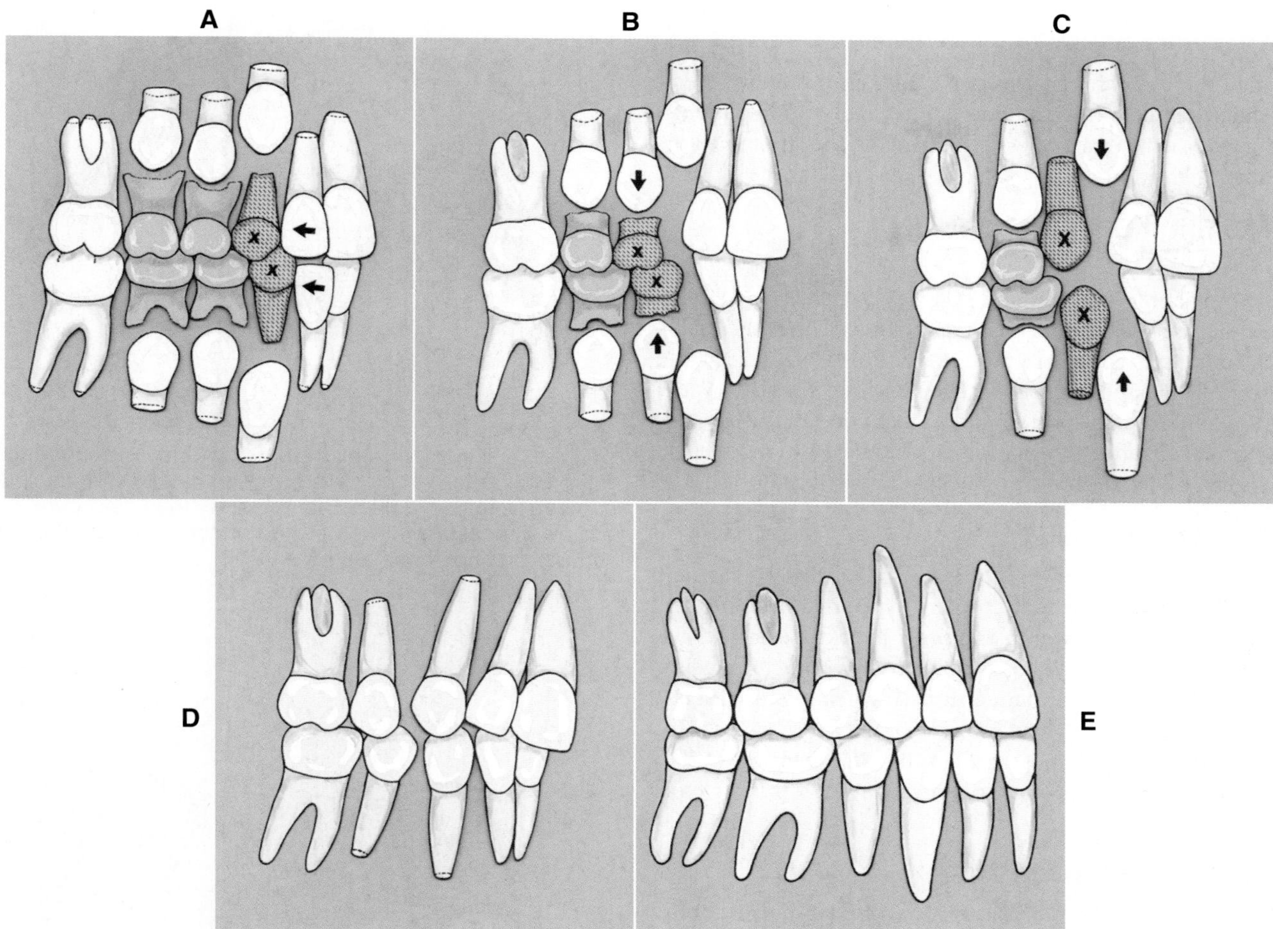

FIG 11-2 Serial extraction protocol. **A,** The removal of the upper and lower deciduous canines *(x)* allows for an improvement in the alignment of the upper and lower incisors. **B,** The removal of the deciduous first molars encourages the eruption of the first premolars. Some clinicians choose to remove the first premolars at the same time to allow the lower canines to migrate posteriorly before emergence. **C,** The removal of the first premolars encourages the eruption and posterior movement of the permanent canines. **D,** The remaining teeth tend to tip toward the extraction sites. The lower incisors often tip lingually as well. **E,** After the lower second premolars near emergence, fixed appliances are used to align the teeth and level the occlusal plane.[1]

Care must be taken to avoid lingual tipping of the lower incisors as well as unfavorable changes in the sagittal position of the maxillary and mandibular dentitions. In addition, the initiation of serial extraction procedures may result in unwanted spacing in the dental arches. Routine serial extraction protocols are also not indicated in situations of extreme skeletal imbalance. These protocols are not recommended in instances of full-blown Class II or Class III malocclusions because of the imbalance in the interarch relationship along with the emerging intraarch problem.

8. What happens if the dental arches are too small to allow for the normal alignment of the teeth?

In instances in which a serial extraction protocol is not appropriate, yet arch space is limited, orthodontic and/or orthopedic expansion may be indicated. Rapid maxillary expansion (RME)[6,7] refers to the use of appliances that result in true orthopedic expansion of the maxilla, in that changes are produced primarily in the underlying skeletal structures rather than by the movement of teeth through alveolar bone. RME not only separates the midpalatal suture, but also affects the circumzygomatic and circumaxillary sutural systems.

A goal of orthopedic treatment initiated in the mixed dentition is to reduce the need for extractions in the permanent dentition through the elimination of arch length discrepancies as well as the correction of bony base imbalances. The original protocol for RME was two turns per day (0.4–0.5 mm of screw expansion), as advocated by Haas.[6] In our practice, a one-turn-per-day (0.20–0.25 mm) protocol is used.[1] Another alternative is "slow maxillary expansion," which refers to having the expander turned once every second or third day.[8]

9. What types of RME appliances are available?

Typically, there are three types of RME devices that are used: the bonded acrylic splint expander in mixed dentition patients and the Haas and Hyrax types for patients in the late mixed or permanent dentition.

BONDED ACRYLIC SPLINT EXPANDER

The acrylic splint type of appliance (Fig. 11-3) that is made from 3 mm thick, heat-formed acrylic (splint Biocryl) has the additional advantage of acting as a posterior bite block because of the thickness of the acrylic that covers the occlusal surfaces of the posterior dentition. The posterior bite block effect of the bonded acrylic splint expander prevents the extrusion of posterior teeth,[9] which is helpful in controlling the vertical dimension.

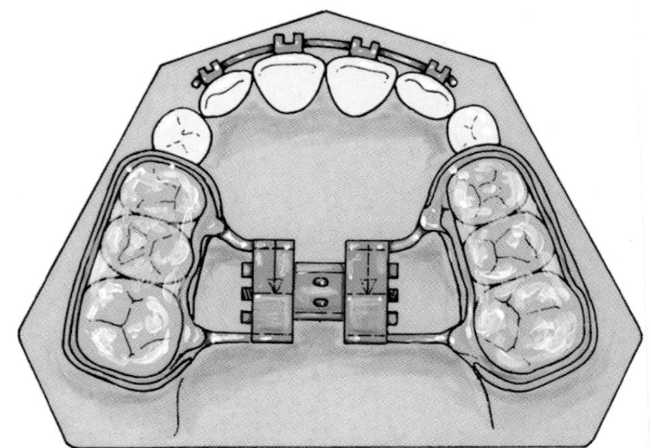

FIG 11-3 The acrylic splint RME appliance is bonded to the primary molars and permanent first molars. The splint is made from 3-mm thick Biocryl rather than cold-cure acrylic. Brackets are often placed on the maxillary incisors for alignment of these teeth.

HAAS EXPANDER

The Haas-type expander[6] (Fig. 11-4) is a tooth- and tissue-borne style of appliance that consists of bands on the upper first molars and first premolars, with a midline jackscrew incorporated in two acrylic pads that closely contact the palatal mucosa. This type of expander is used when maximal skeletal expansion is desired. The purpose of the acrylic pads is to minimize tipping of the posterior teeth. Inflammation of the palatal tissue is an occasional complication with this style of expander.

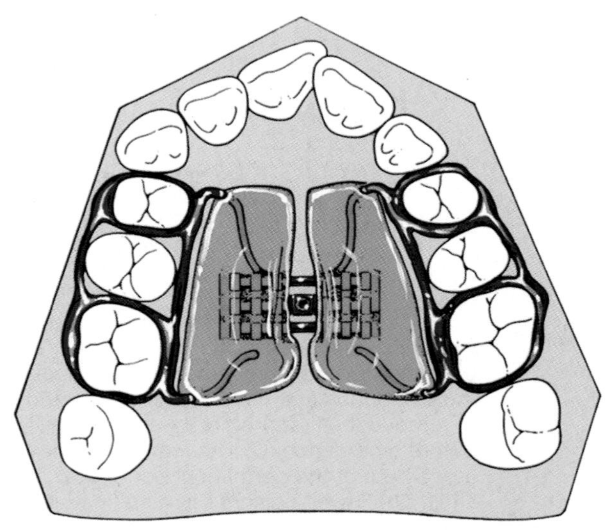

FIG 11-4 The Haas-type expander with an expansion screw incorporated in the palatal acrylic. This design is used in the permanent dentition when maximal skeletal expansion is needed.

HYRAX EXPANDER

The Hyrax-type expander[10] (Fig. 11-5) is a tooth-borne appliance that consists of bands on the maxillary first molars and first premolars, with a jackscrew incorporated in its metal framework. There is no acrylic component to this appliance, making it the most hygienic style of expander. The Hyrax-type expander is more flexible than the two mentioned previously; its use may result in more tipping of the posteriorly teeth laterally.

10. What are the indications for maxillary expansion?

One obvious indication for the use of RME appliances is the existence of a posterior and/or anterior crossbite. Orthopedic expansion is also used for other purposes, including increasing available arch length as well as correcting the axial inclinations of the upper posterior teeth. RME can also be used in the initial preparation of a patient for functional jaw orthopedics, facial mask therapy, or orthognathic surgery. RME may also have a secondary effect of widening the nasal cavity, thus reducing airway resistance and making it easier for some patients to breathe nasally.[11]

11. Can the lower jaw be expanded in the same manner?

No, because a mid-mandibular suture does not exist postnatally. The mandibular teeth usually erupt, however, with a lingual inclination, especially if the maxilla is narrow. Although orthopedic widening of the mandibular dental arch is not possible, the teeth can be uprighted orthodontically with a removable lower Schwarz appliance[1] (Fig. 11-6), especially if the maxilla subsequently is widened by way of RME.

12. Does a Class III malocclusion warrant early treatment?

Class III malocclusions can be treated successfully through early orthodontic and orthopedic intervention. In the instance of a Class III malocclusion that is diagnosed in either the late deciduous or early mixed dentition, the onset of treatment may be earlier than for a Class I patient.[12] The optimal time for beginning treatment (e.g., orthopedic facial mask, chin cup, FR-3 appliance of Fränkel) is coincident with

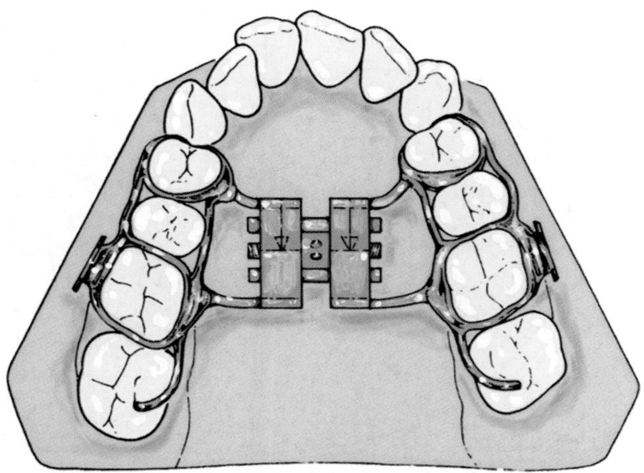

FIG 11-5 The Hyrax-type expander that is the most commonly used design in the early permanent dentition. This design can also be used in mixed dentition patients with bands around the maxillary first permanent molars and wires extending to the lingual of the maxillary deciduous molars.

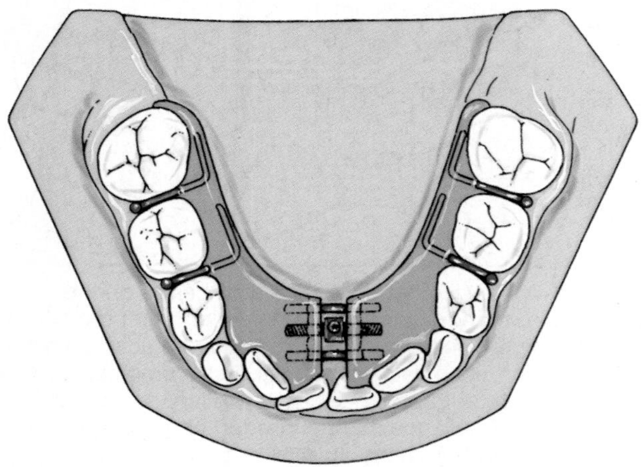

FIG 11-6 The removable lower Schwarz appliance is used for mandibular dental decompensation before orthopedic expansion of the maxilla. Because there is no mid-mandibular suture, the appliance produces tooth tipping rather than bodily movement.

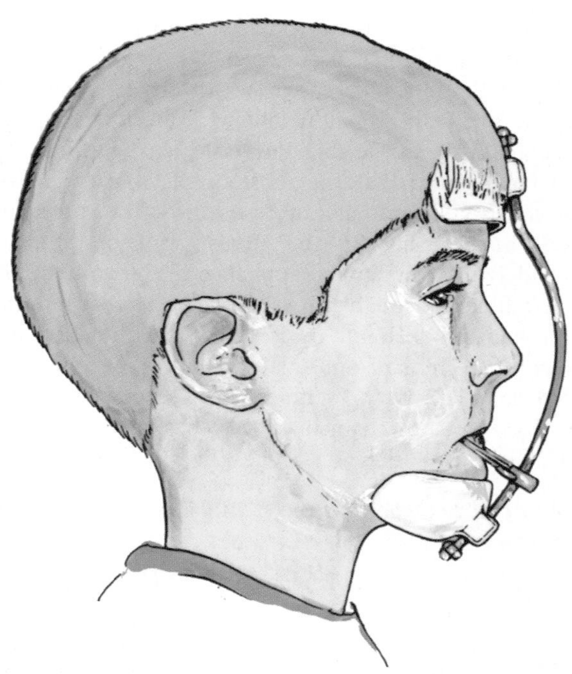

FIG 11-7 The orthopedic facial mask is attached to hooks on a bonded expander by way of strong elastics that produce up to 600 gm of force.

the loss of the maxillary deciduous incisors and the eruption of the permanent central incisors. This earlier intervention obviously will result in a longer period of time between the start of the initial phase of treatment and the end of the comprehensive treatment phase after the permanent dentition has erupted. The early treatment of Class III malocclusions may also be characterized by more than one period of intervention during the mixed dentition.

The most commonly used protocol for young Class III patients is the orthopedic facial mask (Fig. 11-7) combined with a bonded (see Fig. 11-3) or banded expander, to which facial mask hooks are attached. This type of appliance combination has been shown to be effective in causing a forward movement of the maxilla while producing a distal force on the mandible, leading to the resolution of the underlying Class III relationship. These patients should be "overcorrected" during Phase I, with an overjet of at least 4 to 5 mm achieved.[13] Maximizing the vertical overlap of the anterior teeth is also a major treatment objective.

13. Does a Class II malocclusion warrant early treatment?

That depends. Both Class II and Class III malocclusions, if they are severe, can lead to significant social problems during childhood. Thus, if a child has what can be termed a "socially-debilitating" Class II malocclusion (i.e., patients who present with severe neuromuscular, skeletal, or dentoalveolar problems), early intervention is warranted. For the routine Class II patient, however, the timing of treatment is later than has been described previously for Class I and Class III malocclusions.

14. Are all Class II patients treated in the same way?

If the Class II problem is related to a deficiency in mandibular development, a variety of functional jaw orthopedic appliances can be used to correct the sagittal problem, with both skeletal and dentoalveolar adaptations occurring. A delay in the use of functional jaw orthopedics (in patients with Class II malocclusions with mandibular skeletal deficiency) until the late mixed dentition or early permanent dentition period is recommended, because there is a greater growth response with functional appliances when treatment is initiated during the circumpubertal growth period.[14] Ideally, functional appliance therapy (e.g., Herbst, Twin Block, FR-2 of Fränkel) will be followed directly by a phase of fixed appliance therapy to align the permanent dentition.

We have found that the most predictable and effective orthopedic appliance that can be used for the correction of Class II malocclusions is the Herbst appliance, today the most widely used functional appliance in the United States.[1] The mandible is brought forward by the Herbst bite-jumping mechanism, bilateral devices that are attached to the maxillary first molars and mandibular first premolars by bands (Fig. 11-8, *A*) or stainless-steel crowns (our preference). The Herbst mechanism can also be connected to acrylic splints that cover both dental arches (Fig. 11-8, *B*).

15. What approach is used if the Class II problem is in the maxilla?

If a child has a Class II problem characterized by maxillary skeletal or dentoalveolar protrusion, treatment with extraoral traction devices[15,16] may be in order. The most commonly used headgear for such problems is the cervical-pull facebow (Fig. 11-9, *A*), which is attached to the maxillary first molars. This appliance can be used to distalize the maxillary dentition and can also be used as an anchorage device following extraction of two maxillary first premolars. Other appliances, such as the Pendulum or Pendex[17] (Fig. 11-9, *B*), which are not as dependent on patient compliance, can also be used to distalize maxillary molars.

16. Can any other treatments be provided to the Class II patient in the early mixed dentition?

In many patients with a Class II malocclusion identified in the 7- to 9-year-old age range, treatment may be initiated at that time to handle any intraarch problems (e.g., crowding, spacing, flaring); interarch discrepancies (i.e., sagittal Class II problems) may be handled at a later time. In other words, the same protocols (e.g., orthopedic expansion, extractions) that can be used for Class I patients may be initiated in Class II patients with arch length discrepancies; however, the attempt to correct the anteroposterior skeletal relationship is best delayed until the late mixed dentition period in patients with mild to moderate problems.

17. What do you mean by "spontaneous correction" of Class II malocclusions?

An interesting phenomenon occurs in some Class II patients who undergo RME in the early mixed dentition—the spontaneous correction of the underlying sagittal relationship.[18] As long as the maxilla is maintained in a widened relationship relative to the mandible during the transition from the mixed to the permanent dentition, it appears that the patient tends to posture the mandible forward to achieve a better dental interdigitation (as if the teeth act as an endogenous functional appliance). Sometimes the Class II relationship improves over time. If there is a residual Class II problem at the beginning of Phase II, definitive Class II treatment (e.g., Herbst appliance) is initiated.

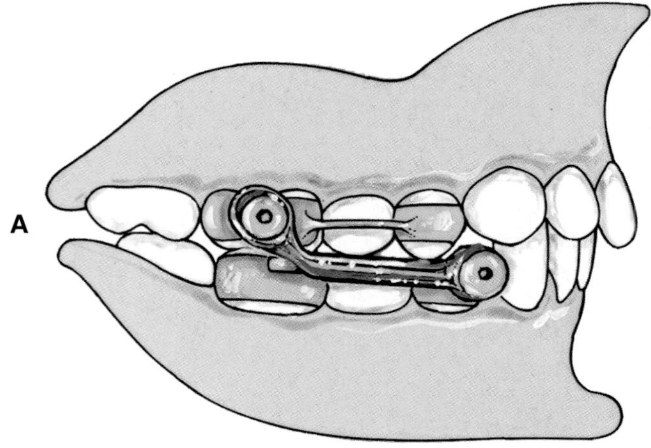

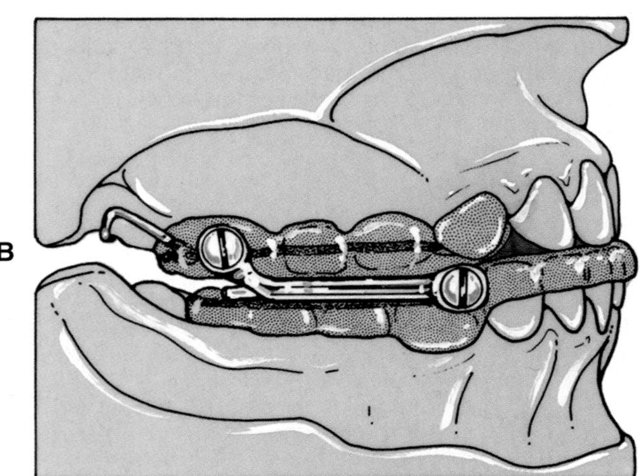

FIG 11-8 **A,** The Herbst appliance with bands on the maxillary and mandibular first premolars and first molars. In other designs, stainless-steel crowns are placed on the maxillary first molars and mandibular first premolars. **B,** The acrylic splint Herbst appliance. The maxillary portion of this type of Herbst appliance can be bonded or removable. The lower splint always is removable.

18. How effective is early treatment in patients with vertical problems such as open bite and deep bite?

Most orthodontists believe that the vertical dimension is the dimension of the face that is the most difficult to correct therapeutically. From a diagnostic perspective, the clinician must differentiate between problems that are primarily dentoalveolar in nature and those that are more skeletally based. An anterior open bite, for example, may be related to a digital sucking habit. The discontinuation of the habit may resolve the problem, with orthodontic treatment progressing smoothly.

Vertical problems that have a significant skeletal component are a challenge. In a growing patient, increasing a short lower facial height may be accomplished most effectively with a growth

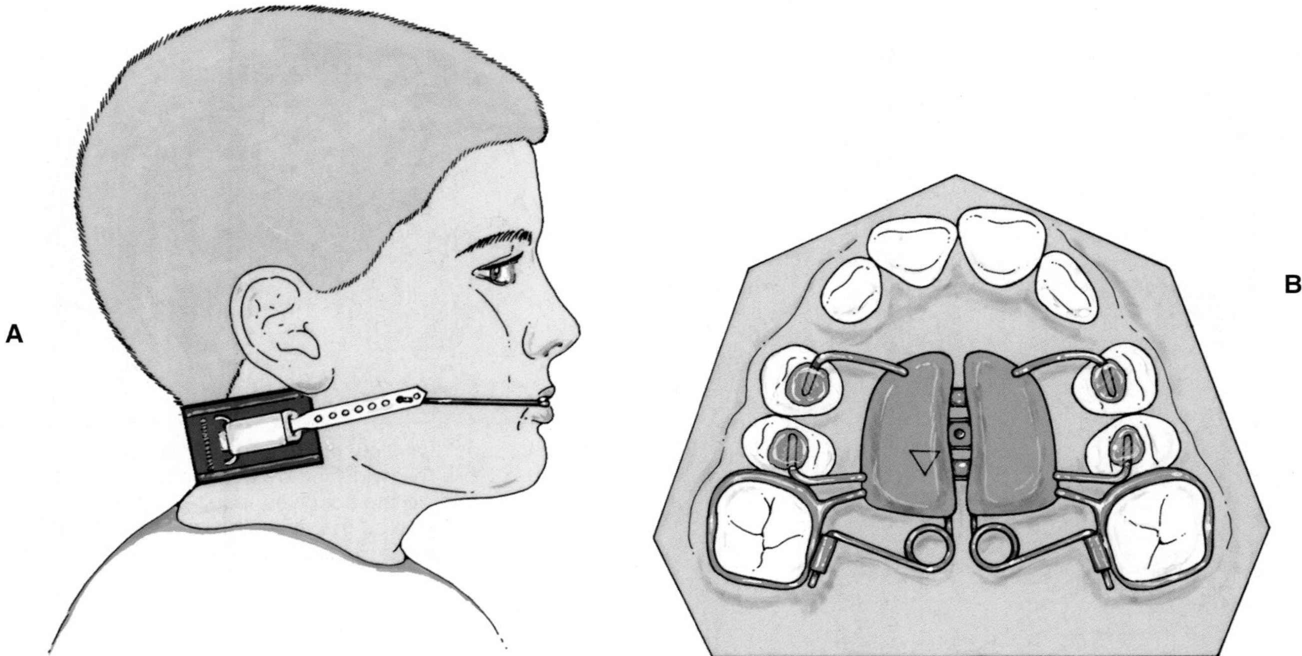

FIG 11-9 **A,** Cervical facebow. The inner bow has adjustment loops that also act as stops against the facebow tubes on the upper first molar bands. The outer bow is longer than the inner bow and typically is connected to an elastic neck strap or to elastics that attach to hooks on a cervical pad. **B,** The Pendex appliance of Hilgers. Locking wires connect the bands on the upper first molars to the acrylic button. These connecting wires are removed after the desired expansion has been achieved.

guidance appliance such as the Twin Block[19] (Fig. 11-10) or the Function Regulator (FR-2) of Fränkel.[20] These types of appliances allow for increased vertical development in the growing patient by opening the bite vertically and allowing eruption of the posterior teeth. In the long-face patient, controlling the vertical dimension has been particularly difficult. For example, the treatment effects of a bonded rapid maxillary expander and vertical-pull chin cup[21] (Fig. 11-11) have been shown to exist primarily in the mixed dentition and not as much in the permanent dentition.[22]

19. What is the duration of a Phase I treatment?

Because treatment is being initiated during a time of skeletal maturation, the provider must have a thorough understanding of craniofacial growth and of the development of the dental arches in order to provide the patient with the most effective and efficient regimen of treatment. Every effort should be made to time the treatment appropriately in order to maximize the treatment benefit in the shortest period of time. Optimally, in the treatment of a mixed dentition patient, there should be a phase of treatment that has a defined duration as well as a predictable outcome. In general terms, an initial phase of treatment usually is approximately *1 year in duration,* followed by intermittent observation during the transition from the mixed to the permanent dentition.

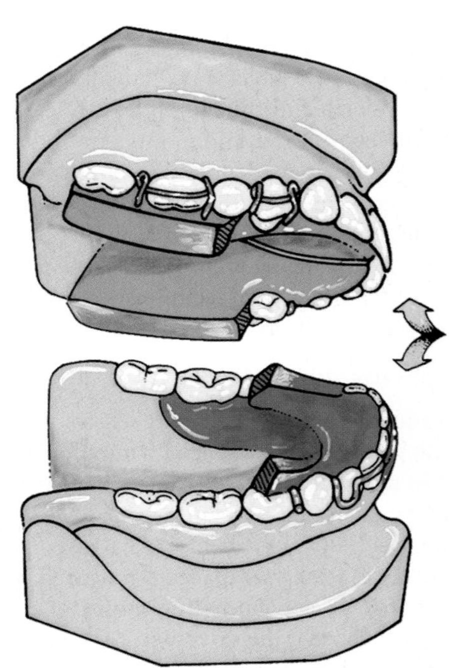

FIG 11-10 View of the modified Twin Block appliance of Clark.[19] Bilateral bite blocks are located posteriorly in the maxillary appliance and anteriorly in the mandibular appliance. These acrylic blocks can be trimmed to allow for posterior vertical development.

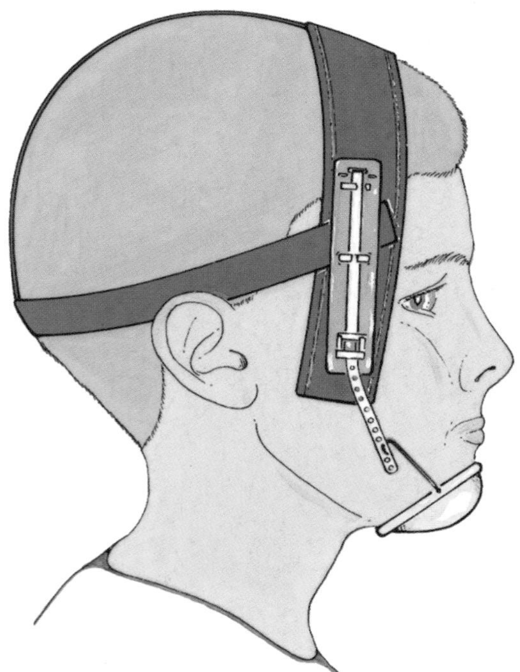

FIG 11-11 Lateral view of the vertical-pull chin cup. The hard acrylic chin cup is attached to the head strap by way of a spring-loaded connector.

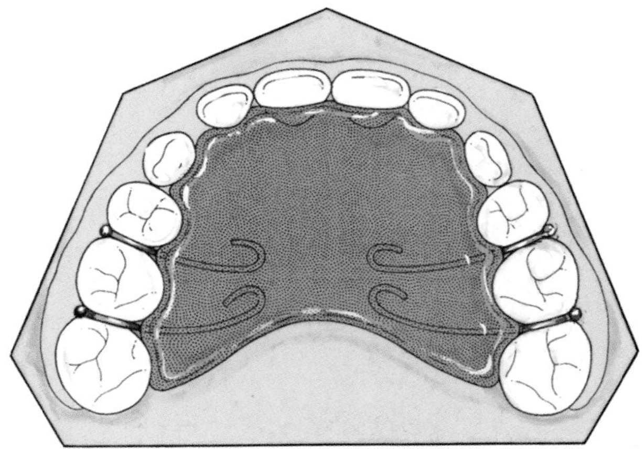

FIG 11-12 Occlusal view of the acrylic maintenance plate that is worn following removal of the rapid maxillary expander to stabilize the achieved result. A labial wire is not used most of the time so that the clinician can determine the relapse potential of the maxillary incisors during the interim period.

20. What happens between Phase I and Phase II?

The time between the initial phase of treatment and the second phase of fixed appliances is termed by us the *"interim period."* Patients typically are given a removable palatal plate (Fig. 11-12), usually without a labial wire. Patients are asked to wear this maintenance plate full-time for at least 1 year and then at night. They are seen every 4 to 6 months until the end of the transition to the permanent dentition when the second deciduous molars become loose. At that point, a transpalatal arch is delivered in about 90% of the patients; about 30% of patients benefit from a lower lingual arch. Fixed appliances are delivered after all of the permanent teeth (except third molars) are erupted or nearing eruption.

21. What occurs during Phase II?

Phase II treatment consists of comprehensive edgewise orthodontic therapy, which is treatment with full appliances. Phase II records are taken and the malocclusion of the patient is reassessed. Even though a patient may have undergone RME during Phase I, it is not unusual (~20% of patients) to have a patient undergo a second round of maxillary expansion if needed, usually with a Hyrax-type of RME appliance. The profile of the patient is examined as well to see if the extraction of permanent teeth is needed. In patients who have undergone either RME alone or RME preceded by a lower Schwarz appliance in our practice, we still extract in about 10% of that patient subgroup.

If the Class II molar relationship still remains at the beginning of Phase II, our appliance of choice is the Herbst appliance combined with fixed appliances and later with Class II elastics. If a residual Class III relationship remains at the beginning of Phase II, facial mask hooks may be added to a Hyrax expander and facial mask therapy is initiated at night. Following the placement of fixed appliances, Class III elastics are worn full-time until the Class III relationship is resolved.

The typical duration of Phase II treatment is about 18 months, but the situation varies. If the patient requires only mild detailing of the occlusion, treatment may take only a year to complete. On the other hand, if extractions are required, the treatment duration may be 18 to 24 months.

22. What are the risks of delaying early treatment in instances in which it is indicated?

In all cases of Class I, Class II, and Class III malocclusions, the loss of growth potential creates a situation in which an otherwise borderline case may be forced into the extraction and/or surgical category. The use of RME, functional appliances, extraoral traction, or facial mask therapy is all dependent on the clinician's ability to take advantage of the growth of a patient. In cases of a tooth size/arch size discrepancy, the greatest risk of delaying treatment is the resultant impaction or ectopic eruption of teeth. In the case of the maxillary canines, an ectopic eruption pattern could lead to loss of the root of the maxillary lateral incisor and/or the need for an exposure to bring the canine into the maxillary arch.

23. Do you have any final comments?

The topic of early treatment continues to be controversial in the orthodontic community, with advocates on both sides of the issue. Part of the controversy is being put to rest, however, as new data emerge from both prospective and retrospective clinical studies of the treatment protocols used on young patients.

The treatment protocols described in this chapter and elsewhere[1] have been used routinely in our practice for nearly three decades. The protocols have been refined over time, but the basic concepts presented here have remained constant. Perhaps the most significant change in our thinking over time has been the treatment of the Class II patient. As described earlier, the treatment of this condition for most patients is delayed until the circumpubertal growth period. Only in those patients with socially handicapping problems is correction of the underlying sagittal problems attempted in the early or mid mixed dentition. We still advocate intervention in the early mixed dentition for patients with Class III problems or tooth-size/arch-size discrepancies.

When we consider the effects of early treatment, it is obvious that the easiest way for a clinician to alter the growth of the face is in the transverse dimension, orthopedically in the maxilla, and dentally in the mandible.[18] Significant success has also been achieved in managing sagittal problems in growing patients. The management of vertical problems of a skeletal nature still remains a significant challenge, whether these conditions are treated early or late.

REFERENCES

1. McNamara JA Jr, Brudon WL: *Orthodontics and dentofacial orthopedics*. Ann Arbor: Needham Press, 2001.
2. Moyers RE, van der Linden FPGM, Riolo ML, McNamara JA Jr: Standards of Human Occlusal Development. Monograph 5, Craniofacial Growth Series, Center for Human Growth and Development. Ann Arbor: The University of Michigan, 1976.
3. Graber TM, Vanarsdall RL Jr, Vig KWL: *Orthodontics: principles and practices*, edition 4. St. Louis: WB Saunders, 2005.
4. Ringenberg QM: Serial extraction: stop, look, and be certain. *Am J Orthod* 1964;50:327-336.
5. Proffit WR, Fields HW Jr., Sarver DM: *Contemporary orthodontics*, edition 4. St Louis: Mosby, 2007.
6. Haas AJ: Rapid expansion of the maxillary dental arch and nasal cavity by opening the mid-palatal suture. *Angle Orthod* 1961;31:73-90.
7. Haas AJ: The treatment of maxillary deficiency by opening the mid-palatal suture. *Angle Orthod* 1965;35:200-217.
8. Hicks EP: Slow maxillary expansion. A clinical study of the skeletal versus dental response to low-magnitude force. *Am J Orthod* 1978;73:121-141.
9. Wendling LK, McNamara JA Jr, Franchi L, Baccetti T: Short-term skeletal and dental effects of the acrylic splint rapid maxillary expansion appliance. *Angle Orthod* 2005;75:7-14.
10. Biederman W: Rapid correction of Class III malocclusion by midpalatal expansion. *Am J Orthod* 1972;63:47-55.
11. Hartgerink DV, Vig PS, Abbott DW: The effect of rapid maxillary expansion on nasal airway resistance. *Am J Orthod Dentofacial Orthop* 1987;92:381-389.
12. McNamara JA Jr: An orthopedic approach to the treatment of Class III malocclusion in young patients. *J Clin Orthod* 1987;21:598-608.
13. Westwood PV, McNamara JA Jr, Baccetti T, et al: Long-term effects of early Class III treatment with rapid maxillary expansion and facial mask therapy. *Am J Orthod Dentofacial Orthop* 2003;123:306-320.
14. Baccetti T, Franchi L, McNamara JA Jr: The Cervical Vertebral Maturation (CVM) method for the assessment of optimal treatment timing in dentofacial orthopedics. *Semin Orthod* 2005;11:119-129.
15. Kloehn SJ: Evaluation of cervical anchorage force in treatment. *Angle Orthod* 1961;31:91-104.
16. Watson WG: A computerized appraisal of the high-pull face-bow. *Am J Orthod* 1972;62:561-579.
17. Hilgers JJ: The pendulum appliance for Class II non-compliance therapy. *J Clin Orthod* 1992;26:706-714.
18. McNamara JA Jr: Maxillary transverse deficiency. *Am J Orthod Dentofacial Orthop* 2000;117:567-570.
19. Clark WJ: *Twin block functional therapy*. London: Mosby-Wolfe, 1995.
20. Fränkel R, Fränkel C: *Orofacial orthopedics with the function regulator*. Munich: S Karger, 1989.
21. Pearson LE: The management of vertical problems in growing patients. In: McNamara JA, Jr, editor: The enigma of the vertical dimension. Monograph 36, Craniofacial Growth Series, Center for Human Growth and Development. Ann Arbor: The University of Michigan, 2000.
22. Schulz SO, McNamara JA Jr., Baccetti T, Franchi L: Treatment effects of bonded RME and vertical pull chin cup followed by fixed appliances in patients with increased vertical dimension. *Am J Orthod Dentofacial Orthop* 2005;128:326-336.

CHAPTER 12

The Invisalign System

Orhan C. Tuncay

Invisalign System is a relatively novel system of moving teeth, but its components are not all necessarily new. The clinician already knows how to make impressions and how to fabricate a suck-down thermoplastic cover over the teeth. It is also known that if the thermoformed plastic does not fit the model or teeth passively, teeth will move enough to accommodate the fit of the plastic. In fact, many orthodontists, when faced with minor relapse of alignment, will advise their patients to seat and press down the old suck-down retainer to realign the teeth. And it works.

The reason we refer to this entire process as a "system" is because the Invisalign System is more than an appliance: it's a mindset. The clinician must treat the patient virtually using the computer images long before touching even a single tooth. This process of predicting what should happen and when requires significant clinical experience.

The best cases for the beginner or occasional user of Invisalign are those with spacing problems devoid of any skeletal disparities. The result is consistently predictable and the process is comfortable. Treatment shown in Fig. 12-1 supports this statement.

The Invisalign System consists of mindset, software, impressions (instead of bracket placement), working with the computer, understanding physical properties and behavior characteristics of the plastic and ensuing force systems acting on teeth, as well as patient management. Just as any other appliance system, Invisalign has many remarkable strengths and many weaknesses. The clinician should know these and plan a treatment strategy accordingly; this strategy includes "treatment objectives."

Clearly, Rome was not built overnight, nor was the edgewise appliance developed overnight, and neither will Invisalign reach its level of perfection overnight. Thus, comparisons of performance to other appliances would be inappropriate. Invisalign is generally used in the adult patient where attrition of the teeth is significant, mutilation is common, and patient desires are not occlusion specific. None of these elements is conducive to assess the outcome of treatment by quantitative means. Instead, the Invisalign-treated case can be judged only qualitatively.

1. Historically, what appliances preceded Invisalign?

Prior to introduction of the Invisalign System, the most widely used appliance was an adjunct to fixed appliances, which was worn once the bands and brackets were removed. The Positioner introduced by Kesling (1945) was originally made out of vulcanite material and aided the settling-in process; but it was also useful in correcting certain tooth positions that could not be finished for one reason or another by fixed appliances.[1] Later, latex became the standard material to manufacture. But even earlier, Remmensnyder had introduced the Flex-O-Tite gum-massaging appliance in 1926 to aid in the treatment of gingival disease.[2] He reported that he was observing tooth movements as a side effect. The first thermoformed plastic sheet to move teeth was invented by Nahoum in 1964.[3] He called it the Dental Contour Appliance. Subsequently it was modified by Sheridan (1993) and called the Essix appliance.[4] Invisalign (1997) takes the principles behind these appliances and manufactures series of Invisalign aligners to move teeth using the CAD/CAM technology.

2. How are Polyvinyl Siloxane (PVS) impressions converted to digital images and subsequently to aligners?

In the manufacture of aligners, a number of imaging technologies have been used. Initially, a laser scanner manufactured by Cyberware was tested, but the undercuts were hard to capture. To improve the speed of image capture, the earlier Invisalign-branded aligners were created from images generated by the destructive scanning process. In this process, layers of 2D images are stacked to form a 3D image. Unfortunately, this technique is lengthy, expensive, and messy. Structured light was a popular method to capture the image of a surface, but it too was not accurate enough; it did not provide enough detail of undercuts and interproximal gaps. Currently, CT scanning is used, avoiding the need for impressions to be poured.

From the images acquired, light-cured polymer molds are manufactured. This process is known as stereolithography (SLA). This series of molds created for each patient is used to thermoform the plastic sheet. Trimming of the plastic is

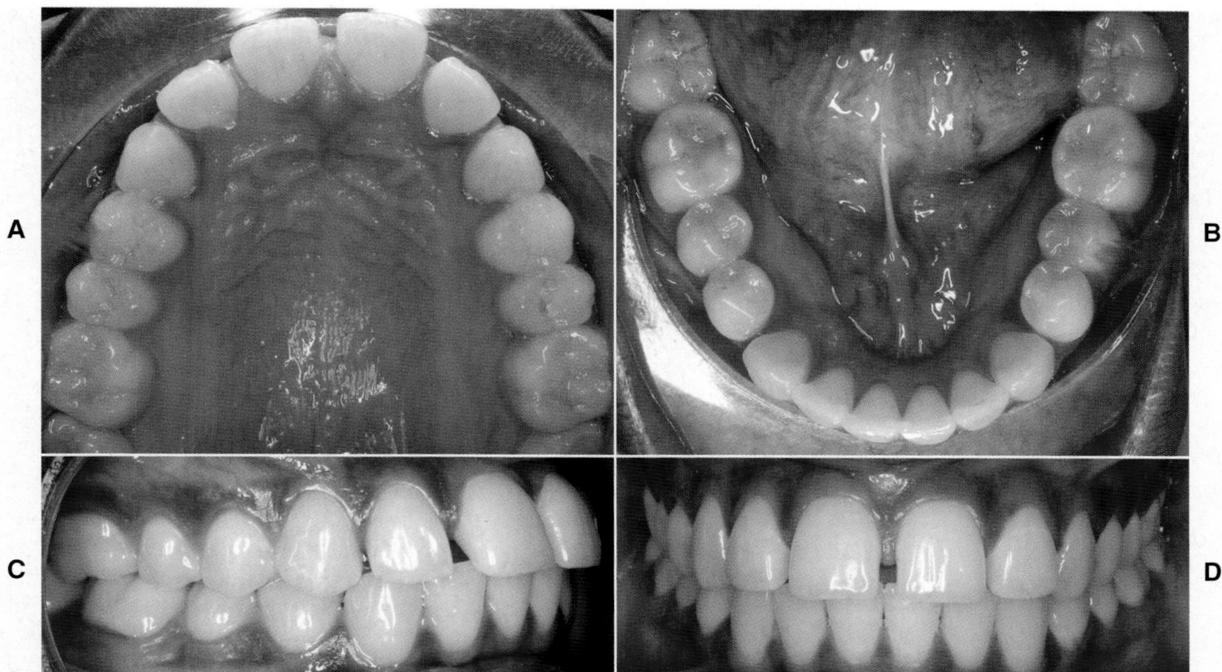

FIG 12-1 **A-E,** This patient exhibits a good posterior occlusion and generalized spacing in the anterior region. These images depict a perfect indication for Invisalign treatment; treatment time will be short and uneventful.
Continued

done by robots, but the final smoothing is still done by hand. Prior to packaging and shipping, Invisalign aligners are disinfected in an ultrasonic bath of disinfectants.

3. What is the process and software involved in creating the Invisalign-branded aligners?

The CT images of PVS impressions are transferred to a special software called "Treat" software.[5] It has a number of components that perform different functions. Initially, imperfections of the impression are smoothed out and then submitted to the ClinCheck technicians. Steps involved in the manufacturing process are:

1. Segmentation (virtual cutting of the teeth)
2. Final setup (the desired end result of orthodontic treatment)
3. Staging (how to incrementally get to the final result)
4. Review (inspection of ClinCheck by the clinician)
5. Fabrication (production of SLA models and thermoforming the plastic to fabricate the Invisalign aligner)

These virtual steps are similar to the manual steps used in the making of wax setups from plaster study casts.

4. What are the force systems generated in the Invisalign aligner that act on each tooth?

This is an area of significant research interest both in fixed appliance systems and with the plastic aligners. Currently, it is not fully understood.[6] Certainly, one could measure the force systems active at the time of insertion of archwires or aligners, but as soon as the appliance is inserted, the measured force systems all change. Practically, our current understanding of orthodontic biomechanics is limited to the first millisecond of tooth movement. Movements of adjacent teeth; the nature of periodontal response to force; precision of brackets, wires, attachments, plastic; and the way the patient handles the hardware all affect the force systems.

5. What are the issues that surround forces generated within the Invisalign aligner over a long duration?

Thermoplastic materials are viscoelastic; thus, their properties are time dependent. Invisalign aligners stretch and fit over the tooth that is programmed to move. While the stretched aligner is trying to move the tooth, it is held at constant strain. In turn, stress relaxation within the plastic sets in and the forces generated by the aligner decrease with time. This process is accelerated in a moist environment.[7]

6. Does thicker aligner material (Ex40) yield better tooth movement?

Increasing the thickness of the aligner material by 0.01 mm from 0.03 to 0.04 mm increases the stiffness of the aligner by one third. This concept is not dissimilar to what is seen in the behavior of orthodontic wires. But clinical trials provide no indication that a thicker aligner is better in finishing a case. Also, the increased thickness does not affect the quality of tooth movement during the active treatment phase.[8] Certainly, as a retainer material, the thicker Ex40 is more robust.

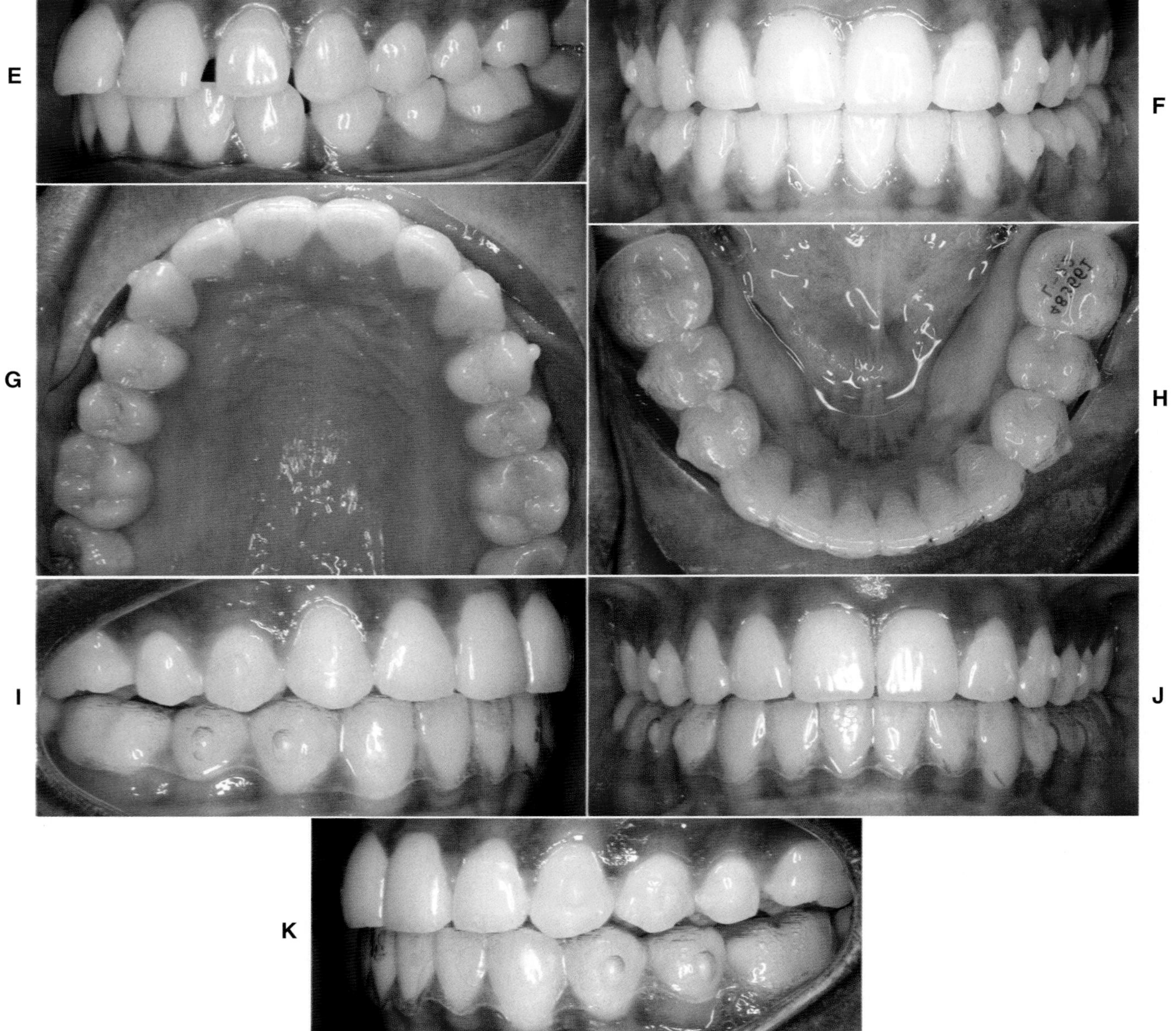

FIG 12-1—cont'd F, Note the improperly placed gingival margin. The overextended tray can strip the gingival tissue away. This is usually due to imperfect registration of the gingival margin in the PVS impression. Another possible error is on the technician's part where the virtual gingival tissue was constructed thinner than it is in real life. During the course of treatment, the clinician or the patient may trim the overextended parts with the aid of common nail trimmers. **G-K,** As can be noted in the images, spaces have closed and the gingival response is very good and devoid of any overgrowth.

7. Can tipping of teeth be controlled in premolar extraction cases?

Tipping of teeth into the extraction space is nearly impossible to avoid, even with fixed appliances.[9] But tipping is exaggerated in the adult. The apices will simply not move very well, especially if the roots of maxillary buccal teeth are in the maxillary sinus (as viewed in the panoramic radiograph). This is because the lining of maxillary sinus does not remodel readily (Fig. 12-2).

Complex attachment designs for teeth adjacent to the extraction site help reduce the tipping, but sectional fixed appliances are necessary almost every time. Another common problem seen after the extraction space is closed is leveling of marginal ridges. First and second molar marginal ridges rarely align properly. The sectional fixed appliance should be fabricated to fix that problem simultaneously as it parallels the roots.

8. What are the weakest elements of aligners?

The foremost frustration is with patient compliance. Even though adults are more cooperative than children, a large percentage of patients do not clock 300 to 400 hours on their aligners. Changing aligners prematurely leads to loss of tracking. But there are no problems reported because of aligners worn longer than 400 hours. Patients who cooperate as prescribed can achieve the ClinCheck movements predictably.

The second most common performance problem is extrusion of teeth, especially the maxillary lateral incisor. But the most recent evidence suggests that this might be due to delayed movements of adjacent teeth, particularly the canines. If the canines do not move, the aligner will not fit well over the laterals and will give the appearance that they are not extruding. Since the canine is a large-rooted tooth, it is prudent to extend the wear time or to significantly slow down the rate of tooth movement on the canine teeth.[10]

The third significant weakness is the aligner's inability to move the root apex, such as in torquing or translational movements.

9. What are the advantages of the Invisalign System over traditional fixed appliances?

- **Esthetics.** Invisalign aligners are undetectable from a distance of 2 feet. Of course, one can remove them at will in anticipation of close encounters or lisping.
- **Comfort.** Traditional pain or soreness associated with fixed appliances is not experienced with Invisalign.
- **Bonding problems avoided.** In patients with amelogenesis imperfecta or prosthetic crowns with porcelain surfaces or bridges, the clinician does not worry about securing brackets onto such surfaces. Also, with the aligner even patients with less-than-perfect oral hygiene do not exhibit white enamel spots or decalcification.
- **Lack of root resorption.** There are no reported studies of noticeable root resorption in patients treated with the Invisalign System. This is probably due to <0.25 mm of tooth movement per tray. This distance does not obstruct the PDL blood flow and avoids formation of necrotic regions.
- **Oral hygiene.** Compared with fixed appliances and untreated control patients, the periodontal tissue health as measured by papillary bleeding score and periodontal pocket depth improves with use of Invisalign during orthodontic treatment.[11]
- **Chair time.** Routine follow-up visits practically take no time. Also, the instruments needed on the tray setup are minimal.
- **No emergencies.** Normally, the Invisalign aligners do not break. But even if they do, the patient need not call the office to schedule an after-hours emergency visit. They simply move to the next aligner.
- **Special patients.** Musicians or athletes benefit greatly from Invisalign. If the aligner interferes with the wind instrument, it can be removed, just as an athlete would. But in most instances the Invisalign trays function as mouthguards.
- **Vertical correction.** The Invisalign aligner can intrude the posterior teeth and close the anterior open bite. Conversely, it can effectively intrude the anterior teeth to open the bite.
- **Bruxism.** The aligner is a good substitute for bite splints. It will also reposition the mandible to read the correct centric relation.
- **Bleaching.** The Invisalign tray may be used for bleaching, but it is critical not to bleach if there are attachments present because color will not change under the attachments.
- **ClinCheck is a diagnostic tool.** The clinician can create innumerable what-if scenarios without messy wax setups and can also fine-tune the desired final tooth positions with overcorrections.[12]

10. What are the considerations for interproximal enamel reduction (IPR)?

The amount of interproximal reduction (IPR) performed with Invisalign should be about the same as with fixed appliances.[13] It is a misconception that one type of appliance needs IPR more than the other. Exceptions aside, IPR should be limited to instances of:

- Bolton's discrepancy
- Need to simulate physiological tooth attrition
- Need to camouflage a skeletal deformity without surgery
- Necessity to alter the tooth morphology

IPR has not been shown to adversely affect dental or periodontal health. Initial concerns of root proximity, caries risk, and the like have not been shown to be valid.[14] Nonetheless, a good depth of enamel must be present so that some of it could be removed. Anterior teeth with peg-shaped morphology are not good candidates for IPR. In the posterior region, it is a good idea to use separators prior to IPR. Separation will allow for better direct vision of the tooth to be reduced. Also, it is best to perform IPR during the course of treatment rather than before the PVS impressions.

To perform good IPR, periapical radiographs are needed, but without such benefit, one may safely remove 0.3 mm from the anterior teeth and 0.6 mm from the posterior.

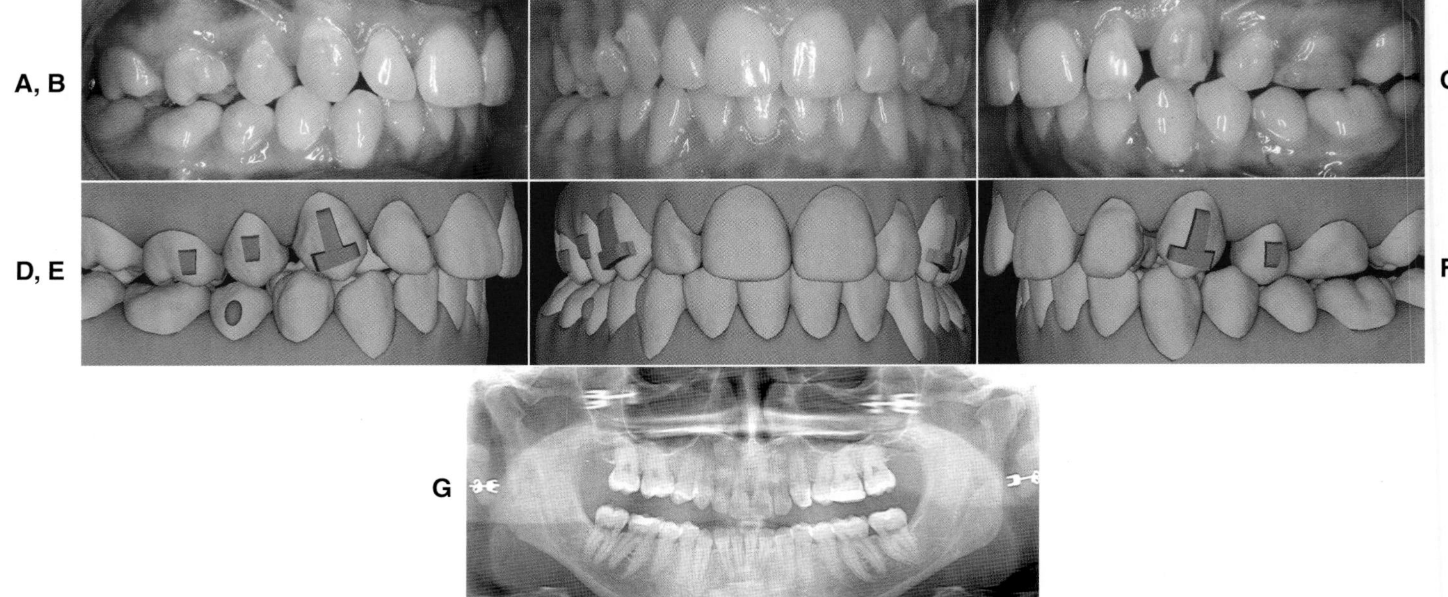

FIG 12-2 **A-F,** In this asymmetrical extraction case (teeth #4 and #12), the "T" attachment minimized tipping of the canine (#11) but the right side molar teeth have tipped into the extraction site. **G,** The panoramic radiograph of this patient reveals that the maxillary sinus floor hinders the movement of molar roots (even with fixed appliances). It is long known, however, that Invisalign cannot move the root apices as effectively as fixed appliances can. This can be seen in the lower incisor region where all the roots are converged. A good finish would be to diverge the lower incisor roots.

REFERENCES

1. Kesling HD: The philosophy of the tooth positioning appliance. *Am J Orthod* 1945;31:297-304.
2. Remmensnyder O: A gum-massaging appliance in the treatment of pyorrhea. *Dent Cosmos* 1926;28:381-384.
3. Nahoum HI: The vacuum formed dental contour appliance. *NY State Dent J* 1964;9:385-390.
4. Sheridan JJ, LeDoux W, McMinn R: Essix retainers: fabrication and supervision for permanent retention. *J Clin Orthod* 1993;27:37-45.
5. Beers A: Invisalign software. In *The Invisalign system*, Berlin: Quintessence, 2006.
6. Cao H, Duong T: Applications of mechanics with Invisalign. In *The Invisalign system.* Berlin: Quintessence, 2006.
7. Tricca R, Chunhua L: Properties of aligner material Ex30. In *The Invisalign system.* Berlin: Quintessence, 2006.
8. Duong T, Derakhshan M: Ex40 material and aligner thickness. In *The Invisalign system.* Berlin: Quintessence, 2006.
9. Tuncay OC: The iatrogenic crowding caused by aligner length/arch length discrepancy. *Clin Rep Tech* 2005 (Fall 1);1:3-5.
10. Nord S: *An exploratory study to identify the conditions that induce loss of tracking in tooth movement with the Invisalign system.* Masters Thesis, Temple University, 2005.
11. Taylor MG, McGorray SP, Durrett S, et at: Effect of Invisalign aligners on periodontal tissues. *J Dent Res* 2003;82:1483.
12. Duong T, Derakhshan M: Advantages of the Invisalign system. In *The Invisalign system.* Berlin: Quintessence, 2006.
13. Miethke RR, Jost-Brinkmann PG: Interproximal enamel reduction. In *The Invisalign system.* Berlin: Quintessence, 2006.
14. Fillion D, Teil II: Vor- und Nachteile der approximalen Schmelzreduktion. *Int Orthod Kieferorthop* 1995;27:64-90.

CHAPTER 13

Treatment of Class II Malocclusions

Richard Kulbersh • Valmy Pangrazio-Kulbersh

Class II malocclusion is not a single entity but results from numerous combinations of both skeletal and dental alveolar components. The earliest description, solely a dental description, was provided by Edward Angle when he defined a Class II malocclusion as characterized by the lower molar in distal position relative to the upper 6-year molar. He further subdivided Class II malocclusions into Class II division 1, characterized by the anterior maxillary teeth being protrusive; and Class II division 2, characterized by two or more maxillary anterior teeth being retroclined. The Class II division 1 was later shown to also be characterized by a retrognathic mandible or a prognathic maxilla with variable vertical dimensions. The Class II division 2 patient was shown to exhibit an orthognathic maxilla, a short and retrognathic mandible, brachyfacial growth pattern, retroclined maxillary central incisors, and a relatively prominent chin, as well as dental deep bite. In later years further assessment of the dental Class II provided information regarding the underlying skeletal components.[1-3]

1. What are the components of a Class II malocclusion?

Utilizing cephalometrics and computer-based statistical evaluation, Moyers et al.[4] determined that Class II patients were divided into six separate horizontal types and five vertical types based upon various skeletal and dentoalveolar characteristics. The six horizontal types are described in Table 13-1.

The five vertical types (Table 13-2) were defined by an assessment of the following four facial planes relative to their normal position:

1. The SN cranial base plane
2. The palatal plane
3. The functional-occlusal plane
4. The mandibular plane

In the transverse dimension, the buccal segments of Class II patients often appear normal. A 3 to 4 mm transverse discrepancy, however, usually exists at the level of the first molar due to a narrow maxillary arch. This is readily observable if the mandible is moved into the Class I relationship at the molar. Further assessment of components of Class II malocclusion in an adolescent population indicated that in a sample of 277 children with a Class II malocclusion, mandibular skeletal retrusion was the most common characteristic. The maxilla was generally either retrusive or well positioned.

2. How can Moyers' differential diagnosis of Class II horizontal and vertical types be used to help us with treatment planning of Class II patients?

Moyers' differential diagnosis of Class II malocclusions allows us to more easily determine the components of the Class II malocclusion problem. It identifies the skeletal problem and the dentoalveolar problem and thus directs our treatment thinking to these specific areas. Treatment planning considerations using Moyers' differential Class II horizontal analysis is summarized, at least in part, in Table 13-3.

In addition to the horizontal considerations addressed in Table 13-3, proper patient treatment also requires assessment of the vertical components. Treatment options for vertical correction in growing patients would include biteblocks and various types of headgear. In non-growing patients, surgical correction options such as LeFort I maxillary impaction and alveolar procedures may be required.

3. What is the prevalence of Class II malocclusions?[3,5]

According to the NHANES III Study, 15% of the U.S. population have an overjet of greater than 4 mm, 38% an overjet of 3 to 4 mm, and 33% Class II occlusal discrepancies. The same frequency for Class II dental characteristics was found in Caucasians, African-Americans and Hispanics. According to McNamara[1], 75% of Class II skeletal discrepancies are the result of mandibular retrognathia.

4. What is the etiology of Class II malocclusion?[6-10]

Class II malocclusion is usually an aberration of normal development and not caused by a pathologic process. It is usually the result of multiple factors that influence growth and development and not from one specific factor. The development of Class II malocclusion, however, may be related to some specific causes, genetic influences, and environmental factors.

TABLE 13-1 The Six Horizontal Class II Types Determined by Moyers et al.

DIAGRAMMATIC REPRESENTATION	DESCRIPTION
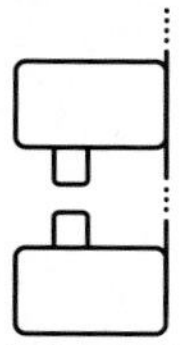	Normal
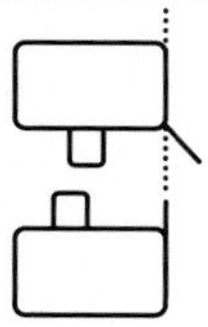	Type A: Maxillary dental protraction
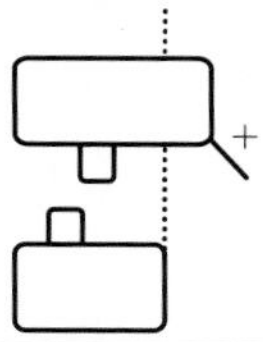	Type B: Maxillary prognathism, dental protraction
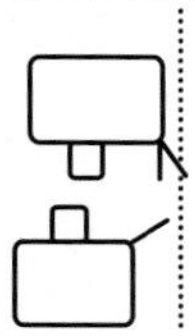	Type C: Maxillary retrognathism with flared or upright incisors, mandibular severe retrognathism with flared lower incisors
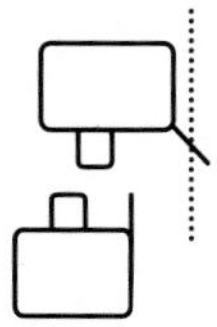	Type D: Maxillary retrognathism with dental protraction, severe mandibular retrognathism
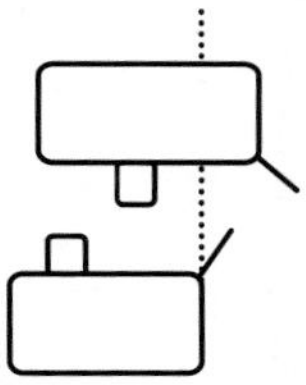	Type E: Maxillary prognathism and dental protraction + mandibular dental flaring
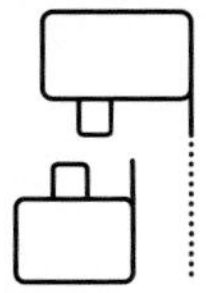	Type F: Mandibular retrognathism

Adapted from Moyers RE, Riolo MS, Guire KE, et al: *Am J Orthod* 1980;78(5):477-494.

Such specific causes as the effect of teratogens on mandibular growth, mandibular deficient syndromes (Pierre-Robin and Treacher-Collins), fetal molding, trauma to the transmandibular junction (TMJ) area during the birth process, childhood fractures of the jaw, and mandibular arthritic problems may all contribute to the development of a Class II skeletal pattern. Less than 1% of orthodontic patients, however, have a disruption in embryological development that can be attributed as the major cause of malocclusion. Genetic influences have been shown to be associated with Class II malocclusions.

Local and environmental factors may also be an issue in the development of Class II malocclusions because of their alteration of the normal physiologic pressures and forces associated with craniofacial growth. These pressures and forces may be disrupted or imbalanced by the effects of abnormal function of the soft tissues. Disruption of normal lip balance such as that associated with lip incompetency may lead to flaring of the upper incisors from an imbalance of labial and lingual musculature. The need to achieve lip–tongue contact for an oral seal during swallowing can cause the lip to retrocline lower incisors

TABLE 13-2 The Five Vertical Class II Types Determined by Moyers et al.

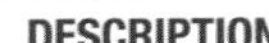

DIAGRAMMATIC REPRESENTATION	DESCRIPTION
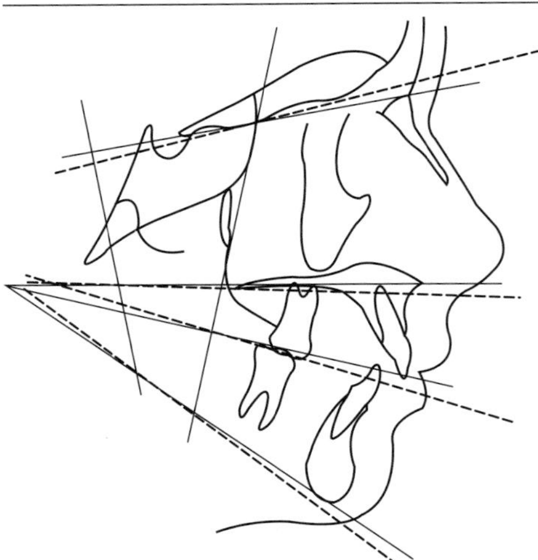 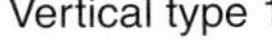 Vertical type 1	Type 1: Mandibular plane steeper than normal, steeper functional occlusal plane, palate tipped somewhat downward, anterior cranial base tipped upward
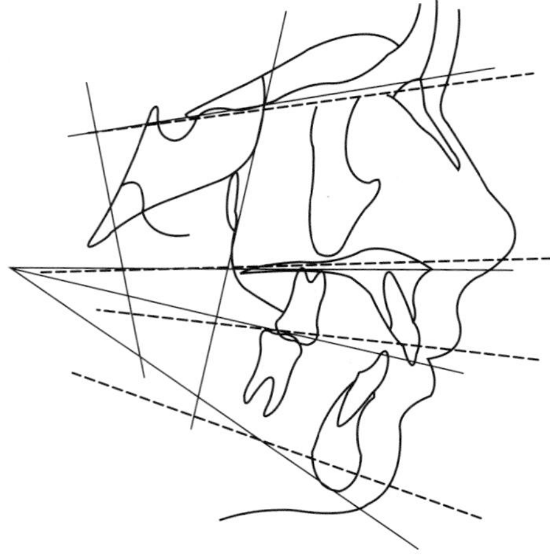 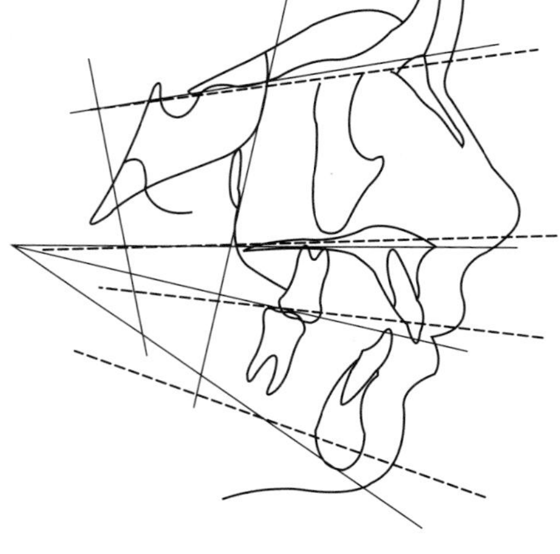 Vertical type 2	Type 2: Mandibular plane, functional occlusal plane and palatal plane are all flatter than normal and are nearly parallel
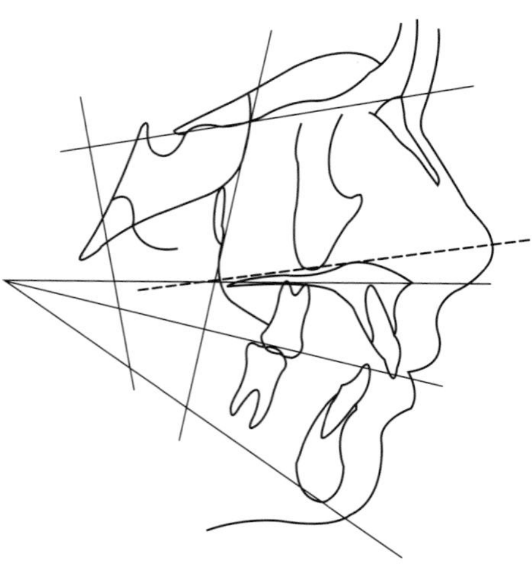 Vertical type 3	Type 3: Palatal plane tipped upward anteriorly

TABLE 13-2 The Five Vertical Class II Types Determined by Moyers et al.–cont'd

DIAGRAMMATIC REPRESENTATION	DESCRIPTION
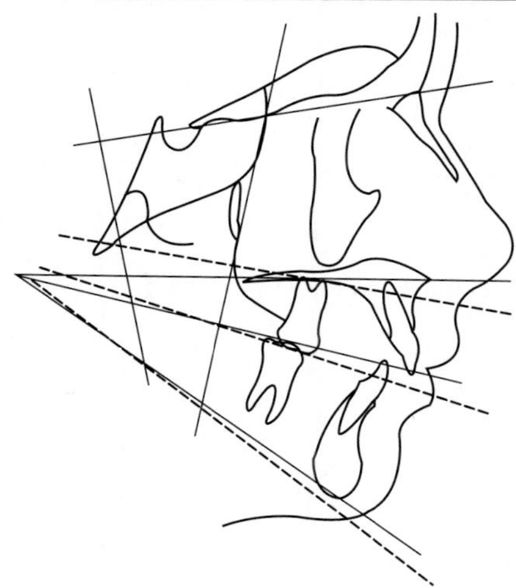 Vertical type 4	Type 4: Mandibular plane, the functional occlusal plane, and the palatal plane are all tipped markedly downward
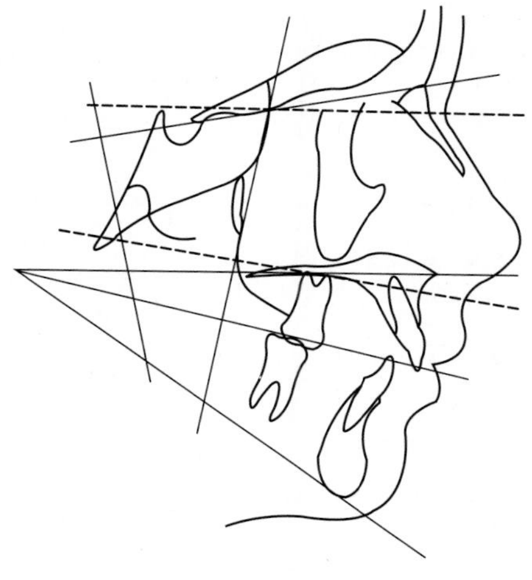 Vertical type 5	Type 5: Palatal plane is tipped downward, cranial base tipped downward

Adapted from Moyers RE, Riolo MS, Guire KE, et al: *Am J Orthod* 1980;78(5):477-494.

and the protruding tongue to flare upper incisors, thus increasing overjet. It has also been speculated that mouth-breathing can cause the opening muscles to place a distal force on the mandible, retarding its growth and rotating the mandible clockwise. In addition, it is thought that finger-sucking habits can produce a Class II division 1 incisal relationship within a Class II or Class I skeletal pattern (Fig. 13-1).

5. What treatment protocols are used to correct Class II malocclusions?

Treatment for Class II malocclusions may involve the following:

- Extra-oral traction
- Distalizing appliances
- Functional jaw orthopedics
- Camouflage
- Surgery

The appropriate protocol for each patient depends upon patient desires and doctor assessment of the exact nature of the Class II problem as well as the orthodontist's treatment protocol preferences.

6. What is extra-oral traction?[3,5,11]

Extra-oral traction is the application of force to the dentition and maxilla through the use of headgears (cervical, occipital, combination) fitted to the skull and attached facebows through which force is directly applied to the dentition, usually through the permanent maxillary first molars. Headgear wear is required for at least 12 to 14 hours per day for 6 to 18 months at a force level of 12 to 16 ounces per side for skeletal modification.

TABLE 13-3 Summarization of Moyers' Differential Class II Horizontal Analysis

TYPE	TREATMENT CONSIDERATIONS
Type A 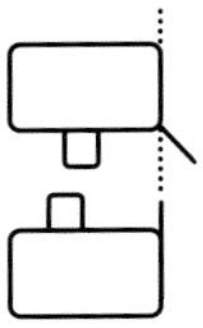	1. Extraction of upper bicuspids + orthodontic retraction and uprighting 2. Distalization of upper dentition into Class I (i.e., headgear, molar distalizers) 3. Surgery: Anterior maxillary alveolar osteotomy setback and uprighting of upper centrals and laterals after extraction of upper bicuspids and orthodontic retraction of canines
Type B 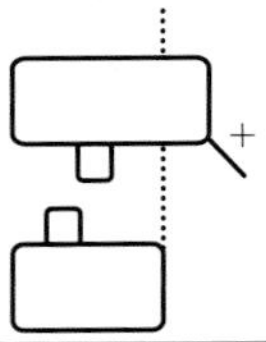	1. Headgear (growing patient) 2. Surgery: maxillary anterior alveolar setback (non-growing patient) with extractions of upper bicuspids
Type C 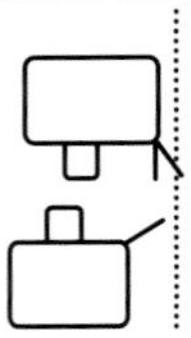	1. Complex skeletal and dentoalveolar considerations 2. Extraction of upper and lower bicuspids, orthodontics + functional appliance 3. Extraction of upper 5/lower 4's, orthodontics to close spaces and upright incisors + surgery: maxillary and mandibular differential advancement
Type D 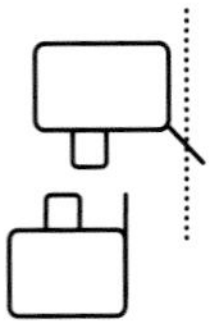	1. Orthodontic + functional appliance (growing patient) 2. Surgery: mandibular advancement (non-growing patient)
Type E 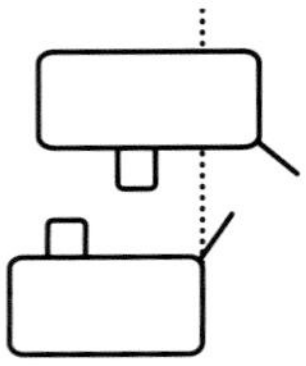	1. Headgear 2. Bimaxillary protrusion-extraction of upper and lower bicuspids 3. Extractions + surgery (non-growing patient)
Type F 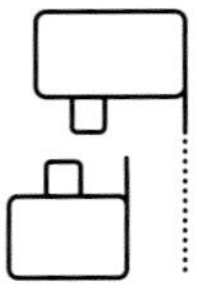	1. Functional appliance (growing patient) 2. Surgery: mandibular advancement (non-growing patient)

Adapted from Moyers RE, Riolo MS, Guire KE, et al: *Am J Orthod* 1980;78(5):477-494.

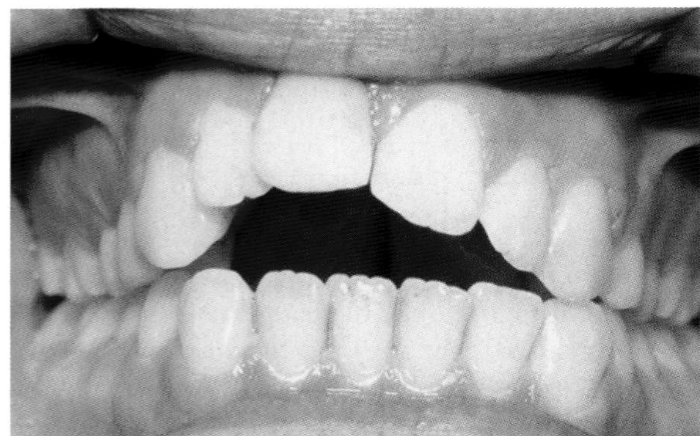

FIG 13-1 Vertical and anteroposterior distortion of maxilla caused by thumb-sucking habit.

Three types of headgear are commonly used depending upon the vertical craniofacial growth pattern: cervical pull headgear for low vertical dimension (Frankfort mandibular plane angle [FMA] $\leq$25), occipital pull headgear (FMA >30) and combination (combi) headgear for cases in which the vector of force application needs to be altered depending upon the desired effect for a specific patient. The various types of headgear and attached facebows are useful in applying forces of appropriate magnitude and direction to the maxilla via the maxillary dentition. The effect of the applied force has an orthopedic effect. It modifies maxillary position by altering its normal downward and forward growth pattern, thus normalizing the Class II to a Class I skeletal pattern (Fig. 13-2).

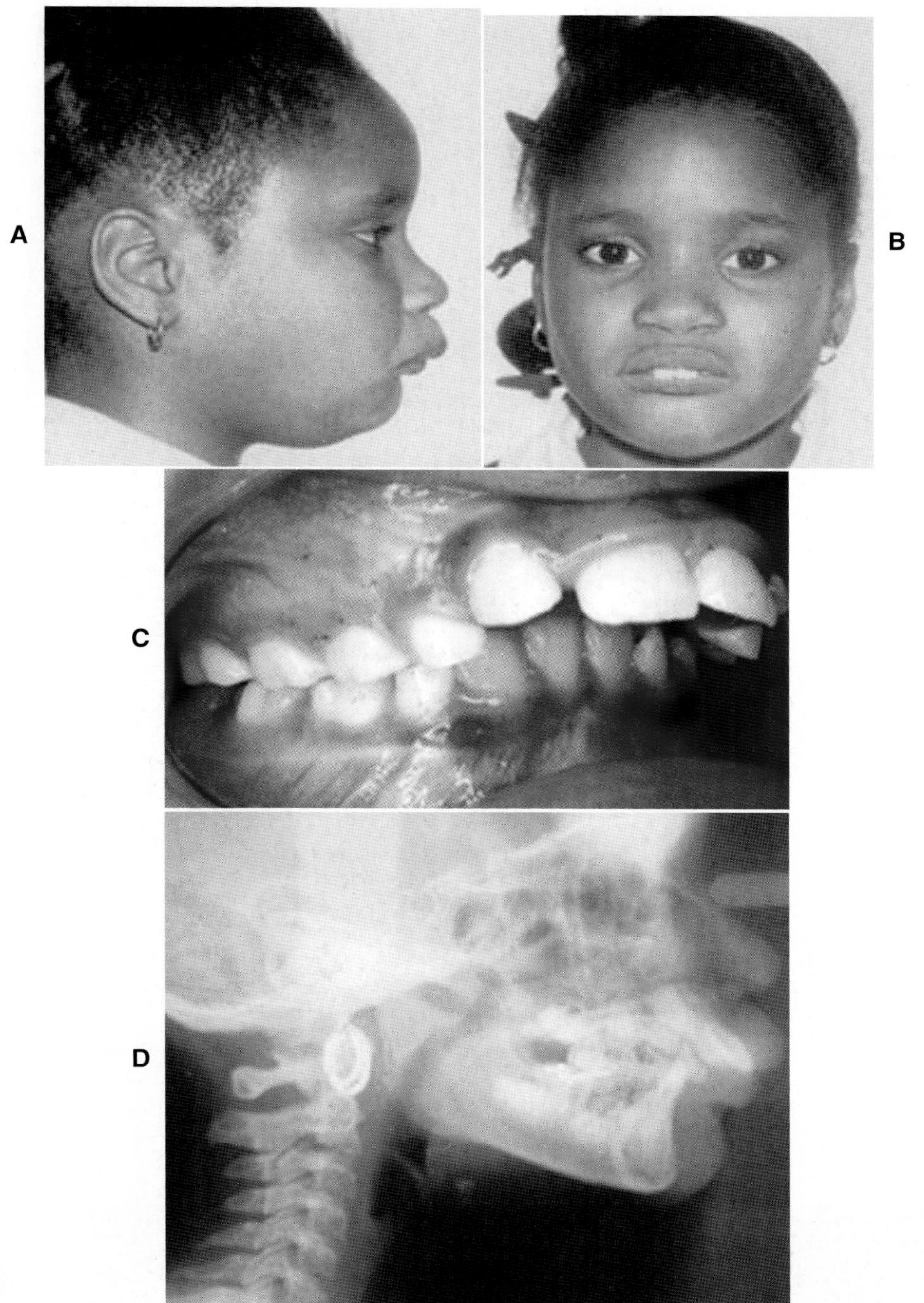

FIG 13-2 Headgear treatment of Class II division 1 malocclusion. **A-D,** Initial photos: facial photos **(A** and **B),** intraoral photo **(C),** and cephalometric radiograph **(D)**.

Continued

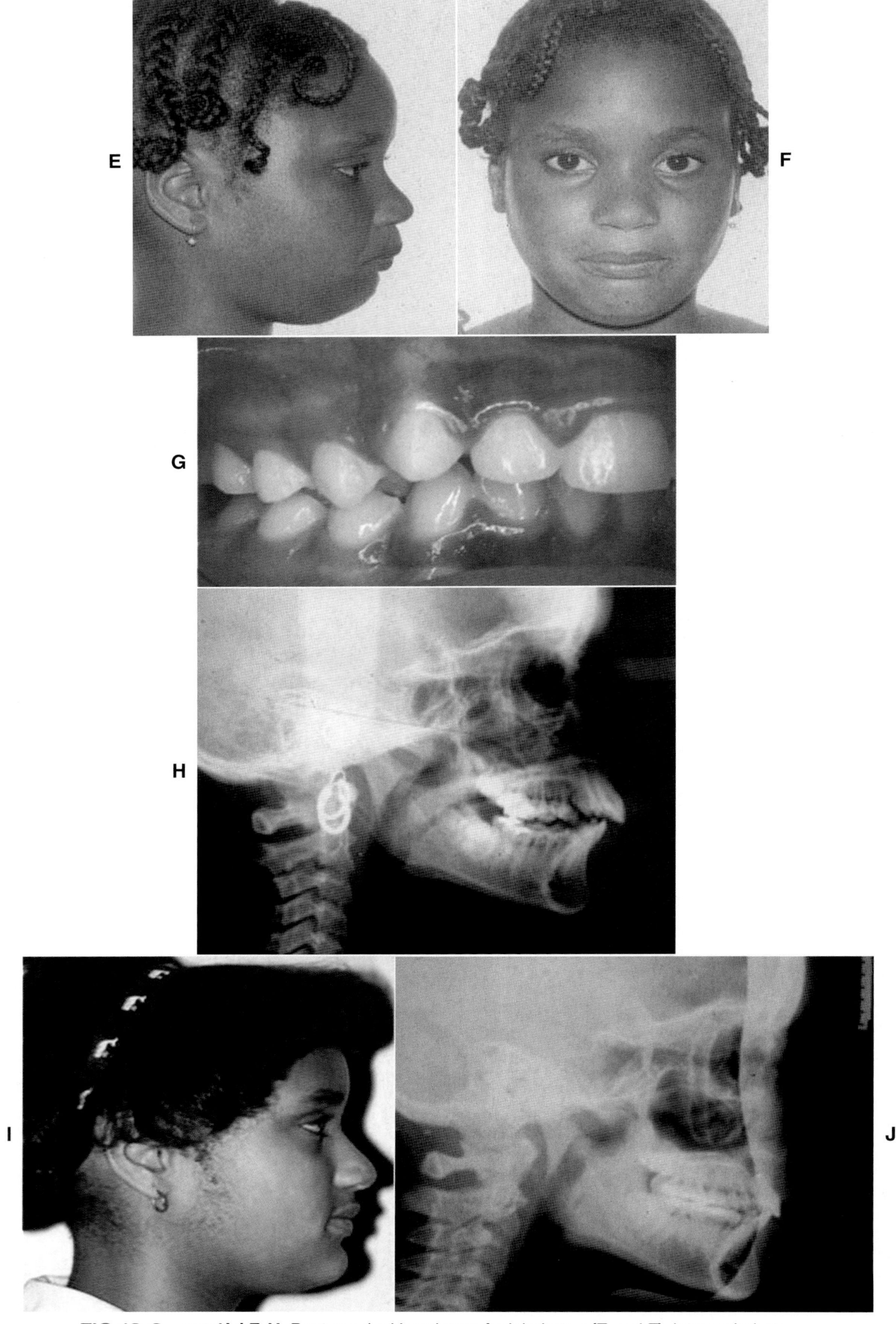

FIG 13-2—cont'd E-H, Post-cervical headgear: facial photos **(E** and **F),** intraoral photo **(G),** and cephalometric radiograph **(H)**. **I** and **J,** Orthodontic treatment with extractions: facial photo **(I)** and cephalometric radiograph **(J)**.

7. What is the distalizing protocol for the correction of Class II?[3,5,11,12]

Molar distalization is used when the Class II problem is dentoalveolar in nature. Molar distalization corrects a dental Class II by moving the maxillary first molar distally into a Class I relationship. Such treatment has no orthopedic effect. Distalizing appliances are usually very effective because they require little, if any, cooperation from the patient. Types of such appliances are:

- Plates
- Pendulum/Pendex (Fig. 13-3)
- Distal jet
- Jones jig
- Jasper jumper

8. What is functional jaw orthopedics?[3,13-15]

Functional jaw orthopedics is the use of appliances that work by forward positioning of the mandible. This results in altering the activity of postural muscles of the craniofacial complex, causing changes in skeletal and dental relationships. The goal is to enhance mandibular growth by allowing the full expression of the genetic potential and encouraging remodeling at the glenoid fossa. The mandible is translated downward and forward by the appliance, with resulting growth at the condyle and posterior surface of the ramus. In animal studies functional jaw orthopedics was shown to increase activity at the lateral pterygoid followed by an adaptive growth response at the condyle. Since the lateral pterygoid activity decreases after 6 to 8 weeks, repeated advancement of the appliance is required. Early correction of Class II dentoskeletal malocclusion with functional jaw orthopedics shows favorable and stable results. Typical results from functional jaw orthopedic therapy show the following:

- Condylar growth during treatment: 1–3 mm
- Fossa displacement, growth and adaptation: 3–5 mm with a dominant vertical vector
- More favorable growth direction: 0.5–1.5 mm
- Withholding of downward and forward maxillary growth: 1–1.5 mm
- Differential upward and forward eruption of lower buccal segments: 1.5–2.5 mm
- Headgear effect: 0.0–0.5 mm

9. When is functional appliance therapy indicated?[16,17]

The primary indication for functional jaw orthopedics is mandibular skeletal retrusion. An abnormal muscular function is also an indication. Functional appliances remove abnormal and restrictive muscular activity that prevents the normal development of the maxilla and mandible as well as appropriate development of the dental arches.

Research has shown that there is an ideal time for functional appliance therapy. Greater mandibular length is obtained when functional appliance treatment is performed during the circumpubertal growth period. Ideally, functional appliance therapy should be started in the late mixed dentition or early permanent dentition followed by Phase II therapy to align the permanent dentition. For some patients who have severe neuromuscular, skeletal, and dentoalveolar problems, treatment may be initiated in the early mixed dentition.

The reason for increased growth response may be related to the synergistic interaction between the change in function, produced by the functional appliance and growth hormone as well as related substances that are in greater quantity during the circumpubertal growth period. In the absence of severe dentoskeletal compensations, functional appliance therapy should be initiated at the beginning of cervical vertebrae maturation stage CS3 to maximize the treatment effects and reduce the need for posttreatment retention.

10. What are the two basic types of functional appliances commonly used today?[5,15,17-24]

The two basic types of functional appliances commonly used today are tooth-borne and tissue-borne appliances. The only tissue-borne appliance is the functional regulator or Frankel II. All other functional appliances, such as the Herbst, Twin Block, Bionator, and MARA (mandibular anterior repositioning appliance) appliance, are considered tooth borne (Fig. 13-4).

The Frankel II appliance is considered a tissue-borne appliance because it uses the buccal vestibule as the main support of the appliance. The Frankel II's vestibular shields and lower labial pads are used to restrain the buccal and labial musculatures that apply pressure and restrict dental and skeletal development. The mandibular musculature is stimulated to reposition the mandible to a functionally anterior position by feedback stimulus from the lingual pad, which is lingual to the lower incisors. Since the appliance is tissue borne, greater flaring of the incisors may be noted. The buccal shields provide spontaneous lateral expansion of the maxillary and mandibular arches caused by pressure elimination from the buccal musculature, thus allowing the tongue to help in arch development. In addition the vestibular shields stimulate additional appositional growth laterally by causing tension on the alveolar periosteum.

The second basic type of functional appliance is the tooth-borne appliance, which uses the dentition as the primary anchor. In this type of appliance, there are more dentoalveolar effects than with the tissue-borne appliance. Increase in mandibular length is expected as well as the potential for some headgear effect. In addition, the maxillary molars usually move distally and the mandibular molars move mesially. The maxillary incisors often tip lingually and mandibular incisors tend to procline. The degree of skeletal and dentoalveolar movement may vary with each type of appliance. Tooth-borne appliances can be fixed or removable. Examples of removable appliances are the Activator, Bionator, and Twin Block. The removable appliances are usually composed of a metal framework with clasps and acrylic. The fixed appliances, on the other hand, such as the MARA and the banded Herbst, are cemented to the teeth, resulting in full-time active forward positioning of the mandible.

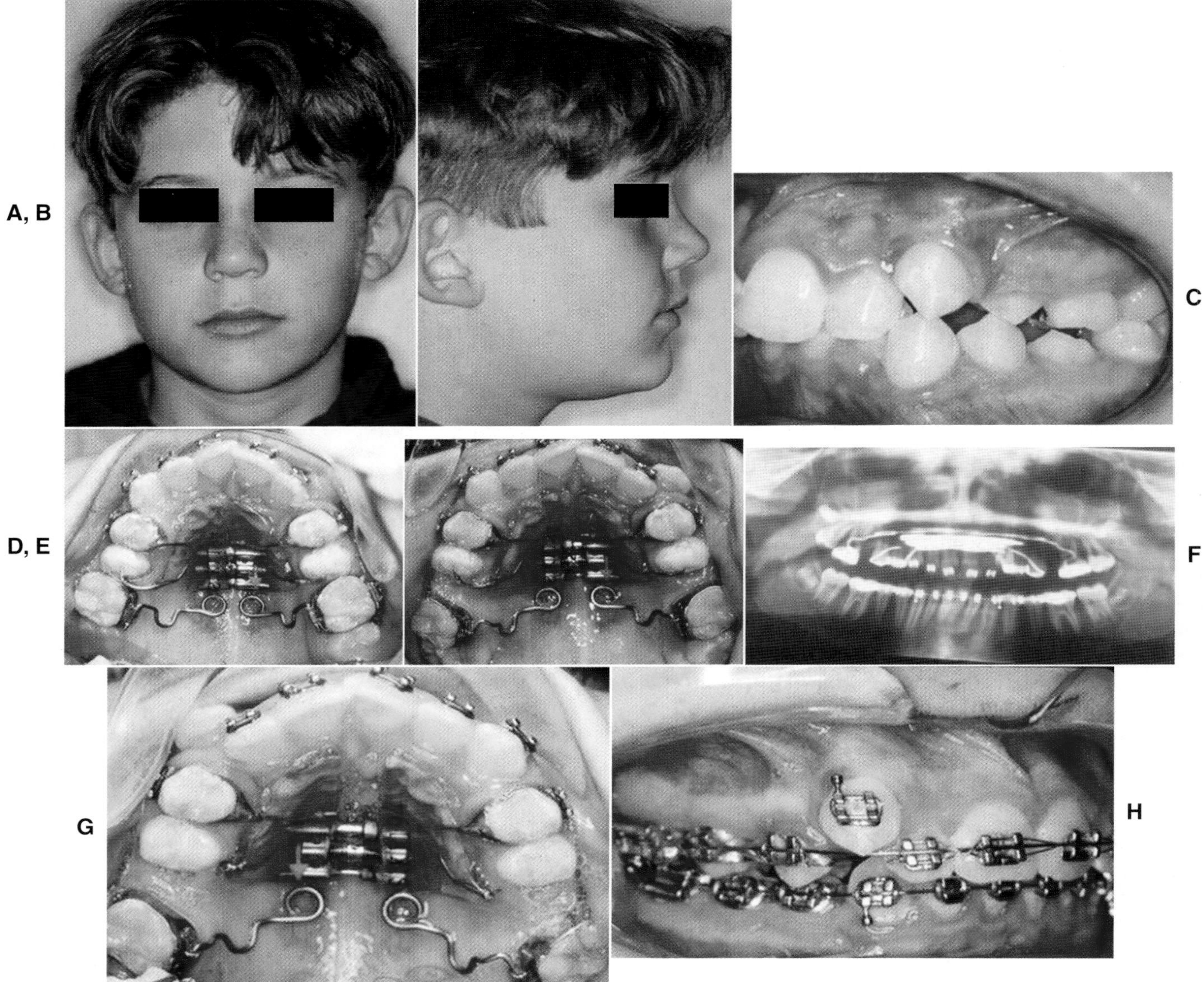

FIG 13-3 Pendex distalizing treatment. **A-C,** Initial photos: facial photos **(A** and **B),** intraoral photo **(C)**. **D,** Pendex appliance in place. **E** and **F,** Note molar distalization. **G,** Pendex arm cut. **H,** Biscuspid alignment.

11. What situations would require orthodontic treatment prior to starting functional jaw orthopedics (FJO)? [5,6,15]

The following four situations usually require orthodontic treatment prior to FJO:

1. **Severe maxillary constriction**—It is often advantageous to expand the maxilla prior to Class II correction to allow the buccal segments to appropriately interdigitate in the final Class I position. This can be done with a rapid palatal expansion appliance prior to FJO.
2. **Deep impinging bite**—In order to allow for forward posturing of the mandible, deep impinging bites should be corrected using a utility arch to intrude, tip, or reposition the incisors.

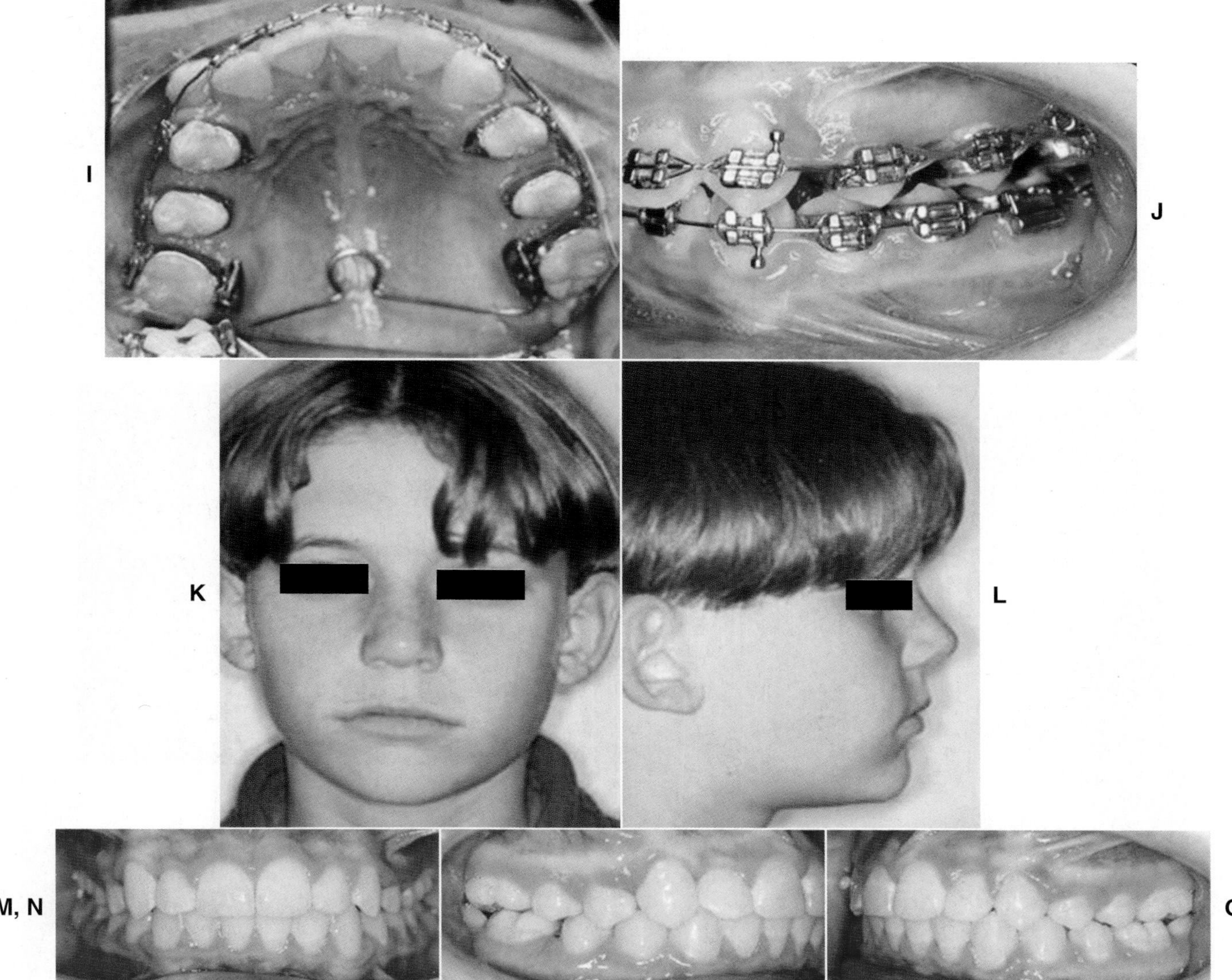

FIG 13-3—cont'd **I** and **J,** Bicuspid distalization. **K-O,** Posttreatment photos: facial photos **(K-L)** and intraoral photos **(M-O).**

3. **Maxillary incisor retroclination and mandibular incisor proclination and spacing**—Over 30% of Class II patients present with maxillary incisors in a retroclined position. This inclination problem must be corrected to allow appropriate mandibular advancement. In addition, flaring as well as spacing of the lower incisors must be corrected to allow for maximum mandibular advancement.
4. **Moderate to severe crowding**—Space supervision or serial extraction may be required depending upon the severity of the upper and lower dental crowding.

12. What is a Twin Block appliance?[5,6,15,18]

The Twin Block is composed of maxillary and mandibular retainer-like acrylic appliances that fit tightly against the teeth and alveolar structures. The upper and lower appliances have two bite blocks, which gives the appliance the name "Twin Block." The upper bite block covers the molars, extending partially to the second bicuspids, and finishing on the mesial with an inclined plane at 70 degrees to the occlu sal plane. The lower bite block usually covers the bicuspids and ends on the distal in a posteriorly directed incline plane just above the second bicuspids (see Fig. 13-4, *D* and *E*).

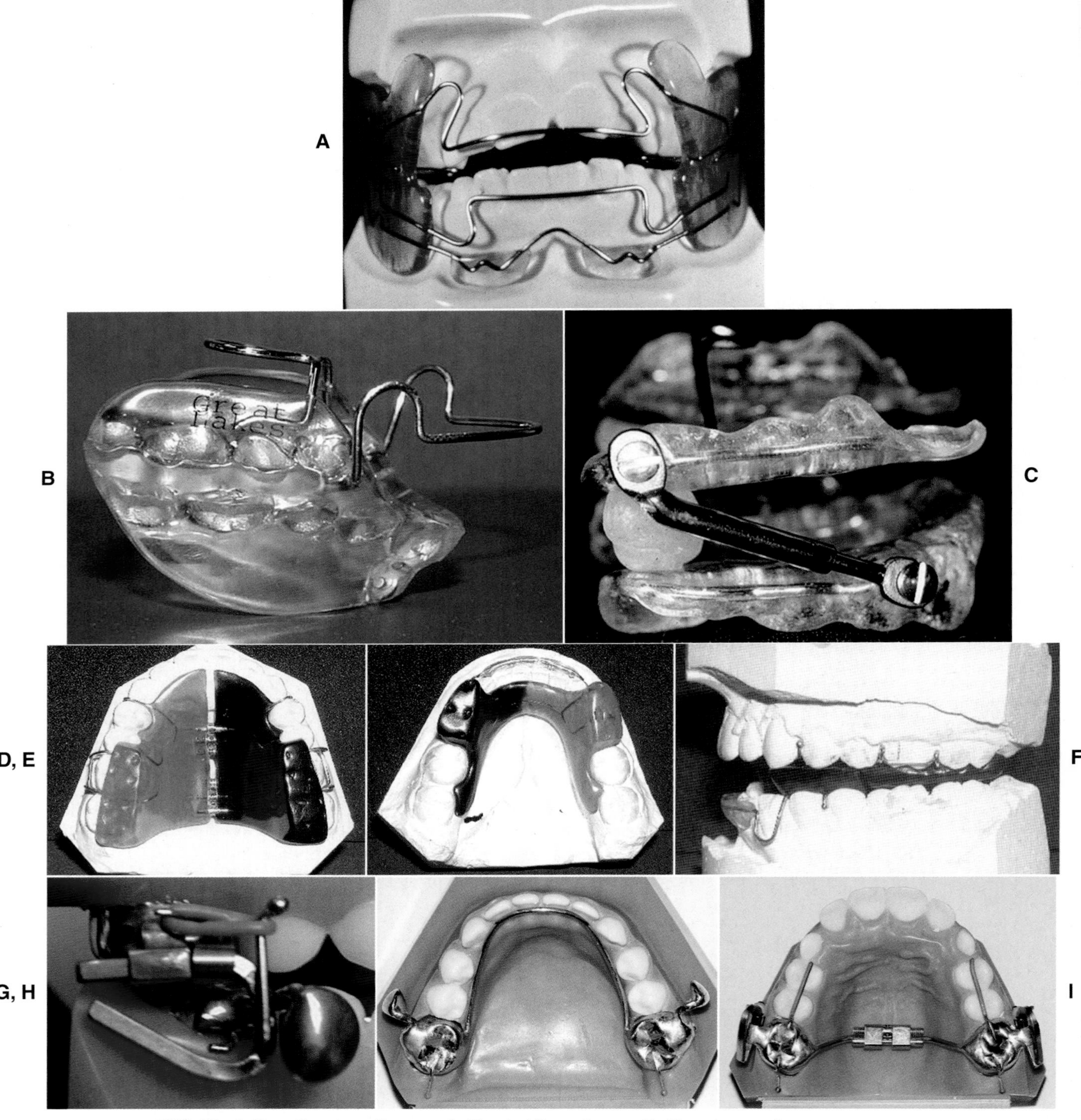

FIG 13-4 Functional appliances. **A,** Frankel II appliance; **B,** Bionator appliance; **C,** removable acrylic Herbst appliance; **D-F,** Twin Block appliance; **G-I,** MARA appliance.

Upon closure the inclined planes contact each other, thrusting the mandible forward. Three-dimensional control is accomplished by selective grinding of the blocks, guided dental eruption, and transverse expansion via a midpalatal jackscrew (Fig. 13-5).

13. What is a Bionator appliance?[5,15]

The Bionator is a tooth-borne appliance that consists of an interocclusal acrylic block with a labial maxillary bow with or without maxillary or mandibular anterior or posterior occlusal coverage. The interocclusal block may have angled flutes to guide the path of eruption of the posterior teeth. Bionators are classified into the following three categories: bionators to open, maintain, or close the bite.

Bionators that open the bite (Fig. 13-6) have eruption grooves in the posterior to allow the dentition to erupt and correct the deep curve of Spee. In addition, occlusal acrylic capping is added to control incisor eruption. Bionators that maintain the bite have acrylic posterior bite blocks that are constructed within the freeway space to prevent tooth eruption. Bionators

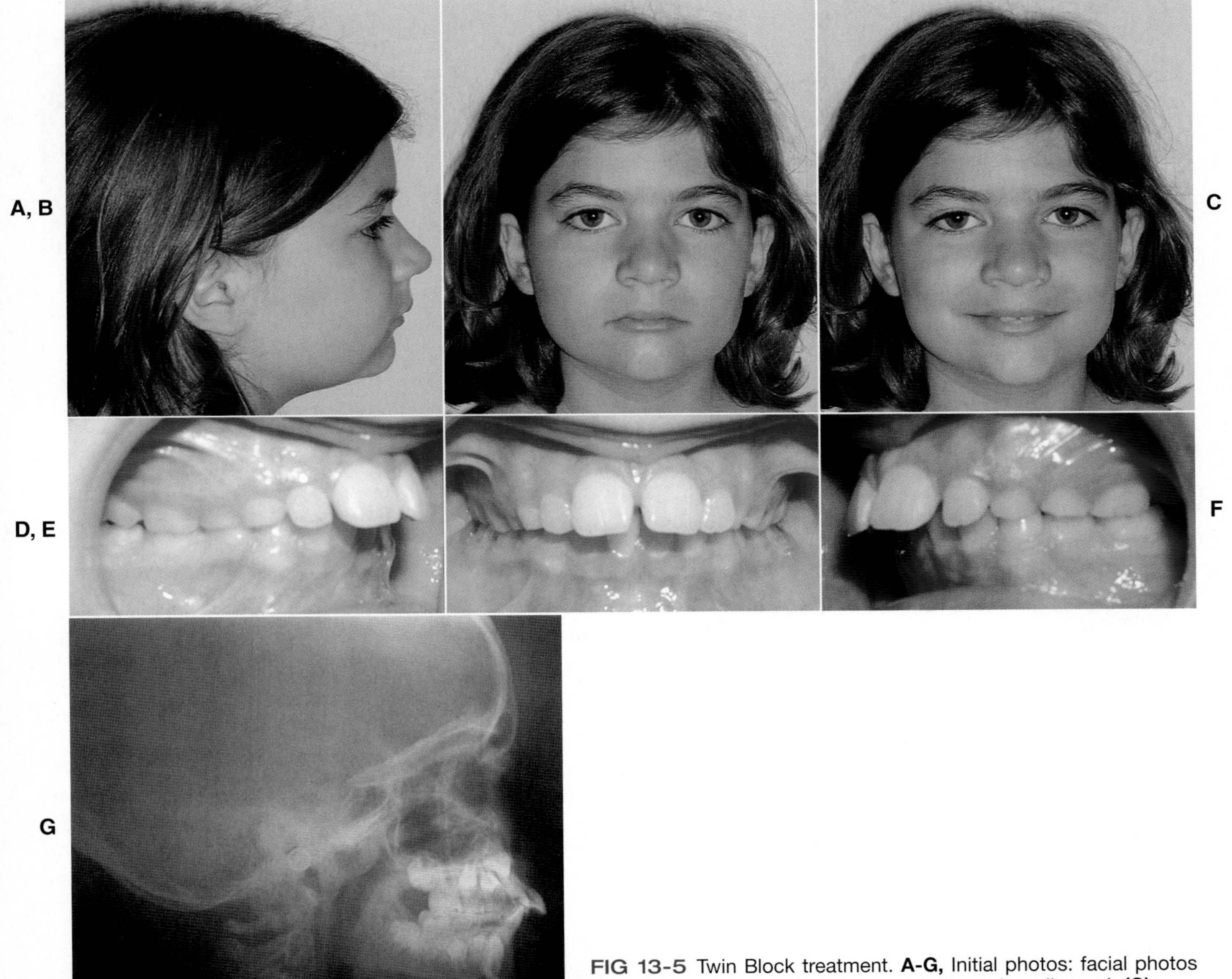

FIG 13-5 Twin Block treatment. **A-G,** Initial photos: facial photos **(A-C)** intraoral photos **(D-F),** and cephalometric radiograph **(G)**.
Continued

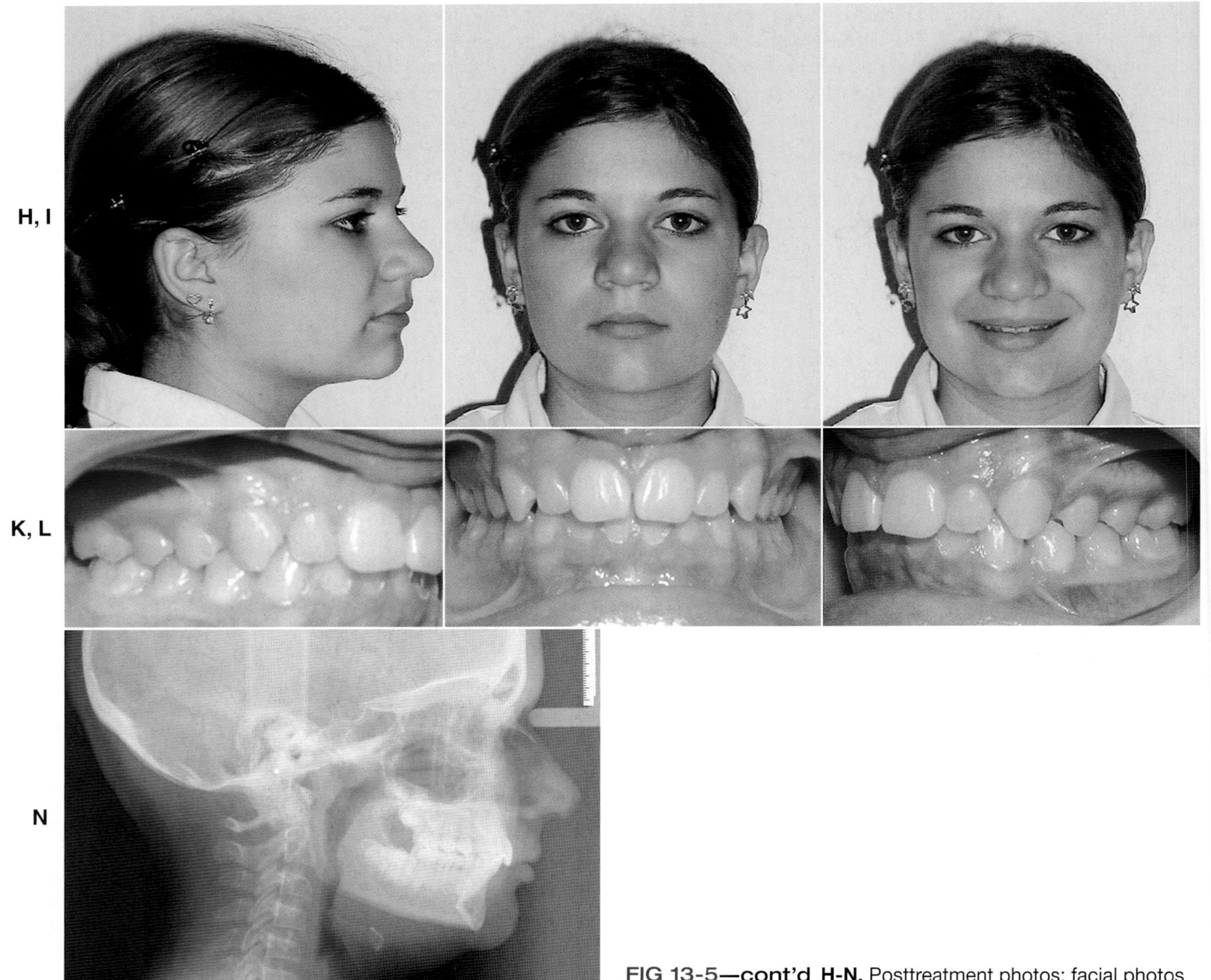

FIG 13-5—cont'd H-N, Posttreatment photos: facial photos **(H-J),** intraoral photos **(K-M),** and cephalometric radiograph **(N).**

to close the bite (Fig. 13-7) have posterior acrylic bite blocks that impinge into the freeway space to stretch the perioral musculature to actively intrude the posterior teeth and allow for vertical ramus growth. The Bionator to close the bite may or may not have lower anterior incisor capping, depending on the absence or presence of an anterior dental open bite.

Wax bite registrations for the Bionator vary depending upon its specific type. The wax registration for the Bionator to open or maintain the bite is taken with the mandible advanced 4 to 5 mm and with an anterior incisor separation of 2 to 3 mm to allow for the incisal capping. The wax registration for the Bionator to close the bite is taken with the mandible advanced 4 to 5 mm and a posterior tooth separation of 5 mm to allow for impingement on the freeway space. Headgear tubes can be added to the Bionator to control either excessive anterior or vertical maxillary growth.

14. What is a Herbst appliance?[5,20]

The Herbst appliance design most frequently used today employs two types of attachment mechanisms to anchor the appliance: stainless-steel crowns and acrylic splints. The stainless-steel crown Herbst features crowns on the maxillary first molars and mandibular first premolars. Pivots soldered to the crowns

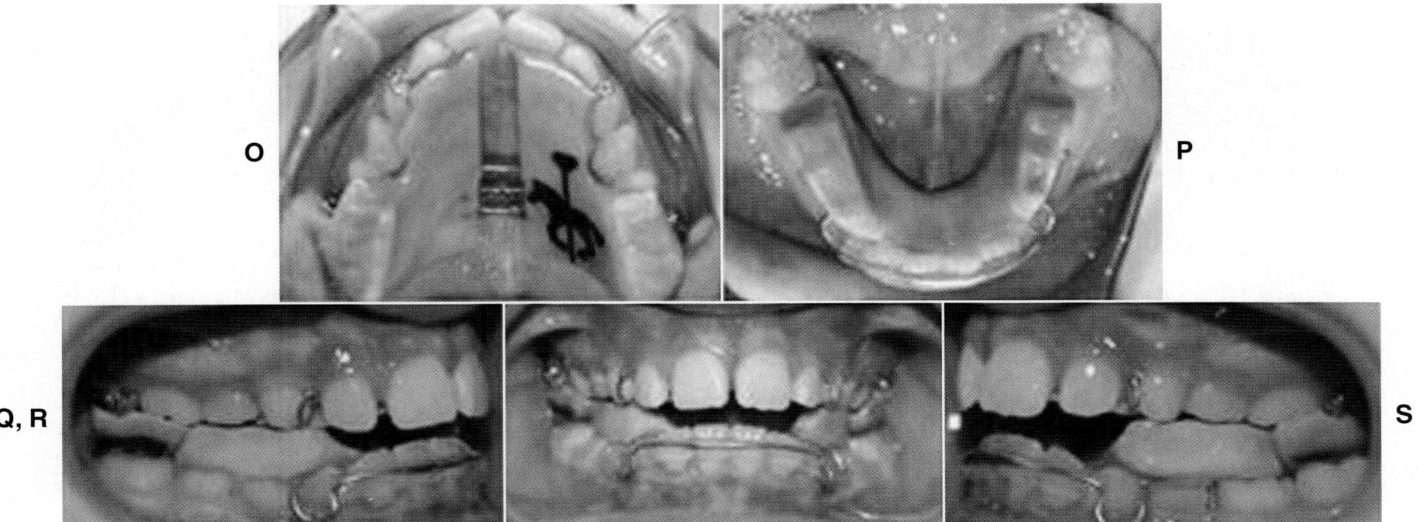

FIG 13-5—cont'd O-S, Twin Block in place.

connect the tube and plunger assembly, with the length of the maxillary tube determining the amount of bite advancement. A lower lingual arch connects the crowns on the mandibular first premolars to bands on the mandibular first molars.

In the second type, the acrylic splint Herbst, an acrylic material 2.5 to 3.0 mm thick is applied over a wire framework (Fig. 13-8). This acrylic splint covers the canines to first molars in the maxillary arch but extends over the complete dentition in the lower arch. As in the banded version, the pivots of the Herbst bite jumping mechanism are soldered to the wire framework adjacent to the mandibular first premolars and maxillary first molars. Anchorage for the Herbst is provided by the acrylic splint/dentition contact, with the maxillary and mandibular sections either cemented or removable.

In both types of Herbst appliances, a Hyrax-type screw may be included to expand the maxilla as the mandible is positioned forward. Step-by-step mandibular advancement is achieved by adding shims to the mandibular part of the bite-jumping mechanism. In addition, vertical eruption of the upper and lower second molars is controlled by either acrylic coverage in the splint-type appliance or wire occlusal stops soldered to the 6-year molar bands in the stainless-steel crown version. Both types of Herbst appliances are worn for 9 to 12 months, after which full fixed appliances are initiated.

15. What is a MARA appliance?[19,21]

The MARA is a tooth-borne functional appliance used to correct Class II malocclusions. There is basically one MARA design. The appliance, however, can be modified to accommodate upper and lower expansion, a transpalatal arch, lower lingual arch, orthodontic appliances, and intrusion mechanics, and it can be used unilaterally in asymmetric cases. The basic MARA design consists of:

- Four crowns on the first molars
- Arms soldered to the lower crowns
- Archwire tubes for upper and lower arches soldered to all first molar crowns
- Elbow tubes soldered to the upper crowns
- Upper elbows shimmed to provide the desired advancement
- Lower lingual arch soldered to lower crowns
- Optional specifications include occlusal holes to assist with crown removal

Upon closure of the mouth, the upper elbow's vertical legs hit the lower arms and the mandible is forced forward. The MARA is effective in treating patients with Class II malocclusion through dental and skeletal changes in the craniofacial complex (Fig. 13-9). The annualized 5.8 mm Class II molar correction is obtained by a 47% skeletal change (2.7 mm) and 53% dental change (3.1 mm). The 2.7 mm skeletal change is completely due to growth of the mandible. The MARA produces increases in mandibular length and in posterior and anterior face height but has no headgear effect on the maxilla. The dental changes are mainly due to the distalization of the maxillary molars (2.4 mm), which accounts for 77% of the total dental correction. Dental changes include distalization of the maxillary molar, slight mesial movement of the mandibular molars, and a slight proclination of the mandibular incisors.

16. Are there variations in clinical response to functional appliance treatment?[6,17]

The effectiveness of functional appliance treatment to correct Class II malocclusions is well reported in the literature. The effect of functional appliance therapy on increasing mandibular size, however, is less well documented. In a systematic review by Cozza et al.[17] evaluating mandibular changes produced by functional appliances, the amount of supplementary growth

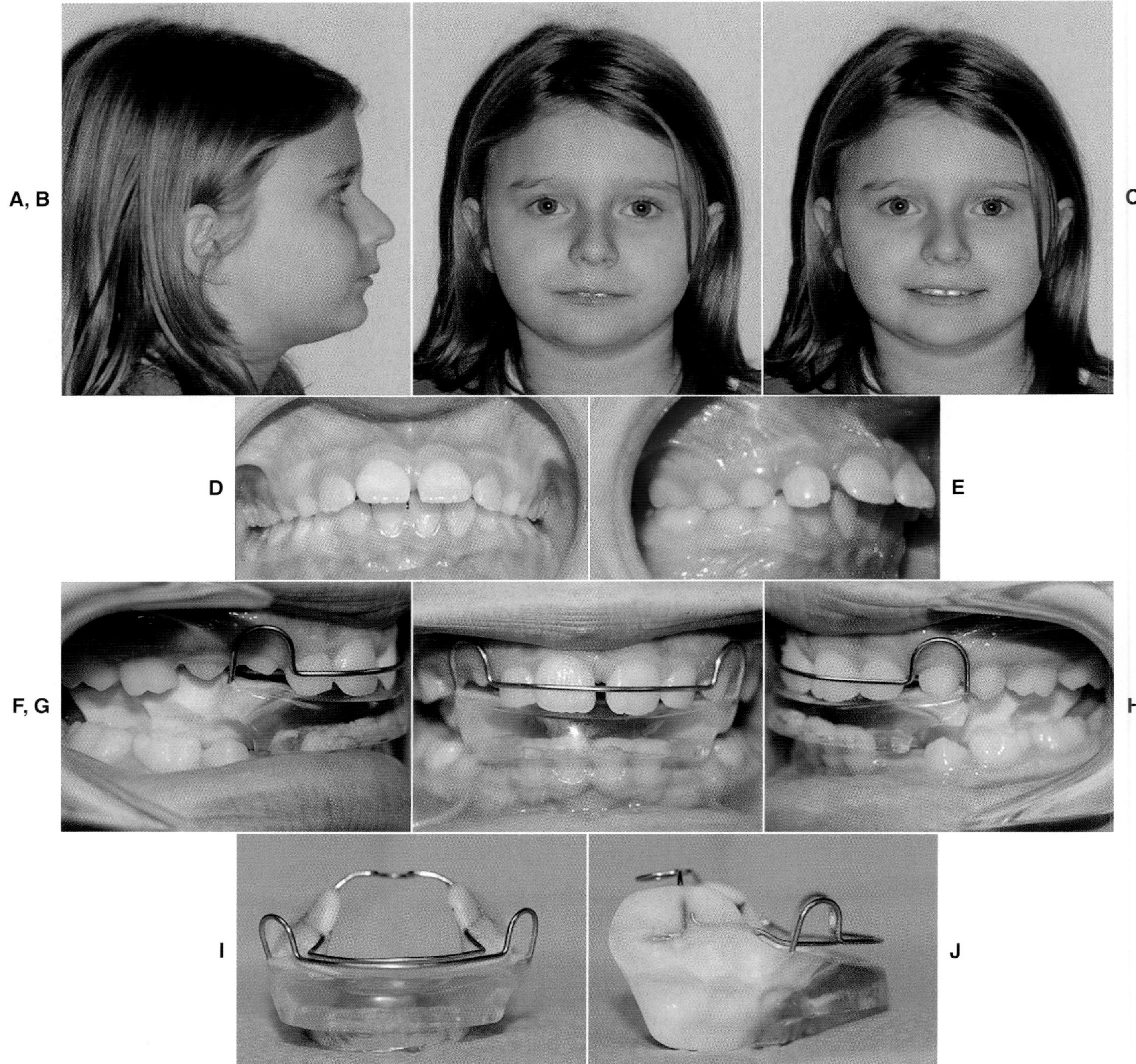

FIG 13-6 Bionator treatment to correct Class II and open the bite. **A-E,** Initial photos: facial photos **(A-C)** and intraoral photos **(D** and **E)**. **F-H,** Bionator appliance intraorally. **I** and **J,** Bionator appliance.

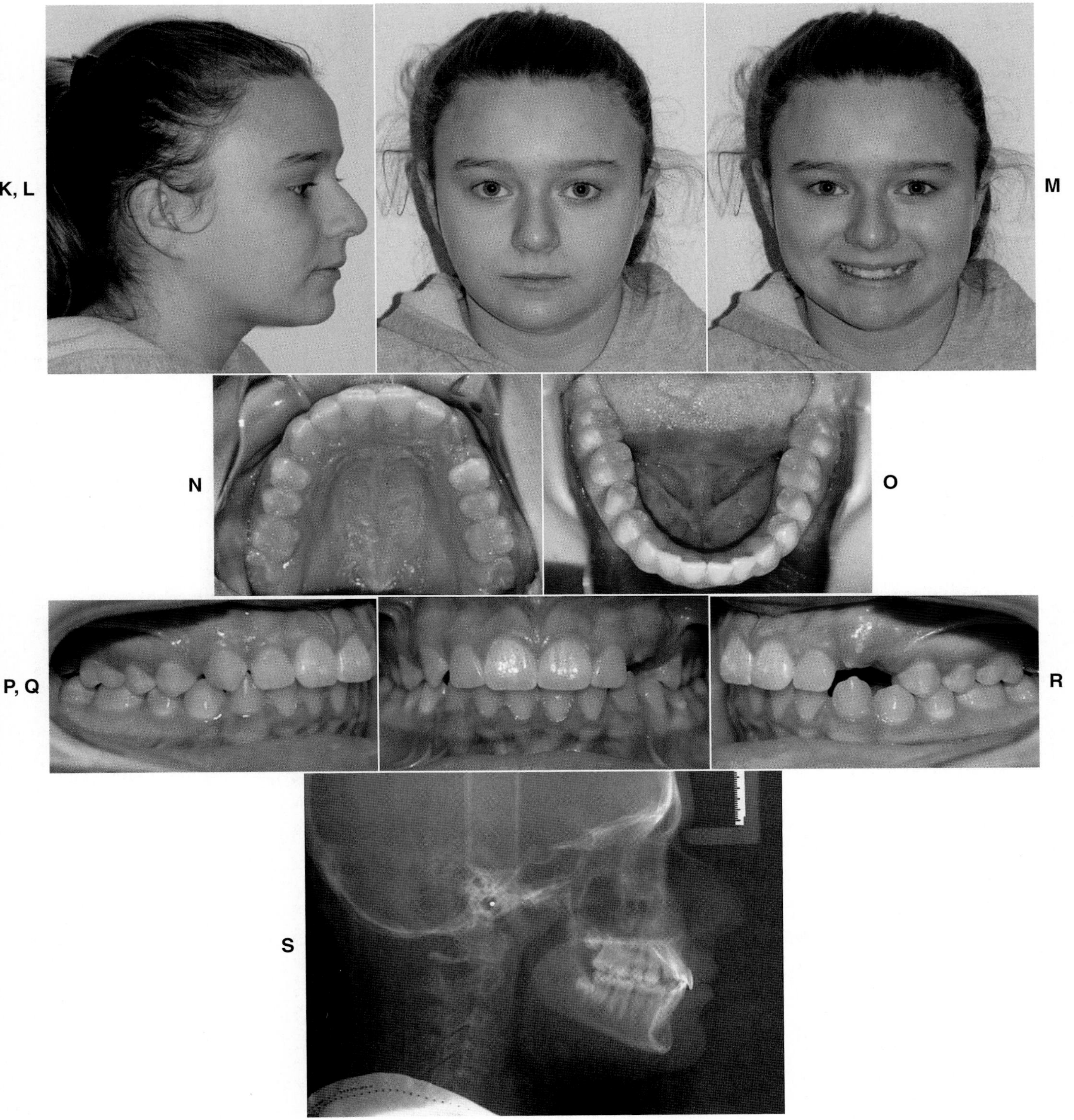

FIG 13-6—cont'd **K-S,** Post-Bionator results: facial photos **(K-M),** intraoral photos **(N-R),** and cephalometric radiograph **(S)**.

Continued

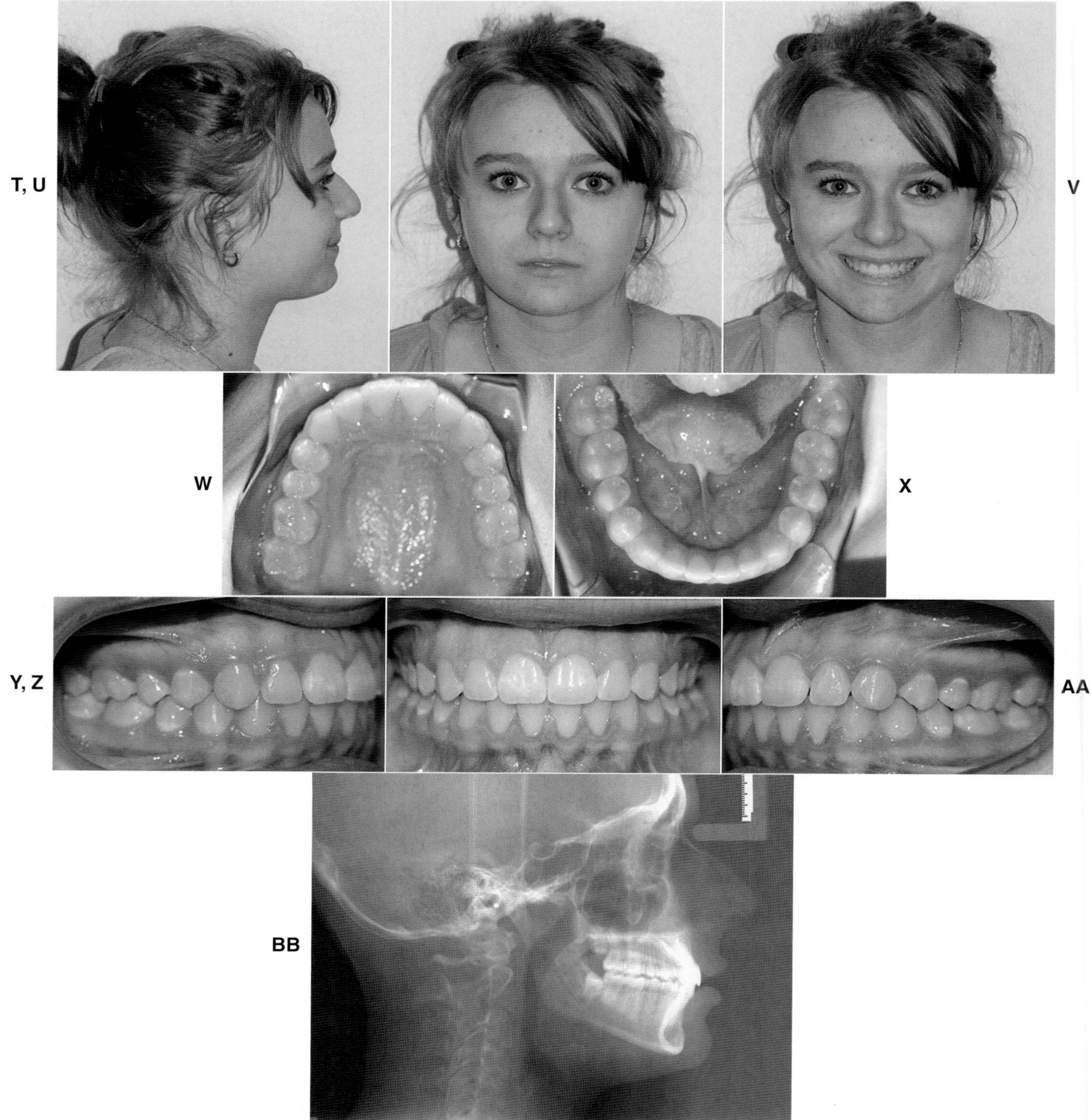

FIG 13-6—cont'd **T-BB,** Post-Bionator and orthodontic results: facial photos **(T-V),** intraoral photos **(W-AA),** and cephalometric radiograph **(BB)**.

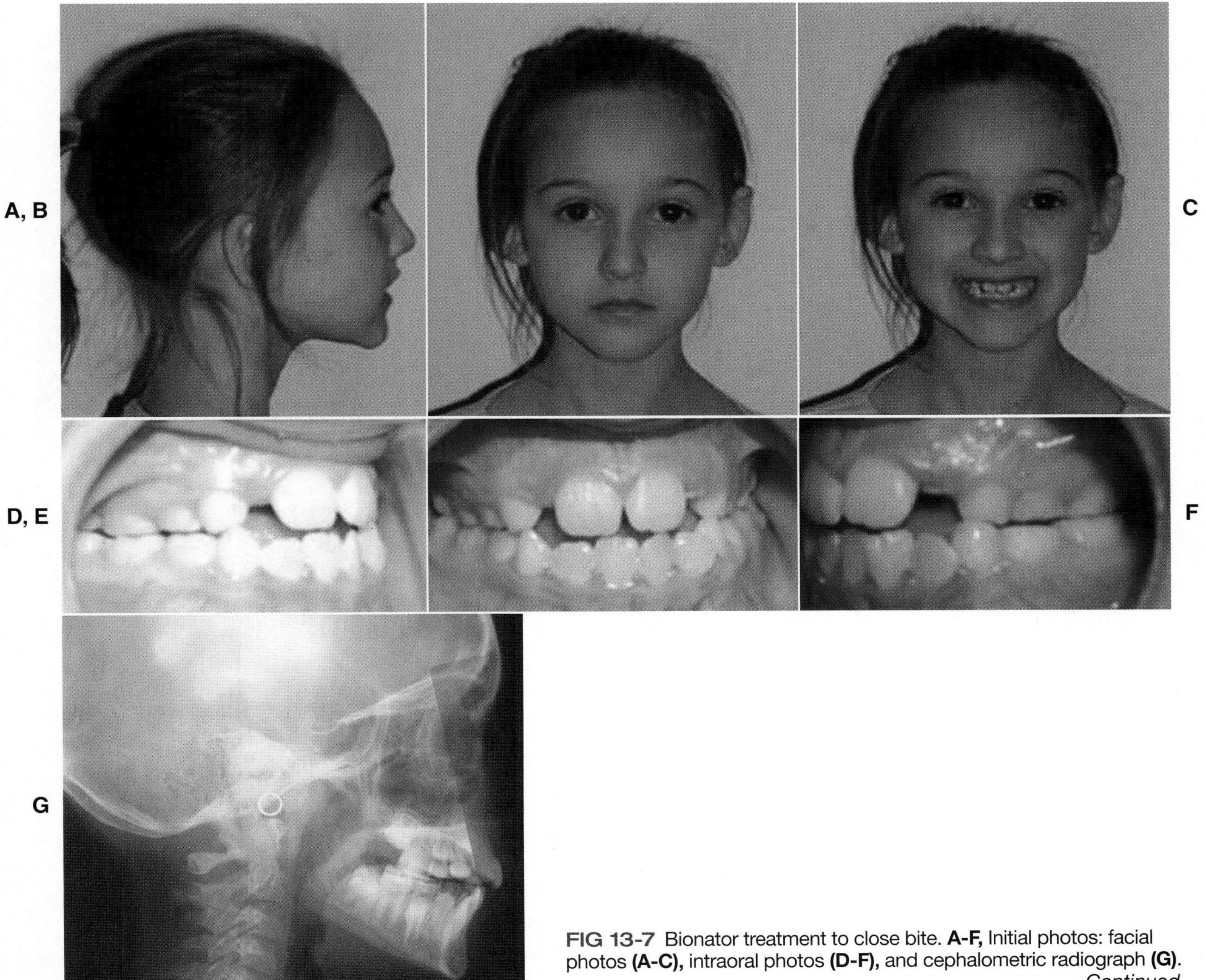

FIG 13-7 Bionator treatment to close bite. **A-F,** Initial photos: facial photos **(A-C),** intraoral photos **(D-F),** and cephalometric radiograph **(G)**.
Continued

of the mandible when compared with untreated Class II controls varied. In Cozza et al.'s review, assessment was difficult because only one third of the studies had any information on skeletal maturity at the time of functional appliance therapy, and it is now a well-known fact that mandibular response is enhanced if functional appliance therapy is carried out during the circumpubertal growth spurt. Tulloch et al.[25] reported that in untreated Class II patients, there is about a 30% chance of favorable change in the Class II relationship, approximately a 50% chance of no change, and a 15% chance the condition will worsen. Functional appliance or headgear treatment has shown a 70% to 80% chance of producing a favorable or highly favorable result and about a 20% chance of no change or a worsening of the Class II. It has also been shown that up to 10% of patients do not respond to functional appliance treatment.

17. Are functional treatment results stable over the long term?[21]

Functional treatment results have been reported to be stable in the long term in a variety of articles. Croft et al.[26] found no significant joint space changes at the end of treatment with the Herbst appliance, thus concluding there would be no relapse caused by mandibular posturing and condylar repositioning. Uner and Gultan[27] found that functional appliance treatment results were

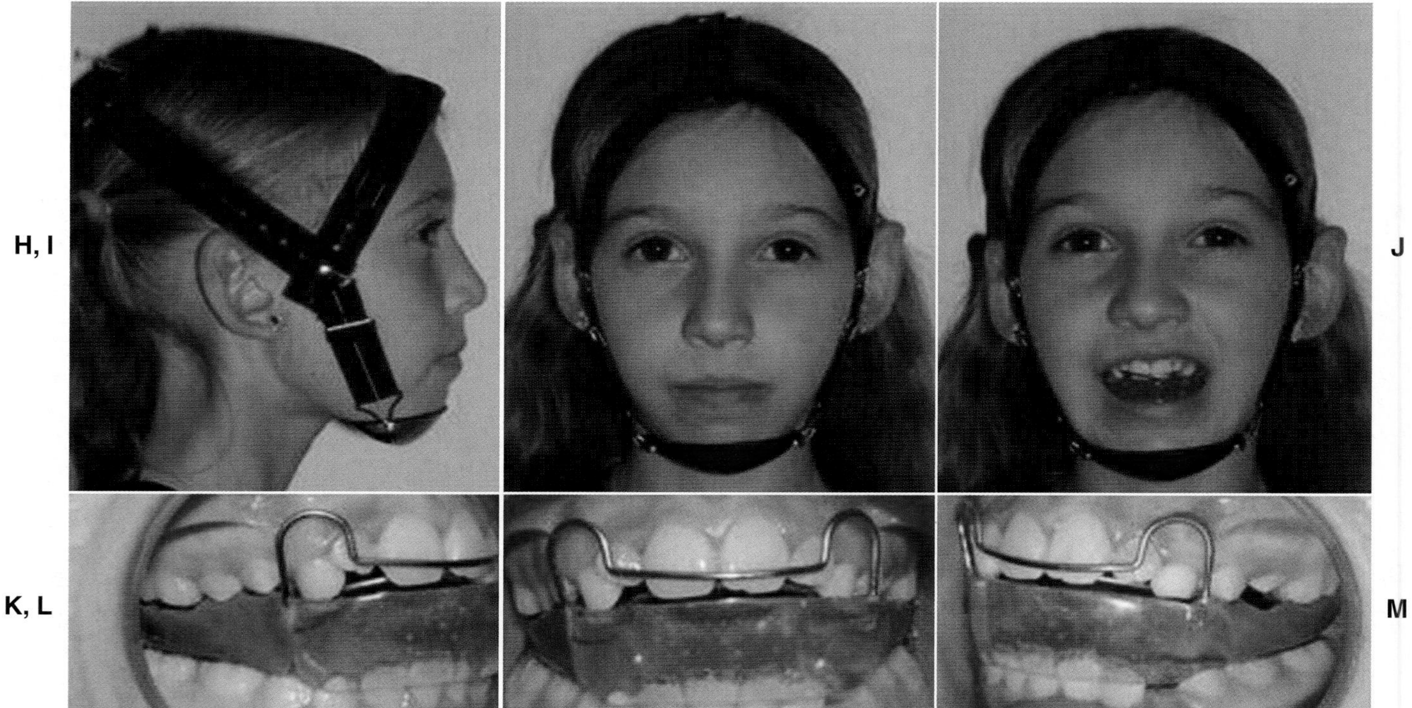

FIG 13-7—cont'd H-M, Bionator treatment with headgear: facial photos **(H-J)** and intraoral photos **(K-M)**.

stable and even improved during retention. Pancherz[28] indicated that stability of functional results was dependent upon finishing the functional appliance phase with good occlusal intercuspation. Berger and Pangrazio-Kulbersh[14] reported that functional appliance patients continued to grow in a favorable direction even after discontinuance of functional appliance therapy and, in addition, the functional results showed stability over time. Functional appliance therapy when initiated at the appropriate patient developmental growth stage has been shown to be stable and to result in the correction of Class II malocclusions.

18. What is Class II camouflage treatment?[6,29]

Class II camouflage treatment is usually considered for patients who are too old for growth modification, have mild to moderate skeletal discrepancies, have reasonably good alignment of teeth, have good vertical proportions, have reasonably good facial esthetics, or have overjet that results more from maxillary protrusion than mandibular retrusion. It is most appropriately used when the patient has a mild Class II skeletal relation with a Class II dental malocclusion. Treatment usually requires the extraction of either upper first bicuspids and lower second bicuspids or only the extraction of upper first bicuspids.

19. What is surgical Class II treatment and when should it be considered?[6,30,31]

Surgical Class II treatment is usually considered when the severity of the discrepancy is so great that neither growth modification nor camouflage treatment can be done to adequately correct the problem. The ultimate decision for surgical Class II correction must include not only the assessment of the treating orthodontist, but also the age, psychological fitness, financial means, and desires of the patient.

Surgical Class II treatment requires the combined efforts of the orthodontist and the oral surgeon. An accurate assessment of the components of the dental and skeletal Class II must be analyzed appropriately and the surgical sites delineated appropriately. The sequencing of this treatment requires presurgical orthodontic alignment and decompensation followed by necessary orthognathic surgery with 6 to 9 months of postsurgical finishing. Excellent surgical outcomes require the joint consultation between all the professionals involved.

Since skeletal Class II problems are most often due to mandibular deficiencies or clockwise rotation of the mandible caused by excessive vertical growth of the maxilla, surgical treatment usually consists of mandibular advancement (66%),

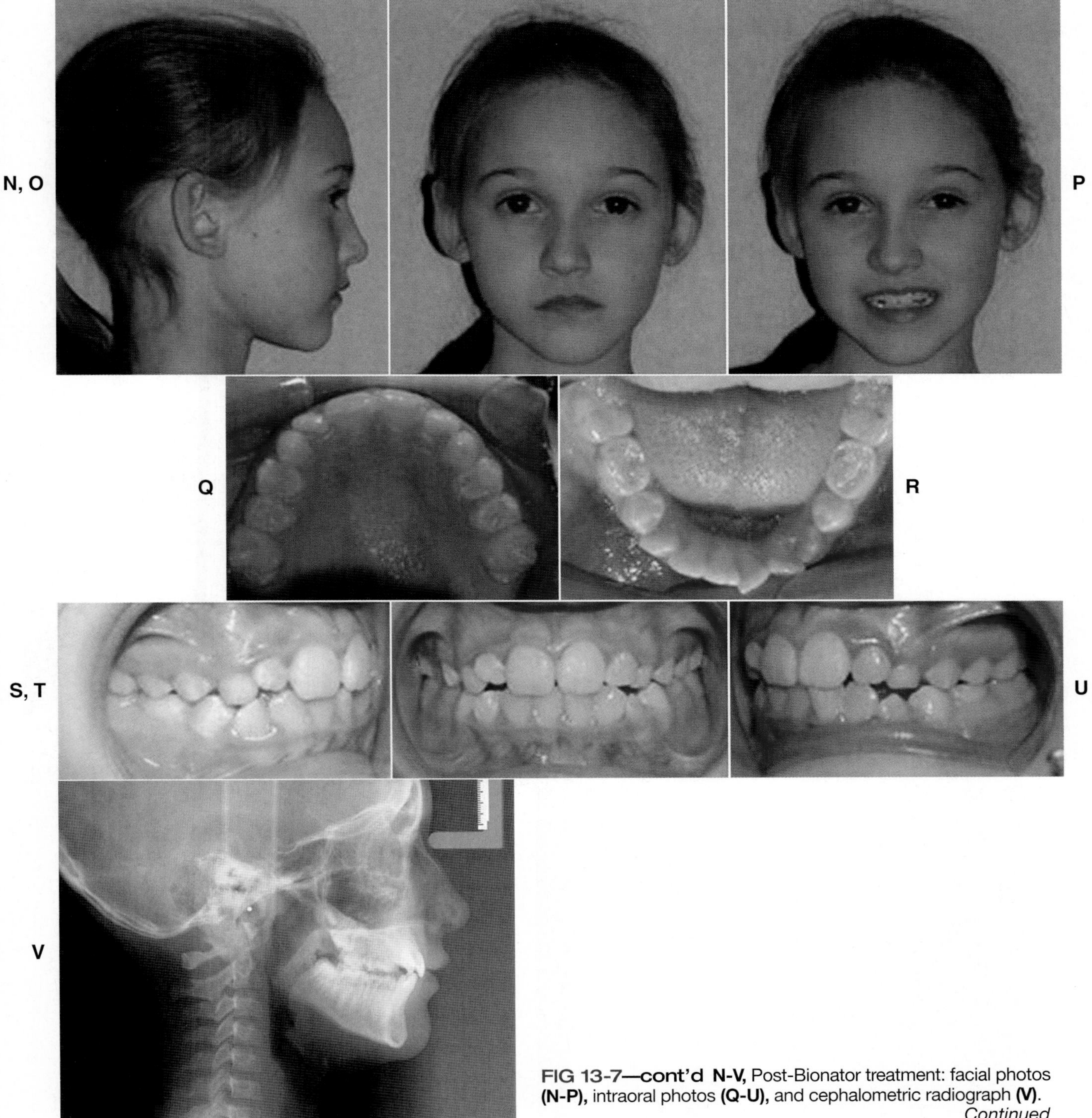

FIG 13-7—cont'd N-V, Post-Bionator treatment: facial photos **(N-P),** intraoral photos **(Q-U),** and cephalometric radiograph **(V).**

Continued

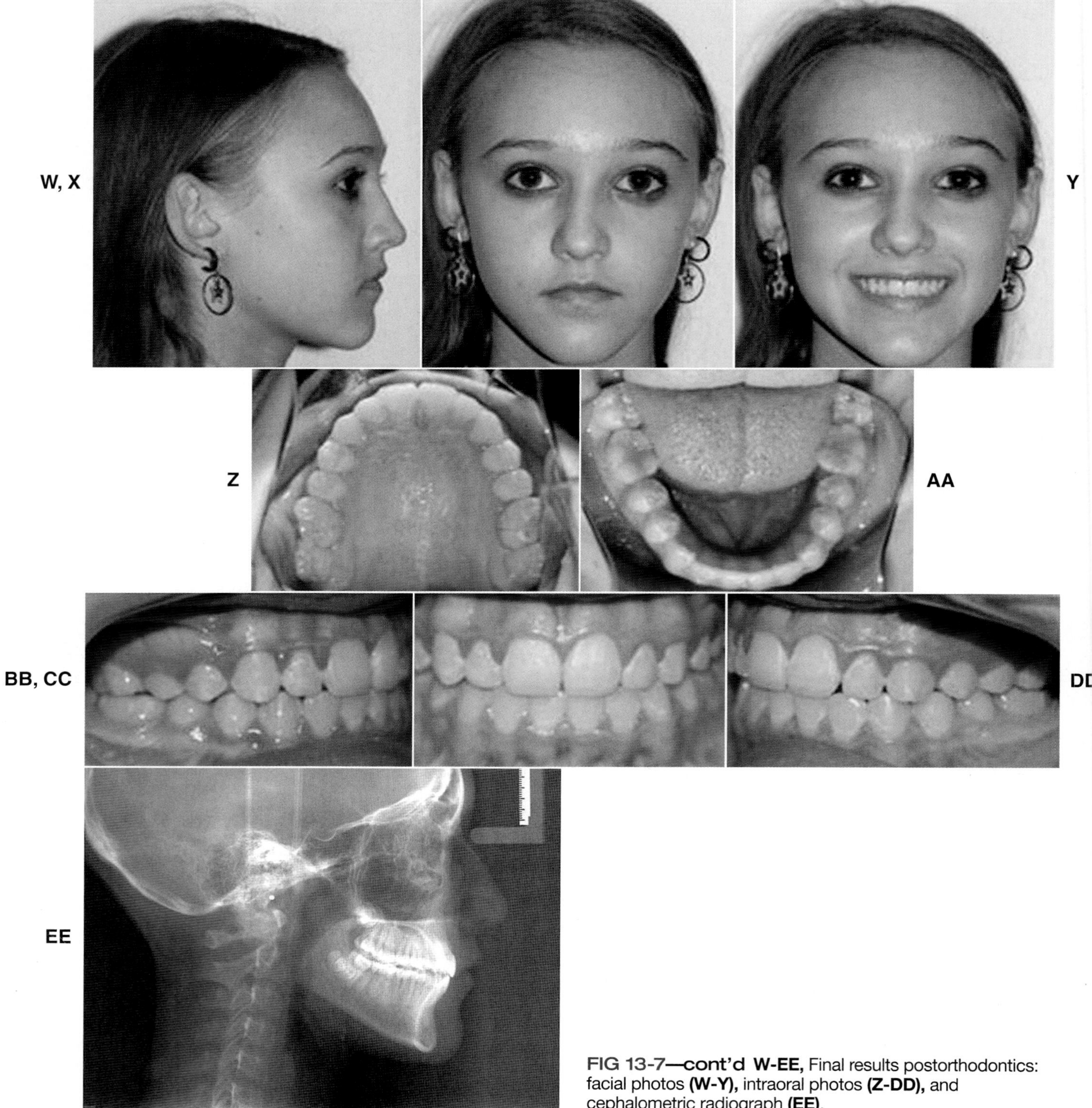

FIG 13-7—cont'd W-EE, Final results postorthodontics: facial photos **(W-Y),** intraoral photos **(Z-DD),** and cephalometric radiograph **(EE).**

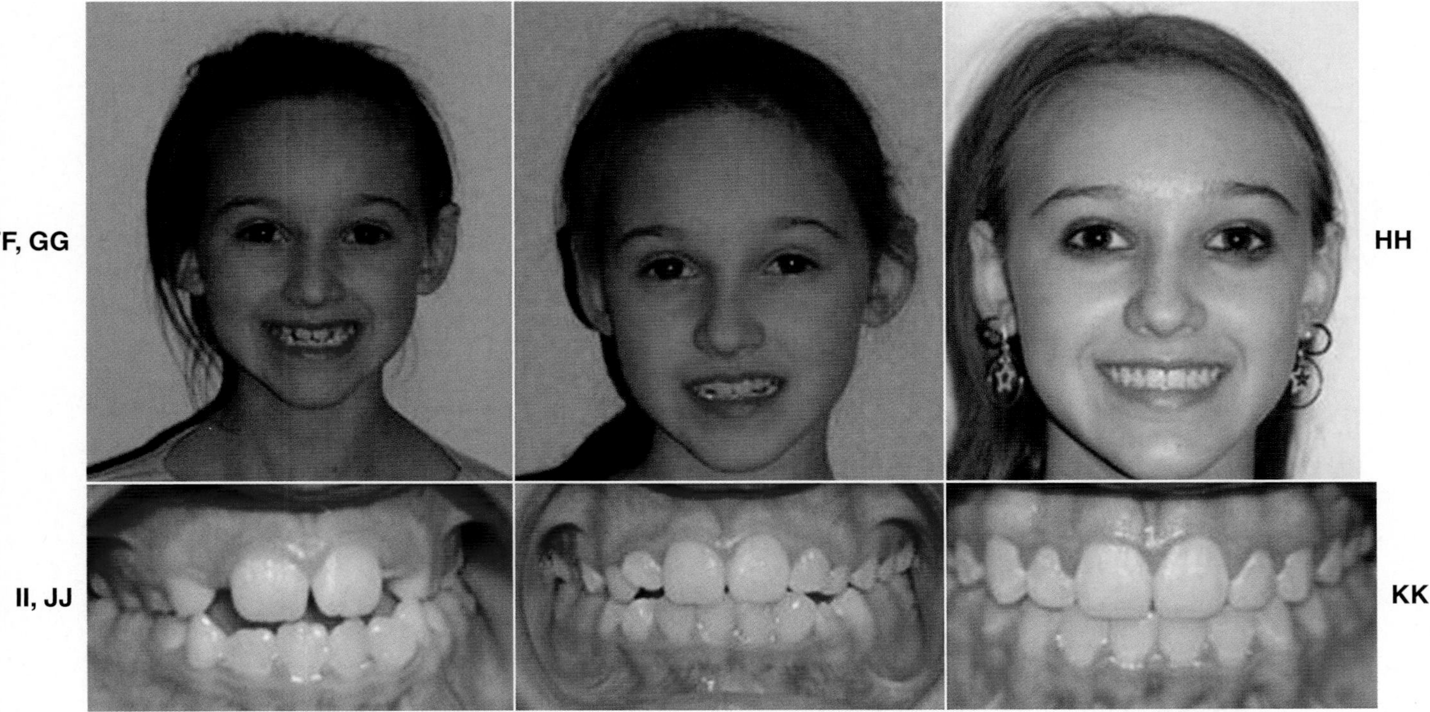

FIG 13-7—cont'd **FF-KK,** Overall treatment comparisons: initial facial and intraoral photos **(FF** and **II),** post-Bionator facial and intraoral photos **(GG** and **JJ),** post-orthodontics facial and intraoral photos **(HH** and **KK)**.

maxillary impaction (15%) or a combination (20%). Larger than 10 mm of overjet in a nongrowing patient usually suggests the need for surgical correction. This is especially true if the lower incisors are protrusive relative to pogonion, the mandible is short, or the anterior face height is long.

20. What is the appropriate timing for orthognathic surgery during growth?[6,30,31]

If there is a significant dentofacial deformity, early orthognathic surgery may improve the health of the patient with regard to speech, airway, anatomy, occlusion, esthetics, TMJ function, masticatory function, and psychosocial factors. In the absence of a severe deformity, however, surgical mandibular advancement before the growth spurt is questionable. When the mandibular growth rate is normal, mandibular advancement can be stable because of continued normal growth of the mandible in its new position. When there is deficient mandibular growth (e.g., progressively worsening mandibular retrusion), the Class II skeletal and dental pattern can be expected to return after surgery as the maxilla continues its normal growth while the mandible continues its deficient growth. In this case additional surgery may be required.

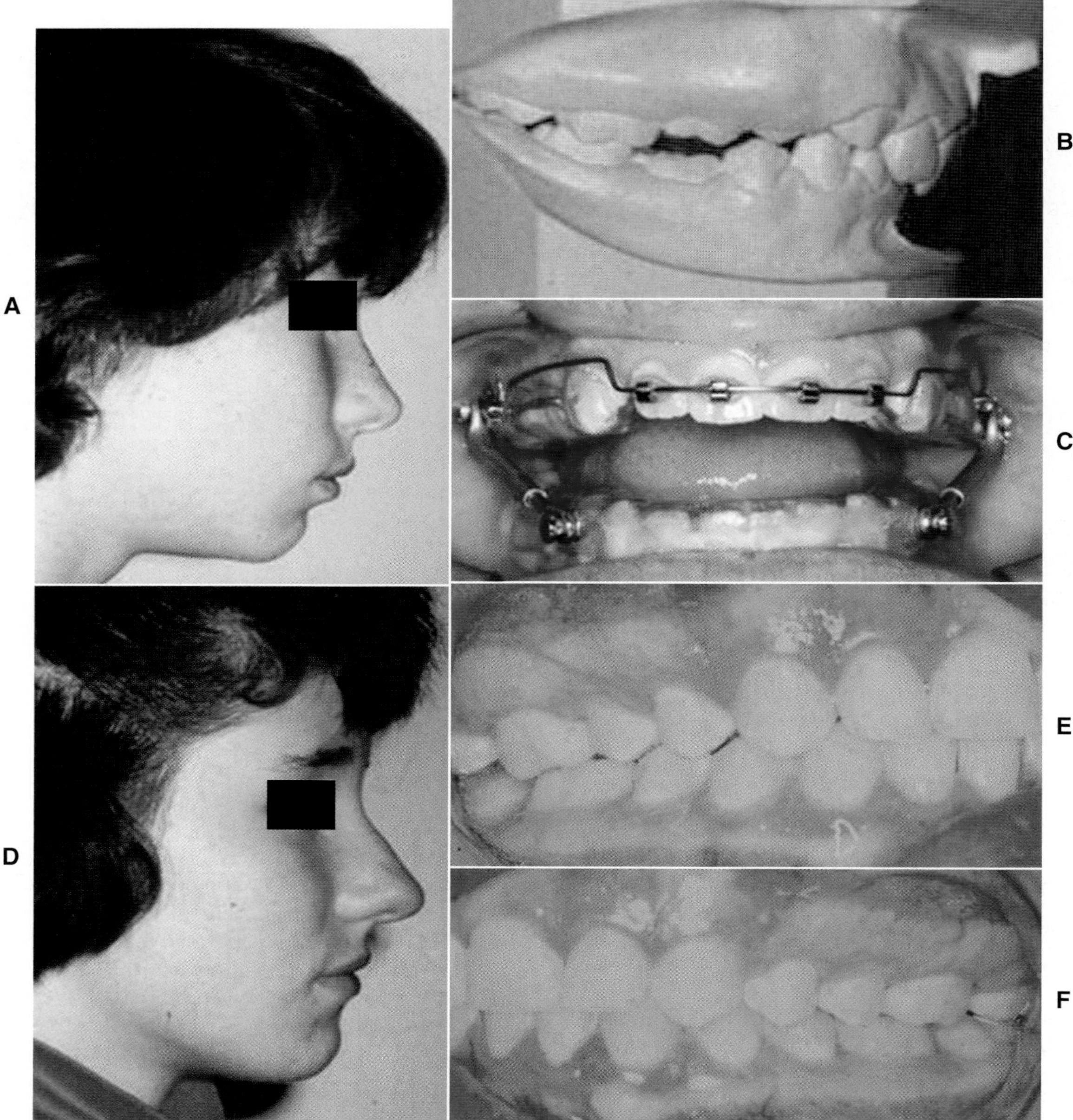

FIG 13-8 Removable acrylic Herbst treatment. **A** and **B,** Initial photos: facial photo **(A)** and cast **(B)**. **C,** Herbst plus upper intrusion arch to flare and intrude incisors. **D-F,** Post-Herbst and orthodontic treatment results: facial photo **(D)** and intraoral photos **(E** and **F)**.

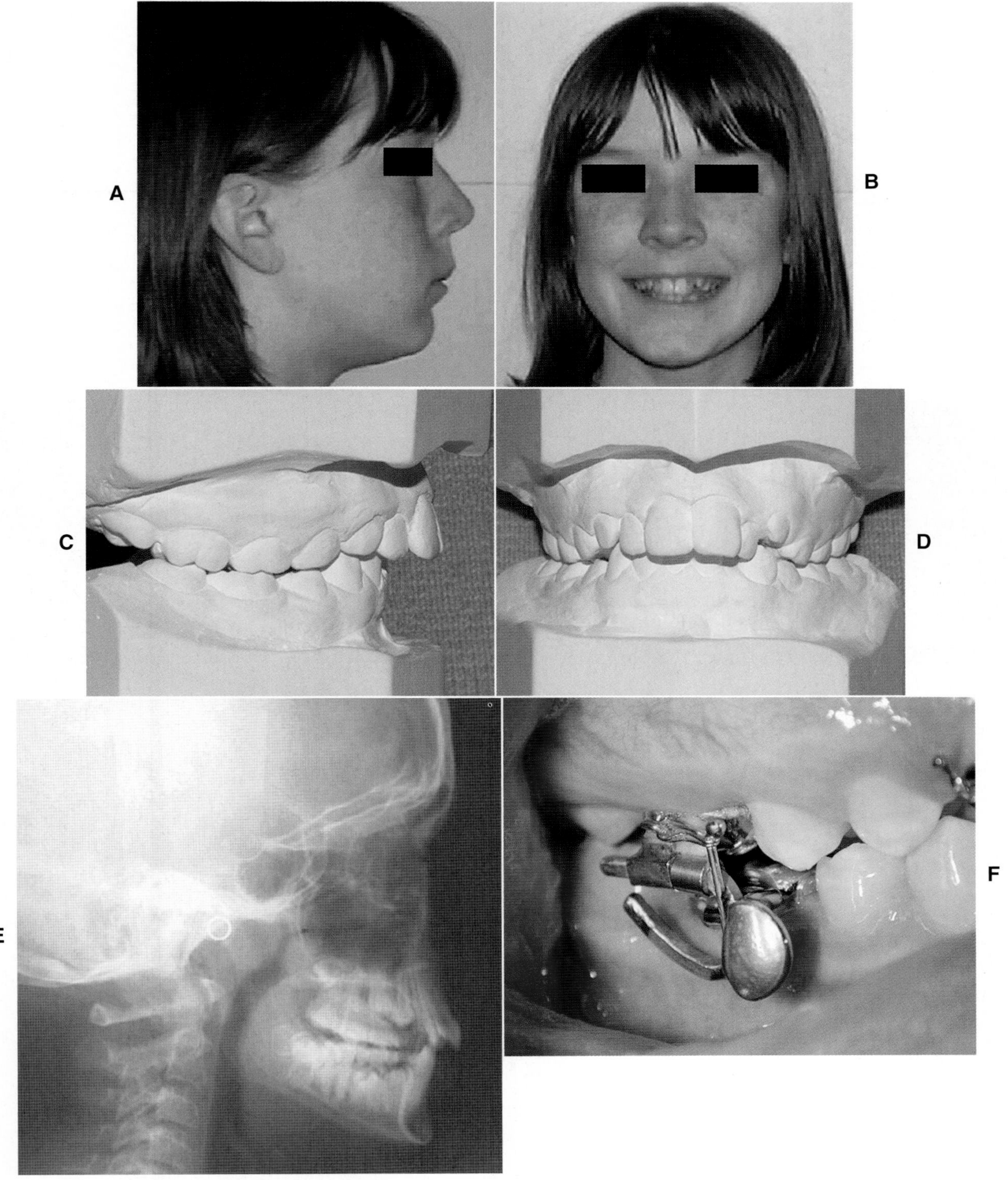

FIG 13-9 MARA treatment. **A-E,** Initial photos: facial photos **(A** and **B),** casts **(C** and **D),** and cephalometric radiograph **(E)**. **F,** MARA appliance in place.

Continued

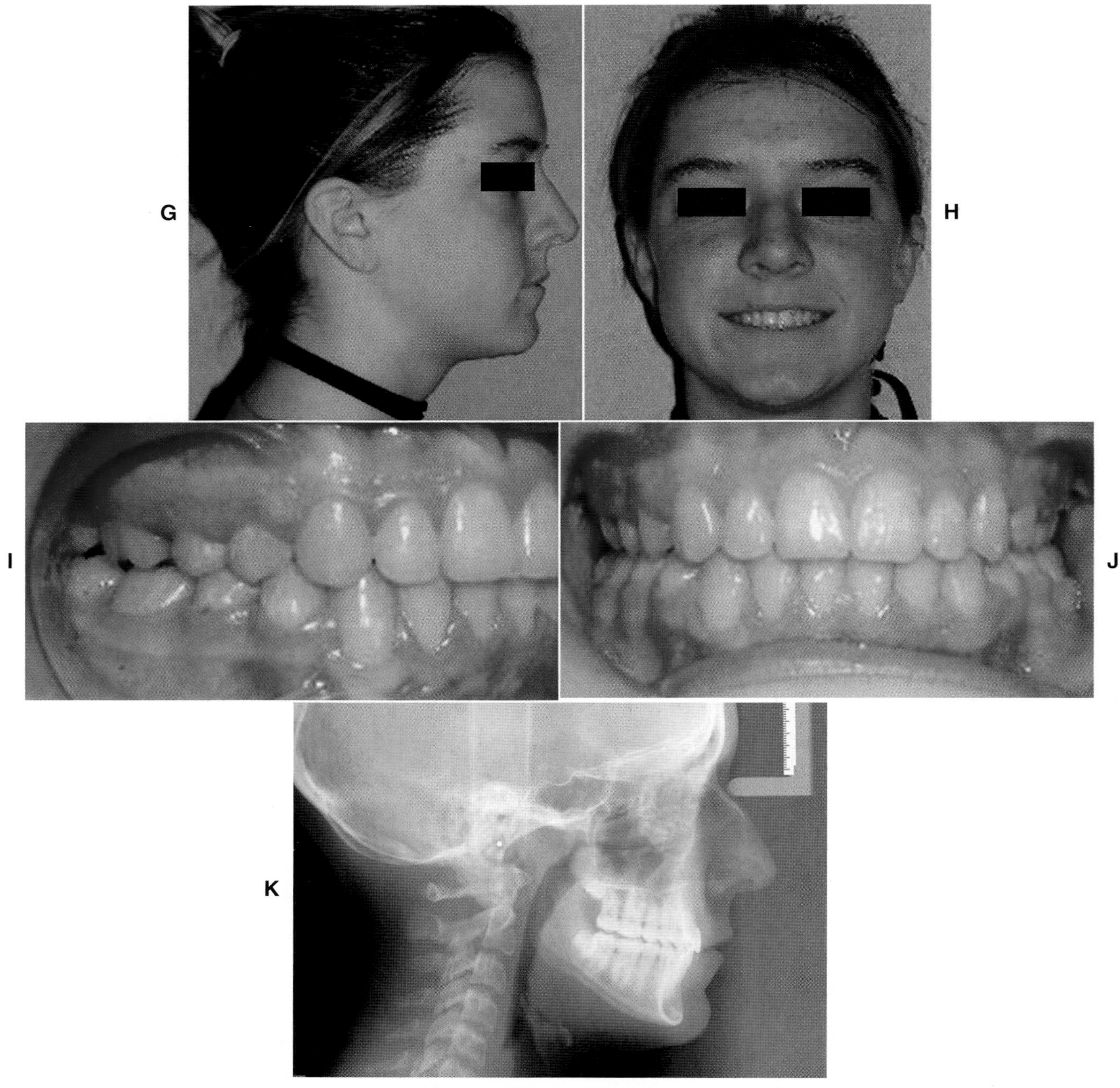

FIG 13-9—cont'd G-J, MARA plus orthodontic treatment final results: facial photos **(G** and **H)** and intraoral photos **(I** and **J)**. **K,** Posttreatment cephalometric radiograph.

REFERENCES

1. McNamara JA Jr: Components of Class II malocclusion in children 8-10 years of age. *Angle Orthod* 1981;51(3):177-202.
2. Baccetti T, Franchi L, McNamara JA, Tollaro I: Early dentofacial features of Class II malocclusions: A longitudinal study from the deciduous through the mixed dentition. *Am J Orthod Dentofacial Orthop* 1997;111(5):502-509.
3. McNamara J, Brudon WL: *Orthodontic and orthopedic treatment in the mixed dentition*. Ann Arbor: Needham Press, 1993.
4. Moyers RE, Riolo MS, Guire KE, et al: Differential diagnosis of Class II malocclusions. *Am J Orthod* 1980;78(5):477-494.
5. McNamara JA, Brudon WL: *Orthodontics and dentofacial orthopedics*. Ann Arbor: Needham Press, 2001.
6. Proffit WR, Fields HW: *Contemporary orthodontics*, edition 3. St Louis: Mosby, 1993.
7. Kjellberg H: Juvenile chronic arthritis. Dentofacial morphology, growth, mandibular function and orthodontic treatment. *Swed Dent J* 1995;109(Suppl):1-56.
8. Mossey PA: The heritability of malocclusion: Part 2. The influence of genetics in malocclusion. *Br J Orthod* 1999;26:195-203.
9. Smith RA: The etiology of angle Class II division 1 malocclusion. *Angle Orthod* 1939;9:15-19.

10. Brezniak N, Arad A, Heller M, et al: Pathognomonic cephalometric characteristic angle Class II division 2 malocclusion. *Angle Orthod* 2002;72(3):251-257.
11. Sfondrini MF, Cacciafesta V, Sfondrini G: Upper molar distalization: a critical analysis. *Orthod Craniofac Res* 2002;5(2): 114-126.
12. Bussick TJ, McNamara JA: Dentoalveolar and skeletal changes associated with the pendulum appliance. *Am J Orthod Dentofacial Orthop* 2000;117:333-343.
13. Shen G, Hagg U, Darendeliler MA: Skeletal effects of bite jumping therapy on the mandible—removable vs. fixed functional appliances. *Orthod Craniofac Res* 2005;8:2-10.
14. Berger JL, Pangrazio-Kulbersh V, George C, Kaczynski R: Long-term comparison of treatment outcome and stability of Class II patients treated with functional appliances versus bilateral sagittal split ramus osteotomy. *Am J Orthod Dentofac Orthop* 2005;127(4):451-464.
15. Graber TM, Vanarsdall RL Jr, Vig KWL: *Orthodontics: current principles & techniques*, edition 4. Philadelphia: Mosby, 2005.
16. Baccetti T, Franchi L, McNamara JA: The Cervical Vertebral Maturation (CVM) method for the assessment of optimal treatment timing in dentofacial orthopedics. *Semin Orthod* 2005;11:119-129.
17. Cozza P, Baccetti T, Franchi L, et al: Mandibular changes produced by functional appliance in Class II malocclusion: A systematic review. *Am J Orthod Dentofacial Orthop* 2006;129:599. e1-12.
18. Clark W: The Twin Block traction technique. *Europ J Orthod* 1982;4:129-138.
19. Allen-Noble P: Clinical management of MARA. Allesee Orthodontic Appliances. February 2002, pp 1-63.
20. McNamara JA Jr., Howe RP, Dischinger TG: A comparison of the Herbst and Frankel appliances in the treatment of Class II malocclusion. *Am J Orthod Dentofacial Orthop* 1990;98:134-144.
21. Pangrazio-Kulbersh V, Berger JL, Chermak DS, et al: Treatment effects of the Mandibular Anterior Repositioning Appliance on patients with Class II malocclusion. *Am J Orthod Dentofacial Orthop* 2003;123(3):286-295.
22. Toth LR, McNamara JA: Treatment effects produced by the Twin-block appliance and the FR-2 appliance of Frankel compared with an untreated Class II Sample. *Am J Orthodontics Dentofac Orthop* 1999;116(6):587-609.
23. Heinig N, Goz G: Clinical application and effects of the Forsus Spring. A study of a new Herbst hybrid. *J Orofac Orthop* 2001;62(6):436-450.
24. 3M US Unitek Forsus Resistant Device. Forsus Fatigue Resistant Device L-Pin Module. Available at: http://solutions.3m.com/wps/portal/3M/en_US/orthodontics/Unitek/solutions/class-II/Forsus-L-Pin/.
25. Tulloch JFC, Phillips C, Koch G, Proffitt WR: The effect of early intervention on skeletal pattern in Class II malocclusion: a randomized clinical trial. *Am J Orthod Dentofacial Orthop* 1997;II1:391-400.
26. Croft RS, Buschang PH, English JD, Meyer R: A cephalometric and tomographic evaluation of Herbst treatment in the mixed dentition. *Am J Orthod Dentofacial Orthop* 1999;116(4):435-443.
27. Uner O, Gultan AS: The changes in orthodontic area after retention period in skeletal Class 2 treated with activator. *Orthodi Dergisi* 1989;2:1.
28. Pancherz H: The Herbst appliance—its biologic effects and clinical use. *Am J Orthod* 1985;87(1):1-20.
29. Mihalik CA, Proffit WR, Phillips C: Long-term follow-up of class II adult treated with orthodontic camouflage: A comparison with orthognathic surgery outcomes. *Am J Orthod Dentofacial Orthop* 2003;123(3):266-278.
30. Wolford LM, Karras SC, Mehra P: Considerations for orthognathic surgery during growth, Part I: Mandibular deformities. *Am J Orthod Dentofacial Orthop* 2001;119(2):95-101.
31. Proffit WR, White RP Jr, Sarver D: *Contemporary treatment of dentofacial deformity*. Philadelphia: Mosby, 2003.

CHAPTER

14

Class III Correctors

Peter Ngan

The skeletal Class III malocclusion is characterized by mandibular prognathism, maxillary deficiency, or a combination of both. These patients may have a retrusive nasomaxillary area and a prominent lower third of the face. Intraorally, patients usually present with a Class III molar relationship and a reverse overjet depending on the severity of the skeletal discrepancy.

Many treatment approaches have been advocated for Class III patients, ranging from early orthopedic intervention to camouflage and definitive surgical intervention. Methods designed to intercept the developing malocclusion have included maxillary expansion and protraction with a facemask, chin cup and fixed orthodontic appliance therapy. In this chapter, an attempt is made to answer a few frequently asked questions related to the use of these Class III correctors, including the indications for treatment, treatment timing, and the response of these appliances to treatment.

1. What is pseudo Class III malocclusion, and how can these patients benefit from early treatment?

Patients with pseudo Class III malocclusion often present with anterior crossbites that are caused by a premature tooth contact or improper inclinations of the maxillary and mandibular incisors (Fig. 14-1). Elimination of the centric occlusion/centric relation discrepancy may avoid abnormal wear and traumatic occlusal forces to the affected teeth, avoid potential adverse growth influences in the maxilla and mandible, and improve maxillary lip posture and facial appearance.[1]

Correction of single or multiple anterior teeth in crossbite can be accomplished by using a fixed or removable appliance with an inclined plane, removable appliance with auxiliary spring, and lingual arch with finger springs (Fig. 14-2).[2]

2. What is a Delaire facemask?

The Delaire protraction facemask is used in the treatment of patients with Class III malocclusion and a maxillary deficiency.[3] Oppenheim[4] was first to suggest that one could not control the growth or anterior displacement of the mandible and suggested moving the maxilla forward in an attempt to counterbalance mandibular protrusion. Petit[5] later modified Delaire's basic concept by increasing the amount of force generated by the appliance, thus decreasing the overall treatment time.

The protraction facemask is made of two pads that contact the soft tissue in the forehead and chin region (Fig. 14-3). The pads are connected by a midline framework and are adjustable through the loosening and tightening of a set screw. An adjustable anterior wire with hooks is also connected to the midline framework to accommodate a downward and forward pull on the maxilla with elastics. To minimize the opening of the bite as the maxilla is repositioned, the protraction elastics are attached near the maxillary canines with a downward and forward pull of 30 degrees to the occlusal plane (Fig. 14-4). Maxillary protraction generally requires 300 to 600 g of force per side, depending on the age of the patient. Patients are instructed to wear the facemask for 12 hours a day.

3. When is facemask therapy indicated?

The facemask is most effective in the treatment of mild to moderate skeletal Class III malocclusions with a retrusive maxilla and a hypodivergent growth pattern. Patients presenting with some degree of anterior mandibular shift on closure and a moderate overbite have a more favorable prognosis (Fig. 14-5, *A-H*). The correction of anterior crossbite and mandibular shift results in a downward and backward rotation of the mandible that diminishes its prognathism (Fig. 14-5, *I-P*).

4. Is expansion necessary for protraction facemask treatment?

Various appliances have been used as anchorage for maxillary protraction, including palatal arches and banded and bonded expansion appliances (Fig. 14-6). Several circummaxillary sutures play an important role in the development of the nasomaxillary complex, including the frontomaxillary, nasomaxillary, zygomaticotemporal, zygomaticomaxillary, pterygopalatine, intermaxillary, ethmomaxillary, and lacrimomaxillary sutures (Fig. 14-7).[2] These sutures are patent until 8 years of age. Patients in the primary and early mixed dentition do not require maxillary expansion for protraction. However, in the mixed dentition, the maxillary sutures become more tortuous and start to fuse together. The use of an expansion appliance

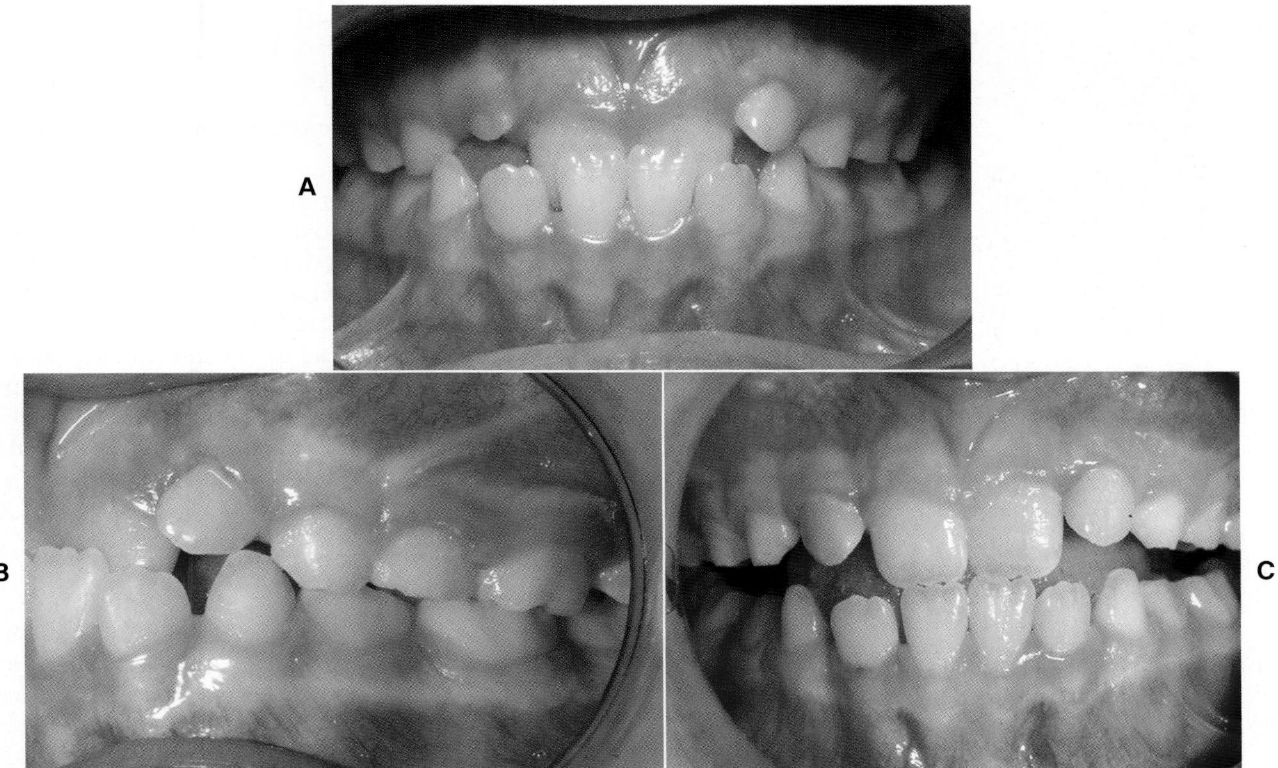

FIG 14-1 **A-C,** Patients with a pseudo Class III malocclusion can often present with an anterior crossbite **(A** and **B)** that can be manipulated back to an end-to-end incisal relationship in centric relation **(C)**.

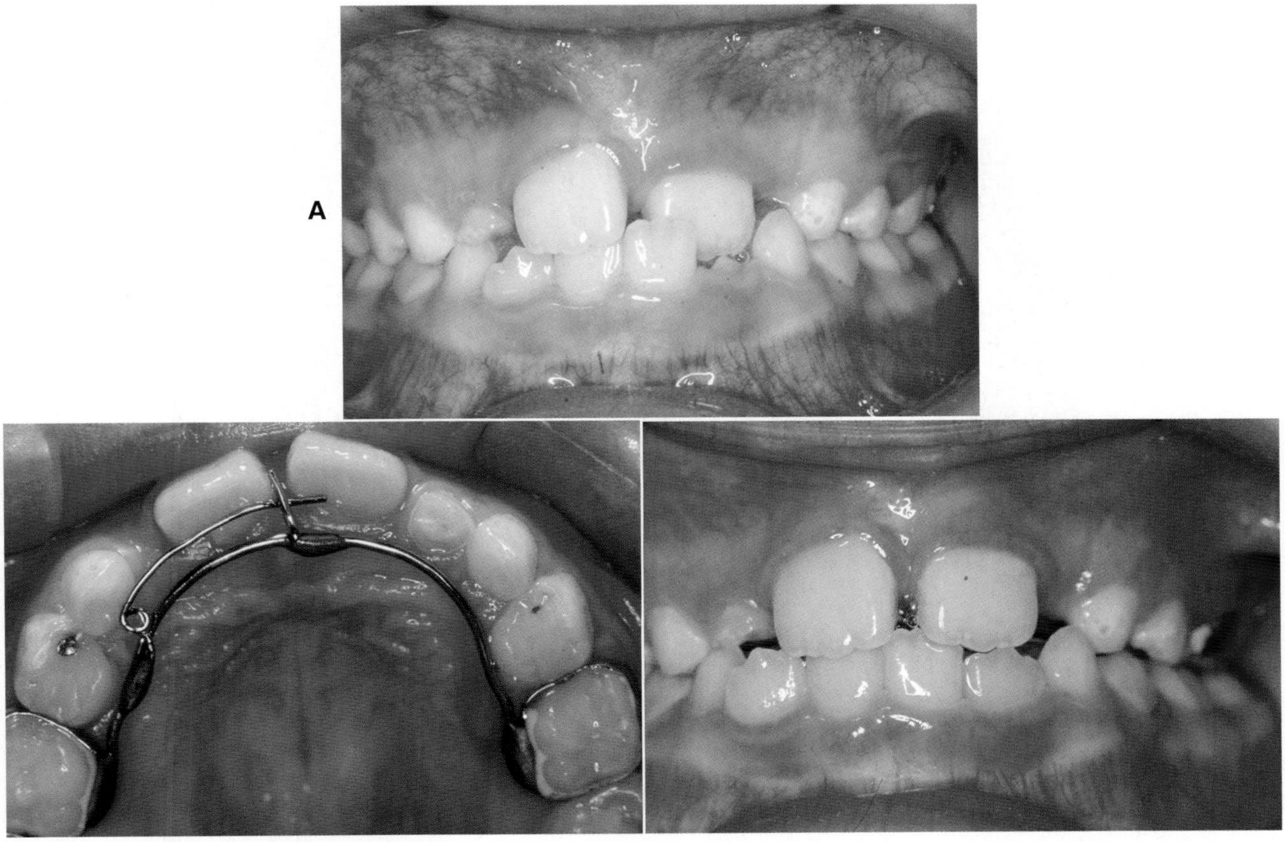

FIG 14-2 **A-C,** Correction of an anterior dental crossbite **(A)** with a fixed lingual arch and finger springs **(B)**. **C,** Posttreatment photo.

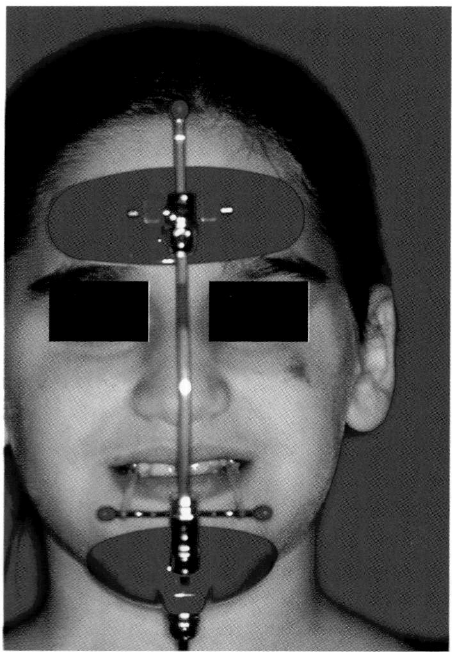

FIG 14-3 The protraction facemask uses the forehead and chin as anchorage to protract the maxilla forward and downward.

can help in "disarticulating" the maxilla and initiate cellular response in the circumaxillary sutures, allowing a more positive reaction to protraction forces.

5. What is the best treatment timing for facemask therapy?

The optimal time to intervene in a patient with early Class III malocclusion is at the time of initial eruption of the maxillary central incisors. A positive overjet and overbite at the end of facemask treatment appear to maintain the anterior occlusion after treatment. Studies have shown that better skeletal and dental response can be obtained in the primary and early mixed dentition rather than in the late mixed dentition. The erupted maxillary first molars provide better anchorage for maxillary protraction. Maxillary protraction is effective through puberty with diminishing skeletal response as the sutures mature.

6. What type of effects can be expected from facemask treatment?

Anterior crossbites can be corrected with 3 to 4 months of maxillary protraction depending on the severity of the malocclusion. Improvement in overbite and molar relationship can be expected with an additional 4 to 6 months of treatment.[6] In a prospective clinical trial, overjet correction was found to be the result of forward maxillary movement (31%), backward movement of the mandible (21%), labial movement of the maxillary incisors (28%), and lingual movement of the

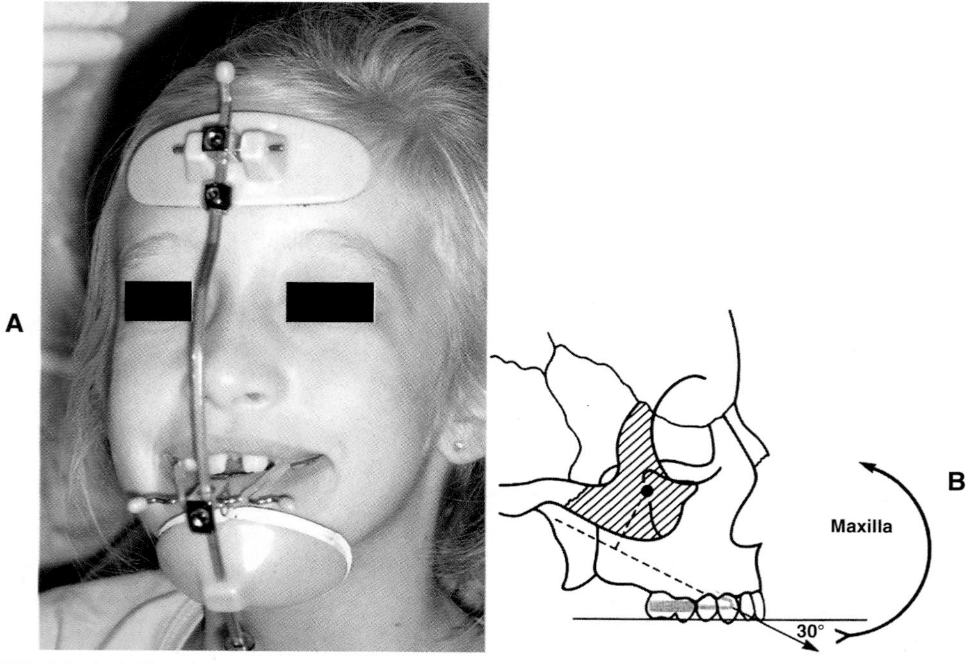

FIG 14-4 **A,** Protraction elastics are attached to the intraoral anchorage appliance near the maxillary canines region with a downward and forward pull of 30 degrees to the occlusal plane. **B,** The force vectors that minimize tilting of the palatal plane.

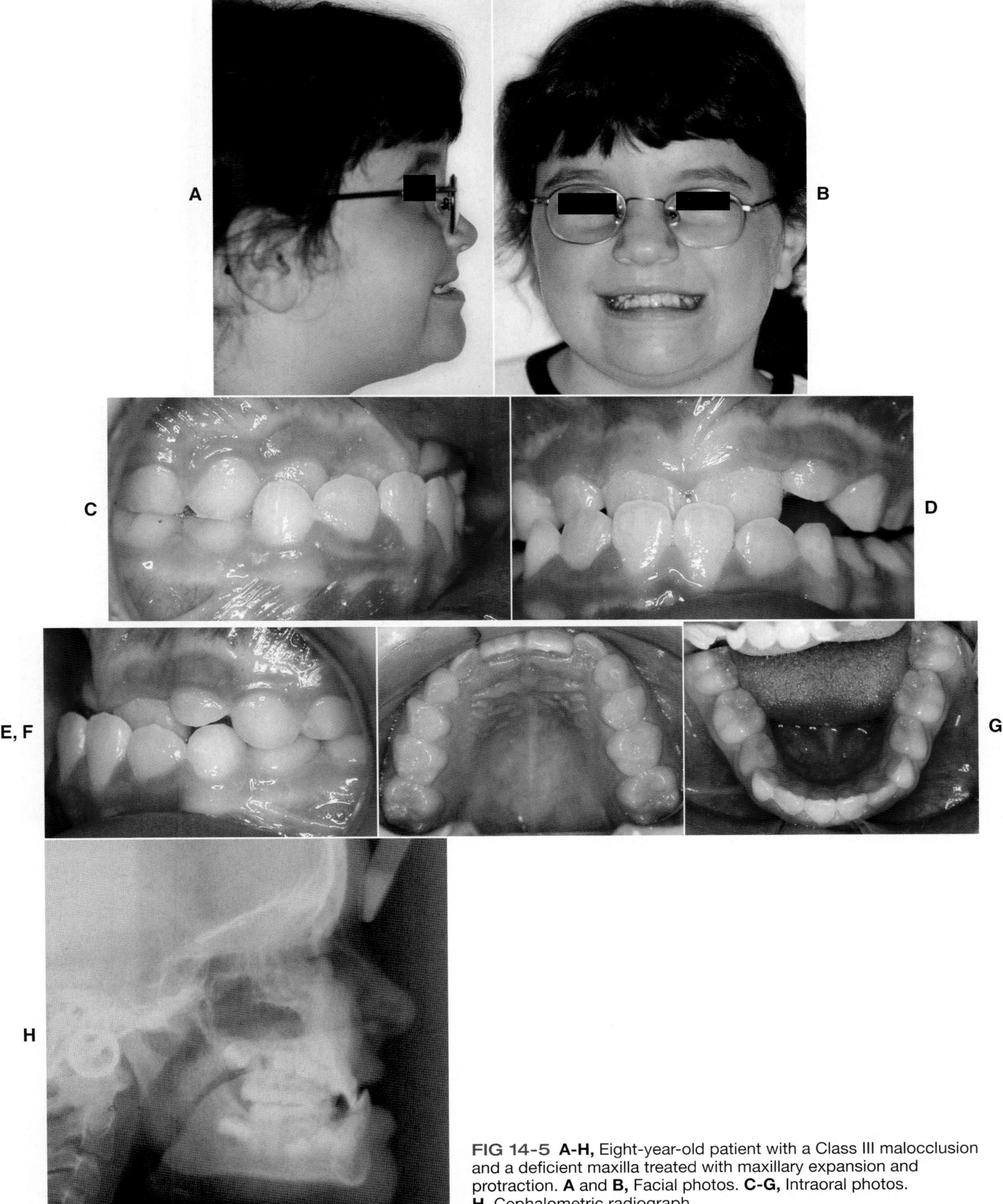

FIG 14-5 **A-H,** Eight-year-old patient with a Class III malocclusion and a deficient maxilla treated with maxillary expansion and protraction. **A** and **B,** Facial photos. **C-G,** Intraoral photos. **H,** Cephalometric radiograph.

Continued

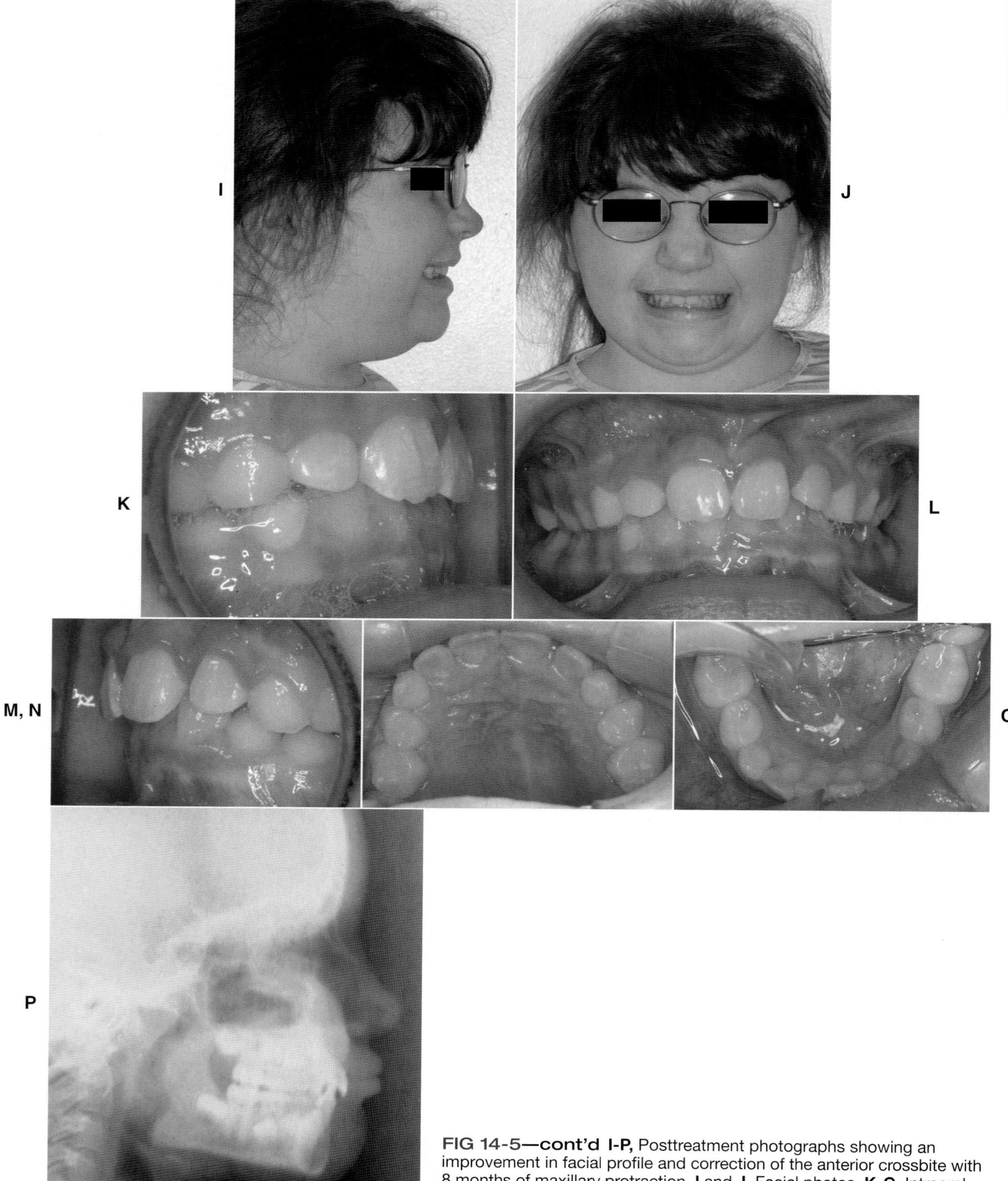

FIG 14-5—cont'd I-P, Posttreatment photographs showing an improvement in facial profile and correction of the anterior crossbite with 8 months of maxillary protraction. **I** and **J,** Facial photos. **K-O,** Intraoral photos. **P,** Cephalometric radiograph.

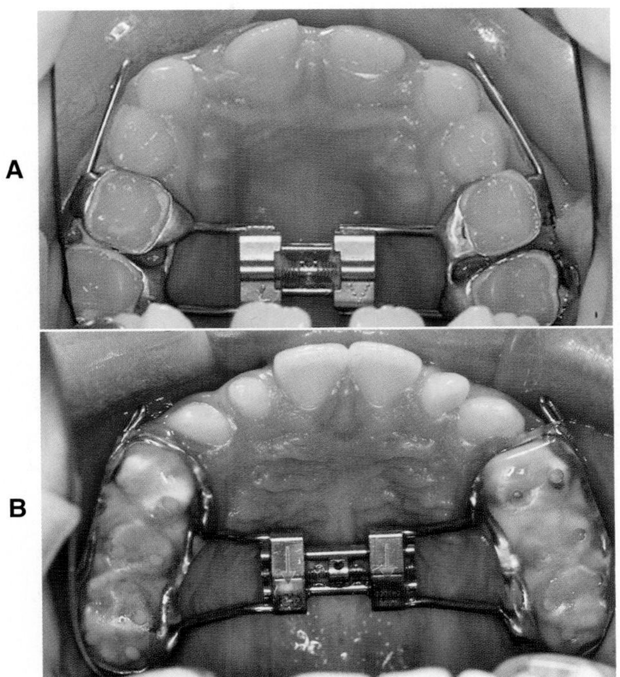

FIG 14-6 **A** and **B,** Rapid palatal expansion appliance used as anchorage for maxillary protraction.

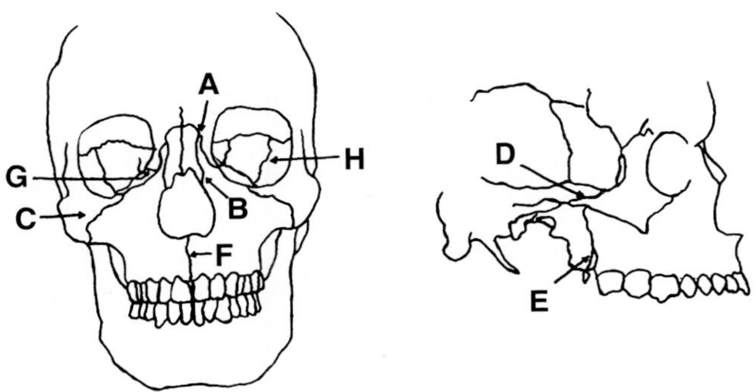

FIG 14-7 Circummaxillary sutures involved in maxillary protraction. *A,* Frontomaxillary suture. *B,* Nasomaxillary suture. *C,* Zygomaticomaxillary suture. *D,* Zygomaticotemporal suture. *E,* Pterygopalatine suture. *F,* Intermaxillary suture *G,* Lacrimomaxillary suture. *H,* Ethmomaxillary suture.

mandibular incisors (20%). Molar relationship was corrected to a Class I or Class II dental relationship by a combination of skeletal movement and differential movement of the maxillary and mandibular molars. Anchorage loss was observed during maxillary protraction with mesial movement of the maxillary molars. Overbite was improved by eruption of the maxillary and mandibular molars. The total face height was increased by inferior movement of the maxilla and downward and backward rotation of the mandible.

Treatment with protraction facemask can also improve the facial profile by decreasing the facial concavity, improving the posture of the lips, and decreasing the retrusive nasomaxillary area.[7]

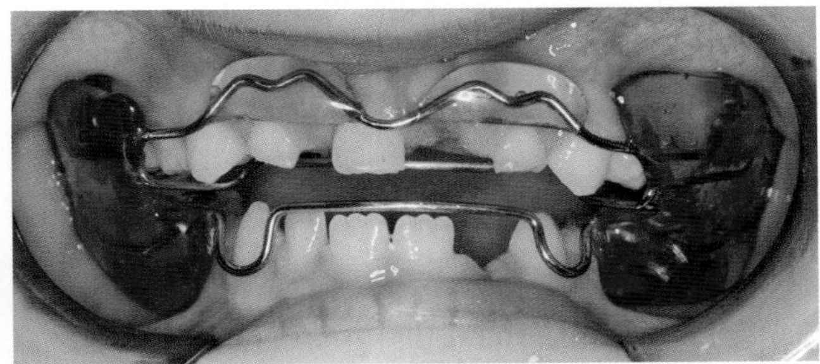

FIG 14-8 Frankel III Regulator used for retention after protraction facemask treatment.

7. Are these treatment results stable long term?

Prospective clinical trials have shown that the effects on the maxilla remained stable for 2 years after facemask treatment.[8] During this growth period, the maxilla and mandible reverted back to the original growth pattern. Long-term studies have shown that treatment is successful in 67% to 75% of the patients.[9,10] The malocclusion can be camouflaged by orthodontic treatment. Patients that reverted back to an anterior crossbite will eventually require surgical treatment when growth is completed. Therefore, an overcorrection of the maxilla to 3 to 4 mm of anterior overjet is recommended for patients who are diagnosed with excessive mandibular growth.

8. Are there variations in clinical response to facemask treatment?

Clinically, the maxilla can be advanced 2 to 4 mm over an 8- to 12-month period of maxillary protraction. The amount of forward maxillary movement is influenced by a number of factors, including age of patient, the use of expansion appliance, the force level, the direction and point of force application, and the treatment time.

In a prospective clinical study, individual variation in the forward movement of the maxilla can vary from −3.5 mm to +6 mm and vertical movement of maxilla varied from −0.5 mm to +2.0 mm with 8 months of maxillary protraction.[11]

9. Is retention necessary after facemask treatment?

Studies have shown that the use of removable appliances such as a Frankel III regulator or a mandibular retractor helps in maintaining the sagittal and transverse correction by facemask and allows muscle adaptation to the new position of the maxilla (Fig.14-8).

10. When should a chin cup be used?

Skeletal Class III malocclusion with a relatively normal maxilla and a moderately protrusive mandible can be treated with a chin cup (Fig. 14-9). It is also indicated in patients when increases in lower anterior facial height are not desired. The objective of this treatment is to provide mandibular growth inhibition and/or redirection and posterior positioning of the mandible.[2]

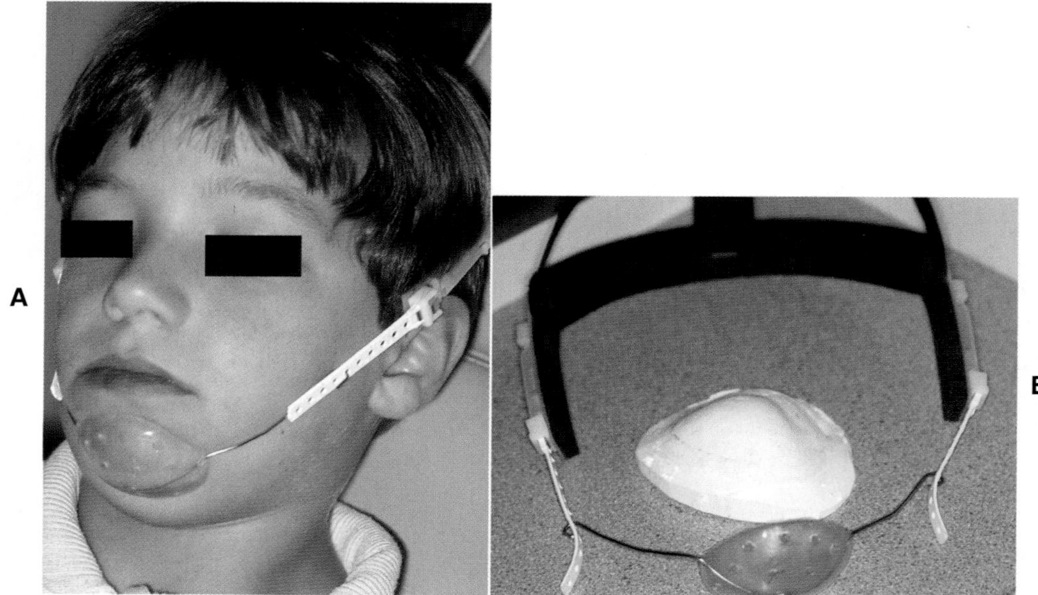

FIG 14-9 **A** and **B,** Chin cup for treatment of patients with Class III malocclusion and protrusive mandible.

11. What is the force magnitude and direction recommended for chin cup treatment?

Chin cups are divided into two types: the occipital-pull that is used for patients with mandibular protrusion and the vertical-pull that is used in patients presenting with a hyperdivergent or long face. An orthopedic force of 600 to 700 g 12 hours per day is recommended. The orthopedic force is usually directed through the condyle or below the condyle (see Fig. 14-9).

12. What type of effects can be expected from chin cup treatment?

The orthopedic effects of a chin cup on a mandible include:

1. Redirection of mandibular growth vertically
2. Backward repositioning (rotation) of the mandible
3. Remodeling of the mandible with closure of the gonial angle

To date, there is no agreement on whether chin cup treatment inhibits mandibular growth. Chin cup treatment has been shown to produce a clockwise rotation of the mandible during orthopedic treatment. However, studies have shown that removal of the chin cup prior to completion of pubertal growth may lead to return of the horizontal growth pattern of the mandible.

13. What is the treatment timing and duration of chin cup treatment?

Patients with mandibular excess can usually be recognized in the primary dentition despite the fact that the mandible appears retrognathic in the early years for most children. Evidence exists that treatment to reduce mandibular protrusion is more successful when it is started in the primary or early mixed dentition. The treatment varies from 1 year to as long as 4 years depending on the severity of the malocclusion. Recent studies have shown that removal of the chin cup before completion of pubertal growth invites treatment relapse because the mandible resumes to a more horizontal Class III growth rate and direction during pubertal growth period. It is recommended that treatment with the chin cup be continued until completion of the pubertal growth period.

14. What is camouflaged Class III treatment?

Patients with mild to moderate skeletal jaw discrepancies can be camouflaged by early orthopedic treatment to move the upper jaw mesially by appliances such as the facemask or position the lower jaw back by appliances such as the chin cup. In the permanent dentition, orthodontic tooth movement can be used to camouflage the underlying jaw differences by proclination of the maxillary incisors or retraction of the mandibular incisors. Fixed appliances with Class III elastics that run from the maxillary molars to the mandibular canines are used to achieve the desired tooth movements. In patients with crowded dentitions or dentoalveolar protrusion, extraction of the mandibular first premolars and maxillary second premolars may be necessary to camouflage the malocclusion (Fig. 14-10).

15. What is surgical Class III treatment?

Class III patients with significant anteroposterior jaw discrepancies that cannot be camouflaged with orthodontic tooth movement will have to be treated surgically. This is usually performed after growth is completed. Depending on the diagnosis, the maxilla may be brought forward with a LeFort I surgical osteotomy procedure and the mandible may be set back with a bilateral sagittal split osteotomy. Presurgical orthodontic treatment is usually necessary to decompensate the dentition and allow maximum jaw movement to obtain optimal facial appearance (Fig. 14-11).

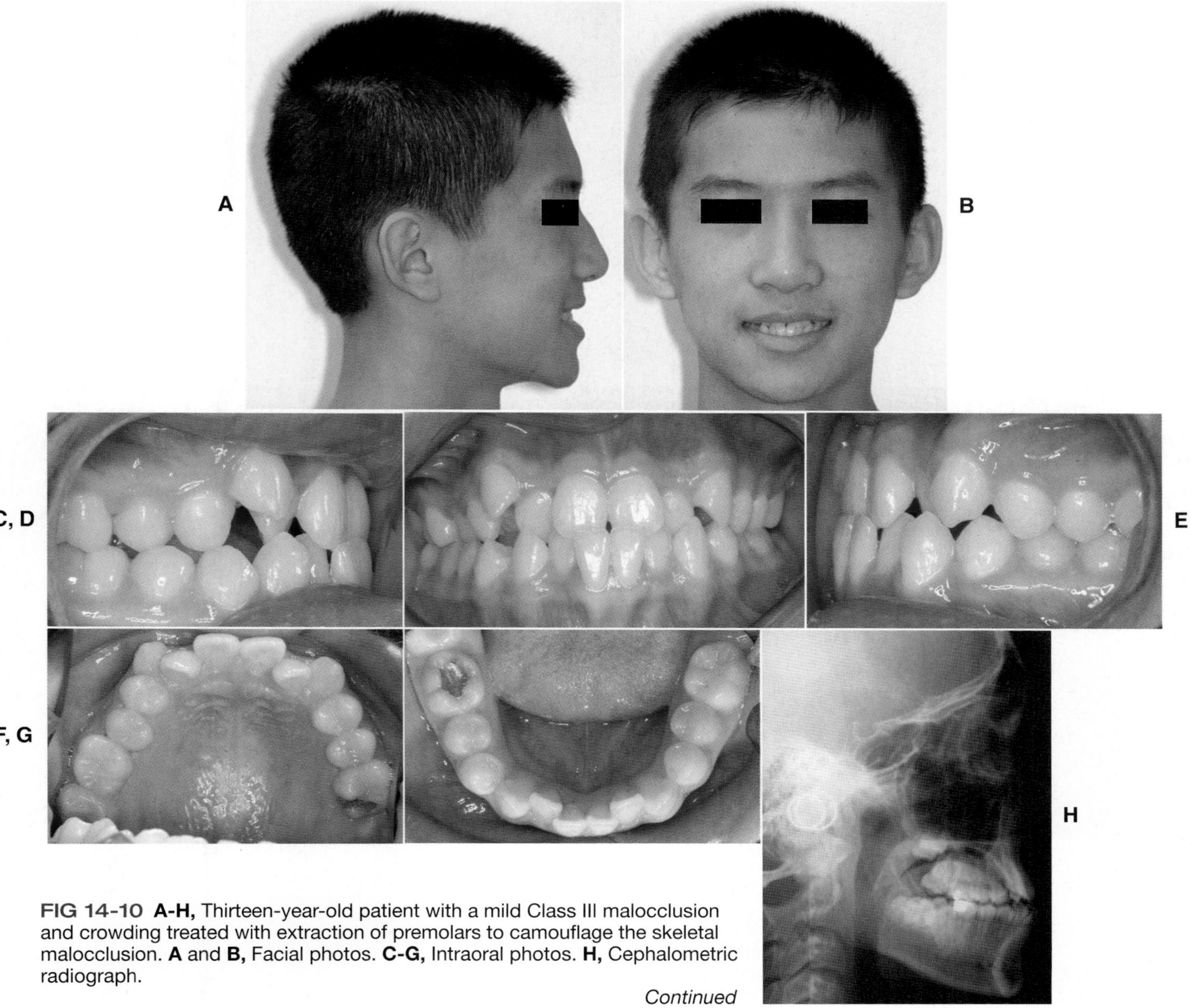

FIG 14-10 A-H, Thirteen-year-old patient with a mild Class III malocclusion and crowding treated with extraction of premolars to camouflage the skeletal malocclusion. **A** and **B,** Facial photos. **C-G,** Intraoral photos. **H,** Cephalometric radiograph.

Continued

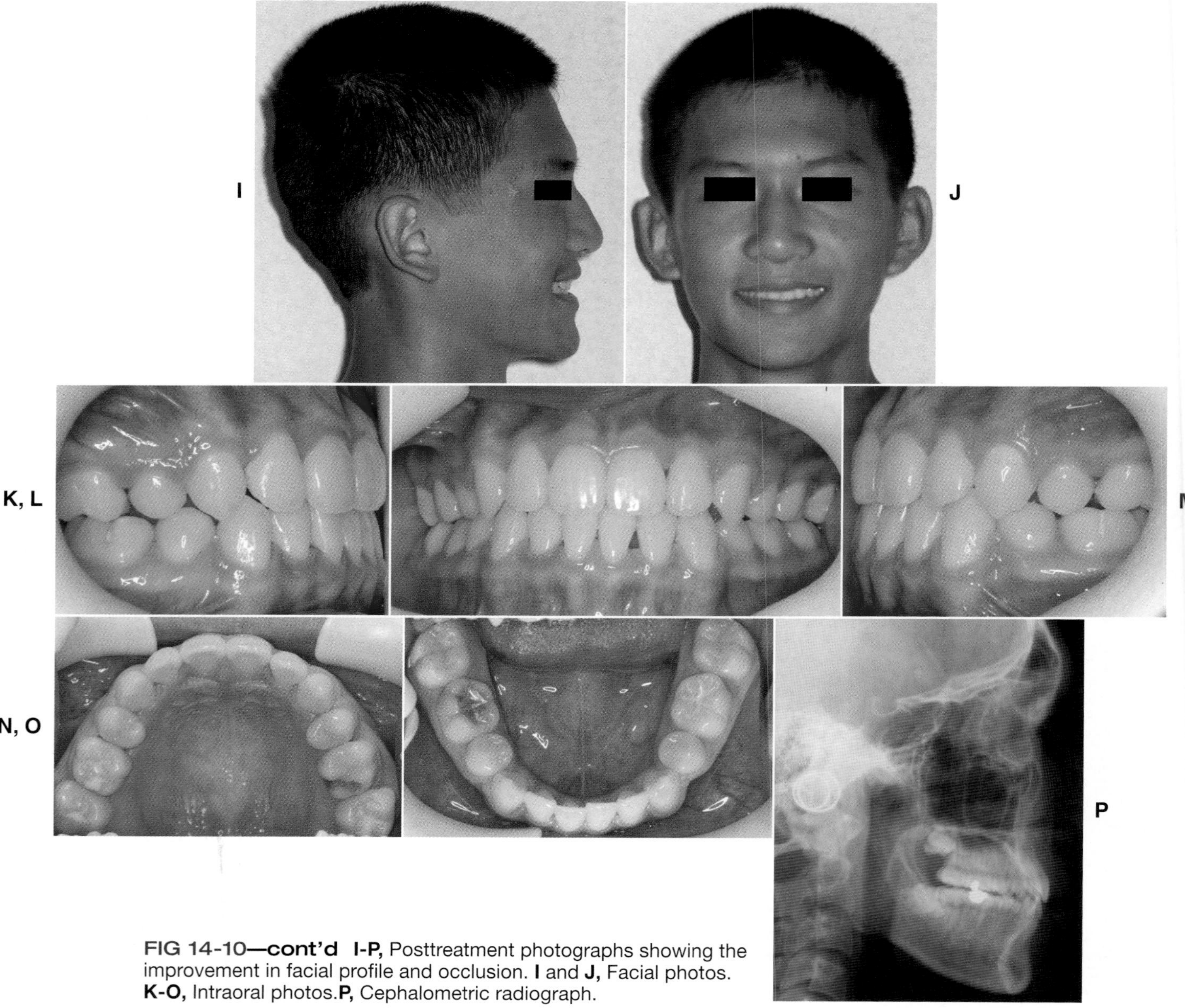

FIG 14-10—cont'd I-P, Posttreatment photographs showing the improvement in facial profile and occlusion. **I** and **J,** Facial photos. **K-O,** Intraoral photos.**P,** Cephalometric radiograph.

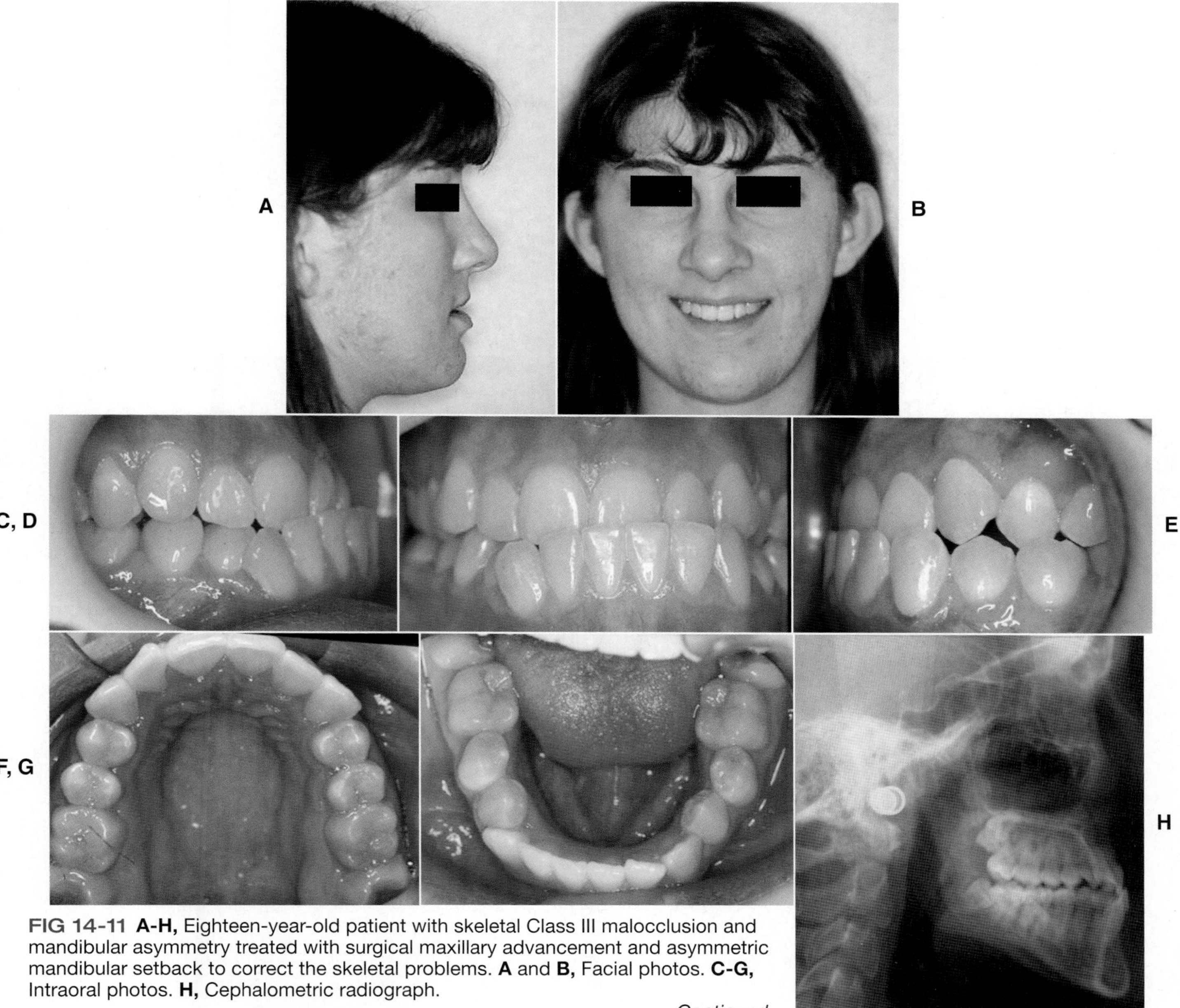

FIG 14-11 **A-H,** Eighteen-year-old patient with skeletal Class III malocclusion and mandibular asymmetry treated with surgical maxillary advancement and asymmetric mandibular setback to correct the skeletal problems. **A** and **B,** Facial photos. **C-G,** Intraoral photos. **H,** Cephalometric radiograph.

Continued

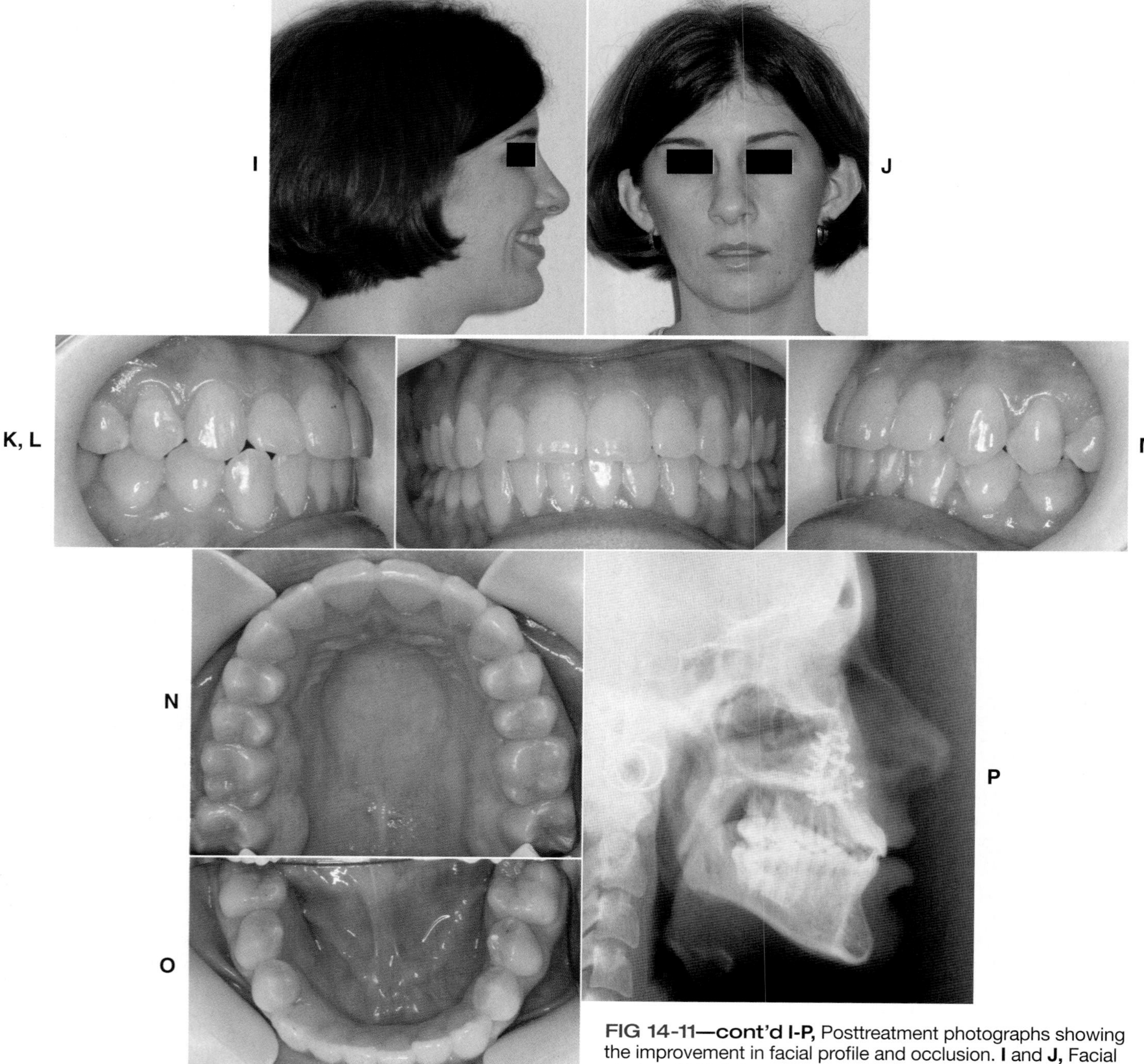

FIG 14-11—cont'd I-P, Posttreatment photographs showing the improvement in facial profile and occlusion. **I** and **J,** Facial photos. **K-O,** Intraoral photos. **P,** Cephalometric radiograph.

REFERENCES

1. Joondeph DR: Early orthodontic treatment. *Am J Orthod* 1993;104:199-200.
2. Ngan P: Treatment of Class III malocclusion in the primary and mixed dentition. In Bishara S. *Textbook of orthodontics.* Philadelphia: Saunders, 2003, pp 375-414.
3. Delaire J: Maxillary development revisited: relevance to the orthopaedic treatment of Class III malocclusions. *Eur J Orthod* 1997;19:289-311.
4. Oppenheim A: A possibility for physiologic orthodontic movement. *Am J Orthod Oral Surg* 1944;30:345-346.
5. Petit HP: Adaptation following accelerated facial mask therapy. In: McNamara JA Jr, Ribbens Ka, Howe RP, editors. Clinical alterations of the growing face. Monograph 14. Craniofacial growth series. Center for Human Growth and Development. Ann Arbor: The University of Michigan, 1983.
6. Ngan P, Hagg U, Yiu C, et al: Treatment response and long-term dentofacial adaptations to maxillary expansion and protraction. *Semin Orthod* 1997;3:255-264.
7. Ngan P, Hagg U, Merwin D, et al: Soft tissue and dentoskeletal profile changes associated with maxillary expansion and protraction headgear treatment. *Am J Orthod Dentofacial Orthop* 1996;109:38-49.
8. Ngan P, Yiu C, Hu A, et al: Cephalometric and occlusal changes following maxillary expansion and protraction. *Eur J Orthod* 1998;20:237-254.
9. Westwood PV, McNamara JA, Baccetti T, et al: Long-term effects of Class III treatment with rapid maxillary expansion and facemask therapy followed by fixed appliances. *Am J Orthod Dentofac Orthop* 2003;123:266-278.
10. Hagg U, Tse A, Bendeus M, et al: Long-term follow-up of early treatment with reverse headgear. *Eur J Orthod* 2003;25:95-102.
11. Ngan P, Hagg U, Yiu C, et al: Treatment response to maxillary expansion and protraction. *Eur J Orthod* 1996;18:151-168.

CHAPTER 15

Minor Tooth Movement

G. Fräns Currier

Isolated tooth movement necessitates that other teeth should not be moved (i.e., anchored). These tooth movements can be within either the maxillary or mandibular arch as either lateral (transverse) or front-to-back (sagittal or anteroposterior) or between the arches, most noticeably transverse or sagittal. Isolated vertical movement such as extrusion or intrusion also necessitates important anchorage considerations so the adjacent teeth do not move.

This tooth movement in the transitional dentition is associated with interceptive orthodontics, whereas in the adult it is adjunctive orthodontics in association with fixed prosthodontics or anterior esthetic restorative dentistry. The most common tooth movement in the primary dentition should be related to the correction of the quadrant posterior crossbite with mandibular shift caused by a narrow maxillary primary intercanine width.

The extraction or discing of selected primary teeth—not permanent teeth unless they are third molars—is often related to certain types of isolated tooth movement. Sometimes the extractions themselves can improve or correct problems as seen with mandibular midline discrepancies or moderate clinical crowding in the 8- to 10-year-old patients, unfavorable pathway of eruption of the permanent canine in the 9- to 11 year-olds, the maxillary midline succedaneous supernumerary tooth in the 7- to 9-year-old, and the uprighting of the permanent second molar in the adult.

Crossbite malocclusions need to be treated in most cases near the time of recognition because of unfavorable asymmetric patterns, anomalous development, or harmful development to the teeth or jaws, including the periodontium. Anterior open bite cases are addressed with the eruption of the permanent eight incisors.

The face's soft tissue profile and esthetic lines, as well as the skeletal pattern seen with the mandibular plane to Frankfort horizontal, are helpful areas of orientation for proper isolated tooth movement.

1. What does minor tooth movement in orthodontics mean compared with major tooth movement?

For some, there is no minor tooth movement. All tooth movement is major. One needs to understand that there is orthodontic tooth movement (and orthodontic force systems, which are lower) compared with orthopedic movement (and orthopedic force systems, which are higher).[1] Lower force systems are usually related to apposition/resorption of the alveolar bone around the tooth/teeth being moved. One can compute these in ounces or in grams (28 grams = 1 ounce).

The current, preferred method for most orthodontic tooth movement is not only on the lighter side, but also in the continuous format.[1,2] One can actually have orthopedic effects (bones moved more than the teeth) with orthodontic forces. An example of this is the quadhelix appliance in the maxillary arch of preschoolers. However, most orthopedic effects are accomplished with higher, or orthopedic, force systems in which the forces applied to the anchor teeth are manifested in the bones.

A better term than minor tooth movement is probably *isolated tooth movement,* in which there is need for a limited amount of orthodontic movement. This also means that other teeth should not be moved; this brings up the concept of anchorage. One does not wish to move the anchor teeth or the orthodontic system is compromised. An example of an anchor unit is a canine-to-canine lingual arch that can be used in the uprighting of a mandibular permanent second molar.

The common term associated with isolated tooth movement in children is *interceptive orthodontics*; it is called *adjunctive orthodontics* when it is associated with adults. It is not associated with first-phase corrective orthodontics where too many movement objectives need to be met. Examples of first phase (usually 12 to 18 months of active therapy) are early treatment of Class II malocclusions with a headgear or a functional appliance and Class III malocclusions with a rapid palatal expander and protraction facemask therapy.[2]

2. When should we first consider orthodontic treatment?

The sequence of maturation of the dentofacial complex is not related to Angle's dental classification of malocclusion, although that helps in classifying treatment problems.[3] That skeletal sequence is the transverse plane (side to side), followed by the sagittal plane (anteroposterior problems), and then the vertical plane (deep bite vs. open bite, or short face syndrome vs. long face syndrome).[4]

In the primary dentition, there is usually no crowding, but there can be shifts of the lower jaw to the left or right as the teeth go into maximum intercuspation of occlusion. The maxillary primary canines can erupt into a constricted intercanine dimension about 15 to 20 months after birth that will not allow the lower arch to fit properly. This usually causes the lower jaw to shift to one side with the dental midlines becoming noncoincident.[5]

If one aligns the midlines of the two arches, it is noticeable that the lower arch cannot fit. One approach and probably the best approach to solve this problem is to expand the maxillary arch. Another approach that involves no isolated tooth movement can be achieved with an occlusal adjustment of the primary canines (i.e., facial of the lower canine and lingual of the upper canine). However, there will be little effect on the lateral overjet of the primary molars.

Expansion of the maxillary arch can be achieved in a variety of ways using either fixed or removable appliances.[6] A removable jackscrew appliance with a biteplane has the limitations of only two turns per week or 0.5 mm of expansion as well as the issue of patient compliance in wearing the appliance. It has no orthopedic effect—only dentoalveolar tipping.

A predictable appliance for use in the preschooler is a quadhelix from the primary second molars. This appliance is an improved biomechanical one from the original "W" appliance. The quadhelix is fabricated to fit passively. Prior to insertion, the appliance is expanded approximately 10 mm in the facial-lingual dimension of the primary second molar and then cemented. By doing this, the appliance can be evaluated in 3- to 5-week intervals. Intraoral activation laterally of a cemented quadhelix is unpredictable. A 10-mm expansion usually gives 5 to 6 mm expansion within a few months. The appliance is left in place for a few months more after getting the proper lateral overjet with no quadrant in crossbite. It is not necessary to remove the appliance to place a passive Hawley for retention. The total length of the quadhelix treatment is usually about 6 to 8 months.

It is not common to have to remove, reactivate, and re-cement a properly expanded quadhelix. This is the most common active appliance in the primary dentition, and it has an orthopedic effect, which means the left and right maxillae also move. This effect is positive, since it increases the chance for the permanent molars to erupt properly.

Another appliance that can be used in the primary dentition is a two-tooth rapid palatal expander appliance (fixed appliance with a screw).[2-6] This fixed RPE can be expanded either once or twice a day. Although appreciable results can be obtained from using the two-tooth RPE, the quadhelix is also the appliance of choice for the treatment of posterior quadrant crossbites in the early to middle transitional dentition. However, upon the eruption of the maxillary first premolars and the presence of a quadrant posterior crossbite, the use of a more rigid appliance that can produce an orthopedic effect should be considered, such as a four-tooth rapid palatal expander. The mechanics related to the RPE are more complex with multiple sutural effects.[7]

The use of coordinated arch wires with light forces in the permanent dentition has been reintroduced into corrective orthodontics for adolescent treatment. The greater the expansion in the posterior portion, the more stable the results. Furthermore, the greater the effect in the middle arch, the greater the increase in arch perimeter.

3. How does one orient the lower arches with posterior crossbites?

The mandibular arch is consistently ovoid or tapered in shape with a midline suture that fuses shortly after birth. In some Class II division 2 malocclusions, the lower arch can be square. There is no orthopedic effect of the left and right mandibular bones used in orthodontics, as the midline fusion occurs so early.[2] However, the facial-lingual inclination of the mandibular posterior teeth (along the long axis of the tooth) helps in the understanding of the treatment of the lower arch. If the posterior permanent teeth lean inward with the crowns toward the tongue and the roots too far to the facial while the lateral overjet is minimal, then there is probably a problem with constriction of the maxillary arch. If one were to upright the lower buccal segments, the result would be a bilateral posterior quadrant crossbite. It is normal to have a mild progressive movement of the roots of the premolars/permanent molars facial to the crowns. All permanent teeth, except the maxillary incisors, are supposed to have their roots facial, or upright, compared with their tooth crowns. These incisors are supposed to have their roots lingual and crowns facial (lingual root torque). This can occur with the mandibular incisors, but it is more variable. The use in individual permanent molar crossbite is the application of cross-elastics. These elastics, usually from the lingual of the maxillary permanent molar to the facial counterpart, present problems with the collateral effect of extrusion of these teeth with the elastics with resultant worsening of the molar relationship.

4. Where does one treat most posterior crossbites?

Crossbites are usually treated in the maxilla. The maxillary arch form can vary by the type of Angle's classification. The common maxillary arch form is ovoid; however, the Class II division 2 malocclusion can present with a square arch form whereas the Class II division 1 malocclusion can present with a tapered arch form. With this Class II division 1 middle arch constriction, as the mandible shifts forward, a bilateral posterior quadrant crossbite will be presented. Therefore, one must be aware that hidden posterior crossbites can occur when the malocclusion is not Class I.[5]

5. Is there more than one type of posterior crossbite from the classic one presented with maxilla lingual and mandible facial?

Yes. The first one, which is not common, has the lower arch completely within the maxilla. It can manifest on one side or both and is called a Brodie bite. The expansion is usually done in the lower arch with a fixed appliance plus a bite plane that helps disarticulate the occlusion. This problem needs early treatment.[5]

The second problem is usually seen later upon the eruption of the permanent second molar. The more common pattern is with the maxillary permanent second molar facial and the less common mandibular permanent second molar lingual. In the maxilla, because of the rhomboid shape of the permanent first molar and the lack of a vertical stop of the malposed permanent second molar, the second molar often needs to be moved distal first and then aligned. Cross-arch elastics are interarch elastics that can make the extrusion problem worse.

Both problems are more difficult to treat than the usual crossbite, which is due to maxillary transverse deficiency. This is due to the vertical dimension that is manifested in these problems.

6. What happens to individual tooth crossbites if left untreated?

If left long enough, abnormal wear patterns appear on the teeth. There can be adverse periodontal responses around the affected teeth. If the quadrant crossbite is left untreated, the growth of the jaw can also be affected adversely.[2]

From an orthodontic tooth movement point of view, the issue becomes more complex. Whatever the orthodontic intervention initially proposed, usually involving more tipping than torque movements, the problem now presents as an issue of arch perimeter and crowding in the area of crossbite. It is necessary to regain the room in the arch prior to correction of the crossbite. This might involve interproximal tooth reduction or discing and/or removal of primary teeth. One should not reduce proximal surfaces of permanent teeth in the transitional dentition in the correction of crossbite. The crossbite problem is now a two-step treatment sequence as opposed to an earlier one-step sequence.

7. If anterior and posterior crossbites exist within the same patient, which crossbite comes first in the tooth movement?

It is usually the posterior quadrant problem involving primary teeth initially. The problem of anterior crossbite of single primary teeth is as rare as a single primary molar crossbite.[8] The anterior quadrant variety of primary incisors is usually a manifestation of a skeletal problem that necessitates a combination of intraoral and extraoral appliances.

If there is a combination of a posterior and anterior crossbite with the same patient, one treats the posterior crossbite first, then the anterior. If you treat the anterior crossbite first, you will lose its correction when the posterior crossbite is corrected.[8] A removable appliance to assist in correction of the anterior crossbite allows retention of the corrected posterior crossbite. The anterior crossbite problem is usually associated with lingual eruption of the maxillary permanent incisors. The permanent lateral incisor is usually more common in crossbite than the permanent central incisor. It is not uncommon for the incisors to erupt lingual in a bilateral expression. The timing of treatment of the permanent incisor crossbite correction is important, and it is related to the stage of eruption and the amount of overbite. Tipping the lingually positioned incisor facially causes the overbite to become more shallow. If the overbite is very shallow initially, the tooth/teeth do not retain well in the corrected position. Therefore, it is more appropriate to treat these incisor crossbites when more overlap is present, so that after the treatment is completed, the occlusion can maintain the correction. Both central incisors or both lateral incisors should be treated at the same time. With increased overbite, there is usually a need for a biteplane to open the bite to allow easier and quicker correction of the crossbite. If there is no anterior slide from centric relation with the incisor crossbite, the prognosis of correction decreases markedly, because a skeletal problem is most likely present.

The problem with correction of permanent incisor crossbites using a removable appliance with finger springs and a bite plane, or a fixed lingual arch with a finger spring, is that the maxillary incisors will not be well aligned after correction. Many times placing brackets from primary canine-to-canine, including the incisors, is needed for proper alignment. This malalignment problem that needs bracket positioning is usually not necessary in the mandibular arch because of the contained arch principal and functioning occlusion.

The removal of the primary canine to gain space for the correction of a permanent lateral crossbite in the maxilla should be limited and treatment should be redirected toward expansion of the buccal segments, space opening with a coil spring for the lateral incisor, and alignment of the primary canine–permanent incisor segment with bracketing. This approach makes the retention of the corrected crossbite much easier than the natural distal angulation of the corrected incisor into the area of the primary canines.

8. What is the problem with these crossbites?

Most early crossbites involve the muscles of mastication and are dental crossbites with shifts, or functional crossbites.[2-5]

Posterior crossbites manifest themselves with curve of Wilson problems (adverse axial inclination of the buccal segments). The posterior teeth are inclined too far facial in the maxilla or too far lingual in the mandible. These are classic signs of the need for maxillary orthopedics, which should be treated early. Because the transverse plane matures the earliest, it is important that it be treated prior to the fusion of the midpalatal suture. The correction of transverse discrepancies later with orthodontics and orthognathic surgery is not as successful or predictable as one would like.

The most common abnormal slide from centric relation in children is related to posterior crossbites with lateral slides and then anterior crossbites later.[6] The pseudo Class III malocclusion with shift is an anterior crossbite malocclusion with a marked slide of 2 to 3 mm. The normal slide in any direction horizontally is 1 mm because of natural skeletal asymmetry, and the normal lateral overjet throughout the occlusion should be about 1 to 2 mm. There is also a pseudo Class III malocclusion that is related to the premature loss of a mandibular primary second molar and the shift of the permanent first molar forward from a Class I molar relationship.

The lack of a slide from centric relation with a crossbite is usually a classic sign of a skeletal problem and should be referred to an orthodontist, especially if the crossbite is in conjunction with a crowding problem; a more complicated intervention is probably needed.

9. What happens if the treatment of crossbite malocclusions does not seem to be working?

Tincture of time certainly helps. Crossbite correction is needed in all types of orthodontics and is usually addressed early in the treatment plan.[1,2,6] If one has isolated cases of the problem and it is taking too long to treat, one needs to step back and reevaluate the treatment plan. There could be problems with the mechanics, problems with cooperation, or problems with the diagnosis. If the diagnosis is not correct, the treatment will not be successful. Crossbites should to be corrected in about 6 months.[2] If treatment time is approaching a year, there is a problem.

10. Does one need an orthodontic database for isolated tooth movement?

Clinicians need to know where they are going. If not, they do not know where they have been. Selected radiographs, photographs, and models with proper analysis will be helpful to plan and implement care.

11. What about the vertical plane and isolated tooth movement?

The vertical plane is the last plane of the face and occlusion to mature and truly manifest itself. It is a complex plane to treat. Bite plane therapy to correct deep bites takes a long time and usually is not as successful as one would like. Dental open bite problems are usually related to digit habits.[9,10] These problems are usually not treated until the permanent incisors erupt. Some open bite/posterior crossbite problems can be treated earlier with patient cooperation. Habit reminder appliances that are removable or fixed, depending upon the specific circumstance, with the use of anterior elastics, are possible in 8- to 10-year-old patients who agree to help stop the habit. Because this appliance attempts to stop an adverse event, it is sometimes considered a mild form of punishment. For these appliances to work, one needs to also use positive reinforcement (praise) in the process of stopping the habit. Usually the tongue is compensatory to the open bite and not the primary etiology. An orthodontic appliance that does not have an active component takes longer to treat with less predictable results. The major mistake made with orthodontic appliances in correction of these open bites is that the habit reminder position at the lingual of the maxillary incisors is too close to the incisors and prevents the future lingual movement of those teeth in the correction of the problem. The presence of diastemata (multiple areas of space vs. diastema for one space) improves the prognosis.

Correction of the anterior open bite associated with speech articulation distortion (age 9 years and older) does not mean that the speech problem will self-correct.[10] These speech problems need to have evaluation prior to correction of the anterior open bite.

12. What does the orientation of the face have to do with isolated tooth movement?

In general, isolated tooth movement is associated with orthodontic treatment plans that involve no planned removal of permanent teeth, except perhaps the third molars.[2,11] Orthodontists should treat to the patient's face.[12] However, the face changes during growth and development. The soft tissue profile does not accurately reflect the underlying hard tissue or bony profile.[13]

13. What are the problems associated with the arches that need to be addressed in the early transitional dentition?

There are two common problems that need to be addressed, both related to ectopic eruption of the permanent lateral incisors and/or the permanent first molars.[2]

The more common problem is the lingual eruption of the mandibular permanent incisors with mild natural expansion of the mandibular primary intercanine width. Because there is usually an incisor liability problem in the lower arch of approximately 5 mm (4-mm wide primary incisors vs. 5 or 5.5 mm wide permanent incisors), anterior clinical crowding should be expected in many cases.[14,15] Natural realignment of the permanent incisors can occur with either discing or removal of the primary canines. In these circumstances, a lingual arch from the permanent first molars with an ideal anterior arch form is usually needed.[16] Lingual arches that are bent to follow the maligned incisors will not allow the natural self-correction of the clinical crowding of these teeth. If one mandibular primary canine has exfoliated early, causing a midline shift, removal of the contralateral primary canine (same tooth on the opposite side) with the placement of a lingual arch can allow the lower midline to self-correct.

Ectopic eruption of the permanent first molar is present in 2% to 3% of occlusions. It is much more common in the maxillary arch. The normal path of eruption of this molar is in a distal-facial pattern. However, the molar can deviate to the mesial and lock itself into the distal surface below the contact of the primary second molar. Conservative intervention is best with limited use of a distalizing orthodontic appliance. Separating springs or deimpacting springs should be used initially and then followed with radiopaque elastomeric separators. Appointments to monitor progress are spaced every 3 to 5 weeks. Discing of the distal of the primary second molars should be limited. Removal of the primary second molar and distal movement of the permanent first molar via a fixed or removable orthodontic appliance is difficult because of patient cooperation, stage of permanent tooth eruption, and anchorage considerations. These orthodontic appliances should be used as a last resort.[17]

After correction of the ectopic permanent first molar, the area near the distal of the primary second molar heals satisfactorily. Only if an endo-perio problem manifests with the primary second molar because of an infected (parulis) or symptomatic circumstance should the primary second molar be removed. Reevaluation concerning distalization mechanics is dependent upon a thorough review of the entire dentofacial complex.[17]

The ectopic position of the mandibular permanent first molar is much less common. This tooth attempts to erupt with a mesial-lingual angulation. Observation/separating/discing/removal/appliance therapy should be considered in that order. This type of ectopic eruption is usually a sign of crowding in the arches that might also be seen in the anterior portion of the arch.

14. How do we treat the mesial angulation tipping of the permanent second molar?

The isolated movements of these teeth would be associated with an occlusion that is normal, except for this problem. If the face or the rest of the occlusion needs to be addressed orthodontically, referral to an orthodontist should be considered.[2] Bilateral molar uprighting creates more stress on the anterior anchorage unit. Combined or individualized uprighting should be done depending upon the features of the dentofacial complex.

The method of uprighting a permanent second molar is not the same for both arches. This problem is usually seen in the lower arch with the loss of the permanent first molar. The permanent second molar is an excellent anchorage unit, so the anterior segment needs to be stabilized to prevent a facial-anterior reciprocal movement of the premolars and canines. Even if the permanent second molar is moderately tipped, usually in a lingual-mesial pattern, the need is still present for anterior cross-arch anchorage with a canine-to-canine lingual arch. If the anchorage units move during the uprighting, the case is compromised. The usual result is an anterior-facial movement of the permanent canine that is very difficult to move back into position.

Active molar uprighting usually takes about 6 to 9 months. However, the tooth needs to be stabilized for a few more months prior to abutment preparations. Restorative preparations are better accomplished on stable, not mobile, teeth.

During molar uprighting, one of the collateral movements of the permanent second molar is extrusion.[17] It is common that the teeth need to be adjusted occlusally during the uprighting. No anterior open bite occlusion should occur in the case. Because most of these cases have anterior deep bite problems, the brackets on the canines need to be placed more gingivally.

The maxillary permanent second molar moves into a position different from that of the mandibular second molar after the loss of the permanent first molar. The maxillary molars rotate more around the larger palatal root with the buccal rotated mesially. Therefore, forces that move it posterior and facial are needed. This means the movement is more of a rotational one as compared with the lower arch. The maxillary arch still should have cross-arch anchorage between the permanent canines. If the permanent canines are too severely angulated to the mesial, a first premolar palatal arch should be considered.

Removable orthodontic appliances to create this type of tooth movement are not as efficient as fixed appliances. Uprighted second molars need fixed retention rather than removable retention to maintain the results. Molar uprighting is usually not associated with removable partial dentures. If the patient stops wearing the retainer or the RPD, the teeth will have a tendency to move back to their original positions.

The use of implants has reduced the number of cases that need molar uprighting. However, the periodontal status and the accompanying marginal bone heights should be considered in the treatment plan.

15. Is there any isolated orthodontic tooth movement the clinician should consider with permanent canines?

Usually the answer is no. However, all cases of unerupted, permanent canines by the age of 9 to 10 years should be palpated. If these teeth cannot be palpated on the facial, they should be assumed to be on the lingual or palatal, or in an unfavorable position.[18] This is a much more common problem in the maxillary arch than the mandibular arch. Most of the time there does not seem to be a major crowding problem in the arches with these cases. The removal of the maxillary primary canine on the affected side should be considered as a method of redirecting the pathway of the unerupted palatal permanent canine. Unfavorable eruption patterns can sometimes be improved with this approach. There is no need to remove the primary canine if there is congenital absence of the permanent lateral incisor on the affected side. The permanent canine will erupt into the position of the lateral incisor and the primary canine will be retained distal to the mesially positioned permanent canine. Future corrective orthodontics can address this problem.

16. Is there any one permanent tooth extraction treatment plan for isolated tooth movement?

There are almost no orthodontic treatment plans involving one permanent tooth.[19] Third molar removal adjacent to second molar uprighting is an exception. Extracting a single permanent tooth in the maxillary arch creates problems associated with crossbites caused by maxillary arch collapse. Extracting a single permanent tooth in the mandibular arch creates lateral overjet problems and anterior deep bite problems. This single extraction sequence results in a tooth-size arch-perimeter discrepancy. This is similar to the tooth-size arch-discrepancy with maxillary peg lateral incisors known as the Bolton discrepancy.[20]

17. What are the isolated tooth movements related to spacing in the arches?

The most common problem is associated with the maxillary midline. There is usually generalized spacing in the maxillary anterior segment between 7 and 10 years of age. This is not true in the lower arch because of the contained arch principle. The maxillary incisor liability problem is usually worse than the mandibular incisor liability problem (7 mm vs. 5 mm). However, the upper arch is not contained unless there is an anterior quadrant crossbite, and there is a generalized facial positioning of the permanent incisor crowns with the roots more lingual as compared with the more upright primary incisors.

The discussion of closing the midline diastema is related to the stage of eruption of the permanent incisors. Usually one does not close the diastema before the eruption of the permanent canines. From tissue emergence to occlusion, the process of tooth eruption usually takes 4 to 6 months. After all four permanent maxillary incisors have erupted, one then estimates the spacing. If the midline diastema is 2 mm or less, the space should close upon the eruption of the permanent canines. If it is larger, the chances of it closing by itself without orthodontic intervention are small.

The one thing a clinician should not do to close this space is to place rubber bands, or elastics, around the two incisors. The elastics will migrate apically, cause loss of the alveolar bone, and may even result in inappropriate loss of these teeth.

It is usually more efficient to close this space with a fixed appliance rather than a removable one. The wire needs to be stiff enough to prevent undue tipping of the incisor crowns, yet allow sliding of the teeth together. In the adult, dark triangles can result if the distance from the alveolar bone height to the apical position of the contact is more than 5 mm after space closure.

A decision relative to frenectomy and orthodontic space closure in this area is related to tooth movement and retention. It is easier to close the space initially and then prescribe the surgical procedure to remove the fibrous band. If the PA radiograph demonstrates an inverted V between the alveolar bone of the two centrals (muscular band), there is probably a greater need to do a surgical procedure. The surgical procedure will remove tissue that will assist in keeping the space closed and prevent the diastema from reopening. The decision to perform a surgical procedure should be discussed prior to orthodontic intervention. To recommend surgical intervention after the isolated movement, without prior information given to the patients and/or parents, is not recommended.

18. What if the permanent incisors erupt in a rotated position?

This problem is often related to either a midline supernumerary tooth that prevents the normal eruption of the affected incisors or trauma and displacement of the primary incisor, usually occurring at the time a child falls down at 2 to 3 years of age.[1,2]

The cause of the rotated permanent incisor should be removed first (i.e., the supernumerary tooth or the ankylosed/traumatized primary incisor). After this, an observation period with radiographic follow-up should occur. This usually takes about 4 to 6 months. If the permanent incisor erupts, but is rotated, a fixed orthodontic appliance should be placed with facial and lingual attachments on the rotated tooth. The specific case might need more extensive bracketing and anchorage, depending upon the situation. However, it is easier to treat early and then retain with a removable appliance with a possible second corrective orthodontic phase to establish a good position in the arch.

Corrected tooth rotations create significant relapse problems in orthodontics. Multiple approaches to address this problem are used, including overcorrection, splinting, and/or supracrestal gingival fiberotomy.[21] The relapse problem is related to transseptal fibers. The fibers near the alveolar bone height need to be resected. This procedure is performed around the affected tooth, except the facial fibers on the tooth, which prevents any possible apical migration of the tissue on the facial of these teeth. A fixed orthodontic appliance needs to be in place and remain in place to act as retention for 4 to 6 months after the surgery. A removable appliance does not effectively maintain a corrected rotated tooth.

19. What about "forced eruption" of a tooth that needs further restorative dentistry?

This is usually related to fractures of anterior teeth. The tooth that needs the extrusion can be treated with a more apical positioning of the bracket.[1,10] One must consider this extrusion as a reduction of a proper crown-root ratio, with a shorter length of the root in the alveolar bone. The relapse potential after the extrusion is apical, so a temporary restoration to maintain the extrusion prior to completion of the restoration should be considered. The lowest forces in orthodontic tooth movement are related to intrusion at 10 to 25 gm per tooth, whereas incisor extrusion is higher so that the bone does not come with the tooth.

20. How does anterior trauma to the dentition affect isolated tooth movement?

Most primary teeth are displaced, not fractured.[1,2] This frequently occurs at the toddler stage, around 2 to 3 years of age, with the incidence the same for boys and girls.

When a permanent tooth is traumatized, the crown is usually fractured. If the tooth is avulsed, it needs immediate replacement and splinting. If possible, bracketing in these cases with a flexible wire positioning the avulsed tooth into position is best. This acts as a semi-rigid splint. Stiff wires can lead to possible ankylosis.

If the permanent incisor is intruded, the bracketing and the placement of a flexible wire allows the tooth to reestablish its normal position much better than waiting and attempting to move the tooth at a later time. The use of vacuum material for holding the newly positioned teeth should be considered.

21. Does the skeletal pattern of the patient affect isolated orthodontic tooth movement?

Yes. There is anterior vertical face height (Nasion [N] to Menton [M]) and posterior vertical face height (either Articulare [Ar] or Condylion [Co] to Gonion [Go]). They do not relate well to each other.[22] In fact, they are usually inversely related with one long and the other short, or vice versa.

If the mandibular plane (Go to Me) as it projects posterior toward the back of the head lies outside the skull, or occiput, the case is described as low angle. These cases are strongly oriented toward nonextraction orthodontic treatment plans.[1,2,23] The mandibular plane becomes even lower with age.

If the mandibular plane intersects inside the skull posteriorly, the case is described as high angle. This type of tooth movement should be viewed as possibly more complex because the posterior teeth have a greater likelihood of overerupting with tooth movement.

The normal or average angle case has the mandibular plane tangent to the skull, or the occiput. It is normal for children under 10 years of age to have a higher value here. In addition to age, the relationship is also affected by race and gender.

22. Does the soft tissue profile of the patient affect isolated tooth movement?

Yes. It depends upon the age and the race of the patient. The younger the patient, the more full the lip position as related to the nose-chin line.[24] If the lips are behind the nose-chin line and the child is 10 years of age or younger, the orientation is toward a non-extraction orthodontic treatment plan. Larger noses or chins allow a more forward position of the lips; this is especially true with a larger chin. The smaller nose projection with a wider face and the positioning of the denture base more anterior usually gives African Americans a fuller lip position. Orthodontic tooth movement affects lip position more with strained or thinner lips compared with unstrained or thicker lips.

The nasolabial angle (from tip of nose along its base to the upper lip) is normally at about a 90- to 110-degree angle (between the positions of an acute and obtuse angle).[25] The more obtuse the angle, the more the case limits the retraction of anterior teeth, so avoid extractions in patients with obtuse nasolabial angles.

23. What happens if one does not wish to perform isolated tooth movement in the practice?

Identify the problem and refer the patient. The relationship between the family dentist and the specialist is symbiotic; the referring doctor needs to be kept informed of the treatment of the patient.

REFERENCES

1. Currier GF: Orthodontic exam and diagnosis. In: Riolo ML, Avery JK: *Essentials for orthodontic practice.* EFOP Press, 2003, pp 264-301.
2. Currier GF: Differential diagnosis and treatment planning in dentofacial orthopedics and orthodontics: Early, middle, and later perspectives. Third International Symposium, Selcuk University on Aesthetics and Function in Dentistry. 2000, August-September, 46-62.
3. Andrews L: The six keys to normal occlusion. *Am J Orthod* 1972;62:296-309.
4. Snodell S, Nanda RS, Currier GF: A longitudinal cephalometric study of transverse and vertical craniofacial growth. *Am J Orthod Dentofacial Orthop* 1993;104(5):471-483.
5. Herman RJ, Currier GF: A retrospective study of the incidence of posterior crossbite and associated orthodontic parameters in primary, transitional, and permanent dentitions. *J Dent Res* 2002;81 (Spec Iss A):A-194.
6. Currier GF, Molloy RB: Correction of posterior crossbite in the transitional dentition with the quadhelix appliance. *Biol Mech Tooth Mov* 2000;333-41.
7. Adkins M, Nanda RS, Currier GF: Arch perimeter changes upon rapid palatal expansion. *Am J Orthod Dentofac Orthop* 1990;97(3):194-199.
8. Housley J, Currier GF: Anterior crossbite malocclusion: Incidence and treatment in the transitional dentition. *J Dent Res* 1999;78:197.
9. Bracket R, Currier GF: Anterior openbite malocclusions. *J Pediatr Dent Care* 2004;10(1):23-26.
10. Currier GF: The smile, the vertical, and time. *J Southeast Soc Pediatr Dent* 1999;5(3):36-39.
11. Nowlin R, Currier GF: Criteria for premolar extraction in orthodontics. *J Dent Res* 1999;78:197.
12. Czarnecki T, Nanda RS, Currier GF: Perceptions of a balanced facial profile. *Am J Orthod Dentofacial Orthop* 1993;104(2):180-187.
13. Formby W, Nanda RS, Currier GF: Longitudinal changes in the adult facial profile. *Am J Orthod Dentofacial Orthop* 1994;105(5):464-476.
14. Revels M, Currier GF, Coury C: Anterior linear and archial analysis in bitemark identification. *J Pediatr Dent Care* 2004;10(1):12-14.
15. Stephens S, Currier GF, Nanda RS: Growth of the dental arches: A longitudinal study from 2 to 22 years. *J Pediatr Dent Care* 2004;10(1):19-22.
16. Gianelly A: Leeway space and the resolution of crowding in the mixed dentition. *Semin Orthod* 1995;1:188-194.
17. Osborn WS, Nanda RS, Currier GF: Mandibular arch perimeter changes with lip bumper treatment. *Am J Orthod* 1991;99(6):527-532.
18. Bishara SE: Impacted maxillary canines: A review. *Am J Orthod Dentofacial Orthop* 1992;101:159-271.
19. Hurd A, Currier GF: Space analysis and prediction in the transitional dentition. *J Pediatr Dent Care* 2004;10(1):33-35.
20. Bolton WA: The clinical application of a tooth-size analysis. *Am J Orthod* 1962;48(7):504-529.
21. Edwards JG: A long-term prospective evaluation of the circumferential supracrestal fiberotomy in alleviating orthodontic relapse. *Am J Orthod* 1988;93:380-387.
22. Bulleigh A, Currier GF, Bursac Z: Vertical tooth-lip positions during growth and development from the frontal and lateral positions. *J Dent Res* 2004;83(Spec Iss A).
23. Wyatt W, Currier GF: Incidence and treatment for congenitally absent permanent teeth. *J Pediatr Dent Care* 2004;10(1):27-29.
24. Blanchette ME, Nanda RS, Currier GF, Ghosh J: Longitudinal growth study of soft tissue facial profile of short and long face subjects. *Am J Orthod Dentofacial Orthop* 1996;109(2):116-131.
25. Fitzgerald JP, Nanda RS, Currier GF: An evaluation of the nasolabial angle and the relative inclinations of the nose and upper lip. *Am J Orthod Dentofacial Orthop* 1992;102(4):328-333.

Phase II: Nonsurgical Adolescent and Adult Cases

CHAPTER 16

Steven D. Marshall • Karin A. Southard • Thomas E. Southard

The majority of patients receiving orthodontic treatment are either adolescents or adults, and the conditions they present with can range from single tooth crossbites to severe dentofacial deformities. When a patient first presents for treatment, identification of all structural and functional jaw and dental problems must be made during the clinical and radiographic examination. These problems occur in all three planes of space and may include significant dental spacing or crowding, dental or skeletal deep bites, anterior or posterior dental or skeletal open bites, anterior or posterior dental or skeletal crossbites, anteroposterior skeletal or dental malrelationships, and asymmetries of the dentition or skeleton. In addition, many patients also present with other dental problems such as mutilated dentitions and periodontal disease.

The goal of orthodontic treatment is always to address the patient's chief complaint through the integration of the best research evidence, the clinician's expertise, and the patient's values (evidence-based orthodontics). A problem-oriented treatment approach must be used to provide an optimal level of care contingent upon the patient's desires and resources.

Orthodontic treatment of adolescent and adult patients may include the use of either removable or fixed appliances. Treatment may include jaw orthopedics to restrict anteroposterior maxillary or mandibular growth, orthopedics to enhance maxillary anteroposterior growth or to accelerate mandibular growth, extraction of permanent teeth to eliminate substantial crowding or to camouflage (mask) an underlying skeletal imbalance, maxillary skeletal expansion or maxillary/mandibular dental expansion, orthognathic surgery, and treatment coordinated with other dental disciplines including cosmetic dentistry, prosthodontics, endodontics, and periodontics.

1. What is a "problem-oriented" approach to treatment?

Based upon a systematic clinical and radiographic examination of the patient, the clinician identifies all structural and functional problems of the jaws and dentition. An exhaustive list of these problems is compiled. From this list and the patient's chief concerns, the goals for treatment are established. Treatment options are composed that address the patient's chief complaint and all problems on the list. Problems that cannot be addressed are considered treatment compromises and must be discussed with the patient.

2. For any patient with an orthodontic problem, what conditions necessitate referral to an orthodontist?

A good rule of thumb is this: if an orthodontic problem exists in a single dimension and can be treated in 9 months or less, it is a problem that generally can be treated in general practice. Such problems include patients in need of space maintenance, single tooth crossbite correction, and Class I mild alignment problems. On the other hand, patients with multi-dimensional malocclusion problems, skeletal imbalances, and problems that take greater than 9 months to treat are generally best referred to an orthodontist. Remember, the goal is to provide the patient with the highest level of care, and orthodontic care provided to the patient must be to the level of the specialist even if that care is provided by a generalist.

The diagnosis of an orthodontic patient follows a logical sequence of evaluation of facial symmetry and proportions, relationship of the jaws, dental arch length, and irregularities of tooth development, tooth position, and intra-oral soft tissues. The following diagnostic criteria will aid in determining if a patient presents with a single dimension or multidimensional orthodontic problem.

FACIAL SYMMETRY AND PROPORTIONS AND RELATIONSHIP OF THE JAWS

Facial symmetry is noted in the frontal view, seen by looking directly at the patient. Mild variation in symmetry from right to left is normal. Landmarks where marked asymmetry can be noted are the eyes, cheekbones, gonial angles of the mandible, occlusal plane, and midline of the chin. The path of opening of the mandible is also evaluated. Opening paths that are not straight or smooth may foretell mandibular asymmetry or temporomandibular dysfunction. Closing path is evaluated to detect the presence or absence of a functional shift of the mandible into centric occlusion. Marked asymmetry of facial structures or presence of a functional shift signifies referral to a specialist.

Vertical and anteroposterior facial proportions are judged in both the frontal and profile views. Significant protrusion or retrusion of the maxilla or mandible are indications for referral. Vertical proportionality is judged by assessing lip competence and the amount of maxillary incisor crown exposure in relaxed pose. Lack of lip competence in a relaxed pose and/or excessive maxillary incisor show are indications for referral.

Transverse proportions are judged intraorally by the presence or absence of posterior crossbite and/or midline discrepancies. Posterior crossbite involving more than two contiguous maxillary teeth is generally skeletal in nature and is an indication for referral.

The amount of incisor protrusion is judged cephalometrically and by evaluation of lip posture and lip function. The presence of mentalis muscle strain on lip closure is an indication of lip incompetence from incisor protrusion. Excessive lip incompetence and incisor protrusion are indications for referral.

IRREGULARITIES OF TOOTH DEVELOPMENT

Unusual delay in the eruption of one or more second bicuspids and/or second molars is not an uncommon finding and can lead to significant malocclusion for the patient. These situations should be monitored and referred for evaluation.

Missing permanent teeth with retained primary teeth adds more complications to the patient's orthodontic problem list and a team approach to the appropriate treatment should be sought.

Tooth size problems commonly occur that prevent ideal Class I occlusion to be obtained. Patients with abnormal incisor widths (e.g., small maxillary lateral incisors) should be referred for further evaluation.

Tooth drift or displacement out of the line of the dental arch signifies eruption path problems. Correction of malposition requires an understanding of the impact on arch form. If malposition is the result of crowding, then correction will require expansion of the arch or gaining space by extraction or selected tooth width reduction. Overexpansion of the dental arch is prone to relapse. Therefore, a diagnosis of tooth malposition must be accompanied by an understanding of the limitations of arch expansion treatment. Cases in which arch expansion will lead to an improper transverse occlusal plane or excessive incisor protrusion should be referred for evaluation by a specialist.

Tooth displacement that results in anterior or posterior crossbite or anterior overjet may be a clue to an underlying discrepancy between the bony bases of the dental arches. Further diagnosis requires cephalometric and/or orthodontic study model evaluation of the alveolar bases to discover intermaxillary skeletal discrepancies.

ANALYSIS OF ARCH LENGTH AVAILABLE

Adolescents still in the late mixed dentition should be evaluated for available leeway space. In general, planned future non-extraction treatment can be facilitated considerably with maintenance of the leeway space in the mandible. There are several published analyses that aid in the determination of arch length available in the late mixed dentition.[1,2]

CLASS I MOLAR RELATIONSHIP

3. A Class I adolescent patient in the late mixed dentition presents with mild mandibular anterior crowding. Assuming that the mandibular second premolars are present but unerupted below the primary second molars, how much space can be gained to spontaneously align the mandibular incisors by placing a lower lingual holding arch (LLHA)? What percentage of Class I molar cases, with mandibular incisor crowding, can be corrected by placing an LLHA before the primary second molars are exfoliated? What is the drawback of using an LLHA?

The primary second molars are wider in mesiodistal dimension than their permanent premolar successors. As a result of this size difference, approximately 3.4 to 5 mm of total space can be gained for alignment of the mandibular anterior teeth by placing an LLHA.[3,4] Studies have shown that 76% of patients can be treated without extraction in the mandibular arch if an LLHA is used to save this excess (leeway) space and the clinician is willing to accept no more than 1 mm of arch length expansion.[5,6] The drawback of using a LLHA is that the leeway space cannot be used by the mandibular first molars to shift mesially into a Class I molar relationship if they are in an end-on position with the maxillary first molars. Thus, in Class II molar relationship or "end-to-end" molar relationship, the use of the leeway space to improve crowding is limited by the amount of mesial movement of the mandibular first molars to gain a Class I molar relationship.

4. What is interproximal reduction (also termed "stripping"), and when could it be used in Class I crowded patients?

Interproximal reduction is the removal of interproximal enamel to make space to align teeth. In primitive humans whose diets consisted of coarse hard foods, interproximal enamel was naturally worn with chewing over time. In theory, this is due to significant movement of teeth and abrasion at interproximal contact points as a result of this tooth movement. In contrast, modern humans with softer diets experience significantly less wear of interproximal enamel over the average human life span. In fact, there is far more enamel present on the sides of human teeth than will ever be worn away during a lifetime of chewing. Therefore, some of this enamel can be removed without detriment to the long-term health of the teeth. Interproximal reduction is a treatment option for Class I malocclusions with crowding of 1 to 5 mm.

However, interproximal reduction requires proper instrumentation and careful technique to maintain adequate tooth enamel and interproximal surface contour. For many years stripping was restricted to anterior teeth. Later, air rotor stripping (or ARS) was introduced to remove interproximal enamel from posterior teeth.[7]

5. What factors are considered in the decision to extract permanent teeth for a Class I patient?

For a Class I patient, the primary consideration for extraction of permanent teeth is the amount of crowding in the dental arch. If there is significant crowding in a dental arch, extraction of permanent teeth is generally considered reasonable. However, other factors must also be considered. In particular, the inclination of the incisors as viewed in the sagittal plane on a cephalometric radiograph, an assessment of the lip posture, and the status of the periodontium should be considered.

If the anterior teeth are inclined severely to the labial and the patient's lips are pushed forward as a result, the option of tooth extraction (even in the presence of less crowding) should be considered. Extraction will permit uprighting the anterior teeth and reduction of lip protrusion. Conversely, if the anterior teeth are inclined to the lingual, tipping these teeth to the labial to increase the dental arch length can allow correction of considerable crowding without extraction. In this case, the periodontium of the mandibular anterior teeth must be assessed with regard to thickness of the attached gingival tissue both incisogingivally and faciolingually. Tipping incisors that are invested in thin attached gingival tissue in an anterior direction can result in loss of periodontium.

6. What factors are considered when choosing which teeth to extract?

Once a decision to extract teeth has been made, dental arch symmetry is an important consideration when choosing which teeth to extract. Generally, in Class I malocclusions, dental arch asymmetries are not severe. The treatment goal is to place the permanent canines in a symmetric position bilaterally relative to the skeletal midline of the arch. As such, extraction choices for Class I molar malocclusions involve two paired teeth in each arch (i.e. two upper first premolars and two lower first premolars). However, significant dental arch asymmetries may call for an asymmetric extraction choice in order to reach a symmetric finished result. In making this decision the choice for upper and lower teeth on each side of the arch should be paired to allow maintenance of the Class I relationship during treatment mechanics to close the extraction spaces (e.g., upper and lower right first premolars and upper and lower left second premolars).

7. Does extraction of four second molars instead of four premolars make sense for a crowded Class I patient?

Premolars are typically extracted when significant crowding and/or protrusion exists in the anterior of the arch. Extraction of mandibular first premolars provides approximately 14 mm of space, allowing alignment of the anterior teeth and/or reduction of their labial inclination. Mandibular second molar extraction (i.e., second molar extraction/third molar replacement[8]) results in only 2.7 mm more arch length compared with controls (2.7 mm less late arch crowding after the third molars have erupted).[9] This amount of space gained from extraction is similar in magnitude to that which could be gained by interproximal reduction. Furthermore, success of the second molar extraction approach depends on third molar eruption path and timing, both of which are not as predictable as the amount of arch length to be gained by interproximal reduction for a particular patient.

CLASS II MOLAR RELATIONSHIP

8. What factors should be considered when making a decision to treat a patient with a Class II molar malocclusion or to refer the patient to a specialist?

The most important factor to consider in a patient with a Class II molar malocclusion is the contribution of intermaxillary jaw position to the interarch Class II relationship of the dentition. Imbalance between the forward growth of the maxilla and the mandible warrants referral to a specialist. Patients who have mild to moderate interjaw imbalance can be treated by the general dentist provided the practitioner has a thorough understanding of facial growth and the application and treatment outcomes of appliances that modify facial growth.

9. If a patient presents with a Class II molar malocclusion and a marked difference in anteroposterior interjaw relationship, what are the major choices for treatment? On what diagnostic criteria are the choices based?

Generally there are only three ways to treat marked anteroposterior differences in interjaw relationships:

1. Orthopedically modifying jaw growth
2. Compensating the position of the dentition within the jaws to mask the discrepancy of the jaws
3. Jaw surgery

Orthopedic treatment is an attempt to modify the growth of the jaw(s) by placing forces against a jaw during facial growth. For instance, a headgear applies a force against the maxilla to restrict its forward growth, and a chin cup applies a force against the chin to restrict the forward growth of the mandible.

Placing dental compensations (masking) is an attempt to camouflage the underlying jaw problem without addressing the skeletal problem itself. Various extraction patterns can be used to move the teeth into more acceptable positions (e.g., reduce overjet) and thereby mask the underlying skeletal problem without actually modifying the jaw position. Surgery is generally used to treat moderate to severe jaw size imbalances in patients whose discrepancies are beyond correction that is obtainable with camouflage or growth modification, or in patients who have completed growth. The decision to use any of these three approaches is based upon many factors, the most important of which are the severity of the jaw imbalance, the severity of the Class II interarch relationship, the growth status of the patient, and the patient's goals.

10. Considering the orthopedic approach to treating Class II malocclusions caused by small mandibles, do functional appliances (Bionators, Activators, Frankels, Herbst, Twin Block, etc.) grow mandibles beyond their inherent length?

There is no evidence that functional appliances increase mandibular growth beyond that normally achieved by the patient in the long term. This conclusion was reached by the American Association of Orthodontists Council on Scientific Affairs after conducting a systematic review of the orthodontic literature.[10] In the short term, functional appliances do accelerate growth of the mandible. Years ago, this acceleration of growth was misinterpreted as true growth enhancement. However, later studies showed that, following this initial growth acceleration, mandibular growth of control subjects eventually caught up to that of patients treated with functional appliances. In other words, long-term functional appliances do not significantly increase mandibular length.

11. If functional appliances do not cause mandibles to grow more than they would normally grow, then how do they work? In other words, how do functional appliances correct a Class II molar relationship?

Functional appliances are effective in moving teeth (dentoalveolar effect).[11-13] With the use of mandibular propulsive functional appliances such as an Activator, Bionator, Twin Block, or Herbst appliance, the mandible is postured forward, the condylar head is distracted out of the glenoid fossa, and the musculature and other soft tissues are stretched. As the stretched soft tissues try to pull the mandible back, the effect of the functional appliance is to increase the labial inclination of the mandibular incisors, reduce the labial inclination of the maxillary incisors, and move the posterior teeth in the alveolar process bone toward an interarch Class I relationship. The increased labial inclination of the mandibular incisors can be of concern, especially if a patient's mandibular incisors are labially inclined before initiation of functional appliance treatment. In addition, there is some restrictive effect on the forward growth of the maxilla with the use of mandibular propulsive functional appliances.

12. What is the effect of a headgear in correcting a Class II molar relationship?

A high-pull headgear—that is, a headgear with the force vector directed toward the top and back of the head—has the effect of restricting downward and forward growth of the maxilla while the mandible grows forward. Also, the maxillary molars are retracted distally and their eruption is slowed. Both effects will improve an interarch Class II molar relationship toward a Class I molar relationship. A cervical-pull headgear, with the force vector directed from the molar teeth down and back toward the cervical vertebrae, also restricts the forward growth of the maxilla and retracts the maxillary molars distally, which will improve the interarch molar relationship from Class II to Class I.[14-16]

13. Does growth modification for a Class II patient with mandibular propulsive appliances result in a different profile change compared with growth modification with a headgear appliance?

Earlier claims that the profile improvement with mandibular propulsive appliances occurs by greater forward movement of the chin in profile have not been substantiated. Profile outcomes that occur when treating an interjaw discrepancy with growth modification appear to be similar whether mandibular propulsive or headgear type appliances are used.[17]

14. How are orthodontic elastics used in treating Class II molar malocclusion?

With Class II elastics, usually worn from the maxillary canines to the mandibular molars, the maxillary teeth tend to be moved posteriorly while the mandibular teeth tend to move anteriorly. The effect is to change a Class II canine and molar relationship toward a Class I relationship. In addition, Class II elastics tend to tip the patient's occlusal plane in the sagittal view, such that the posterior aspect tips superiorly and the anterior aspect tips inferiorly.

15. What are molar distalizing "non-compliance" appliances? How are they used in Class II molar malocclusions?

A problem with using headgears, elastics, and removable functional appliances is the need for patient cooperation. The patient must be motivated to wear these appliances. In an attempt to eliminate the need for patient cooperation, a variety of non-compliance appliances were developed for correction of Class II malocclusions. For the most part, these appliances consist of an acrylic button overlaid on the anterior palate and connected with a rigid wire to the maxillary second premolars. The acrylic button and premolars act as the anchorage unit and offer resistance to springs driving the first molars distally.

These appliances (Pendulum, Distal Jet, etc.) do distalize maxillary molars. However, for every action, an equal, but opposite, reaction occurs. With the use of these appliances, as the molars are forced distally, the premolars (and anterior teeth) are driven mesially.[18-20] Study after study has pointed to the same problem with these appliances. After the molars are distalized to a Class I relationship, they must be held there while the premolars and anterior teeth (which have been pushed anteriorly) must be gathered and brought back. To accomplish this, headgears or elastics must again be worn—defeating the original purpose of using a "non-compliance" appliance.

16. An adult Class II patient (Class II molars and canines) presents with a convex profile, excessive overjet, and a moderately retrusive lower jaw. The patient lacks profile concerns and does not wish to consider orthognathic surgery to move the mandible forward and correct the Class II dental relationship. What extraction patterns might be considered to obtain Class I canines, proper overbite and overjet, and a stable interdigitation of the posterior teeth, as well as to mask the underlying skeletal discrepancy?

The goal will be to provide space to move the maxillary canines from a Class II relationship to a Class I relationship and to eliminate the patient's overjet. Extraction of the maxillary permanent first premolars would permit this. In this approach, the anchorage provided by the roots of the permanent maxillary second premolars and molars will be reciprocally pitted against the anchorage provided by the canines and incisors during space closure, allowing distal movement of the canines into Class I interarch relationship and improvement of incisor overjet.

An alternative approach is the extraction of the maxillary second premolars. This extraction pattern would be indicated for a relatively mild Class II malocclusion. With extraction of maxillary second premolars, the anchorage provided by the roots of the maxillary permanent molars is pitted against the anchorage provided by the roots of the first premolars, canines, and incisors during space closure. Less distal movement of the maxillary canines and incisors will result. This is often desirable when maximum incisor retraction is not required.

17. What other extraction patterns could be considered in treating an adult Class II patient?

If a non-growing adolescent or adult patient presents with a Class II molar malocclusion and significant lower incisor crowding or labial inclination, other extraction patterns can be considered. If, in addition to extraction of the maxillary first premolars, the mandibular first premolars are also extracted to provide room to retract the mandibular canines and align the mandibular incisors, correction of the Class II canine relationship becomes difficult. In a Class II malocclusion, the maxillary canines are already anterior to the mandibular canines in their interarch relationship. Retracting the mandibular canines will necessitate retracting the maxillary canines even farther distally to gain Class I occlusion. In some instances this will not be possible, and at the end of treatment the patient will still have Class II canines and excess overjet.

One alternative approach is to remove two maxillary premolars and one mandibular incisor. This allows retraction of maxillary canines while holding mandibular canines essentially in their pretreatment position in the lower dental arch. The mandibular crowding and/or labial inclination are improved by the 5 to 6 mm of space gained by the mandibular incisor extraction.[21] This approach reaches the treatment goal of improved (Class I) canine function and leaves the patient with incisor overjet that is improved from the pretreatment condition but is not ideal.

Another possible extraction pattern for this type of malocclusion includes maxillary first premolars and mandibular second premolars. This pattern is often considered in patients with a "full step" Class II molar relationship—that is, a molar relationship in which the maxillary molar mesiobuccal cusp is seated, interproximally, between the mandibular second premolar and first molar. Whereas the goal with extraction solely of maxillary first premolars is to obtain Class I canines and Class II molars, the goal with extraction of maxillary first premolars and mandibular second premolars is to obtain Class I canines and Class I molars. If mandibular second premolars are extracted, space closure in the mandible generally results in retraction of the mandibular canines to the point where the patient may finish treatment with Class II canines and excess overjet. However, end-on Class II molar relationship may be effectively treated with extraction of mandibular second premolars,

CLASS III MOLAR RELATIONSHIP

18. What are the effects of wearing a high-pull chin-cup in a growing Class III patient?

A high-pull chin-cup applies a backward and upward force against the chin. This vector of force is useful in growing Class III patients with excessive mandibular growth. The anteroposterior effects include a restriction of forward mandibular growth while simultaneously allowing the maxilla to continue its forward growth. The result is improvement in the abnormal Class III molar and canine relationship. Vertically, the anterior face height is decreased with treatment.[22,23]

19. What are the effects of wearing a reverse-pull face mask in a growing Class III patient?

A reverse-pull face mask applies a forward and downward force to the front of the maxilla. This vector of force is useful in growing Class III patients with deficient maxillary forward growth. The skeletal effects of the reverse-pull face mask include forward maxillary movement plus downward and backward rotation of the mandible. The result is improvement in the abnormal Class III molar and canine relationship. The dental effects include maxillary incisor labial inclination and mandibular incisor lingual inclination. The result is improvement (creation) of overjet.[24-26] Timing (age of treatment) can markedly affect the outcome and amount of dental correction, with late correction producing more dental effects (less skeletal change with more incisor labial inclination) and early treatment producing a greater skeletal effect (more skeletal change with less incisor labial inclination). Maintenance of the correction may require a growth modification appliance (chin-cup) until growth is complete.

20. How are orthodontic elastics used in treating Class III molar malocclusion?

With Class III elastics, usually worn from the mandibular canines to the maxillary molars, the mandibular teeth tend to move posteriorly while the maxillary teeth tend to move anteriorly. The effect is to change a Class III canine and molar relationship toward a Class I relationship. In addition, Class III elastics tend to tip the patient's occlusal plane, in the sagittal view, such that the posterior aspect tips inferiorly and the anterior aspect tips superiorly.

21. An adult Class III patient (Class III molars and canines) presents with an underbite and a moderately strong lower jaw. The patient lacks profile concerns and does not wish to consider orthognathic surgery to correct the Class III interarch relationship. What extraction patterns might be considered to obtain Class I canines, proper overbite and overjet, and a stable intercuspation of the posterior teeth, as well as to mask the underlying skeletal discrepancy?

In this case, the goal will be to provide space to move the mandibular canines back (distally) from a Class III relationship into a Class I relationship and to retract the lower incisors back into a normal overjet relationship. Extraction of the permanent first premolars would permit this—the anchorage provided by the roots of the permanent second premolars and molars will be reciprocally pitted against the anchorage provided by the canines and incisors during space closure. This will generally result in the mandibular canines and incisors moving distally more than the mandibular posterior teeth move mesially, and the goals would be achieved. However, care must be taken not to move the mandibular canine teeth too far distally into a Class II relationship with the maxillary canines. For this reason, extraction of the second premolars should be considered as an option and may offer a better alternative for a relatively mild Class III patient. With extraction of mandibular second premolars, the anchorage provided by the roots of the permanent molars is pitted against the anchorage provided by the roots of the first premolars, canines, and incisors during space closure. Less distal movement of the mandibular canines and incisors will result.[27] In the case of a relatively severe Class III patient who may not have profile concerns, camouflage treatment with extraction may not be possible because of the limits of lower incisor retraction in the region of the mandibular symphysis.

22. What other extraction patterns could be considered in treating an adult Class III patient?

With extraction of only mandibular premolars, the canines can be corrected to a Class I relationship. However, the molars will still remain Class III. Another extraction pattern option is to extract the maxillary second premolars in addition to the two mandibular premolars. With this option, the canines can be corrected to a Class I relationship, and the maxillary molars may be moved mesially into a Class I molar relationship. The risk of extracting premolars in the maxillary arch is that, during space closure, the maxillary canines can be retracted distally, making correction of the Class III canine relationship even more difficult.

OPEN BITES AND CROSSBITES

23. What is the difference between dental and skeletal anterior open bites? What is the difference in how they are treated?

An anterior open bite exists when a gap is present between the anterior teeth while in occlusion. A dental (functional) anterior open bite exists when there is an anterior open bite while in occlusion but the vertical proportions of the face and jaws, the skeletal proportions, are normal. The cause of a dental anterior open bite is usually of functional origin, either continued thumb-sucking or habitual posturing of the tongue in the open bite space. The cause is not tongue-thrusting during swallowing because we do not swallow for long enough periods each day to cause tooth movement.[28] A psychological approach should first be attempted in treating an adolescent with a thumb habit. If ineffective, a tongue crib may be fabricated and inserted across the palate to interfere with the habit. An effective means of retraining the tongue in cases of tongue posturing is the use of tongue spurs attached to the anterior of an LLHA. If the tongue or thumb habit can be corrected, the anterior teeth will usually commence erupting until the open bite closes.

When the maxilla grows downward more than the mandibular ramus lengthens, the mandible will be rotated downward and backward. The result will be a skeletal anterior open bite where only the molars are in contact and the lips must be stretched to close. Treatment of a developing skeletal anterior open bite will consist of trying to either decrease the vertical descent of the maxilla or decrease eruption of the molars. High pull headgears, vertical pull headgears, biteplates, biteplates with repelling magnets in the posterior, exercises (chewing gum), and even LLHAs can all help reduce or correct a developing skeletal open bite. In adults, surgery (maxillary impaction osteotomy) may be necessary to close a skeletal open bite, although recent case reports have found that intrusion of the posterior teeth using skeletal anchorage screws may be effective.[29]

24. What is the difference between a posterior dental and skeletal crossbite? What is the difference in how they are treated?

A posterior dental crossbite exists when the maxilla and mandible relate properly to each other but the teeth in the opposing arches are tipped buccally or lingually into a crossbite. Usually, if one or two posterior teeth are in crossbite, it is a dental crossbite, but not always. A better way to diagnose a dental crossbite is to ask the question, "If any occlusal shifts are removed, and if the posterior teeth are uprighted, what will happen to the crossbite?" If the answer is that the crossbite is greatly improved or eliminated, then the crossbite was a dental crossbite. Treatment of a dental crossbite follows the logic of the diagnosis. Posterior teeth are simply uprighted. Correction of a dental crossbite may necessitate the patient wearing a biteplate in order to provide interarch space for banding or bonding and to permit opposing molar cusps to cross during correction. Depending on the degree of supraeruption of the molars in crossbite, occlusal adjustment may also be necessary if the bite is opened significantly during treatment.

A posterior skeletal crossbite exists when the maxilla and mandible do not relate properly in the transverse dimension. In this instance, the posterior teeth may be tipped buccally or lingually in the body's attempt to compensate for the underlying transverse skeletal discrepancy. However, if any occlusal shifts are removed, and if the posterior teeth are uprighted, the crossbite will worsen in the case of a skeletal crossbite. Skeletal crossbites should be treated by addressing the underlying transverse skeletal problem. Most frequently, the skeletal problem is a narrow maxilla, and the treatment involves increasing the basilar maxillary width by lateral expansion. A Hyrax jackscrew appliance is the most common technique for lateral expansion of the midpalatal suture. The younger the adolescent, the greater the chance for successful maxillary expansion. In older children and in adults, maxillary skeletal expansion may not be possible without surgical assistance to reduce the bony resistance to expansion.[30]

SPECIAL CONSIDERATIONS

25. What are some indications for extraction of a single mandibular permanent incisor?

Case types for extraction of a single mandibular incisor[21] include:

- Class I with moderate to severe lower anterior crowding without deep bite
- Class III tendency with good buccal occlusion, lower incisor crowding without deep bite
- Class I with anterior tooth size discrepancy (mandibular anterior excess)
- Class II with mandibular anterior crowding and two maxillary teeth extracted
- Class I with one mandibular incisor extracted (treat nonextraction); may need to perform interproximal reduction on maxillary teeth
- Class I with one mandibular incisor missing with moderate/severe mandibular anterior crowding (treat with one additional lower incisor extraction and two maxillary extractions)

26. How can a patient with missing maxillary lateral incisors be treated?

There are two options. The first would be to open spaces for prosthetic replacement of the maxillary lateral incisors. The second is to close spaces while protracting the posterior teeth and substitute the maxillary canines for laterals and the maxillary first premolars for canines.

The ideal situation for prosthetic replacement of the laterals exists when the patient is Class I in both the molars and canines and when there is ideal occlusal intercuspation, ideal overbite, and ideal overjet. In this ideal case, orthodontics is not even needed. If everything is ideal but the maxillary canines have erupted into the lateral spaces, the maxillary canines need to be retracted distally into a Class I position as the spaces are opened. The lateral incisors can then be restored as pontics in a fixed partial denture, a removable partial denture, or as implants.

The ideal situation for substitution of the maxillary canines as lateral incisors exists when the patient is a full-step Class II at the molars and premolars; there is ideal occlusal intercuspation, overbite, and overjet; both canines have erupted into the missing lateral incisor position; and where both canines look like lateral incisors. In this ideal case, orthodontics is not even needed. If a Class II molar interarch relationship exists but is less than a full-step Class II, the maxillary posterior teeth will usually need to be brought forward into a Class II molar relationship. This may be accomplished with Class III elastics, a reverse-pull headgear, or use of skeletal orthodontic anchorage. Also, if the canines do not resemble lateral incisors, cosmetic dentistry may be required to make them look like laterals.

27. When should teeth be extruded? What is meant by "extrusion to extraction"?

Teeth are extruded for a variety of reasons. For example, in the case of trauma to a maxillary central incisor, the tooth may be fractured below the level of the alveolar crest. Although a crown extension surgical procedure may be performed to provide an adequate biologic width for restoration, the result may be unacceptable esthetically if the patient has a high smile line and the crown extension results in a more apical gingival margin on the fractured central incisor. Crown lengthening can be done using orthodontic extrusion in combination with a supracrestal fiberotomy to extrude the root fragment. Additional gingival and/or osseous surgical procedures may be needed after extrusion. If it is desirable to bring down gingival or osseous tissues, the tooth can be extruded initially without the supracrestal fiberotomy. Later, the fiberotomy procedure can be done to aid in stabilizing the extrusion. In addition, postextrusion surgery may be needed to fine-tune gingival heights and contours.

Another reason is to extrude teeth prior to implant placement. This procedure is termed *extrusion to extraction.* In this instance a tooth may have been deemed hopeless because of periodontic or endodontic status of the tooth. If the tooth is simply extracted, the alveolar process will collapse, making implant placement difficult even with bone grafting. By orthodontically extruding the tooth first, before extraction, both bone and soft tissue are developed in the future implant site with a result of improved prosthetic bone and soft tissue contours for the prosthesis.[31,32]

28. What is skeletal anchorage, and how is it used in orthodontics?

Again, for every action, an equal, but opposite, reaction exists. Newton's third law poses a problem in orthodontics, where frequently the desired movement of one tooth is pitted against the undesired movement of other teeth. These latter teeth are termed the *anchor teeth*. For instance, in a Class II patient, it may be desirable to move the maxillary canines distally following extraction of the maxillary first premolars. However, if a force (e.g., an elastic) is applied from the canine back to the molars, then not only will the canine be moved distally (desirable movement), but also the molars will tend to move mesially (undesirable movement, or *anchorage loss*). To overcome anchorage loss, headgears (or in some cases elastics) have traditionally been incorporated to restrain this mesial molar movement. However, these appliances require significant patient cooperation.

In 1945, the first attempt to eliminate this need for patient compliance, through the use of skeletal orthodontic anchorage, was made at The University of Iowa.[33] Skeletal anchorage consists of attaching surgical mini-screws or implants directly to the mandible, maxilla, or zygomatic arch. With a portion of the plate protruding through the mucosa, it is used as an attachment and for anchorage. As opposed to using teeth as anchorage, these auxiliaries undergo very little reciprocal movement. With temporary anchorage devices acting as skeletal anchorage, teeth may be translated, rotated, extruded, and intruded without undesirable reciprocal effects.[34-37]

29. In adult patients, orthodontic treatment frequently involves the family dentist, the orthodontist, and other dental specialists. What is the normal sequence of treatment in adults, and what is the most important aspect of treatment?

The key to adult multidisciplinary treatment is communication. The family dentist (restorative dentist) is the end-point of the patient's care and all treatment should be directed toward helping that doctor achieve an excellent result. The family dentist is at the center of the treatment hub, and all communications regarding the patient should be coordinated with that doctor.

The dentist, orthodontist, and other dental specialists should work as a team to first diagnose and create a treatment plan for the patient. A diagnostic "wax-up" of the final occlusion should be fabricated to establish the treatment goal. The restorative dentist must answer the question, "Where do I need the patient's teeth in order to restore them?" The orthodontist must answer the question, "Can I, through dental tooth movement or orthognathic surgery, move the teeth into the requested position?"

Disease control should be instituted. The level of caries activity should be assessed and active caries removed. Teeth requiring extensive restorative treatment, such as crowns, should generally receive provisional restorations until orthodontic movement is complete. Active periodontal disease should be assessed and treated. Although periodontal surgery to help control disease can be desirable, bone removal should usually be minimized until orthodontic tooth movement is complete. Hopeless teeth should be extracted unless "extruding to extract" in an effort to save alveolar bone. Teeth requiring endodontic treatment should be treated, if they are to be retained.

During orthodontic treatment the patient's level of hygiene should be closely monitored and treated. The patient should receive regular dental check-ups and cleanings from the family dentist, and the orthodontist should provide regular progress updates, especially as the time for removal of braces nears. Once the restorative dentist and orthodontist have determined that the teeth are in the desired position, the braces are removed. Retention must be immediately instituted to maintain the teeth in the corrected position.

REFERENCES

1. Moyers RE: *Handbook of orthodontics*, edition 3. Chicago: Year Book Medical Publishers; 1974, pp 369-379.
2. Staley RN, Kerber RE: A revision of the Hixon and Oldfather mixed-dentition prediction method. *Am J Orthod* 1980;78:296-302.
3. Nance H: The limitations of orthodontic treatment. I. Mixed dentition diagnosis and treatment. *Am J Orthod Oral Surg* 1947;33:177-223.
4. Brennan M, Gianelly A: The use of the lingual arch in the mixed dentition to resolve incisor crowding. *Am J Orthod Dentofacial Orthop* 2000;117:81-85.
5. Gianelly A: Leeway space and the resolution of crowding in the mixed dentition. *Semin Orthod* 1995;1:188-194.
6. Moyers RE, van der Linden FPGM, Riolo ML, et al: Standards of Human Occlusal Development, Monograph No. 5, Craniofacial Growth Series, Ann Arbor, MI: Center for Human Growth and Development, the University of Michigan, 1976.
7. Sheridan JJ: Air rotor stripping update. *J Clin Orthod* 1987;21(11):781-788.
8. Witzig J: *The clinical management of basic maxillofacial orthopedic appliances, volume 1. Mechanics*. Chicago: Year Book Medical Publishers, 1987, p 213.
9. Richardson M, Mills K: Late lower arch crowding: the effect of second molar extraction. *Am J Orthod Dentofacial Orthop* 1990;98:242-246.
10. Huang G, English J, Ferguson D, et al: Ask Us—Functional appliances and long-term effects on mandibular growth. *Am J Orthod Dentofacial Orthop* 2005;127:271-272.
11. Aelbers C, Dermaut L: Orthopedics in orthodontics. I. fiction or reality—a review of the literature. *Am J Orthod Dentofacial Orthop* 1996;110:513-519.
12. Dermaut L, Aelbers C: Orthopedics in orthodontics: fiction or reality. A review of the literature—Part II. *Am J Orthod Dentofacial Orthop* 1996;110:667-671.
13. Pancherz H: The Herbst appliance: a powerful Class II corrector. In Nanda R, editor. *Biomechanics in clinical orthodontics*. Philadelphia: WB Saunders, 1997.
14. Firouz M, Zernik J, Nanda R: Dental and orthopedic effects of high-pull headgear in treatment of Class II, Division 1 malocclusion. *Am J Orthod Dentofacial Orthop* 1992;102:197-205.
15. Baumrind S, Korn D, Isaacson RJ, et al: Quantitative analysis of the orthodontic and orthopedic effects of maxillary traction. *Am J Orthod* 1983;83:384-398.
16. Kirjavainen M, Kirjavainen T, Hurmerinta K, Haavikko K: Orthopedic cervical headgear with an expanded inner bow in Class II correction. *Angle Orthod* 2000;70:317-325.

17. Sloss E, Southard K, Qian F, et al: A comparison of soft tissue profiles following treatment with headgear or Herbst appliances. *Am J Orthod Dentofacial Orthop* (in press).
18. Ghosh J, Nanda R: Evaluation of an intraoral maxillary molar distalization technique. *Am J Orthod Dentofacial Orthop* 1996;110:639-646.
19. Chaqués-Asensi J, Kalra V: Effects of the pendulum appliance on the dentofacial complex. *J Clin Orthod* 2001;35(4):254-257.
20. Ngantung V, Nanda R, Bowman S: Post treatment evaluation of the distal jet appliance. *Am J Orthod Dentofacial Orthop* 2001;120:178-185.
21. Kokich V, Shapiro P: Lower incisor extraction in orthodontic treatment. *Angle Orthod* 1984;59(2):139-153.
22. Deguchi T, Kuroda T, Minoshima Y, Graber TM: Craniofacial features of patients with Class III abnormalities: growth-related changes and effects of short-term and long-term chin cup therapy. *Am J Orthod Dentofacial Orthop* 2002;121:84-92.
23. Wendell PD, Nanda R, Sakamoto T, Nakamura S: The effects of chin cup therapy on the mandible: a longitudinal study. *Am J Orthod* 1985;87:265.
24. Ngan P: Biomechanics of maxillary expansion and protraction in Class III patients. *Am J Orthod Dentofacial Orthop* 2002;121: 582-583.
25. Ngan P, Hagg Yiu C, Wei S: Treatment response and long-term dentofacial adaptations to maxillary expansion and protraction. *Semin Orthod* 1997;3:255-264.
26. MacDonald K, Kapust A, Turley P: Cephalometric changes after the correction of Class III malocclusion with maxillary expansion/facemask therapy. *Am J Orthod Dentofacial Orthop* 1999;116:13-24.
27. Kim T, Kim J, Mah J, et al: First or second premolar extraction effects on facial vertical dimension. *Angle Orthod* 2005;75: 177-182.
28. Proffit W, Mason R: Myofunctional therapy for tongue-thrusting: background and recommendations. *J Am Dent Assoc* 1975;90:403-411.
29. Kuroda S, Katayama A, Takano-Yamamoto T: Severe anterior open-bite case treated using titanium screw anchorage. *Angle Orthod* 2004;74:558-567.
30. Marshall S, Southard K, Southard T: Early transverse correction. *Semin Orthod* 2005;11(3):130-139.
31. Mantzikos T, Shamus I: Forced eruption and implant site development: soft tissue response. *Am J Orthod Dentofacial Orthop* 1997;112(6):596-606.
32. Mantzikos T, Shamus I: Case report: forced eruption and implant site development. *Angle Orthod* 1998;68(2):179-186.
33. Gainsforth BL, Higley LB: A study of orthodontic anchorage possibilities in basal bone. *Am J Orthod Oral Surg* 1945;31: 106-117.
34. Roberts WE, Nelson CL, Goodacre CJ: Rigid implant anchorage to close a mandibular first molar extraction site. *J Clin Orthod* 1994;28:693-704.
35. Southard T, Buckley M, Spivey J, et al: Intrusion anchorage potential of teeth versus rigid endosseous implants: a clinical and radiographic evaluation. *Am J Orthod Dentofacial Orthop* 1995;107:115-120.
36. Liou E, Pai B, Lin J: Do mini-screws remain stationary under orthodontic forces? *Am J Orthod Dentofacial Orthop* 2004;126:42-47.
37. Miyawaki S, Koyama I, Inoie M, et al: Factors associated with the stability of titanium screws placed in the posterior region for orthodontic anchorage. *Am J Orthod Dentofacial Orthop* 2003;124:373-378.

CHAPTER

17 Adult Interdisciplinary Orthodontic Treatment

Valmy Pangrazio-Kulbersh

Increased awareness of the importance and benefits of a healthy dentition and a pleasant smile are motivating adults to seek orthodontic treatment more so now than in the past. Presently, the amount of orthodontic treatment rendered to adults comprises 30% of the orthodontic practice. The desire for a better smile is not only being patient generated, but general dentists are also becoming more knowledgeable about the possibilities of adult tooth movement to facilitate the establishment of function and health to the different components of the stomatognathic system.

Interdisciplinary treatment is calling for more orthodontic interaction with the other specialties to obtain more optimum results in the restoration of often broken-down adult dentitions. The advent of new technology, such as esthetic brackets, invisible braces, new orthodontic wire alloys, and better brackets designed to reduce friction and speed up tooth movement, are also an incentive to attract more adults to seek orthodontic treatment.

1. What are the major differences between adult and adolescent treatment?[1-6]

These differences are as follows:

- Adult orthodontic treatment is usually initiated by the general dentist requesting the establishment of occlusal harmony (Fig. 17-1, *A* and *B*).
- The lack of craniofacial growth offers no advantage or disadvantage to the orthodontic treatment.
- Periodontal disease is present in about 80% to 90% of the adult patients (Fig. 17-1, *C-E*)
- There is a high incidence of missing permanent teeth.
- Increased tooth mobility; this is a consequence of a change in occlusal scheme and loading as a result of the uncontrolled dental shifting caused by the mutilated dentitions and/or periodontal disease.
- The lack of long-term stability resulting from periodontal problems requires a different approach to retention.
- The increased prevalence and incidence of temporomandibular joint (TMJ) disorders requires a careful approach to the change in occlusal scheme.
- The use of segmental orthodontic treatment mechanics and differential forces should be considered when the crown-to-root ratio is unfavorable.
- Most adults are concerned with esthetics and the appearance of braces. The use of less conspicuous orthodontic appliances like ceramic brackets, lingual orthodontics, and Invisalign should be considered.
- Motivation for treatment in adults comes from the pursuit of esthetic changes or to restore a broken-down dentition or alleviate functional problems (e.g., TMJ dysfunction). The psychological response to treatment varies with the initial motivation. Those patients seeking treatment to improve function are more likely to have a better psychological response than those who are expecting an impact in others by their perceived change in facial appearance.
- Most adults require a multidisciplinary treatment plan to adequately restore esthetics and function.

2. What are the goals of adult orthodontic treatment?[1-3,6,7]

The objectives of adult orthodontic treatment are:

- To achieve improved function, stability, and esthetics
- To eliminate occlusal interferences and trauma to reduce tooth mobility and promote periodontal healing
- To obtain better bone and gingival architecture
- To establish proper tooth position and improve the plane of occlusion for prosthodontic rehabilitation
- To achieve harmony between teeth and TMJ function
- To address the patient's chief complaint, which is usually related to dental and facial esthetics

3. What are the contraindications for adult orthodontic treatment?[8-12]

- The presence of advanced local and/or systemic diseases such as bone, metabolic, or endocrine and renal disorders could adversely affect tooth movement and bone turnover. The use of bisphosphonates, calcitonin, and ibuprofen has a negative effect on the rate of tooth movement.
- The presence of active periodontal disease contraindicates orthodontic tooth movement, since it could accelerate the process of periodontal problems and concomitant tooth loss.
- Patients with significant root resorption and poor crown-to-root ratio may not benefit from orthodontic treatment.

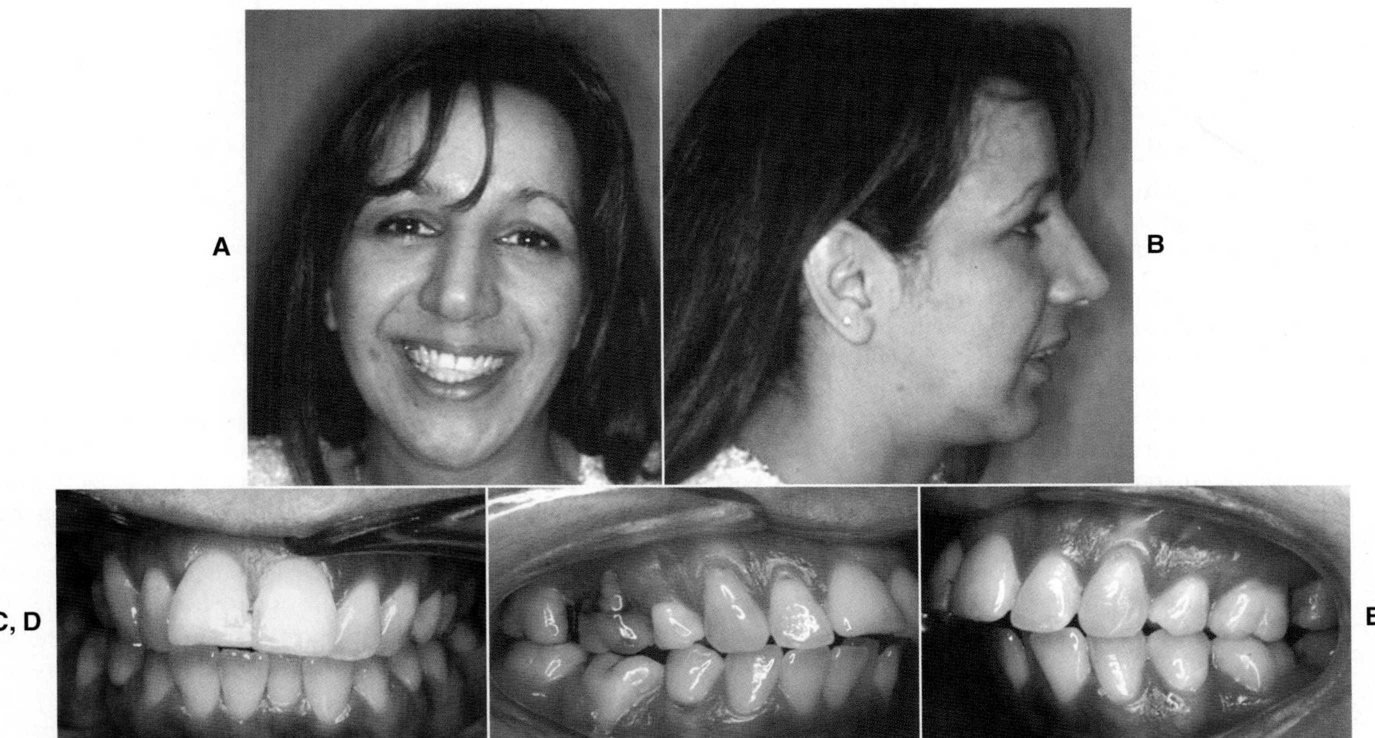

FIG 17-1 Adult patient seeking orthodontic treatment. Note the complexity of the malocclusion. **A** and **B,** Pretreatment facial photos depicting the skeletal imbalance. **C-E,** Intraoral photos show the dental and periodontal problems in this adult patient.

- When patient compliance with long-term retention and follow-up prosthetic rehabilitation is not present, orthodontic treatment should not be initiated.
- Because of the high incidence of osteopenia and osteoporosis in adults over 50 years of age, a bone mass density test could be prescribed to screen for bone disorders that can lead to alveolar bone loss and loss of teeth.

4. What are the effects of orthodontic treatment on the periodontal tissues?[13-17]

- The elimination and control of inflammation before and throughout orthodontic treatment is imperative to ensure the health of the supporting tissues. Clinical studies have demonstrated that teeth with reduced periodontal support, in the absence of inflammation, can undergo tooth movement without compromising the periodontal status.
- Reduction of pocket depth and probing in orthodontically moved teeth in adults as well as maintenance of a minimal band of attached gingiva can be accomplished with orthodontic treatment.
- A free gingival graft is recommended when minimum amount of attached gingiva is present and when the tooth movement is directed toward the thin gingival tissue. When tooth movement is confined to the alveolar support, no harmful effects on the surrounding tissues are to be expected.
- Adults have an increased prevalence of root resorption during orthodontic treatment. The use of light forces is recommended to avoid the formation of hyalinized areas and to expedite tooth movement.

5. What kind of periodontal therapy should be instituted before, during, and after adult orthodontic tooth movement is initiated?[18]

- The elimination of inflammation that rapidly deteriorates the periodontium is essential prior to the initiation of tooth movement. Plaque and inflammation control should continue throughout orthodontic therapy and afterwards.
- Scaling, root planing, open flap surgery, and gingival grafting should be done prior to the commencement of orthodontic treatment.
- Recontouring osseous surgery should be postponed until after orthodontic treatment. The architecture of the bone will change with the tooth movement and possibly less bone recontouring may be necessary after orthodontic treatment.
- Bone grafting procedures to increase alveolar width and height in an edentulous area through which tooth movement is to occur, should be done prior to orthodontic treatment. Bone grafting for implant placement could be done 6 months prior to debanding or postponed until treatment completion.

- Equilibration of occlusal interferences that may arise during treatment should be done at each appointment as necessary to avoid periodontal breakdown and excessive tooth mobility from occlusal trauma.

6. Which orthodontic records are necessary for proper diagnosis and treatment planning of the adult orthodontic patient?[19-21]

Because of the complexity of factors among which the malocclusion is included, a careful evaluation of the patient, including a thorough medical history, chief complaint, and psychological evaluation, is necessary to properly integrate those factors with the ones related to the actual dental treatment. The standard orthodontic record consists of:

- **Facial photographs** (frontal with lips in repose, frontal smiling, profile with lips in repose). This will provide important information about the soft tissue drape of the face, such as lip length and competency, soft tissue chin prominence, nose prominence and slope, amount of gingival display, midline deviations, and overall facial proportionality.
- **Cephalograms** (lateral and frontal).
- **Panoramic x-rays and full mouth periapical surveys** to evaluate for bony, dental, and periodontal pathologies as well as anatomy of the roots.
- **Submental x-ray and TMJ tomograms** may be necessary to diagnose skeletal asymmetries and TMJ pathology.
- **Models mounted in centric relation** will help to detect a CO-CR slide, which is imperative before the commencement of orthodontic treatment. Roth has suggested that even in the absence of obvious signs or symptoms of TMJ dysfunction, adult patients, specifically those with mutilated dentitions, should undergo splint therapy to eliminate muscle splinting and to avoid treatment planning from a false mandibular position.

7. What is the sequence of adult orthodontic treatment?[22]

Once the diagnosis and treatment plan have been established, a treatment sequence should be considered as follows:

1. Emergency relief of pain—this step, in many instances, will precede the gathering of orthodontic records and follow-up diagnosis.
2. Therapy of soft tissue lesions
   - Hygiene instructions
   - Scaling and root planning
   - Correction of inadequate restoration
   - Root resection and endodontic treatment
3. Treatment of the lesions of the attachment
   - Flap surgery and root planning
   - Guided tissue regeneration
   - Autogenous keratinized mucosal or connective tissue grafts
   - Orthodontic therapy
   - Occlusal adjustment
   - Myofunctional therapy
4. Provisional stabilization and retention
5. Reevaluation for further therapy (e.g., extraction of nonrestorable teeth)
6. Completion of periodontal treatment
7. Final occlusal adjustment
8. Restorative prosthetic dentistry
9. Continued periodontal care

8. What are the treatment options for adult patients?[23]

Limited tooth movement and comprehensive orthodontic treatment can be considered when treatment planning an adult orthodontic case. The severity of the malocclusion and treatment goals should be considered when selecting the treatment.

Limited tooth movement is carried out either with removable or partial fixed orthodontic appliances and is aimed at specific treatment goals. In most instances, limited tooth movement is considered as an adjunct to the overall oral rehabilitation of the patient.

Comprehensive orthodontic treatment aims to the correction of malocclusion as a whole and has the potential to modify the complete occlusal scheme as required.

9. What are the specific problems that can benefit from limited tooth movement treatment?[24]

Limited tooth movement is indicated to reposition the dental units in a specific quadrant to facilitate prosthetic replacements of missing teeth and to improve periodontal health and dental esthetics. Molar uprighting to improve parallelism of the abutments, to create appropriate pontic space, or to facilitate implant replacement of missing teeth can be accomplished with limited orthodontic treatment. Forced eruption to facilitate preparation of the root for crown placement or to create bone through the occlusal movement of the tooth for implant placement can also be accomplished with partial orthodontic treatment. Correction of spacing, crowding, rotations, and dental crossbites can be accomplished with either fixed or removable orthodontic appliances.

10. What are the diagnostic considerations when treatment planning for molar uprighting?[25]

A thorough evaluation of the occlusion and skeletal characteristics of the patient is indicated.

Molar uprighting is best accomplished with limited treatment when an acceptable occlusion with anterior guidance and cuspid rise is present and in patients with a normal vertical dimension. Patients with dolichocephalic faces are not good candidates for molar uprighting, which necessitates distalization of the molar crown. This type of tooth movement further increases the vertical dimension with concomitant development of a dental open bite.

11. What are the types of tooth movements that could be considered for molar uprighting?[26-28]

Molar uprighting can be accomplished by:

- Distalization of the crown
- Mesialization of the root
- A combination of both

In many instances, mesial movement of the bicuspids that have drifted distally into the edentulous area may be necessary. When indicated, complete space closure of the edentulous space using temporary anchorage devices should also be considered. When only a single tooth is to be uprighted, the clinician has the option of choosing between removable or fixed orthodontic appliances. A removable appliance with a finger spring mesial to the tooth to be uprighted will tip the tooth distally without vertical or transverse control. Because of this limitation as well as the dependence on patient cooperation, removable appliances are not widely prescribed.

Partial fixed orthodontic appliances are more effective in controlling tooth movement in three planes of space (Fig. 17-2). When uprighting a molar, standard brackets can be used on the anchoring teeth (cuspids and bicuspids) and a double buccal tube placed on the molar to be uprighted. The double buccal tube allows for the placement of an auxiliary uprighting spring when necessary. Periodic occlusal adjustment and root planing of the tooth being uprighted is recommended to avoid trauma from occlusion, excessive tooth mobility, and pain as well as to promote periodontal healing.

Another important treatment consideration is the disposition of the third molar. The presence of an antagonist, the occlusion, and type of tooth movement planned will dictate the fate of the third molar. The demand for anchorage would be part of the appliance design and selection. A lingual cuspid-to-cuspid fixed retainer or temporary anchorage devices (temporary implants) could be used when stabilization of the anchoring teeth is necessary (Fig. 17-3).

12. What is the retention protocol after molar uprighting?[25,26]

The uprighted teeth should be retained until the placement of the prosthetic device. The retention can be accomplished with an intracoronal stabilization bar or a rigid stainless steel wire bonded to the teeth neighboring the edentulous area. The preparation for the bridge or the placement of the implant should be postponed until the reappearance of the lamina dura around the uprighted tooth. This usually takes place 8 to 12 weeks after the tooth has reached its final position.

13. What is forced eruption?[29]

Forced eruption is defined as the orthodontic tooth movement in the coronal direction through the application of continuous forces to create changes in the architecture of the soft tissue and bone. This procedure facilitates the conservative management of non-restorable teeth. Forced eruption helps restore the "biological width," allowing the restoration to be placed away from the epithelial attachment, thus preventing periodontal inflammation and breakdown. To maintain a healthy periodontium, 3 to 4 mm of tooth length is needed occlusal to the alveolar crest.

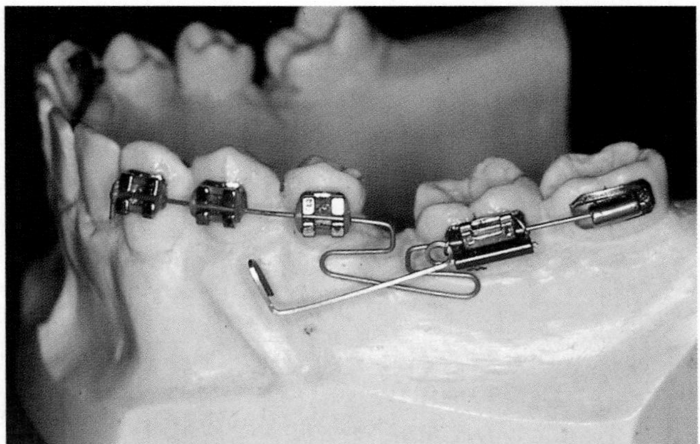

FIG 17-2 Typical appliance assembly for molar uprighting. Note auxiliary spring to aid in the uprighting.

14. How is forced eruption accomplished?[29,30]

Forced eruption can be done slowly to promote bone remodeling in periodontally compromised teeth or to protect the integrity of the pulpal tissues and avoid root damage.

The coronal movement of the tooth elicits bone formation and soft tissue recontouring. This improves the overall esthetics of the final restoration even when crown lengthening with osseous surgery is needed for placement of the crown.

Endodontically treated teeth can be extruded with heavier forces and more rapidly. Bone recontouring does not take place as readily, obviating in some cases the need for osseous surgery, especially when the forced eruption is combined with circumferential sulcus fiberotomy before and weekly during the tooth movement.

The retention period after forced eruption is approximately 2 to 6 weeks to allow for the rearrangement of the principal fibers of the periodontal ligament. The healing of the periodontal tissues dictates the time of placement of the final restoration. The practitioner should be aware that the restoration will have a longer taper from the occlusal to the gingival margin due to the smaller dimension of the root surface being exposed. Careful attention should be given to the contour of the restoration to obtain good esthetics and gingival health (Figs. 17-4 and 17-5).

15. What are the orthodontic considerations for the correction of dental alignment?[31-33]

The correction of crowding, spacing, rotations, crossbites, and tipped teeth is indicated not only for esthetic reasons, but also to facilitate restorative procedures and maintain oral health. Crowding and rotations are the result of tooth size/arch length discrepancies. The creation of spaces in the dental arches to correct these problems can be obtained through flaring of the anterior teeth, transverse expansion of the dental arches, interproximal enamel reduction, or extractions. Approximately

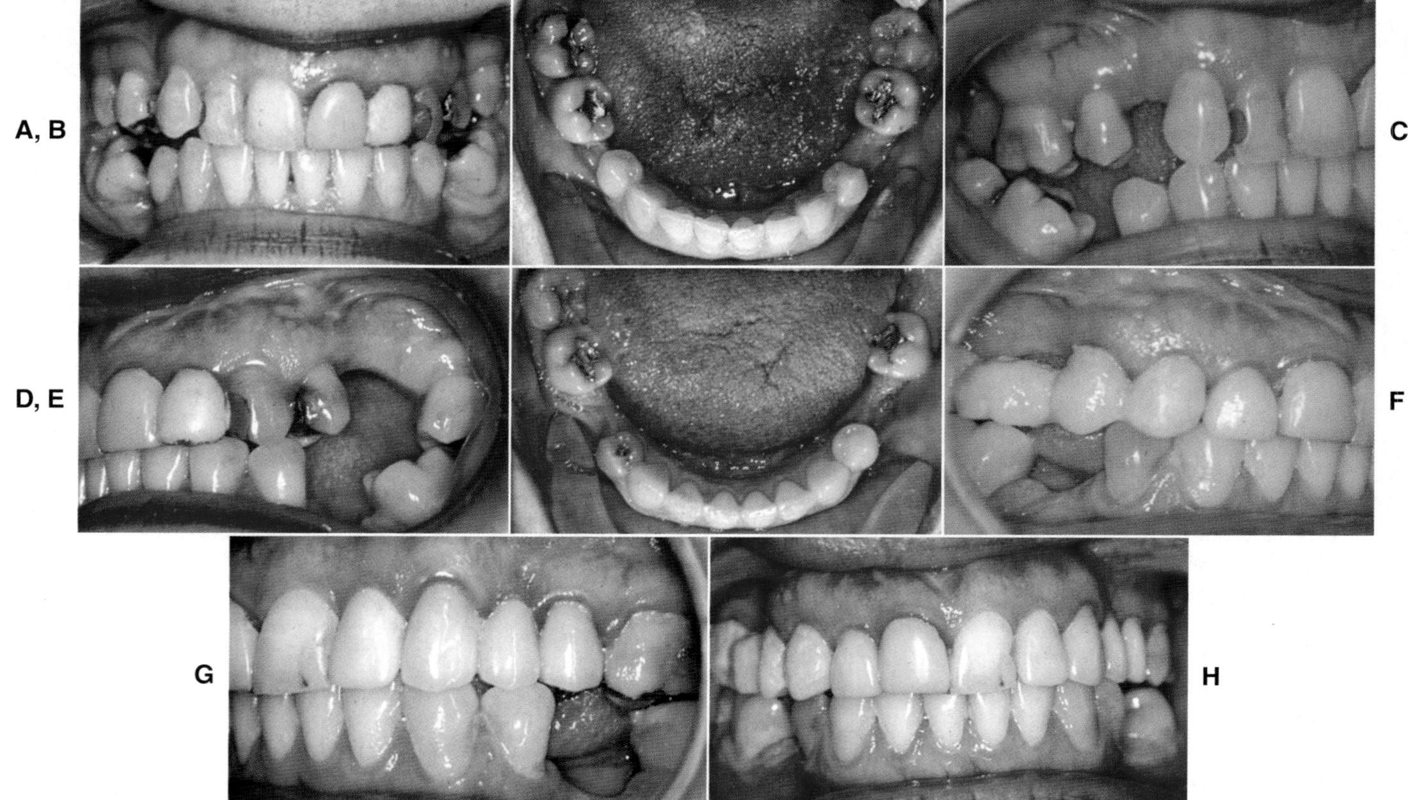

FIG 17-3 Bilateral lower molar uprighting. **A-D,** Pretreatment intraoral photos. **E-H,** Posttreatment intraoral photos. Note the extraction of the lower right third molar to facilitate distal crown movement.

0.5 mm of enamel can be removed from the mesial and distal surfaces of the upper anteriors for a total of 4 to 5 mm. Because of the smaller diameter of the lower anterior teeth, less reduction is possible.

Before embarking in the closure of excessive maxillary or mandibular anterior spacing, a careful evaluation of the etiologic factors should be considered. Arch length/tooth size discrepancies, loss of teeth, presence of CO-CR discrepancies produced by posterior interferences, periodontal disease, abnormal labial frenum or abnormal interseptal bone architecture, presence of supernumerary teeth, and habits like tongue thrust or nail-biting could be involved in the etiology of this malocclusion. The recognition and elimination of the etiologic factors is essential to select the appropriate mechanotherapy.

The correction of crowding, rotations, spacing, crossbites, and tipped teeth, in the presence of an acceptable occlusion, can be accomplished with partial fixed orthodontic treatment or with Invisalign® treatment.

16. When is comprehensive orthodontic treatment indicated for the adult patient?[22,32,34,35]

Adults with mutilated dentitions and/or periodontal disease have a history of dental neglect that has contributed to the malocclusion. Dental and functional compensations that have taken place during a prolonged period usually result in a complex malocclusion. The elimination of the structural and functional malocclusions often requires the use of full orthodontic appliances. The use of osseous integrated implants and temporary anchorage devices is rapidly expanding the scope of orthodontic treatment for adults. Comprehensive orthodontic treatment, designed to change the entire occlusal scheme of the adult patient, can be performed successfully because of innovations in orthodontic appliance design, orthodontic wires made with new alloys that deliver lighter and more continuous forces, and periodontal, prosthetic, and surgical advances that give the adult patient excellent esthetic and functional results.

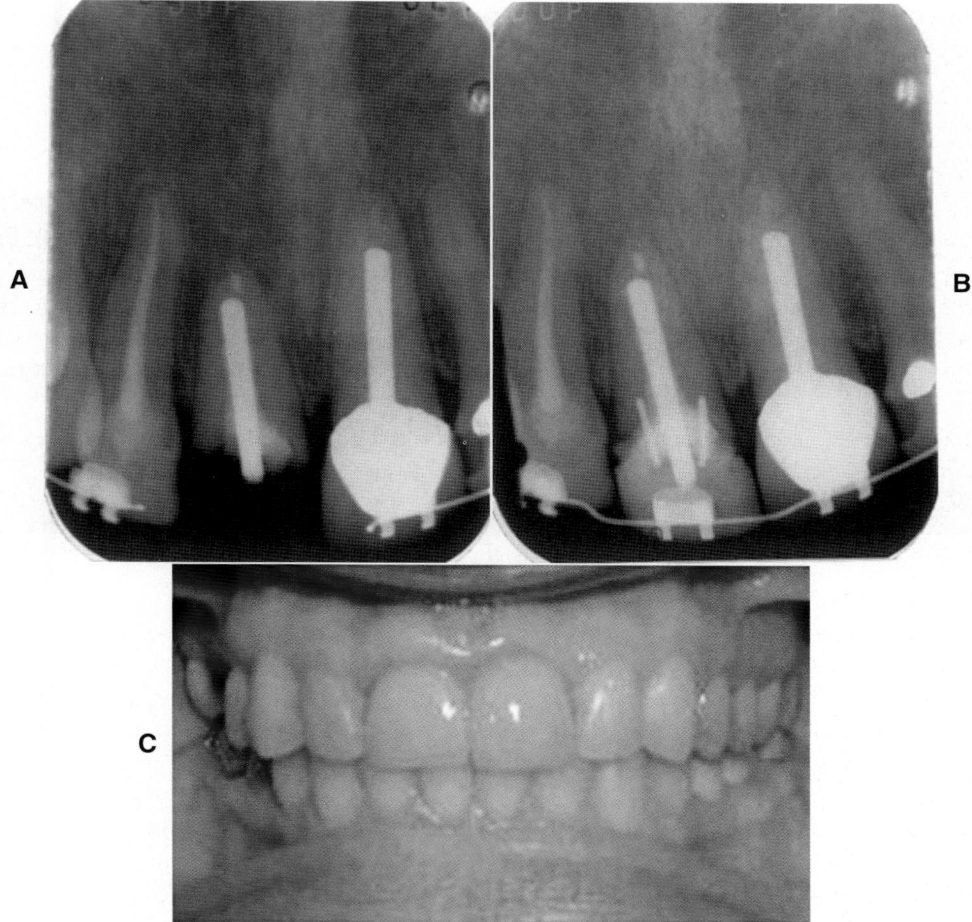

FIG 17-4 Forced eruption of the upper right central to facilitate crown preparation. **A,** Pretreatment periapical radiograph. **B,** Posttreatment periapical radiograph. **C,** Posttreatment intraoral photo.

The ultimate goal of comprehensive adult orthodontic treatment should be the attainment of Andrews'[35] six keys to normal occlusion and to restore health and harmony of the different components of the stomatognathic system.

17. What are the retention considerations after adult orthodontic treatment?[36,37]

Permanent splinting of periodontally compromised teeth is advisable after adult tooth movement. The replacement of missing teeth should be done 3 to 6 months after the removal of the fixed orthodontic appliances. Delaying their replacement can cause the loss of tooth alignment and bite collapse. The retainers should be designed to maintain tooth position in three planes of space. In partially edentulous patients, an acrylic bite block should be incorporated into the extraction site to maintain the edentulous space and prevent extrusion of the opposite tooth. Invisible plastic retainers offer increased esthetics and comfort as well as protection against parafunctional habits.

18. When should orthognathic surgery be considered for the adult patient?[38,39]

Adult patients with severe skeletal deformities in any of the three planes of space should be considered for combined orthodontic and surgical treatment (Fig. 17-6).

The indication for surgery is also determined by the lack of availability for growth modification treatment, the effect of tooth movement on facial esthetics and periodontal health, anatomy of the palate and the symphysis, other functional and anatomical limitations, as well as patient cooperation and length of treatment. The role of the orthodontist is to remove the dental compensations caused by the skeletal deformity and to coordinate the upper and lower dental arches to facilitate the surgical coordination of the skeletal bases. Rigid fixation has made the surgical procedures more stable and acceptable to patients. The success of orthognathic surgery is dependent on knowledge of basic orthodontic and surgical principles as well as the interaction and communication among all practitioners

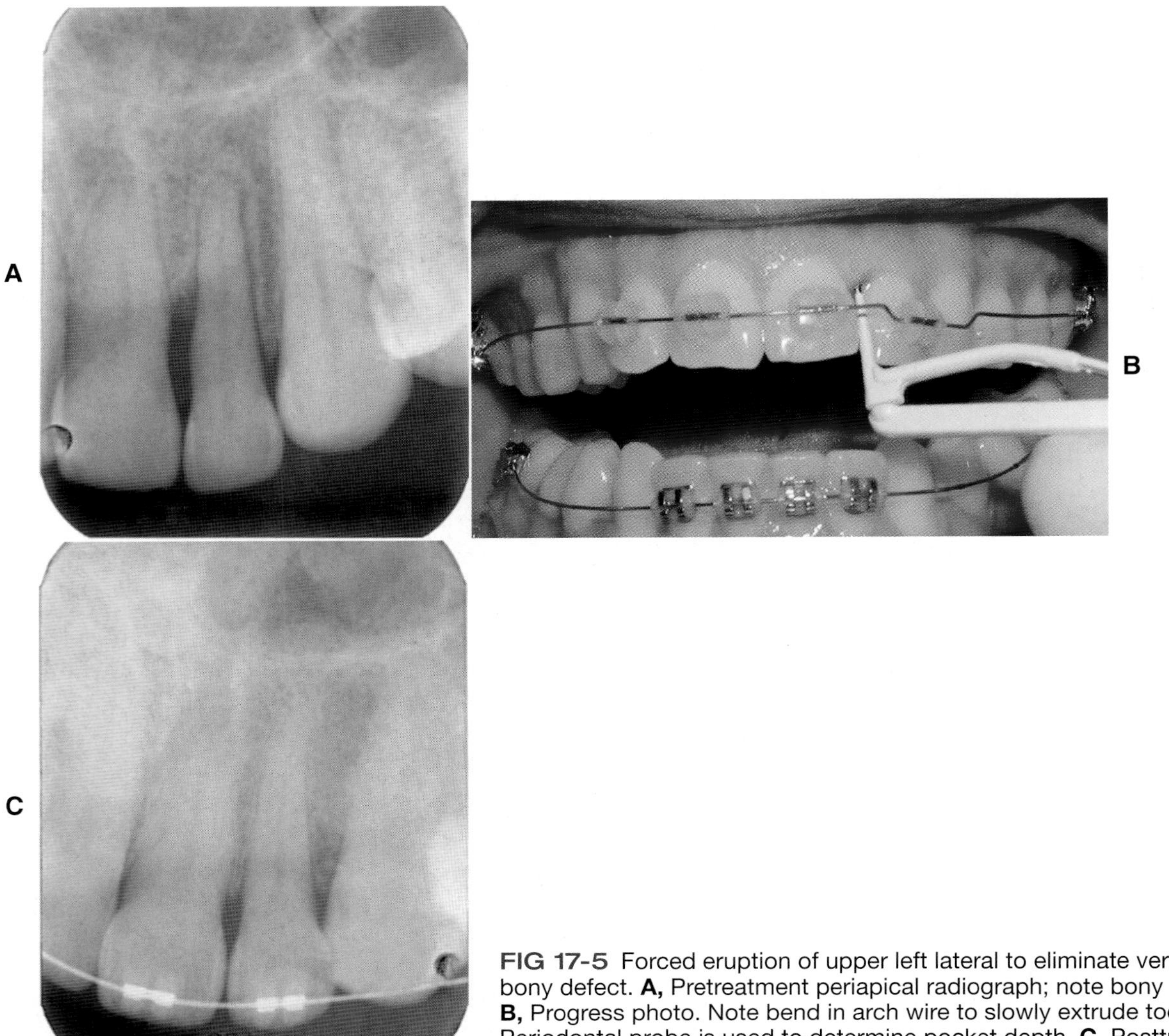

FIG 17-5 Forced eruption of upper left lateral to eliminate vertical bony defect. **A,** Pretreatment periapical radiograph; note bony defect. **B,** Progress photo. Note bend in arch wire to slowly extrude tooth. Periodontal probe is used to determine pocket depth. **C,** Posttreatment periapical radiograph shows elimination of vertical bony pocket.

involved in the final restoration of the esthetic function and psychological well-being of the patient.

19. What are the orthodontic considerations that relate to patient's dental esthetics?[40-49]

Over the last decade, advances in dental materials have expanded the restorative procedures available to today's clinicians, especially in regard to esthetic dentistry. Orthodontists are in a unique position to participate in the "smile design" of the adult patient by properly positioning the anterior teeth to facilitate the placement of esthetic restorations (Fig. 17-7).

The relationship between extraoral and intraoral structures is essential to dental esthetics. The three structures that compose the smile—the lips, the gingiva and the teeth—must have a harmonious relationship for an acceptable esthetic appearance.

If excessive maxillary spacing is present because of tooth size discrepancy, orthodontic treatment to redistribute the space is indicated. Consideration for space allocation needed for the proper restorative sizing of the incisors is essential. The esthetic success of the final restorations will be totally dependent on the prerestorative orthodontic dental repositioning.

In cases in which the excessive spacing is due to dental shifting into an edentulous space (e.g., missing maxillary lateral incisor), orthodontic repositioning should be done to open the appropriate amount of space as well as to obtain root parallelism to facilitate implant placement (Fig. 17-8). The minimum amount of space needed for the placement of an implant to replace a maxillary lateral incisor is 6 mm at the root level. This allows for a minimum of 1 mm space mesial and distal to the implant.

The presence of a "black triangle" between the anterior teeth, specifically the central incisors, is considered to be esthetically unpleasant to many patients (Fig. 17-9). This space usually appears after the correction of overlapped incisors, where the dental papillae did not develop. Interproximal reduction of the mesial surface of the central incisors is recommended to reduce the triangular space. Also, reducing the

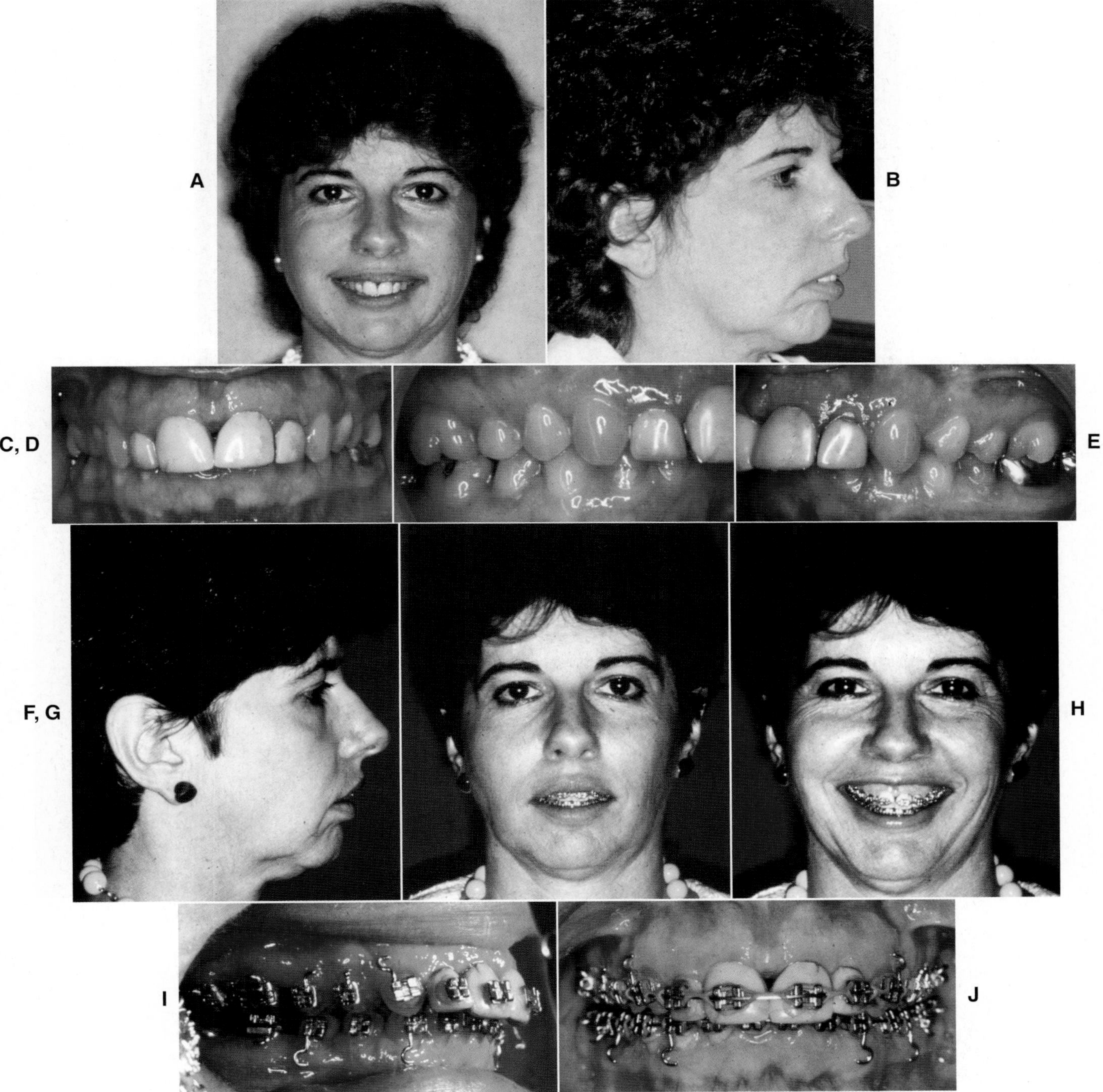

FIG 17-6 Orthognathic surgical treatment of a severe dentoskeletal Class II malocclusion characterized by maxillary vertical excess, mandibular retrognathia, and maxillary constriction. **A-E,** Pretreatment photos. **F-J,** Presurgical preparation.

Continued

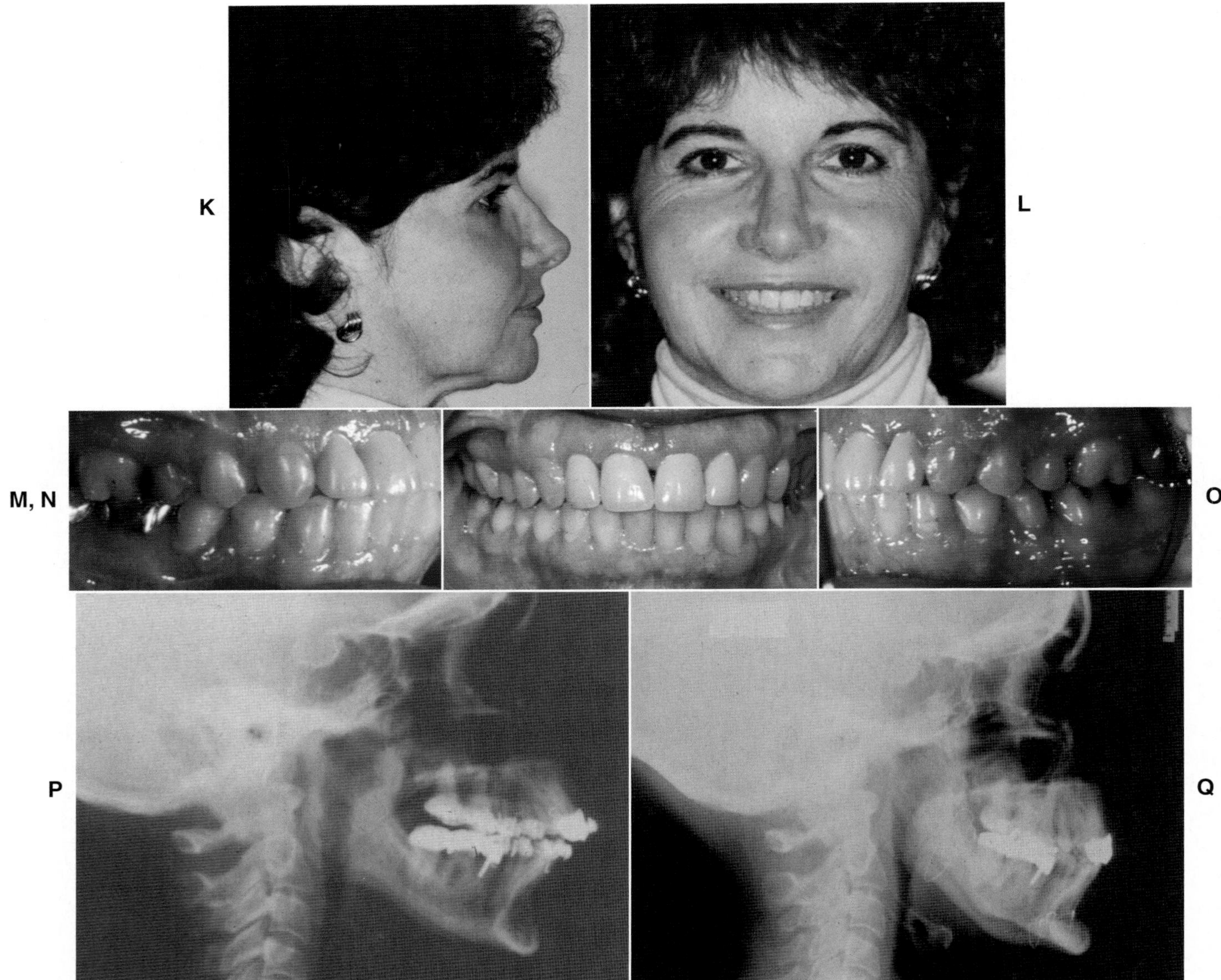

FIG 17-6—cont'd K-O, Posttreatment results after LeFort I maxillary impaction, mandibular sagittal split advancement, and advancement genioplasty. **P** and **Q,** Comparisons of pretreatment and posttreatment cephalograms.

distal tip of the roots of the central incisors will approximate the crowns gingivally, decreasing the size of the space. When this is done, recontouring of their incisal edges may be necessary. Extrusion and intrusion of teeth, especially in the anterior region of the upper arch, could be considered for leveling of the gingival margins. Intrusion will produce apical migration of the gingival border and extrusion will bring the level of the gingival tissue toward the occlusal plane. Adjustment of the incisal edges either with equilibration or veneers is recommended when considering these types of tooth movement. Recently high gingivectomy with lasers has been used for this purpose (Fig. 17-10).

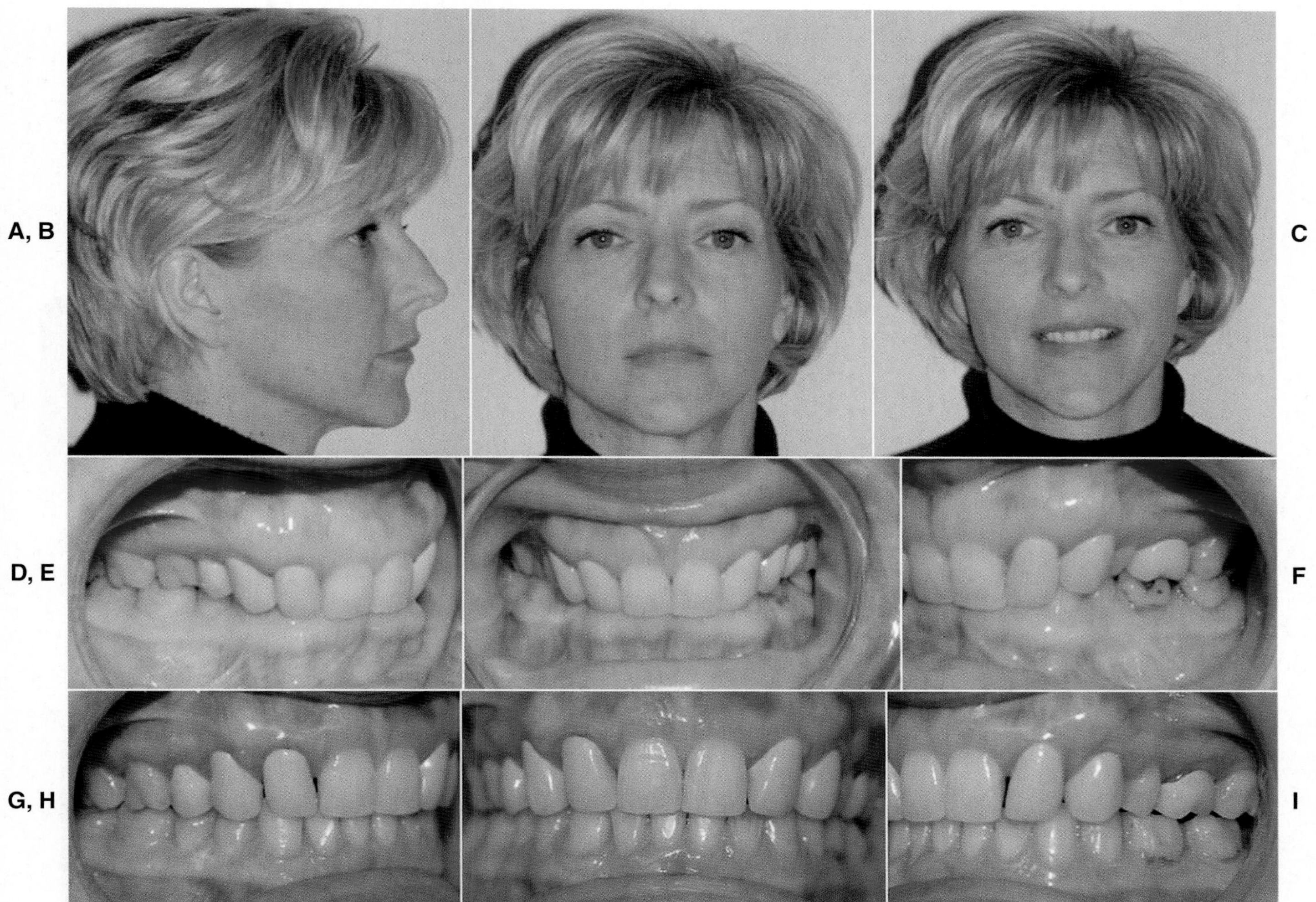

FIG 17-7 Comprehensive orthodontic treatment to intrude the upper and lower incisors and to obtain clearance for crown restorations on severely abraded anterior teeth. **A-F,** Pretreatment presentation. **G-I,** Postorthodontic occlusion prior to restorations.

Continued

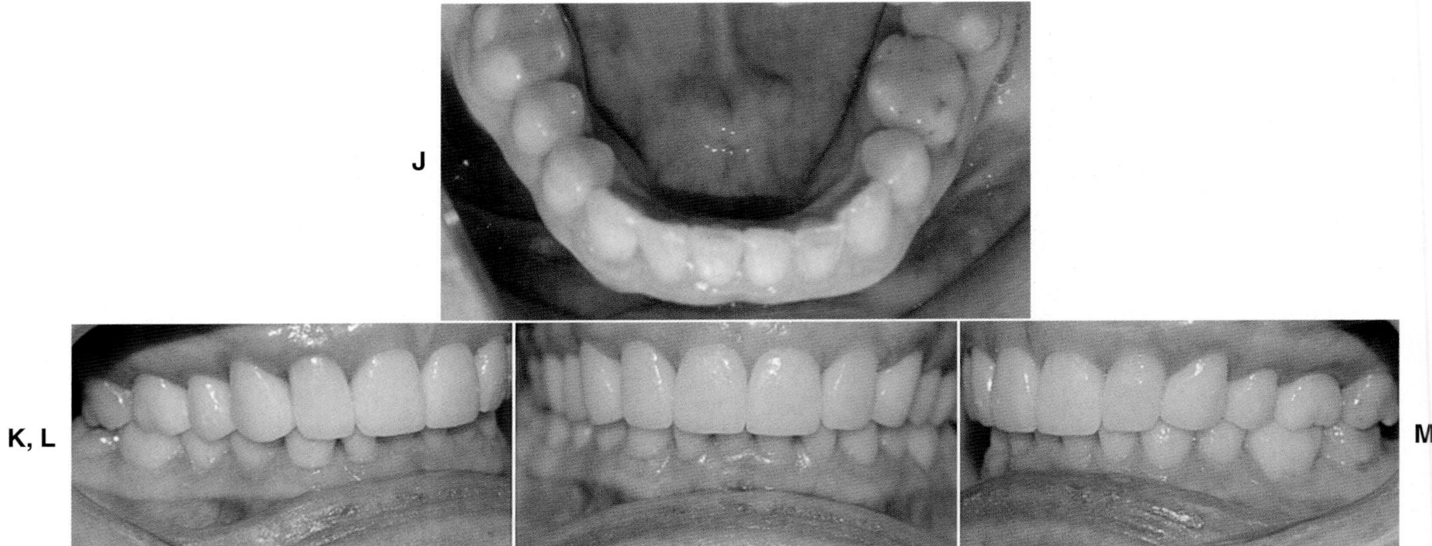

FIG 17-7—cont'd J, Occlusal view of lower arch. Note abrasion of lower dentition. **K-M,** Final result.

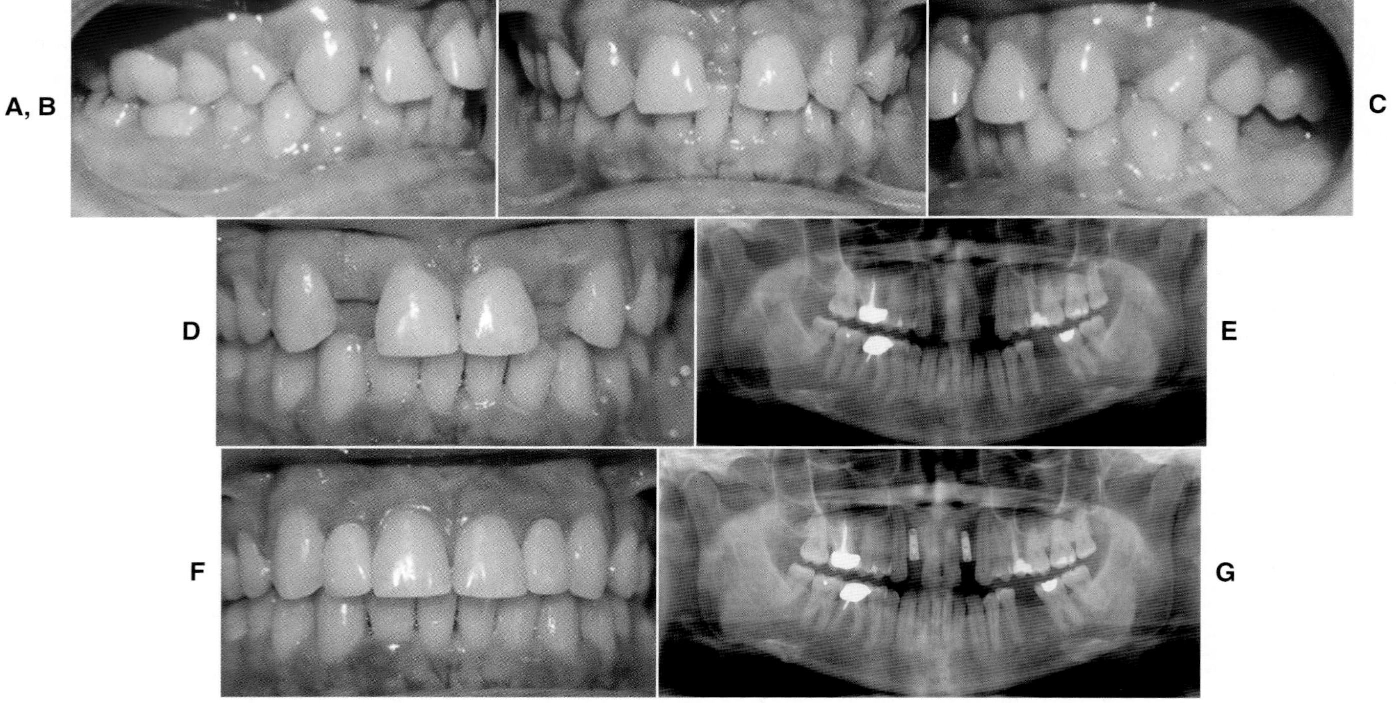

FIG 17-8 Orthodontic preparation for implant replacement of upper lateral incisors. **A-C,** Pretreatment intraoral photos. **D** and **E,** Postorthodontic preparation. Note root positioning to facilitate implant placement. **F** and **G,** Postimplant placement results.

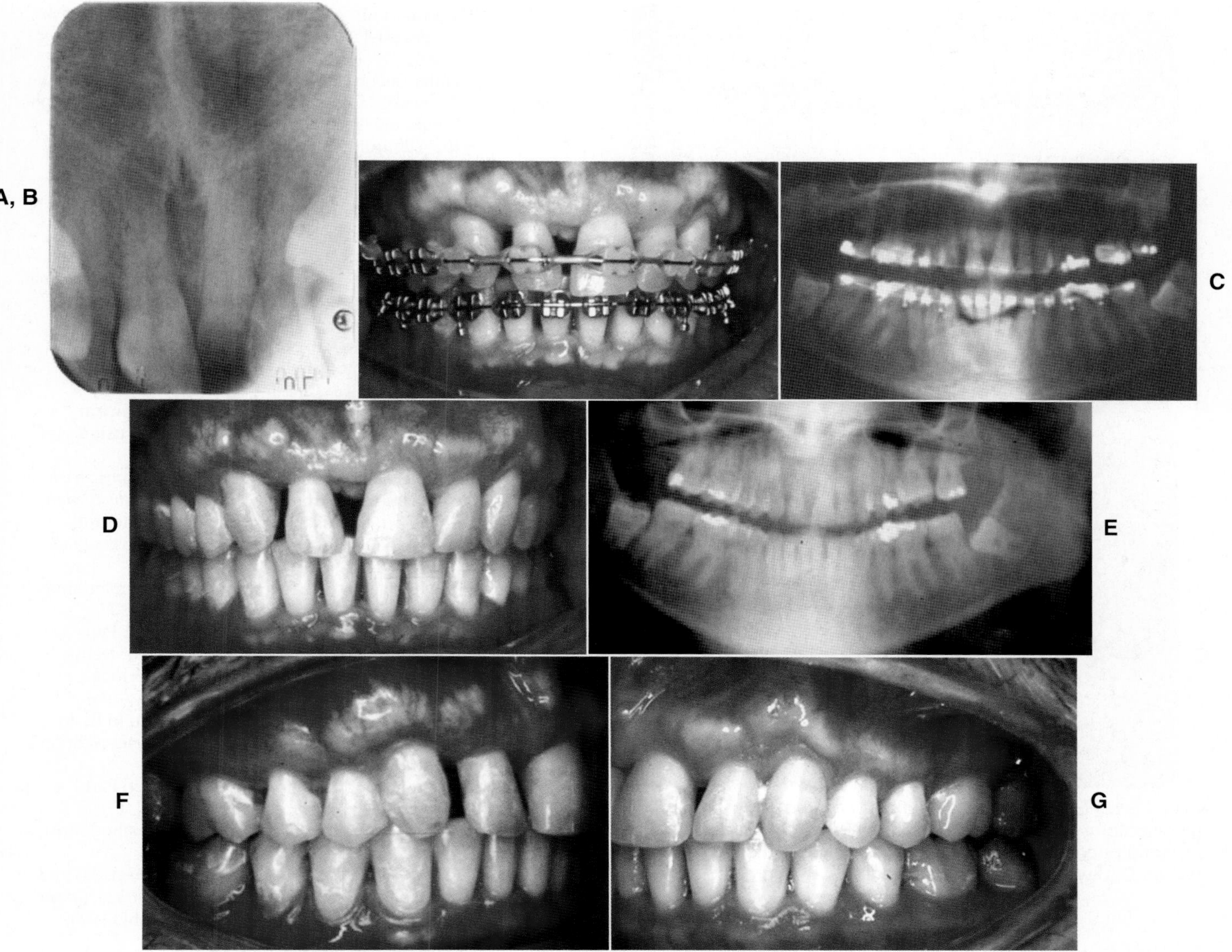

FIG 17-9 Orthodontic treatment to facilitate space redistribution after extraction of the severely decayed upper right central incisor. The lateral incisor was moved into the central space. Esthetic restoration would reshape the lateral as a central incisor. **A,** Pretreatment radiograph. **B** and **C,** Orthodontic preparation. Extraction of the upper left decayed first molar and space closure was also accomplished. **D-G,** Final results.

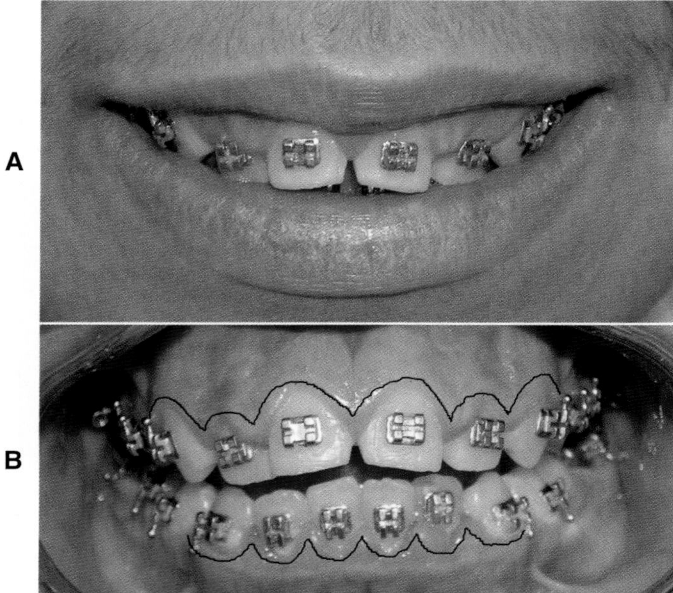

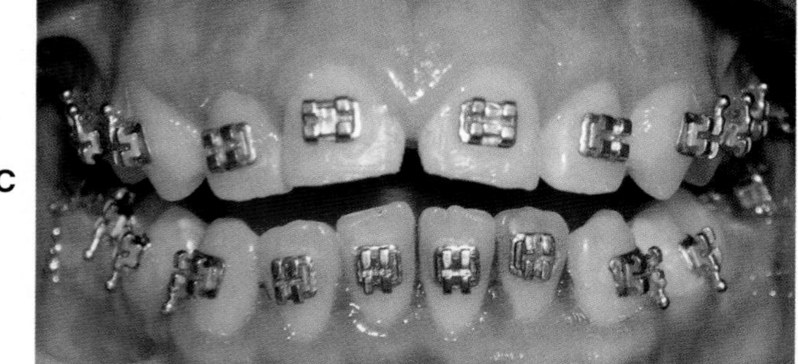

FIG 17-10 Excessive gingival display corrected with high gingivectomy to improve the "gummy" smile. **A,** Pretreatment intraoral photo. **B,** Gingival markings to guide in contouring of tissue. **C,** 3 weeks postsurgical result.

REFERENCES

1. Kuhlberg A, Glynn E: Treatment planning considerations for the adult patients. *Dent Clin North Am* 1997;41(1):17-27.
2. Matthews DP, Kokich VG: Managing treatment of the orthodontic patient with periodontal problems. *Semin Orthod* 1997;3(1):21-38.
3. Roberts EW, Hartsfield JK Jr: Primary management of congenital and acquired compensated malocclusions: Diagnosis, etiology and treatment planning. *IDA J* Summer 1996.
4. Phillips C, Bennett ME, Broader HL: Dentofacial disharmony: Psychological status of patients seeking a treatment consultation. *Angle Orthod* 1998;68(6):547-556.
5. Barrer G: The adult orthodontic patient. *Am J Orthod* 1977;72:617-640.
6. Boyd RL, Leggott PJ, Quinn RS, et al: Periodontal implications of orthodontic treatment in adults with reduced or normal periodontal tissues versus those of adolescents. *Am J Orthod* 1989;96(3):191-198.
7. Thilander B: Indications for orthodontic treatment in adults. In Thilander B, Ronning O, editors: *Introduction to Orthodontics.* Stockholm: Tandlakarforlaget, 1985.
8. Chanavaz M: Screening and medical evaluation of adults, absolute and relative contraindications for invasive dental procedures. *J Indiana Dent Assoc* 1999;78(3):10-17.
9. Roberts WE, Garetto LP, Arbuckle GR, et al: What are the risk factors of osteoporosis? Assessing bone health. *J Am Dent Assoc* 1991;122(2):59-61.
10. Payne JB, Reinhardt RA, Nummikoski PV, Patil KD: Longitudinal alveolar bone loss in post-menopausal osteoporotic/osteopenic women. *Osteoporos Int* 1999;10(1):34-40.
11. Zachrisson BU: Clinical implications of recent orthodontic—periodontic research findings. *Semin Orthod* 1996;2(1):4-12.
12. Ong MA, Wang H-L, Smith FN: Interrelationship between periodontics and adult orthodontics. *J Clin Periodont* 1998;25(4):271-277.
13. Artun J, Urbye K: The effect of orthodontic treatment on periodontal bone support in patients with advanced loss of marginal periodontium. *Am J Orthod Dentofacial Orthop* 1988;93(2):143-148.
14. Polson A, Caton J, Polson AP, et al: Periodontal response after tooth movement into infrabony defects. *J Periodontol* 1984;55(4):197-202.
15. Melsen B, Agerback N, Eriksen J, Terp S: New attachment through periodontal treatment and orthodontic intrusion. *Am J Orthod Dentofacial Orthop* 1988;94(2):104-116.
16. Zachrisson BU: Periodontal changes during orthodontic treatment. In McNamara Jr JA, Ribbens KA, editors: *Malocclusion and the periodontium.* Michigan Growth Series, Center for Human Growth and Development. Ann Arbor: University of Michigan, 1989, pp 43-66.
17. Dorfman HS: Mucogingival changes resulting from mandibular incisor tooth movement. *Am J Orthod* 1978;74:258-277.
18. Wennstrom JL, Stokland BL, Nyman S, Thilander B: Periodontal tissue response to orthodontic movement of teeth with infrabony pockets. *Am J Orthod Dentofacial Orthop* 1993;103(4):313-319.
19. Pangrazio-Kulbersh V: Adult orthodontic treatment. In Riolo ML, Avery JK, editors: *Essentials for orthodontic practice*, edition 1. Grand Haven, MI: EEOP, 2003, pp 510-532.
20. Roth RH: Functional occlusion for the orthodontist, Part I. *J Clin Orthod* 1981;15(1):32-51.
21. Roth RH, Rolfs DA: Functional occlusion for the orthodontist, Part II. *J Clin Orthod* 1981;15(2):100-123.
22. Vanarsdall RL, Musich DR: Adult orthodontics: Diagnosis and treatment. In Graber TM, Vanarsdall RL: *Orthodontics: current principles and practice*, edition 2. St Louis: CV Mosby; 1994, pp 750-836.
23. Roberts WE: Adjunctive orthodontic therapy in adults over 50 years of age, clinical management of compensated, partially edentulous malocclusions. *J Indiana Dent Assoc* 1997;76(2):33-41.
24. Roberts WE, Hartsfield JK: Multidisciplinary management of congenital and acquired compensated malocclusions. *J Indiana Dent Assoc* 1997;76(2):42-51.
25. Tulloch JF. Uprighting molars as an adjunct to restorative and periodontal treatment in adults. *Br J Orthod* 1982;9(3):122-128.
26. Roberts WW, Chacker FM, Burstone CJ: A segmental approach to mandibular molar uprighting. *Am J Orthod* 1982;81(3):177-184.
27. Hom B, Turley P: The effects of space closure of the mandibular first molar area in adults. *Am J Orthod* 1984;85(6):457-469.
28. Tuncay OC, Biggerstaff RH, Cutcliffe JC, Berkowitz J: Molar uprighting with T-loop springs. *J Am Dent Assoc* 1980;100(6):863-866.
29. Pontonero R, Celenza F, Ricci G, Carnevale G: Rapid extrusion with fiber resection: A combined orthodontic—periodontic treatment modality. *Int J Period Restor Dent* 1987;7(5):31-34.
30. Stevens B, Levine RA: Forced eruption: A multidisciplinary approach for form, function and biologic predictability. *Comp Contin Educ Dent* 1998;19(10):994-1004.

31. Hohlt WE, Hovijitra S: Multidisciplinary treatment of anterior spacing by orthodontic and prosthodontic management. *J Indiana Dent Assoc* 1999;76(3):18-23.
32. Gianelly AA: *Bidimensional technique theory and practice.* Rapid City, SD: Fenwyn Press, 2000, pp 229-256.
33. Sheridan JJ, Ledoux PM: Air-rotor stripping and proximal sealants. *J Clin Orthod* 1989;23(12):790-794.
34. Bishara SE: *Textbook of orthodontics.* Philadelphia: WB Saunders, 2001, pp 494–531.
35. Andrews LF: The six keys to normal occlusion. *Am J Orthod* 1972;62(3):296-309.
36. Bishara SE, Treder JE, Damon P, Olsen M: Changes in the dental arches and dentition between 25 and 45 years of age. *Angle Orthod* 1996;66(6):417-422.
37. Zachrisson BU: Third generation mandibular bonded lingual 3-3 retainer. *J Clin Orthod* 1997;19(9):562-583.
38. Epker BN, Fish L: *Dentofacial deformities: integrated orthodontic surgical correction.* St Louis: CV Mosby, 1983.
39. Proffit WR, Fields H Jr: *Contemporary orthodontics*, edition 3. St Louis: CV Mosby, 2000.
40. Spear FM, Matthezus DM, Kokich VG: Interdisciplinary management of single tooth implants. *Semin Orthod* 1997;3(1):45-72.
41. Roberts WE, Baldwin JJ: Pre-prosthetic alignment of a compensated Class II malocclusion in a partially edentulous adult case. *Stud Orthod* 2000;3(1):1-6.
42. Kokich VG: Esthetics: The orthodontic-periodontic restorative connection. *Semin Orthod* 1996;2(1):21-30.
43. Salama N, Salama M: The role of orthodontic extrusive remodeling in the enhancement of the soft and hard tissue profiles prior to implant placement: A systematic approach to the management of extraction site defects. *Int J Period Restor Dent* 1993;13(4):312-333.
44. Chu SJ, Karabin S, Mistry S: Short tooth syndrome: Diagnosis, etiology, and treatment management. *J Calif Dent Assoc* 2004;32(2):143-152.
45. Spear FM: Interdisciplinary esthetic management of anterior gingival embrasures. *Adv Esth Interdisc Dent* 2006;2(1):20-28.
46. Kokich VG, Spear FM, Kokich VO: Maximizing anterior esthetics: An interdisciplinary approach. In McNamara Jr JA, editor: *Frontiers in dental and facial esthetics.* Ann Arbor: Needham Press, 2001, pp 1-18.
47. Kokich V: Esthetics and anterior tooth position: An orthodontic perspective, Part III: Mediolateral relationships. *J Esth Dent* 1993;5(5):200-207.
48. Kokich V: Esthetics and anterior tooth position: An orthodontic perspective, Part II: Vertical position. *J Esth Dent* 1993;5(4):174-178.
49. Kokich VG: Maxillary lateral incisor implants: Planning with the aid of orthodontics. *J Oral Maxillofac Surg* 2004;62 (9 suppl 2):48-56.

CHAPTER 18

Implants in Orthodontics

Brody J. Hildebrand

As one of the oldest specialties in dentistry, orthodontics has seen several periods of radical transformation. New theories, new devices, and new ways of treatment have often dramatically changed the way orthodontists move teeth or jaws. From bracket development such as edgewise slots, bondable adhesives, ceramics, and self-ligating brackets to NiTi wires, coils, and rapid palatal expanders, all the way through LeFort osteotomies and distraction osteogenesis, the world of orthodontics is radically different from what the founding fathers might remember.

Orthodontics is once again poised for greater and more efficient treatment, less reliance on patient cooperation, and possibly even less need for surgical interventions. Temporary implantation of material to gain a mechanical advantage during orthodontic treatment will undoubtedly be one of the great transformers of orthodontics in the early portion of the 21st century. Knowledge of the history of implants as well as various implant types available to practitioners is critical in being able to provide patients with the best and most up-to-date technical materials available for orthodontic treatment with temporary implant anchors (TIAs).

1. What is the history of implants in dentistry?

The history of implantable material in the oral cavity goes back several millennia. There are reports of items such as seashells, precious stones, ivory, and bone being used as implants.[1,2] In the Middle Ages, wealthy persons might attempt to implant a less-fortunate person's tooth for a fee. Recent implantable materials include Vitallium, ceramics, Zirconia, stainless steel, titanium alloys, and pure titanium, among many other compounds.

In the mid 1960s, P.I. Brånemark made famous the body's ability to accept and bond to titanium, a process coined *osseointegration*.[3] Andre Schroeder was another pioneer in the development of surface and design modifications in the development of predictable dental implants.[4] These changes shortened the healing time from 6 months to several weeks and effectively allowed for the realistic use of implants in orthodontics.[5-7] Currently the most predictable and acceptable implant material is commercially pure titanium with some type of subtractive surface treatment (Fig. 18-1).[8-10]

2. What is the history of implants in orthodontics?

Attempts to use implants in orthodontic treatment can be traced back to the early 1900s[11] with some reports coming from the late 1800s. Certainly, several of the attempts in the early 1900s can be seen as a valiant yet unsuccessful efforts at implantable anchorage.[12] However, with the advent and success of the titanium implant, the speed of research in both animal and human models accelerated. The 1980s saw a rise in the use of endosseous implants in orthodontics by clinicians such as Gray, Turley, Shapiro, Roberts, and others.[13-17]

The first mention of implant osseous anchorage in the palate was by Triaca[18] in 1992. The Straumann and Brånemark companies developed the only two available palatal implants in the United States. Intermaxillary fixation screws began to be used during the late 1980s and into the early 1990s. Widespread development and use outside the United States has led to the development and acceptance of TIAs on a global scale. These TIAs are now marketed by both traditional implant companies as well as orthodontic supply companies.

3. Why would one consider implants for orthodontic treatment?

Implants are useful in orthodontic treatment for the very fact that orthodontists rely exclusively on anchorage to move teeth.[19] Force values are applied to a tooth in order to move that tooth through the alveolar process.[20] In order for forces to be effective they must be applied and countered.[21] This promotes a response in the periodontal ligament that allows for bone remodeling to occur on the pressure side and deposition of bone to occur on the tension side of the tooth.

Force transfer is less than complete when the anchor teeth experience movement themselves.[22-25] With implants, this loss of force transfer can often be avoided due to the stationary nature of the implant, and not the mobile nature of the tooth, as the anchor. In addition, when the mechanics rely heavily on the cooperation of the patient and the patient is less than enthusiastic about complying, treatment progress can be hindered.[26] Osseointegrated implants provide a stable, secure, and absolute anchorage.

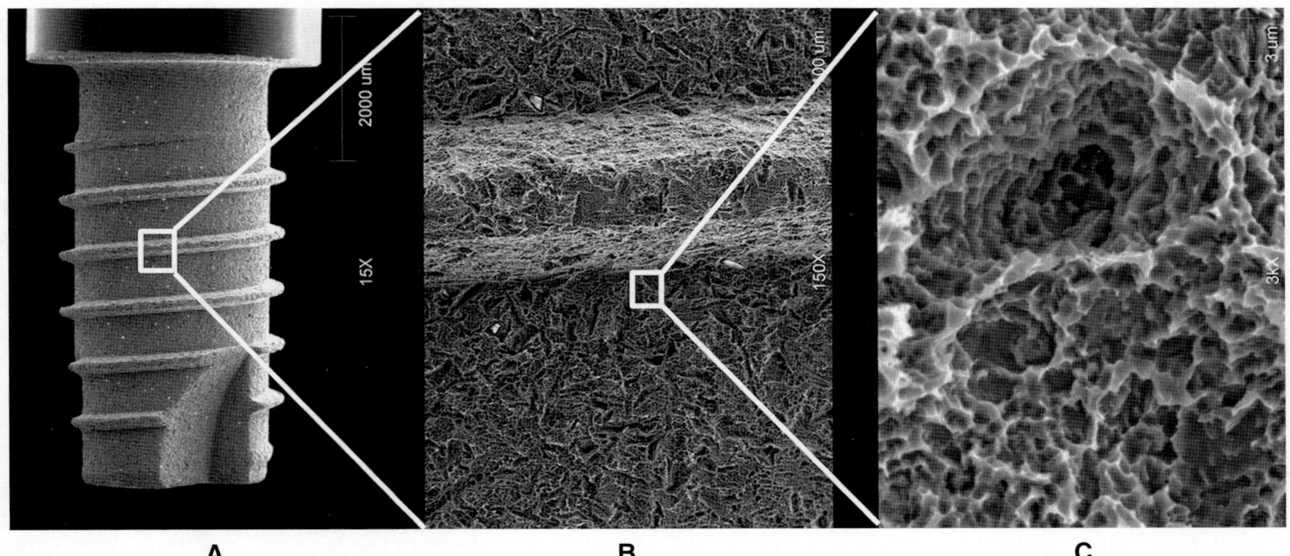

FIG 18-1 **A,** SEM implant surface (15X). **B,** SEM of roughened surface implant (150X). **C,** SEM of macro and micro roughness of SLA surfaced implant (3000X). This provides the architecture for the bone to be directly laid down on the implant surface.

BENEFITS OF IMPLANTS IN ORTHODONTICS

4. What are some of the advantages of using implants for orthodontic treatment?

Implants allow clinicians:

- The ability to treat patients that might not otherwise have been treated.
- The ability to avoid some unpopular and complex mechanical devices such as headgear.
- The ability to move teeth with less round tripping, less incidental tooth movement, and fewer unintended consequences.
- The ability to shorten treatment time by allowing the force application to be more accurately directed toward the teeth that need to be moved.
- The ability to use lower force levels because force values are not lost on movement of anchorage units and force vectors can be more ideally in line with centers of rotation.
- The ability to correct malocclusions in patients who have negative treatment responses or unexpected rates and directions of growth.
- The opportunity to treat borderline or even mild surgical candidates without the associated cost, trauma and time involved with orthognathic surgical intervention.

5. What are some of the disadvantages of using implants for orthodontic treatment?

A disadvantage of using implants can be the cost, the procedure involved, and possible complications encountered. With all types of implants, cost should be addressed. When a surgeon's office is placing an implant, there is usually a fee for placement as well as for removal. This fee will vary depending on the cost of the materials as well as the variation in location. Even if an implant is to be placed by the orthodontist, a fee may still be considered necessary for financial as well as for procedural purposes.

The procedure, although often espoused to be "minor," should still be thought of as a surgical procedure. Nonsurgical correction of patients traditionally considered surgical patients is promising but has not been verified with adequate long-term results; thus, the ability to maintain the end treatment result is not completely confirmed. Finally, the complications that may arise from placing an implant into a tooth or with the movement of a tooth into an implant would be less than desirable. Complications with every device an orthodontist uses should always be considered a disadvantage.

6. What are some of the considerations in regard to specific treatment mechanics?

When any orthodontic implant is used, force vectors need to be appropriately applied and delivered.[27-29] Depending on the type of implant placed, the mechanics applied to the implant and the positioning of the implant may vary. For example, when attempting to retract anterior teeth, consideration should be given to the existing vertical and horizontal position of the teeth to be moved. If the maxillary anterior teeth exhibit an excessive vertical overlap (deep bite), retraction and intrusion from a mini-implant placed higher in the buccal vestibule would be appropriate, as would attachment of the retraction force close to the bracket of the teeth to be retracted. This would provide not only a posterior force vector, but also a vertical force vector. The creation of a counter-clockwise rotational force around the center of rotation of the anterior segment would intrude the maxillary anterior segment as it is retracted.[30]

If the maxillary anterior teeth exhibit a shallow or negative vertical overlap (open bite tendency), retraction from a mini-implant placed closer to the gingival margin of the teeth would be appropriate, as would the attachment of the retraction force to a hook extending a distance off the wire. This would place the retraction force higher into the vestibule and thus retract in a more horizontal vector to help correct the open bite. With palatal implants, the teeth themselves can either be moved with the use of activation from the implant or locked down as anchors to move adjacent teeth with traditional mechanics.[31]

7. How can implants benefit orthodontics beyond traditional mechanics?

Implants may release *some* of the constraints that Newton's Third Law holds on the orthodontist when working with tooth-borne anchorage. Of course, Newton's Third Law still applies, but the resultant force on the implant releases the other teeth from force application and hence movement. Newton's First Law gains greater importance in that teeth that are not "in motion" will likely stay put. Depending on the implant system and mechanics, a greater expression of the force applied results in more accurate torque control and movement of the teeth to be moved.

Implants also allow the orthodontist to treat patients who may have an inadequate number of teeth to act as anchors (Figs. 18-2 to 18-4). At times these patients are the ones most desperately in need of orthodontic treatment in order to save existing teeth and prepare the mouth appropriately for restorative modalities.[32] Implants give the practitioner the option to treat patients that might not be physically capable or compliant when using patient-dependent auxiliary devices. The treatment of patients with compromised maxillary and mandibular dentition can be more easily handled with proper planning for implant and the possible use of implants during treatment. Implants make traditional treatments easier and open treatment options for these underserved populations of our dental community.

8. Should we consider implants in more orthodontic treatments?

Whether or not an individual practitioner decides to consider implants as an option in treatment plans that are "more routine" is entirely up to the practitioner's desire. If implants can aid treatment, decrease morbidity of teeth, and increase the effectiveness of the bracket system, then most certainly they should be considered for use in any complex treatments that are not being featured on an "extreme makeover" edition.

One might argue that using implants is too invasive to consider using for routine application because of the surgical procedure. Many practitioners could counter that the use of a

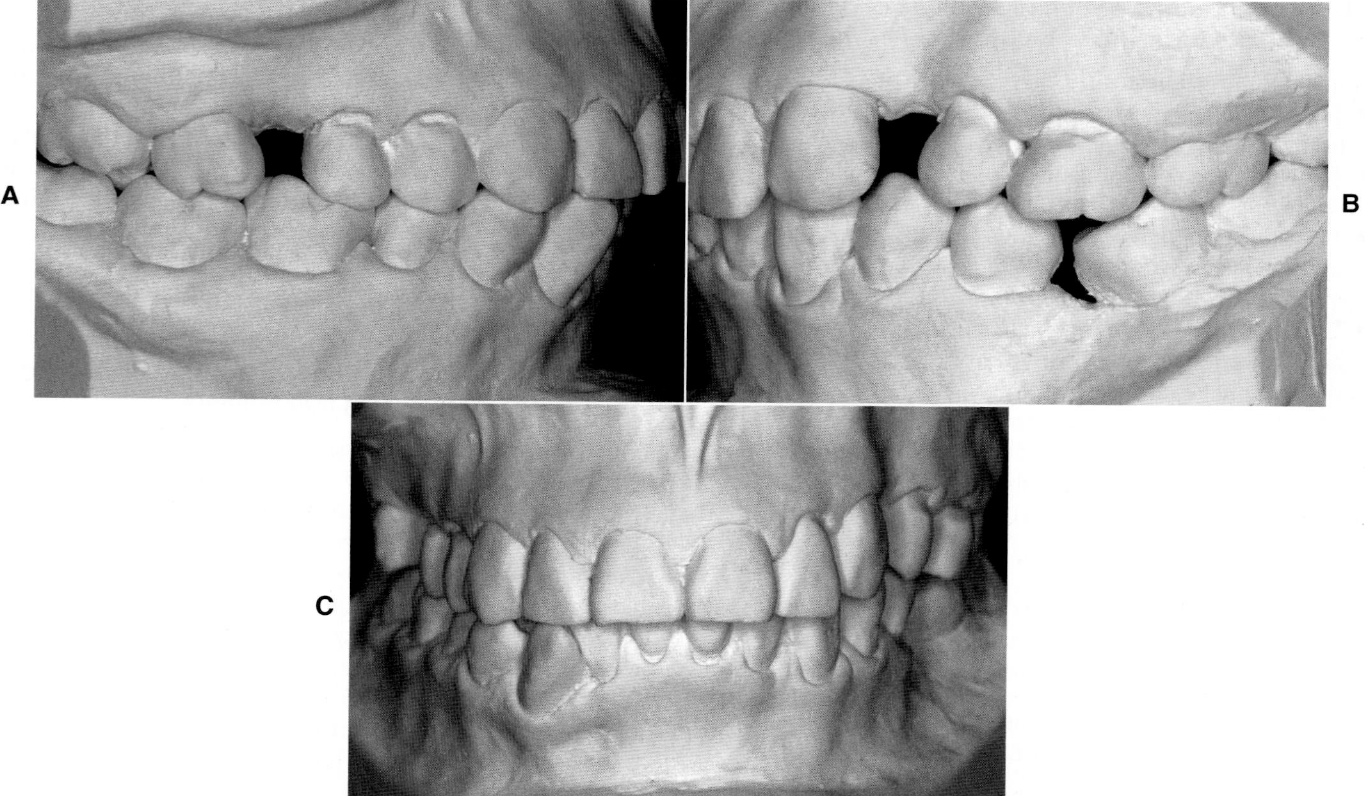

FIG 18-2 A-C, Adult patient with compromised maxillary and mandibular dentition caused by long-standing loss of teeth, supereruption, crowding, midline shifts, and angulation problems.

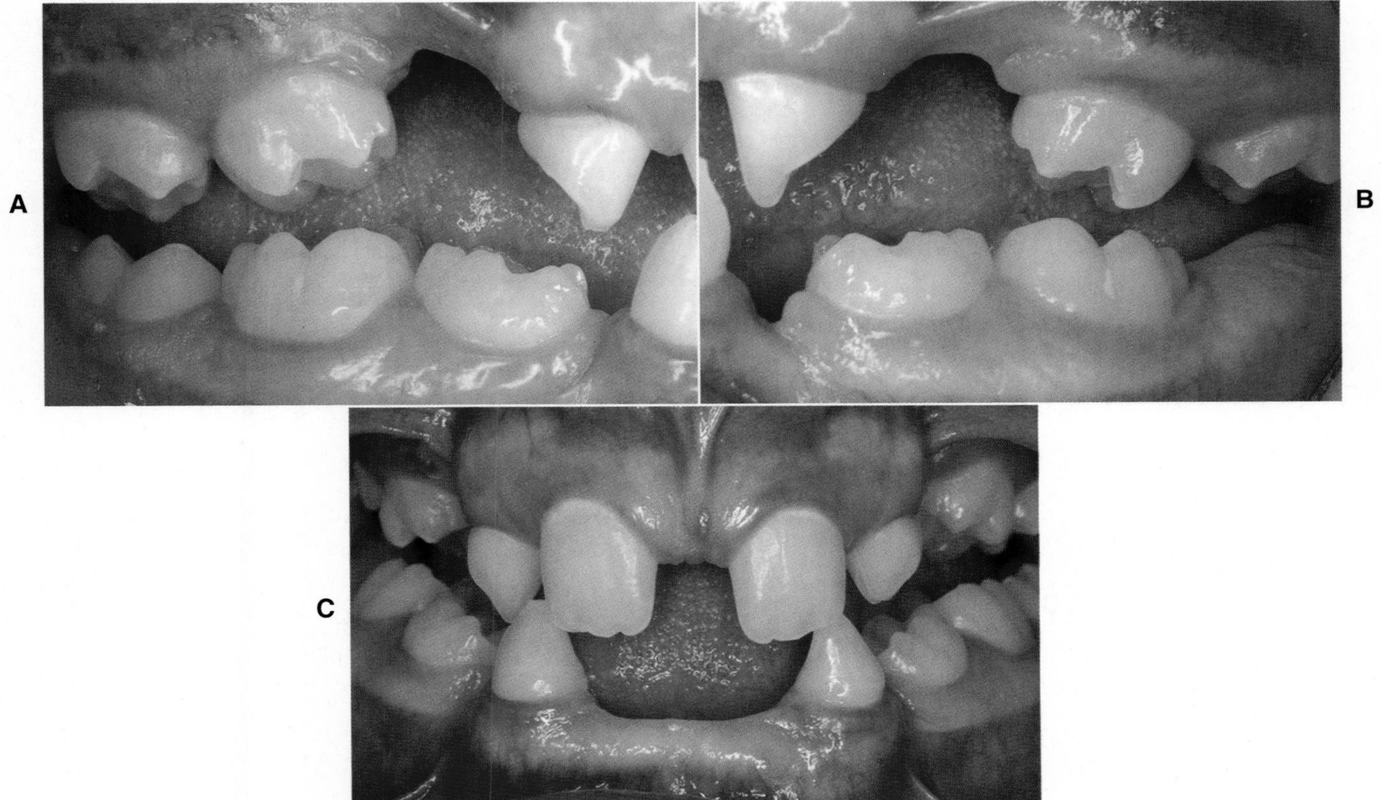

FIG 18-3 **A-C,** Adolescent patient with compromised maxillary and mandibular dentition caused by congenital failure of eruption and the resultant atrophic ridges, spacing, diastema, and angulation problems.

transpalatal arch (TPA) and headgear is much more invasive, certainly more taxing on the patient, and obviously affecting the patient in a far greater way than the placement of some form of temporary implant. Where the line is drawn should not be relative to the *perceived* "invasiveness" or a *claimed* "extraneous" application of dental materials.

DENTAL IMPLANTS (FIG. 18-5)

9. What is the impetus behind, the advantages of, and the disadvantages of dental implants being used for orthodontics?

The idea of dental implant usage in orthodontics is to use a proven dental restorative modality to secure anchorage when other anchorage modalities are not available or less effective. Dental implants bond to the bone through osseointegration and thus serve as the ultimate anchor to resist forces when moving teeth.[33] The obvious advantage is that reciprocal movement is minimal, and thus force distribution is concentrated on the teeth requiring movement (Fig. 18-6).[34]

The disadvantages of dental implants hinge around their cost, surgical procedure, and site availability. Dental implants are relatively expensive to purchase and even more expensive to place. Surgical placement also necessitates that an area of bone be available that can hold the large-size titanium screws, traditionally 4+ mm in diameter. It is important that 1 mm of bone be present on the buccal, lingual, mesial, and distal of the implant. Usually these implants are placed with the intention of being restored after orthodontic treatment. Care should be taken to ensure that the implant will be in the correct position for proper crown shape and size for the prosthodontist or restorative dentist (Fig. 18-7).[35]

When an edentulous site is not available, the only viable option is the retromolar pad and ascending ramus (Fig. 18-8). This site is often difficult to access surgically and often leaves the implant fixture in a less-than-ideal position or angulation. The clinician is also somewhat limited in the ability to use this anchor for maxillary movements. When done properly, implants do offer the orthodontist the ability to work with a fantastic anchor for orthodontic treatment.[36]

10. What is the surgical process involved?

Dental implants require definitive knowledge of ridge anatomy, augmentation protocols, and sinus structures as well as neurovascular considerations. The surgical procedure includes local anesthesia and, at times, sedation. Each implant system has its own predetermined drill sequence that must be followed, depending on the implant size to be placed. The placement of dental implants is generally done by an experienced periodontist or oral surgeon.

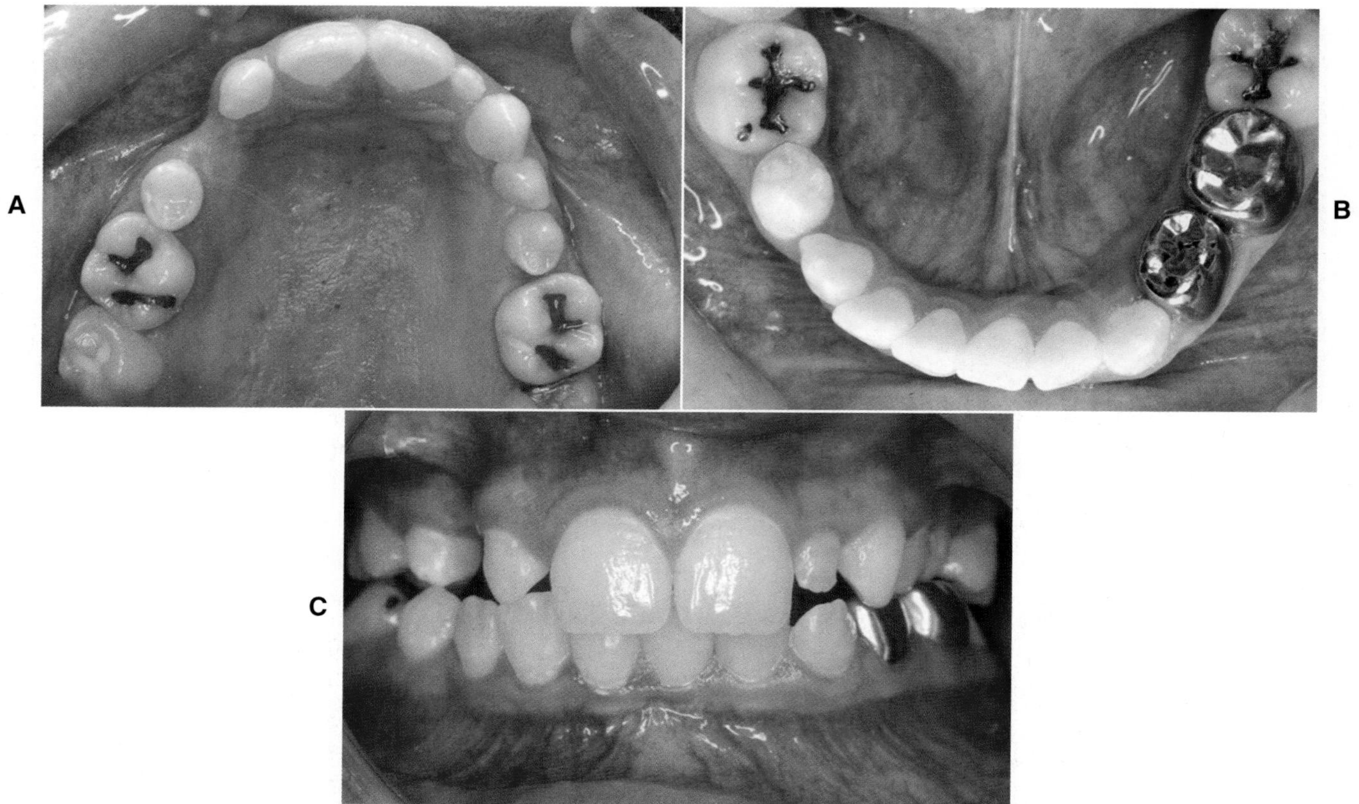

FIG 18-4 A-C, Adolescent patient with compromised maxillary and mandibular dentition caused by congenital failure of eruption and idiopathic condylar resorption, spacing, and angulation problems.

PALATAL IMPLANTS (FIG. 18-9)

11. What is the impetus behind, the advantages of, and the disadvantages of the palatal implant for orthodontics?

Palatal implants were conceived as a way to use the body's acceptance of titanium implants without being constricted by the availability of edentulous sites or the ascending ramus.[37,38] Bone is more than adequate in the palate, and the lack of anatomic structures that would limit placement is extremely attractive.[39] Palatal implants provide the best of the predictability of dental implants coupled with the ready availability of bone and a lack of compromising structures. The applications of force vectors is widespread and adjustable during treatment. Palatal implants are quite impressive in their ability to correct open bite, Class II, Class III, and debilitated dentitions. A single palatal implant can also be used in instances of intrusion, retraction, or midline rotations where numerous mini-implants may be required (Fig. 18-10).[40]

Although a palatal implant is excellent for controlling movement of maxillary teeth, it does have the limitation of being ineffective in controlling intrusion of mandibular teeth. Although the surgical placement of this implant is much simpler than that of a dental implant, there is a definite need to use local anesthetic in the palate. A final consideration is that the palatal implant requires an impression of the implant and a lab procedure, much in the same way a transpalatal arch or rapid palatal expander.

12. What is the surgical process involved for the palatal implant?

The surgical procedure for placing a palatal implant is similar to that of placing a dental implant, although much less demanding. Without root structures, sinus cavities, nerve bundles, and large blood vessels to avoid, the midpalatal suture is almost ideal for placement of implants. The major consideration when placing the palatal implant is to avoid use in the midpalate of young children. If treatment with a palatal implant is necessary, a paramedian placement would suffice. In some instances, two palatal implants can be used.

Local anesthesia is necessary for the entire palate. The drill sequence consists of a tissue punch, a round bur, and the single site preparation drill. Some type of controlled torque delivery system would be recommended to prepare the site. The implant is placed and then left to osseointegrate for 6 to 12 weeks. Removal is completed after treatment with an implant trephine.

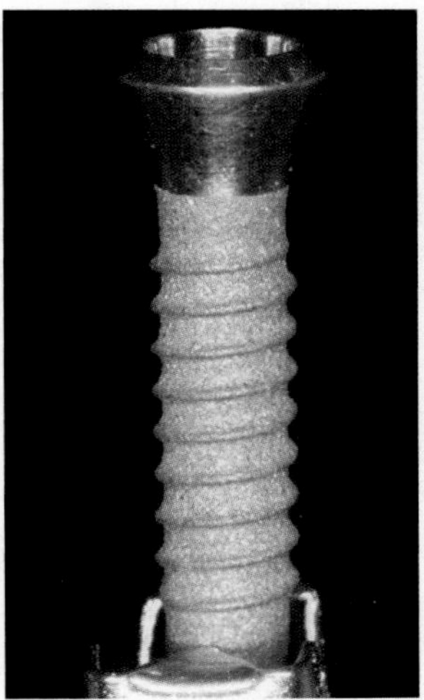

FIG 18-5 Conventional dental implant.

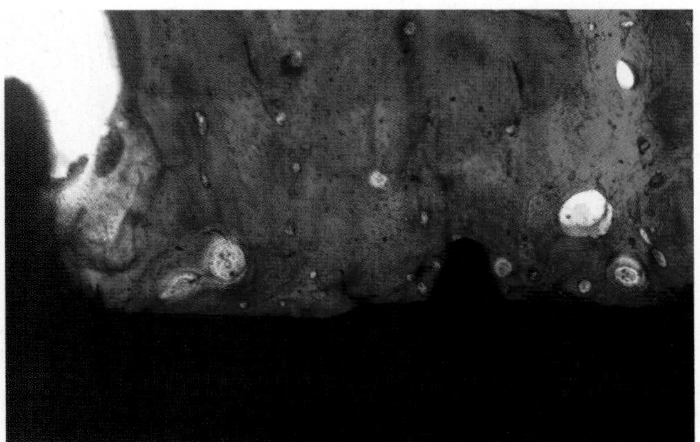

FIG 18-6 Histological section of osseointegrated orthodontic implant surface. Close and complete adaptation of the bone to the implant surface allows for a stable anchorage point to resist forces required to move other teeth.

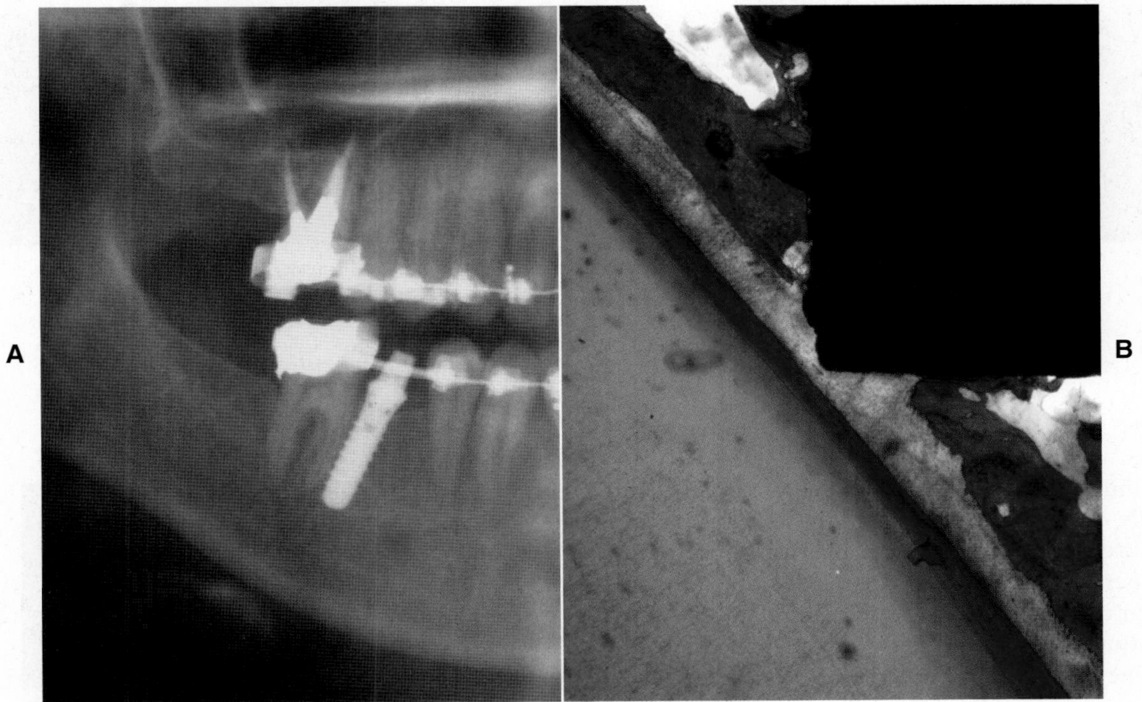

FIG 18-7 **A,** Dental implants placed before orthodontic treatment is complete may be done so without knowledge of the determined final position of a tooth. **B,** This could pose a hindrance to the final orthodontic alignment of the dentition, the restorability of the implant, and even the survivability of the tooth.

MINI-IMPLANTS (FIG. 18-11)

13. What is the impetus behind, the advantages of, and the disadvantages of mini-implants for orthodontic treatment?

Mini-implants are much in demand primarily because of their simplicity. It is this fact alone that has propelled them to the forefront of the implant-assisted orthodontic discussion. They are versatile and small, require little in terms of hardware, and are easily removed. When used in multiples, the orthodontist can retract, protrude, intrude, and extrude single teeth or entire segments of teeth. They can also provide anchorage in many of the instances that dental and palatal implants are capable of doing (Fig. 18-12).[41,42]

Many of these same advantages are also disadvantages. They may fail to provide anchorage for an extended time,

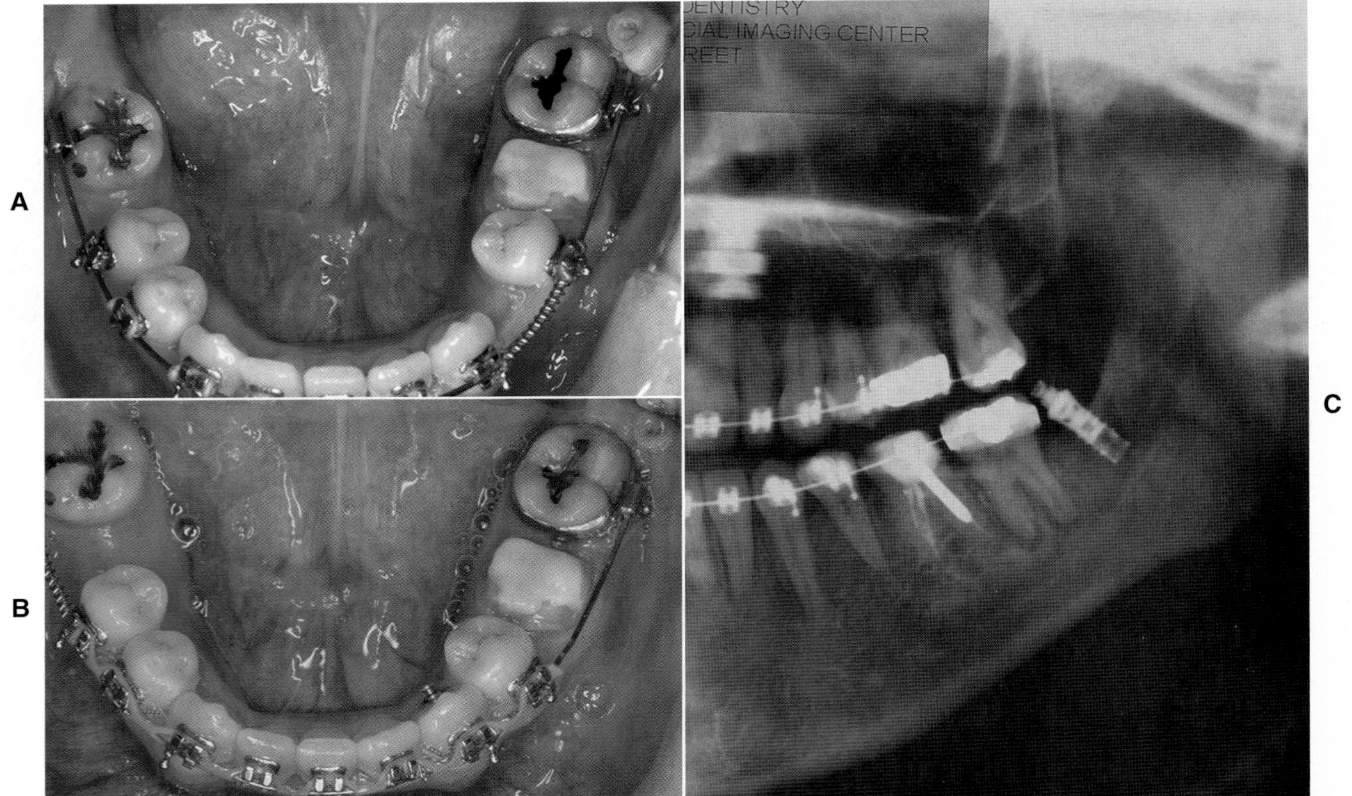

FIG 18-8 **A** and **B,** Dental implants placed in the retromolar area can be used in a number of different methods to retract, intrude, and level arches without loosing anchorage of key teeth. In this instance the left second molar needed to be distalized and then serve as a primary anchor for arch rotation to close spaces and shift the midline. **C,** Radiographic view of implant site.

their proximity to root structures should be watched, and they usually do not have the capability to resist forces in different directions once they are placed. In addition, a large number of mini-implants are needed for more complex movements. A failure of a mini-implant, as well as the inability to place the implant in the desired location because of neurovascular structures, anatomy, or hard/soft tissue deficiencies are all possibilities. Unfortunately, often the failure of an implant in a strategic site might stall treatment until the bone has healed enough to place another mini-implant.[43]

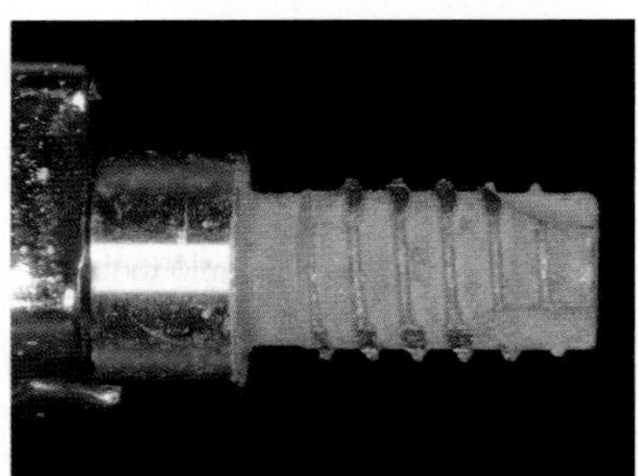

FIG 18-9 Palatal implant.

14. What is the surgical process involved?

The surgical process of placing most mini-implants is relatively straightforward. The debate over whether local anesthetic is necessary is still ongoing. Many surgical procedures are completed with a very strong topical anesthetic. There are times that this will not suffice, so clinicians that attempt the procedure with topical anesthetic should, at the very least, be equipped to provide local anesthetic when it is warranted. It is important to note that unwanted soft tissue poses a significantly higher risk of failure and infection for mini-implants. Placement in the palate can be achieved, although the risk of dislodgement from tongue forces does need to be considered.

Each individual implant system has its own drill set. Various systems call for a tissue puncture followed by a pilot drill slightly smaller than the mini-implant to be placed. Some smaller implant systems are "drill-free" and thus small enough to be placed through the cortical plate and into the alveolar bone without the pilot drill. Removal is typically done by reversing the

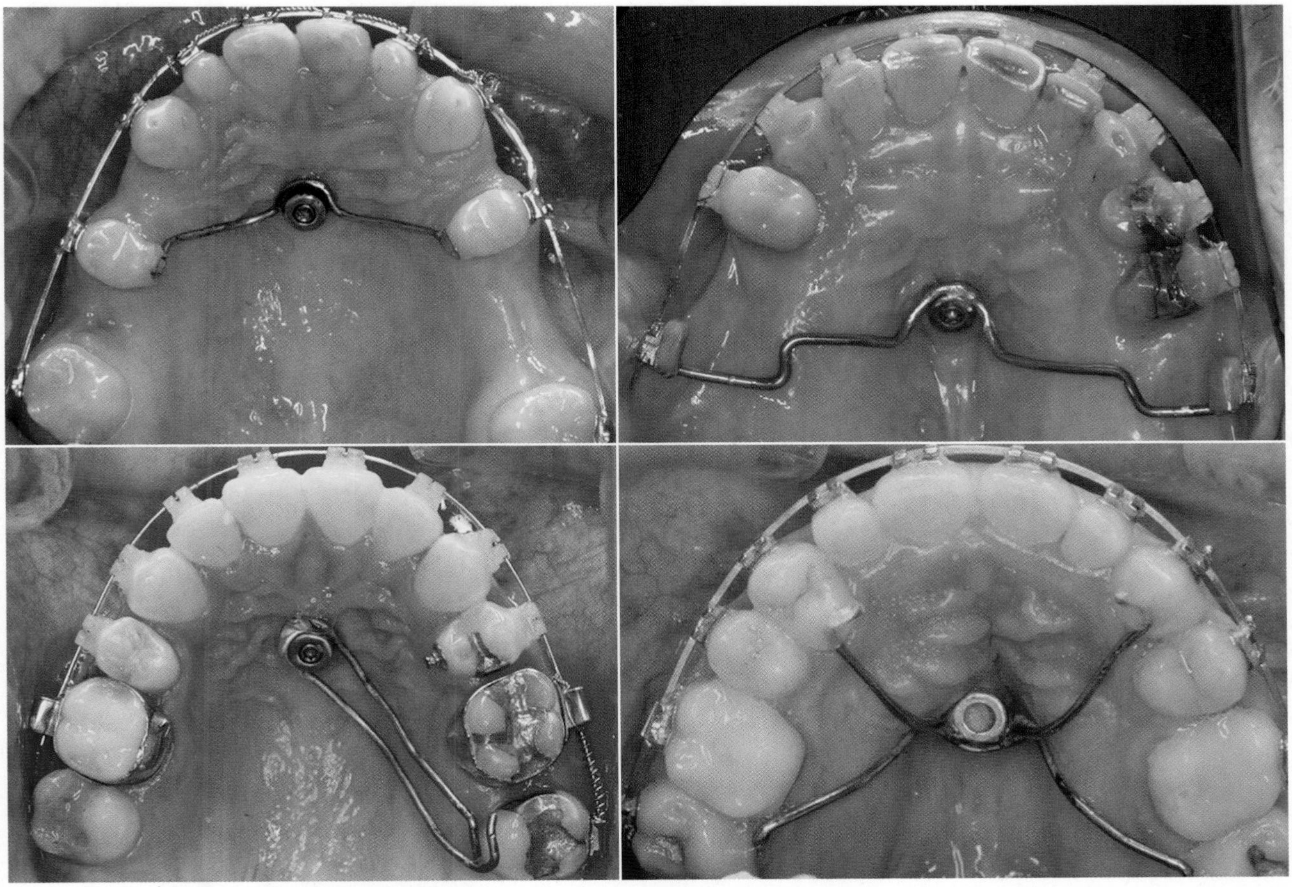

FIG 18-10 **A,** Palatal implant to stabilize arch and serve as anchor for movement of anterior teeth. **B,** Palatal implant to serve as leveling, intruding force, and retraction of maxillary anterior teeth. **C,** Palatal implant first used to distalize second molar and later to act as anchor for retraction of maxillary arch. **D,** Palatal implant used to intrude maxillary premolars and molars in an open bite patient.

inserting device. These implants do not integrate as completely as dental implants and thus may break free without a problem. If the implant does integrate, the risk of fracture is present when smaller implants are in place. A trephine would be necessary to fully remove any implant that does not easily come out or fractures.

SURGICAL PLATES

15. What is the impetus behind, the advantages of, and the disadvantages of surgical plates for orthodontic treatment?

Surgical plates have been used for orthodontic treatment to avoid structural contraindications with the mini-implants. Their advantage is the ability to provide anchorage while avoiding the problems that tooth roots, unattached gingiva, and sinus cavities pose for mini-implants. Surgical plates can be placed in the buccal mucosa of both the maxilla and mandible. Many systems use the maxillary cheek bones and zygomatic buttress as attachment sites.[44]

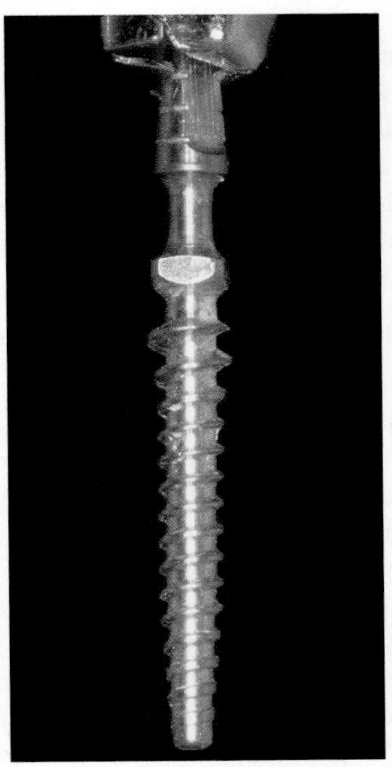

FIG 18-11 Mini-implant.

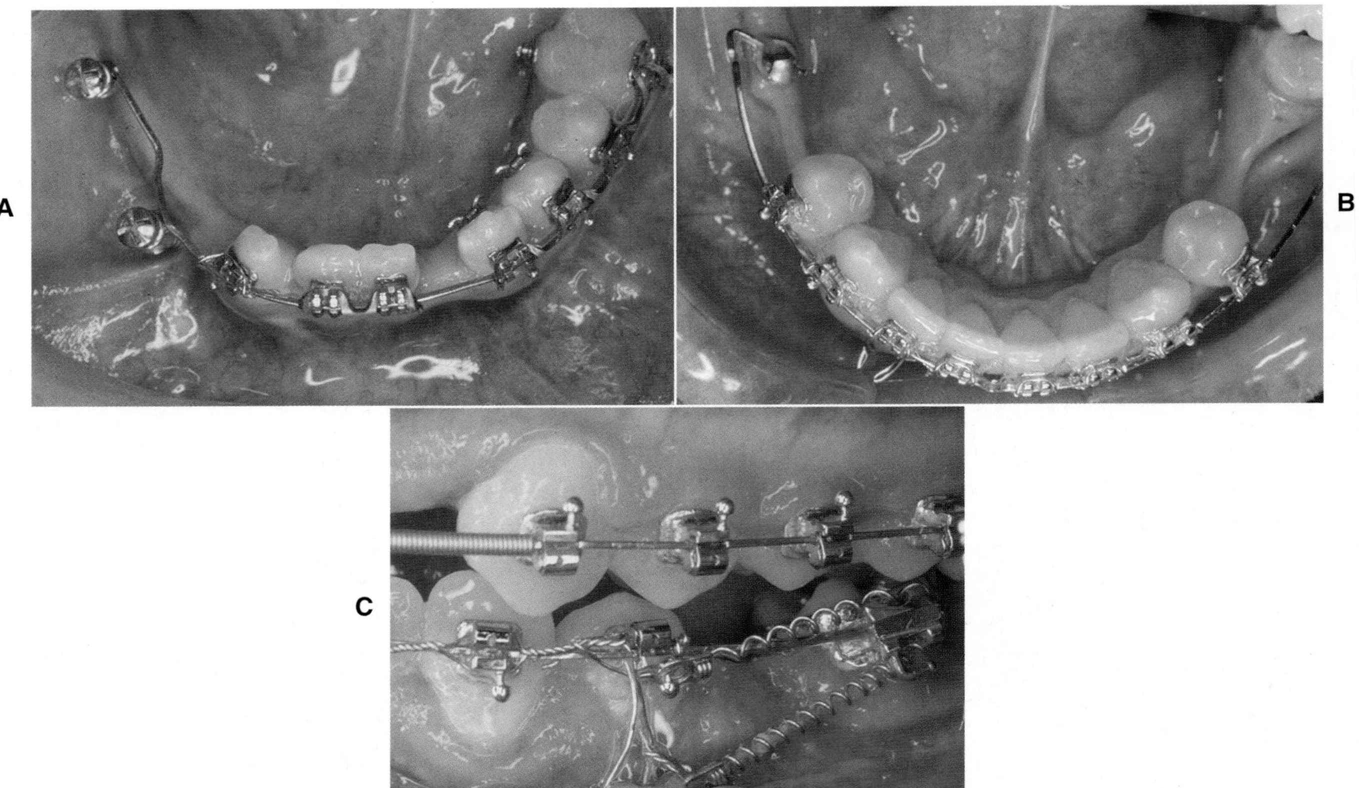

FIG 18-12 **A** and **B,** Mini-implant used to act as arch former and retractor of mandibular anterior teeth. **C,** Mini-implant used to protract mandibular molar.

Some of the disadvantages with the surgical plates are related to the surgical procedure itself. Obviously, with this type of implantable anchorage, a full-thickness flap and sutures would be required after surgical plate placement. Most clinicians will not find placement in the palatal vault a viable option. Lingual placement in the mandible is also not a likely option. Force vectors would need to be carefully considered, since most of the surgical plate attachment heads are deeper in the buccal vestibules. Removal would also require a surgical flap coupled with sutures.

16. What is the surgical process involved?

Surgical procedures for orthodontic plates almost exclusively require that a soft tissue flap is reflected. Obviously, local anesthetic and knowledge of suturing protocols are required. Plates are attached with any number of small screws depending on the shape, size, and location. Most of these screws do not need pilot drills for placement. Removal will require a flap to be raised to gain access and reversing torque on the screw heads holding the surgical plate in place. The surgeon would suture the flap for healing after removal. There is the chance that some bone could grow over parts of the plates, but this is usually removed easily if present.

FUTURE DIRECTIONS

17. What is the future of orthodontics and implants?

Implants will most certainly be used by a greater number of orthodontic clinicians in the years to come. As more and more orthodontic programs adopt implant-assisted orthodontic treatment into their clinical, research, and didactic curriculums, the proportion of clinicians comfortable with and willing to use TIAs will undoubtedly rise. Implants may not be the panacea for all orthodontic treatments, but they do afford the clinician the ability to treat their complicated, uncooperative, and anchorage-challenged patients with greater ease, less time, and simpler mechanics.

18. What are some of the future developments that we shall see with regard to implants for orthodontics?

Implants will continue to develop for orthodontic use, but design changes will most likely be limited to small specific items on the mini-implants. Dental implants will likely not change in response to any orthodontic usage. Although the onplant is rarely used today, the palatal implant's shape

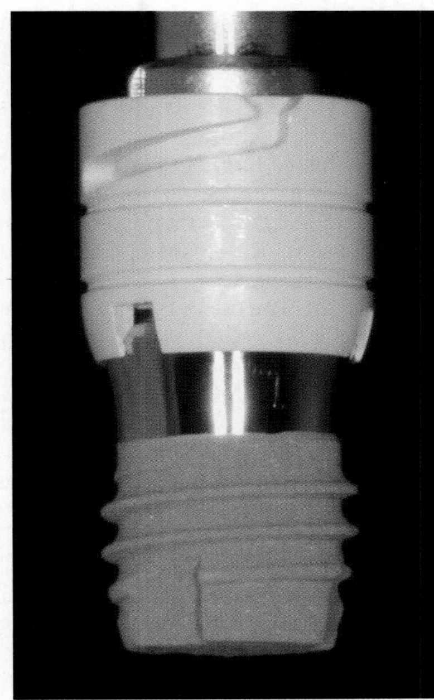

FIG 18-13 The latest palatal implant (due in 2007).

will remain fairly constant. The larger palatal implant is necessary for attachments, and this size difference also gives rise to its increased surface area and thus greater strength (Fig. 18-13)

As for mini-implants, thread pitch, intraoral implant top configuration, and surface treatments should dominate most of the advancements in the near future.[45] Survival rates of these implants would be greatly enhanced with roughened, and/or bioactive surfaces. Some feel a greater amount of osseointegration is a disadvantage for removal, but this may be more of a concern with only the smallest mini-implants because of the possibility of fracture. Most likely the greatest advances will come in the increase in survival percentages, not only initially, but throughout the course of force application, as well as a decrease in length of mini-implants.[46,47] Materials may change slightly but implant history has continually shown that commercially pure titanium is the most biocompatible and successful material to date.[48]

19. What are some of the legal implications when using implants in an orthodontic practice?

Probably the most overlooked item in relation to the application of implants in orthodontics is the legal implication. In a litigious society, one cannot afford to dismiss or ignore this aspect. When complications arise, there will be times when the qualifications of practitioners and their ability to handle complications will be reviewed. Even orthodontists that simply use implants are not immune from inclusion in legal entanglements. When negative outcomes occur because of the surgical placement, the orthodontic utilization, or the final result, litigation is a possibility.

In addition, any orthodontist who is placing implants should be certain that they are covered for these specific procedures by either their malpractice carrier or that of the institution where they are performing such procedures. Orthodontists that place implants should be certain of the basic surgical considerations that an experienced periodontist or oral surgeon would take. In addition, basic knowledge of many of the surgical aspects of this area of dentistry should be reviewed, including anesthesia, anatomical considerations, and proper preoperative and postoperative precautions.

20. Will implant-assisted orthodontic treatment become the standard of care?

Implant-assisted orthodontics will not become the absolute standard of care, just as rapid palatal expansion, cervical pull headgear, or nickel titanium wires are not the absolute standard of care. There are so many options and techniques available to orthodontists for treatment that to say one specific anchorage modality will become the standard of care is not plausible.

Implants will, however, become much more commonplace in orthodontic practices, simply by their ability to allow the practitioner to work faster with fewer anchorage concerns, rely on less patient cooperation, and tax the existing dentition to a lesser degree. Implants hold great promise for future orthodontic generations and will likely change the scope of our understanding and application of orthodontic treatment in ways we cannot foresee even today.

REFERENCES

1. Becker MJ: Ancient "dental implants": a recently proposed example from France evaluated with other spurious examples. *Int J Oral Maxillofac Implants* 1999;14(1):19-29.
2. Ring ME: A thousand years of dental implants: a definitive history—part 1. *Compend Contin Educ Dent* 1995; (10):1060, 1062, 1064 passim.
3. Brånemark PI, Adell R, Breine U, et al: Intra-osseous anchorage of dental prostheses. I. Experimental studies. *Scand J Plast Reconstr Surg* 1969;3(2):81-100.
4. Schroeder A, Pohler O, Sutter F: [Tissue reaction to an implant of a titanium hollow cylinder with a titanium surface spray layer]. *SSO Schweiz Monatsschr Zahnheilkd* 1976;86(7):713-727.
5. Thomas KA, Cook SD: An evaluation of variables influencing implant fixation by direct bone apposition. *J Biomed Mater Res* 1985;19(8):875-901.
6. Carlsson L, Rostlund T, Albrektsson B, Albrektsson T: Removal torques for polished and rough titanium implants. *Int J Oral Maxillofac Implants* 1988;3(1):21-24.
7. Brunski JB: Biomechanical factors affecting the bone-dental implant interface. *Clin Mater* 1992;10(3):153-201.
8. Buser D, Schenk RK, Steinemann S, et al: Influence of surface characteristics on bone integration of titanium implants. A histomorphometric study in miniature pigs. *J Biomed Mater Res* 1991;25:889-902.
9. Cochran DL, Schenk RK, Lussi A, et al: Bone response to unloaded and loaded titanium implants with a sandblasted and acid-etched surface: a histometric study in the canine mandible. *J Biomed Mater Res* 1998;40(1):1-11.

10. Lohmann CH, Sagun R Jr, Sylvia VL, et al: Surface roughness modulates the response of MG63 osteoblast-like cells to 1,25-(OH)(2)D(3) through regulation of phospholipase A(2) activity and activation of protein kinase A. *J Biomed Mater Res* 1999;47(2):139-151.
11. Gainsforth B, Higley L: A study of orthodontic anchorage possibilities in basal bone. *Am J Orthod Oral Surg* 1945;31:406-416.
12. Beder OE, Eade G: An investigation of tissue tolerance to titanium metal implants in dogs. *Surgery* 1956;39:470-473.
13. Roberts WE, Smith RK, Zilberman Y, et al: Osseous adaptation to continuous loading of rigid endosseous implants. *Am J Orthod* 1984;86(2):95-111.
14. Roberts WE, Helm FR, Marshall KJ, Gongloff RK: Rigid endosseous implants for orthodontic and orthopedic anchorage. *Angle Orthod* 1989;59(4):247-256.
15. Gray JB, Steen ME, King GJ, Clark AE: Studies on the efficacy of implants as orthodontic anchorage. *Am J Orthod* 1983;83(4):311-317.
16. Shapiro PA, Kokich VG: Uses of implants in orthodontics. *Dent Clin North Am* 1988;32(3):539-550.
17. Turley PK, Kean C, Schur J, et al: Orthodontic force application to titanium endosseous implants. *Angle Orthod* 1988;58(2): 151-162.
18. Triaca A, Antonini M, Wintermantel E: Ein neues Titan-Flachschrauben-Implantat zur orthodontischen Verankerung am anterioren Gaumen. *Informationen aus der orthodontischen Kieferorthopaedie* 1992;24:251-257.
19. Reitan K: Behavior of Malassez' epithelial rests during orthodontic tooth movement. *Acta Odontol Scand* 1961;19:443-468.
20. Frost HM: Mechanical determinants of bone modeling. *Metab Bone Dis Relat Res* 1982;4(4):217-229.
21. Reitan K: Biomechanical principles and reaction. In Graber, techniques, Philadelphia: W.B. Saunders, 1975.
22. Chen J, Chen K, Garetto LP, Roberts WE: Mechanical response to functional and therapeutic loading of a retromolar endosseous implant used for orthodontic anchorage to mesially translate mandibular molars. *Implant Dent* 1995;4(4):246-258.
23. Akin-Nergiz N, Nergiz I, Schulz A, et al: Reactions of peri-implant tissues to continuous loading of osseointegrated implants. *Am J Orthod Dentofacial Orthop* 1998;114(3):292-298.
24. Chen J, Esterle M, Roberts WE: Mechanical response to functional loading around the threads of retromolar endosseous implants utilized for orthodontic anchorage: coordinated histomorphometric and finite element analysis. *Int J Oral Maxillofac Implants* 1999;14(2):282-289.
25. Trisi P, Rebaudi A: Progressive bone adaptation of titanium implants during and after orthodontic load in humans. *Int J Periodontics Restor Dent* 2002;22(1):31-43.
26. Bartsch A, Witt E, Sahm G, Schneider S: Correlates of objective patient compliance with removable appliance wear. *Am J Orthod Dentofacial Orthop* 1993;104:378-386.
27. Smith RJ, Burstone CJ: Mechanics of tooth movement. *Am J Orthod* 1984;85:294-307.
28. Stewart CM, Chaconas SJ, Caputo AA: Effects of intermaxillary elastic traction on orthodontic tooth movement. *J Oral Rehabil* 1978;5:159-166.
29. Dougherty HL, Beazley WW: A biodifferential system of facebow mechanics. *Am J Orthod* 1976;70:505-516.
30. Kim TW, Kim H, Lee SJ: Correction of deep overbite and gummy smile by using a mini-implant with a segmented wire in a growing Class II Division 2 patient. *Am J Orthod Dentofacial Orthop* 2006;130:676-685.
31. Park HS, Kwon TG, Kwon OW: Treatment of open bite with microscrew implant anchorage. *Am J Orthod Dentofacial Orthop* 2004;126:627-636.
32. Odman J, Lekholm U, Jemt T, Thilander B: Osseointegrated implants as orthodontic anchorage in the treatment of partially edentulous adult patients. *Eur J Orthod* 1994;16:187-201.
33. Brunski JB, Moccia AF Jr, Pollack SR, et al: The influence of functional use of endosseous dental implants on the tissue-implant interface. I. Histological aspects. J Dent Res 1979;58: 1953-1969.
34. Higuchi KW, Slack JM: The use of titanium fixtures for intraoral anchorage to facilitate orthodontic tooth movement. *Int J Oral Maxillofac Implants* 1991;6:338-344.
35. Goodacre CJ, Brown DT, Roberts WE, Jeiroudi MT: Prosthodontic considerations when using implants for orthodontic anchorage. *J Prosthet Dent* 1997;77:162-170.
36. Roberts WE, Marshall KJ, Mozsary PG: Rigid endosseous implant utilized as anchorage to protract molars and close an atrophic extraction site. *Angle Orthod* 1990;60:135-152.
37. Wehrbein H, Merz BR, Diedrich P, Glatzmaier J: The use of palatal implants for orthodontic anchorage. Design and clinical application of the orthosystem. *Clin Oral Implants Res* 1996;7(4):410-416.
38. Wehrbein H, Glatzmaier J, Yildirim M: Orthodontic anchorage capacity of short titanium screw implants in the maxilla. An experimental study in the dog. *Clin Oral Implants Res* 1997;8(2):131-141.
39. Wehrbein H, Merz BR, Diedrich P: Palatal bone support for orthodontic implant anchorage–a clinical and radiological study. *Eur J Orthod* 1999;21(1):65-70.
40. Wehrbein H, Merz BR: Aspects of the use of endosseous palatal implants in orthodontic therapy. *J Esthet Dent* 1998;10(6): 315-324.
41. Kanomi R: Mini-implant for orthodontic anchorage. *J Clin Orthod* 1997;31:763-767.
42. Ohmae M, Saito S, Morohashi T, et al: A clinical and histological evaluation of titanium mini-implants as anchors for orthodontic intrusion in the beagle dog. *Am J Orthod Dentofacial Orthop* 2001;119:489-497.
43. Papadopoulos MA, Tarawneh F: The use of miniscrew implants for temporary skeletal anchorage in orthodontics: A comprehensive review. *Oral Surg Oral Med Oral Pathol Oral Radiol Endod* 2007;103(5):e6-15.
44. Umemori M, Sugawara J, Mitani H, et al: Skeletal anchorage system for open-bite correction. *Am J Orthod Dentofacial Orthop* 1999;115:166-174.
45. Berens A, Wiechmann D, Dempf R: Mini- and micro-screws for temporary skeletal anchorage in orthodontic therapy. *J Orofac Orthop* 2006;67:450-458.
46. Cheng SJ, Tseng IY, Lee JJ, Kok SH: A prospective study of the risk factors associated with failure of mini-implants used for orthodontic anchorage. *Int J Oral Maxillofac Implants* 2004;19:100-106.
47. Wiechmann D, Meyer U, Buchter A: Success rate of mini- and micro-implants used for orthodontic anchorage: a prospective clinical study. *Clin Oral Implants Res* 2007;18:263-267.
48. Morais LS, Serra GG, Muller CA, et al: Titanium alloy mini-implants for orthodontic anchorage: Immediate loading and metalion release. *Acta Biomater* 2007;3(3):331-339.

Mini-Screws and Palatal Implants for Orthodontic Anchorage

CHAPTER 19

Marc Schätzle

Anchorage is one of the limiting factors in orthodontics, and its control is essential for successful orthodontic treatment. The term *orthodontic anchorage* was first introduced by Angle[1] and later defined by Ottofy.[2] Orthodontic anchorage denoted the nature and degree of resistance to displacement of teeth offered by an anatomic unit when used for the purpose of tooth movement. The principle of orthodontic anchorage has been implicitly explained already in Newton's Third Law (1687) according to which an applied force can be divided into an *action* component and an equal and opposite *reaction* moment. In orthodontic treatment, reciprocal effects must be evaluated and controlled. The goal is to maximize desired tooth movement and minimize undesirable effects.

Basically, each tooth has its own anchorage potential as well as a tendency to move when force is applied toward the tooth. When teeth are used as anchorage, the inappropriate movements of the anchoring units may result in a prolonged treatment time and unpredictable or less-than-ideal outcomes.

Orthodontic anchorage is oriented to the quality of the biological anchorage of the teeth. This is influenced by a number of factors, such as the size of the root surfaces available for periodontal attachment, the height of the periodontal attachment, the density and structure of the alveolar bone, the turnover rate of the periodontal tissues, the muscular activity, the occlusal forces, the craniofacial morphology and the nature of the tooth movement planned for the intended correction.[3] To maximize tooth-related anchorage, techniques such as differential torque,[4] placement of roots into the cortex of the bone,[5] and distal inclination of the molars[6,7] may be used. If the periodontal anchorage is inadequate with respect to the intended treatment goal, additional intraoral and/or extraoral anchorage may be needed to avoid negative effects. Although the teeth are the most frequent anatomic units used for anchorage in orthodontic therapy, other structures such as the palate, the lingual mandibular alveolar bone, the occipital bone, and the neck are also alternatives.

Additional anchorage such as extraoral and intraoral forces are visible and compliance dependent and are associated with the risk of undesirable effects such as tipping of the occlusal plane, protrusion of mandibular incisors, and extrusion of teeth.

Implants, mini-screws, and ankylosed teeth, as they are in direct contact with bone, do not possess a normal periodontal ligament. Consequently, they do not move when orthodontic forces are applied[8] and hence can be used for "absolute anchorage" that is independent of the patient's compliance.

The aim of this chapter is to present skeletal anchorage to be integrated into orthodontic treatment as "absolute anchorage," thereby avoiding the disadvantages listed previously.

1. Historically, what kind of anchorage devices preceded mini-screws and palatal implants ?

The first known attempt to achieve skeletal anchorage was made in 1945 by Gainsforth and Higley.[9] They placed vitallium screws in the ramus of dog mandibles and then immediately applied elastics from the screw to the maxillary arch wire in order to tip or retract the canines (Fig. 19-1). Tooth movement was successfully

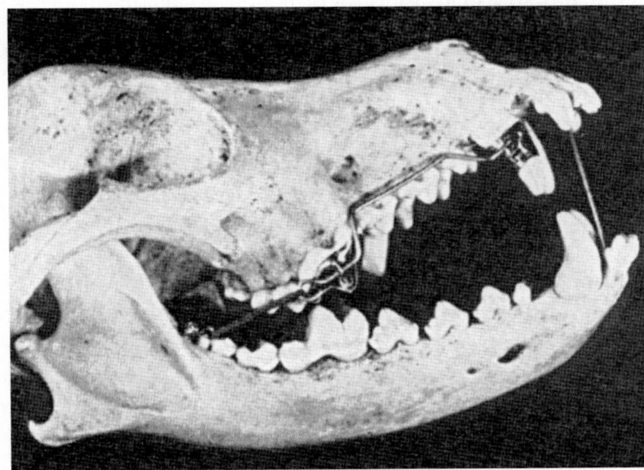

FIG 19-1 Skull of dog with orthodontic appliance using vitallium screw anchorage. Force is applied through traction of the elastic that connects two hooks. The arch wire is welded to the canine band and slides freely in the perforated buccal flange of the molar overlay. (From Gainsforth BL, Higley LB: *Am J Orthod Oral Surg* 1945;31:406-416.)

accomplished in two cases, but an effective force could not be maintained longer than 1 month in any case. This may have been due to infection and the immediate loading of the screw.

Later, skeletal anchorage systems evolved from two lines. One line originated from dental implants, which have a solid scientific base of clinical, biochemical, and histological studies. The other one developed from screws used in traumatology and orthognathic surgery.

Linkow[10] reported using blade implants as anchorage to retract teeth with rubber bands; however, long-term results were never presented. Later Ödman et al.[11] and Shapiro and Kokich[12] suggested using endosseous implants. This resulted in the development of specially designed implants to the retromolar area[13] and to the palatal site of the maxilla introduced by Triaca et al.[14]

The other category developed from surgical screws. The first clinical report of the use of a temporary anchorage device (TAD) appeared in 1983, when Creekmore and Eklund[15] used a vitallium bone screw to treat a patient with a deep overbite. The screw was inserted into the anterior nasal spine; 10 days after its placement, the screw was used to intrude the upper incisors by an elastic thread from the screw to the incisors. Kanomi[16] first described a mini-implant specially designed for orthodontic use.

2. How can the skeletal anchorage be classified?

Currently available skeletal anchorage devices can be classified either as biocompatible or biological. Ankylosed teeth are biological anchorage units.

Biocompatible skeletal TADs can be further subclassified based first on the nature of mechanical retention in the bone (modification of surgical fixation methods), such as fixation wires,[17] fixation screws,[15] fixation screws in combination with mini-plates[18] and mini-screws.[16] The second basis is the biological osseointegration such as endosseous prosthetic implants[11,12] (Fig. 19-2). Since orthodontic patients do not usually display edentulous alveolar bony ridges for the insertion of an implant, special implants for orthodontic anchorage purposes were developed for the retromolar[13] and palatal areas.[14]

From a clinical point of view, it is relevant whether implants are to be used only as TADs or subsequently to be used as abutment for supporting prosthetic appliances. These aspects determine insertion sites, implant types, and dimensions, as well as type of orthodontic anchorage. Moreover, the fact that these devices may have to be placed in a growing patient is of particular importance.

Another device, the Onplant®,[19] placed subperiostally, is a smooth titanium disc with a hydroxyapatite-coated surface that is supposed to connect to the bone. Because of the submerged installation, the monitoring of the healing process of these Onplants may be troublesome and their osseointegration may be questioned.[20]

3. What is the definition of temporary anchorage devices?

A TAD is a device that is placed into bone in order to enhance orthodontic anchorage. They either support the anchorage teeth or act by themselves as the anchorage element/unit. They are temporary and are subsequently removed after use. They can be located on the bone surface (transosteal), under the periosteum (subperiosteal), or inside the bone (endosteal) and can be fixed to bone either mechanically (cortically stabilized) or biologically (osseointegration). It should also be pointed out that dental implants placed for the purpose of supporting prosthesis, regardless of the fact that they may be used for orthodontic anchorage, are not conceptually considered TADs since they are not removed after orthodontic treatment. Importantly, the incorporation of dental implants and TADs into orthodontic treatment makes *absolute anchorage* possible, which has been defined in terms of implants as showing no movement (no anchorage loss) as a consequence of reaction forces.[21]

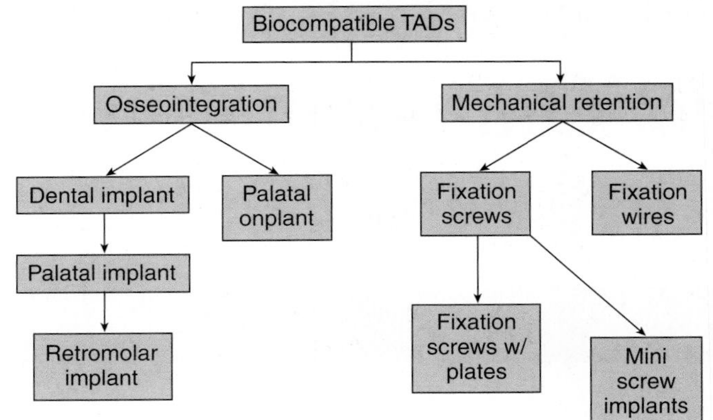

FIG 19-2 Biocompatible temporary anchorage devices. (From Cope JB. *Semin Orthod* 2005;11:3-9.)

4. Where can implants used as temporary anchorage be placed?

Since orthodontic patients do not normally display edentulous alveolar bony ridges for the insertion of an implant, implants for orthodontic anchorage must be placed in areas other than the usual topographical locations foreseen for the replacement of missing teeth. Besides the installation of orthodontic anchorage implants into the retromolar area of the mandible,[13,22] the midsagittal palatal region[14,19,23] had initially been proposed.

Incomplete closure of the median palatal suture during childhood and early adolescence, however, prevents placement of orthodontic implants into the midsagittal region of fully grown adolescents and adults because of possible developmental disturbances of the palatal suture.[23,24] The paramedian insertion site is therefore a potential alternative in young patients. Furthermore, the exact site chosen for palatal implants should be carefully evaluated to avoid perforations of the inferior nasal turbinate.[23]

5. Where can mini-screws or similar devices be placed as temporary anchorage?

The introduction of small temporary orthodontic anchorage devices such as mini-screws (<2 mm) in various lengths[16,25] and titanium pins,[26] as well as L-shaped mini-plates with the long arm exposed into the oral cavity[18] and the zygomatic anchors[27] both fixed by bone screws, offered new additional insertion sites: the interradicular septum,[16,26] the supra-apical and infra-zygomatical area,[16,18,25,27] and the mandibular symphysis.[25]

Through an analysis of panoramic radiographs and computed tomographic (CT) images, adequate bone for mini-screw placement exists primarily in the maxillary (mesial to first molars) and mandibular (mesial and distal to first molars) posterior regions. Typically, adequate interradicular bone distance was found more than halfway down the root length, which is likely to be covered by movable mucosa.[28,29] Inability to place mini-screws in attached gingiva may necessitate design modification or oblique insertion direction to decrease soft-tissue irritation.[29,30] The absence of keratinized mucosa around mini-screws significantly increases the risk of infection and failure.

6. What kind of imaging measures are recommended prior to palatal implant insertion?

Presurgical dental CT and/or lateral cephalograms have been recommended to evaluate vertical bone volume of the hard palate, which determines whether palatal implants can be used. Examinations of the palate have shown that the vertical bone volume commonly decreases posteriorly.

Dental CT of the alveolar process is well established for the evaluation of the alveolar bone volume before implant placement.[31] It can also be used to assess the hard palate and is currently the most accurate tool for measuring the vertical bone volume at this site. Bernhart et al.[32] found the greatest mean of about 6 to 9 mm posterior to the foramen incisivum in the midsagittal plane. To avoid the midpalatal suture, the suitable area for implant placement is located 6 to 9 mm posterior to the foramen incisivum and 3 to 6 mm paramedian. If the suitable bone volume for an insertion of implants is defined as 4 mm or more, Bernhart et al.[32] found that 95% of the patients in their study had enough bone vertically for accommodating palatal implants with a length of 4 mm, which correlates with the clinical experience of Schiel et al.[33] However, a preoperative diagnostic evaluation is recommended in order to avoid perforation of the inferior nasal turbinate.

Wehrbein et al.[34] insisted on obtaining precise information for the intended implant site before placing palatal implants to avoid perforations of the nasal cavity. For this purpose, in lateral cephalograms the vertical bone volume along the palatal suture was evaluated presurgically. Since these are already used for orthodontic diagnosis and treatment planning, patients are spared from additional radiation exposure.

The vertical bone level in the anterior and middle thirds of the hard palate is at least 2 mm higher vertically than seen on lateral cephalograms. A safety margin of at least 2 mm is recommended when planning treatment on the basis of lateral cephalograms to avoid potential complications.[34] But it must be considered that even though some implants are projecting beyond the nasal floor in lateral cephalograms, they can cause false-positive results and could not be related to actual penetrations into the nasal cavity (Fig. 19-3).[35]

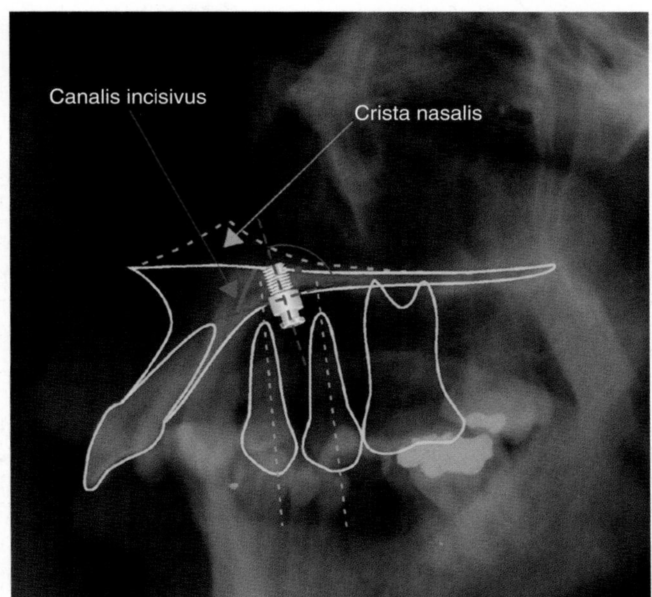

FIG 19-3 Most palatal implants are installed satisfactorily when the location of entry into the cortical bone is at the anteroposterior level of the maxillary first and second premolars—perpendicular to the palatal surface.[62] (From Männchen R, Schätzle M: *Clin Oral Implants Res* [submitted].)

7. Are imaging measures needed prior to mini-screw insertion?

A panoramic radiograph, normally available from pretreatment diagnostic records, is usually sufficient for establishing the insertion areas outside the alveolar process. Where a mini-screw is to be inserted into the alveolar process, a periapical radiograph taken with an acrylic or putty-based template serves as a guideline for establishing the exact height and orientation of the mini-screw.[17]

In addition, devices such as an adjustable surgical guide,[36] the use of a surgical stent[37] or the surgical index[38,39] have also been proposed for evaluating the proper insertion site.

8. Do palatal implants placed in the midpalatal suture have an effect on the transverse maxillary growth?

During normal growth, maxillary expansion in the transverse direction is a result of two processes: appositional remodeling of the alveolar processes and growth in the midpalatal suture. It has been estimated that growth in the maxillary width is an average of 3 mm between ages 10 and 18 years.[40] Therefore, the question arises if implantation of an orthodontic anchorage in the midpalatal suture has an effect on the normal transverse growth.

It has been shown in an experimental study[41] that the placement of a palatal implant in the midpalatal suture has a restricting effect on the transverse maxillary growth.

Deficient transverse maxillary growth may also cause maxillary arch length discrepancies leading, for example, to upper canine impaction. To prevent possible restriction in normal transverse maxillary growth, insertion of palatal implants paramedially in growing individuals is recommended.

Furthermore, placement of implants in the midpalatal suture in growing patients may be contraindicated because of the questionable quality of bone in that area.[42] On the other hand, the paramedian region of the anterior palate is highly stable from the growth point of view.[43]

9. Do palatal implants have an influence on the vertical growth of the maxilla and its dentition?

The most important vertical growth changes occur through displacement and cortical drift. By implant placement in the palate, the sutural lowering of the maxillary complex as well as the apposition at the orbital floor and at the infrazygomatic crest will not be affected; however, the resorptive lowering of the nasal floor and the increase of the alveolar bone height of the maxilla may be influenced. Björk and Skieller[40] measured the mean degree of growth from the age of 4 to adulthood. During this time the nasal floor drifts 4.6 mm caudally and the height of the maxillary alveolar bone increases 14.6 mm. Assuming that about one third of these growth changes take place from the age of 12 years to adulthood, that implies a residual vertical growth of about 1.5 mm in the palate and about 5 mm in the alveolar bone (both by drift).

As discussed before, osseointegrated implants are in direct contact with bone, do not possess a periodontal ligament, and behave like ankylosed teeth. Therefore, a palatal implant would remain 1.5 mm behind its surrounding bone whereas an implant placed in the alveolar bone would produce an infraocclusion of 5 mm in the same time. Consequently, a palatal implant directly or indirectly attached to teeth would lead to an infraeruption of a single tooth, several teeth, or the whole upper dentition, respectively.

Finally, it must be remembered that palatal implants as TADs just remain 1 to 2 years in situ. Thus, potential vertical growth impairment is likely to be limited to values of less than 1 mm.

10. When can the palatal implants be loaded after surgical replacement?

In some cases there is a premature loss of the implant prior to orthodontic load. This loss may be caused by the lack of sufficient primary stability. An insufficient primary stability, which is one of the most critical factors in osseointegration, causes an inappropriate healing and a possible premature loss of the implant.[44,45]

Following the placement of an endosseous implant, primary mechanical stability is gradually replaced by biological, secondary stability (Fig. 19-4). The transition from primary mechanical stability, provided by the implant design, to biological stability, provided by newly formed bone as osseointegration, occurs during early wound healing.[46] There is, therefore, a period of time during healing in which osteoclastic activity has

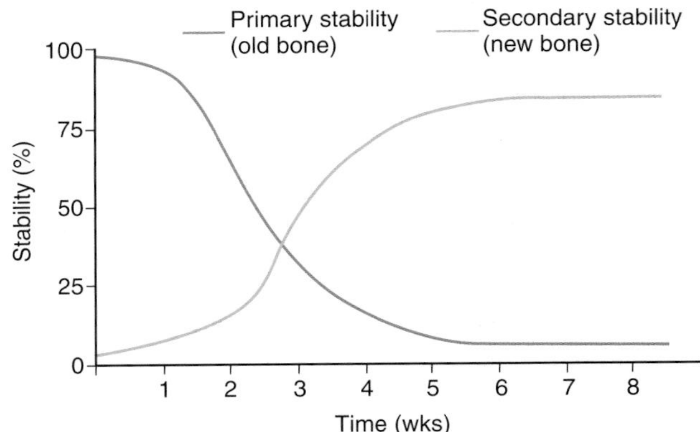

FIG 19-4 Changeover from primary stability created at the time of implant placement to secondary stability created by deposition of new bone (osseointegration) in humans. (From Raghavendra S, Wood MC, Taylor TD: *Int J Oral Maxillofac Implants* 2005;20:425-431).

decreased the initial mechanical stability of the implant but the formation of new bone has not yet occurred to the level required to maintain implant stability.

In orthodontic treatment the placement of an implant as an absolute anchorage device facilitates and accelerates the therapy[47] despite an inactive waiting time of at least 3 months after insertion.[24,48-50] Even though there are several studies that have reported a successful outcome of early or immediate loaded conventional dental implants placed in the alveolar ridge,[51-56] there is a lack of reliable data about adequate healing time in the palatal region. However, there is some evidence that the healing time of 12 weeks, as recommended by the producer, could be reduced.[57]

11. What is the clinical procedure and loading time schedule for palatal implants?

The patient's stress during implantation is reduced by applying a minimally traumatic surgical technique. Under palatal local anesthesia, the palatal mucosa is perforated to the cortical bone using a mucosal punch and removed with an elevator or a curette.

After smoothing the exposed bone surface to prevent the profile drill from slipping, the center of the implant site is marked with a round bur. The implant bed is then prepared to the required depth using a series of pilot and twist drills. The drilling axis perpendicular to the bone surface is defined based on the presurgical cephalometric analysis. While the insertion site is prepared, intermediate drilling and cooling of the drilling channel continuously with precooled physiological saline or Ringer's solution should be performed. The implant is then hand-installed as far as possible, and a ratchet is used to tighten the implant to its final position.

The implant is covered with the healing cap to prevent the inner screw well of the implant from clogging up and from being covered by hyperplastic mucosal tissue. After insertion, the palatal Orthosystem® implant is allowed to heal in situ for 12 weeks during which it should not be loaded.

12. What is the clinical procedure for mini-screws?

The mini-screws are inserted into areas that are not blocked by the roots. There are situations, although rarely, where minor tooth movements are necessary to create adequate space to facilitate mini-screw insertion between the roots.

Only a small amount of local anesthetic solution is needed for the mini-screw installation, since it is not necessary to achieve a profound anesthesia of the teeth. When anesthetizing the mucosa, the needle can probe and measure the mucosal thickness to help determine the appropriate length of the mini-screw.

After the mucosa is cleaned with chlorhexidine, the intended mini-screw site is marked with a probe. Further procedures depend on the characteristics of the mini-screw to be used. When a self-drilling screw is used, the insertion is done directly through the mucosa. With the insertion of a self-tapping mini-screw, a bed is first drilled with a low-speed contraangle handpiece under saline solution irrigation followed by the implant installation. The mini-screw is then inserted manually with a screwdriver or hand-driver with a torque gauge.

Following insertion, the head of the mini-screw remains outside the mucosa in the attached gingiva, with the base of the head resting on, but not compressing, the mucosa.

If the intended installation site for the mini-screw is in the movable mucosa, an incision has to be performed to prevent soft-tissue roll-up around the drill or the mini-screw, respectively.

13. What happens after root injury from mini-screws?

Insertion of mini-screws in the alveolar process between roots of teeth is a critical procedure. Even if preventive measurements are taken, such as apical radiograph before insertion of the screw, root damage can occur. In an experimental study,[41] at least three roots were damaged by the mini-screws. In all cases, the same observations were made on the radiographs and the histological slides: a defect was seen in the root, but an almost complete repair of the cementum lining the root occurred in a period of 18 weeks and started, at the earliest, 12 weeks after the screw was removed.

14. What is the loading time schedule for mini-screws?

The majority of the publications on this issue are case reports and technical descriptions. A systematic review of the loading time for mini-screws[58] shows that forces ranging from 150 to 500 g immediately after insertion of the screws have been successfully used. A waiting time of at least 2 weeks is recommended by some studies before loading the screws with a force of 100 to 400 g.

Two experimental studies[59,60] and a recent clinical study[61] maintain that immediate loading can be performed without loss of stability. Finally, it must be kept in mind that the short waiting period is sufficient for healing but not for osseointegration.

15. How can the palatal implants be loaded?

Depending on the clinical situation and the orthodontic treatment plan, palatal implants can be loaded either indirectly or directly. Indirect loading[23] means that the teeth act as an anchorage unit, indirectly stabilized by the palatal implant to avoid anchorage loss. This is achieved with a transpalatal arch (TPA) (Fig. 19-5, *A*).

In direct anchorage, the force systems act directly between the teeth to be moved and the implant[62] (Fig. 19-5, *B*).

16. How can the mini-screws be loaded?

The mechanics used in relation to the application of mini-screws depends on whether the mini-screw is being used as direct or indirect anchorage. For direct anchorage, the line of action of the force has to pass through the mini-screw. If the line of action of the force does not pass through the mini-screw, as would be the case of a power arm, a force away from the mini-screw long axis would be generated, thereby creating a moment that results in a shearing force. Since these mini-screws are not osseointegrated, a shearing force would likely lead to screw loosening and failure. For indirect anchorage, the mini-screw can be ligated to a tooth or a group of teeth via a full-sized rectangular stainless-steel wire. The tooth or group of teeth stabilized with the mini-screw can then be used as absolute anchorage.[17]

17. Do palatal implants remain stable under orthodontic loading, and what is the reaction in the adjacent bone?

Despite small dimensions, orthodontic palatal implants must stay positionally stable under orthodontic loading in order to serve as absolute anchorage. Therefore, osseointegration is needed.

Osseointegration was first defined on a histological basis only as direct contact between an implant surface and bone without interposed soft tissue at light microscopic level.[63] However, complete (100%) bone connection to the implant may not occur. Instead of the histologic definition of osseointegration, a stability-based definition has been proposed. Osseointegration was then defined as "a process whereby clinically asymptomatic rigid fixation of alloplastic material is achieved, and maintained, in bone during functional loading."[64]

Histologic examination of the bone specimens around explanted human palatal orthodontic implants revealed that osseointegration is maintained during long-term orthodontic loading. The percentage of implant-to-bone contact in the removed implants was an average of 75% (range between 34% and 93%)[65] showing comparable results as osseointegrated prosthetic endosseous implants yielding at least 60% of bone implant contact.[66]

Palatal implants, however, should not only fulfill prosthetic stability, but must also withstand the stress and strain applied during orthodontic treatment. But there are substantial differences between orthodontic forces and occlusal loading. Orthodontic

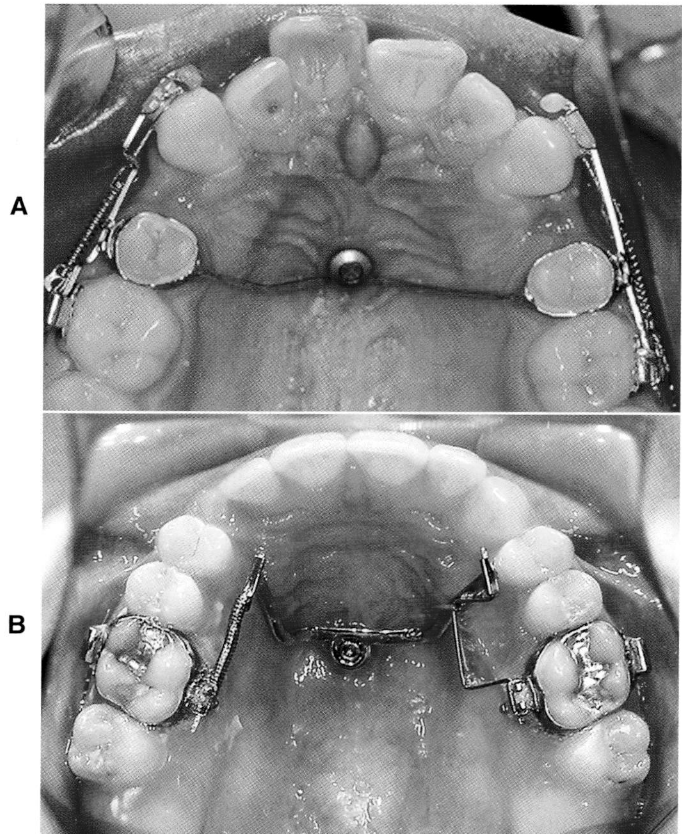

FIG 19-5 **A,** Indirect anchorage. **B,** Direct anchorage. (**A** from Wehrbein H, Merz BR, Diedrich P, Glatzmaier J: *Clin Oral Implants Res* 1996;7:410-416. **B** from Büchter A, Wiechmann D, Gaertner C, et al: *Clin Oral Implants Res* 2006;17:714-722.)

forces are continuous and horizontal; occlusal loads, in contrast, are discontinuous and mainly in a vertical direction.

The effect of orthodontic loading to the adjacent bone of the implant is of great interest, especially when an implant is used after the intended orthodontic treatment for prosthetic purposes. The applied forces should not have a negative impact on the periimplant bone and should therefore not impair the long-term prognosis as a prosthetic abutment.

In a study by Melsen and Lang,[8] specially designed oral implants were inserted in monkeys and, after healing, subjected to well-defined continuous loading. This study supports the theory that apposition of bone around an oral implant is the biological response to a mechanical stress below a certain threshold, whereas loss of marginal bone or complete loss of osseointegration may be the result of mechanical stress exceeding a certain force magnitude.

18. Do mini-screws remain stable under orthodontic loading?

Even though mini-screws have been used in recent years in orthodontics, it is still not clear if they remain absolutely stationary under loading. There is only one study to determine any movement of mini-screws.[67] In 7 out of 16 examined patients, the mini-screws tipped and were extruded and did not remain stable under orthodontic loading. In an animal study, mini-screws with as little as 5% bone contact at the bone-implant interface successfully resisted orthodontic force.[68] Thus, despite the fact that mini-screws increase anchorage, they do not remain absolutely stationary throughout orthodontic loading.

19. What is the clinical procedure after completion of the orthodontic treatment with palatal implants?

Palatal implants are usually removed after completion of the orthodontic treatment. By means of a system-compatible trephine, the peri-implant bone is separated from the device. Then the implant may be explanted together with the surrounding bone by slow rotations with an extraction forceps. As a variation, the implant-bone-contact may be broken by turning the ratchet used for seating the implant counterclockwise. After explanation, possible oral-nasal communication must be verified and treated if necessary. Full recovery at the original anchorage site may be observed 3 to 4 weeks after implant removal.

20. What is the clinical procedure after completion of the orthodontic treatment with mini-screws?

The removal procedure is usually completed uneventfully and the mini-screws are often removed with topical anesthesia, or at most, local anesthesia. The custom-made screwdriver of the manufacturer is used to unscrew the mini-screw. In the rare case where the mini-screw is so tight that it is difficult to unscrew, just the act of attempting to unscrew the mini-screw usually causes local microfractures or bone remodeling sufficient to loosen the mini-screw after a few days. No soft tissue closure is necessary.

21. What is the success rate of palatal implants?

Even though palatal implants have been used in orthodontic treatment for more than 10 years,[23] only one prospective study of nine patients exists to demonstrate successful osseointegration and stability in all patients.[34] More recently a subjective report of 40 Orthosystem palatal implants was published[69] and indicated a 92% success rate of osseointegration.

A recent clinical study[70] reported that only 1 (1.5%) out of the 67 successfully osseointegrated palatal implants that were loaded actively and/or passively for approximately 19 months failed. This report documented success rates for palatal implants after orthodontic loading comparable to those reported for conventional oral implants.[71,72]

REFERENCES

1. Angle EH: *Treatment of malocclusion of teeth*, edition 7. Philadelphia: S. S. White Dental Manufacturing, 1907.
2. Ottofy L: *Standard dental dictionary*. Chicago: Laird and Lee, 1923.
3. Diedrich P: Different orthodontic anchorage systems. A critical examination. *Fortschritte der Kieferorthopädie* 1993;54:156-171.
4. Burstone CJ: The segmented arch approach to space closure. *Am J Orthod* 1982;82:361-378.
5. Ricketts RM: Bioprogressive therapy as an answer to orthodontic needs. Part II. *Am J Orthod* 1976;70:359-397.
6. Begg PR, Kesling PC: The differential force method of orthodontic treatment. *Am J Orthod* 1977;71:1-39.
7. Tweed CH: The applications of the principles of the edgewise arch in the treatment of malocclusions. *Angle Orthod* 1941;11:12-67.
8. Melsen B, Lang NP: Biological reactions of alveolar bone to orthodontic loading of oral implants. *Clin Oral Implants Res* 2001;12:144-152.
9. Gainsforth BL, Higley LB: A study of orthodontic anchorage possibilities in basal bone. *Am J Orthod Oral Surg* 1945;31:406-417.
10. Linkow LI: The endosseous blade implant and its use in orthodontics. *Int J Orthod* 1969;7:149-154.
11. Ödman J, Lekholm U, Jemt T, et al: Osseointegrated titanium implants—a new approach in orthodontic treatment. *Eur J Orthod* 1988;10:98-105.
12. Shapiro PA, Kokich VG: Uses of implants in orthodontics. *Dent Clin North Am* 1988;32:539-550.
13. Roberts WE, Marshall KJ, Mozsary PG: Rigid endosseous implant utilized as anchorage to protract molars and close an atrophic extraction site. *Angle Orthod* 1990;60:135-152.
14. Triaca A, Antonini M, Wintermantel E: Ein neues Titan-Flachschrauben-Implantat zur orthodontischen Verankerung am anterioren Gaumen. *Informationen aus Orthodontie und Kieferorthopädie* 1992;24:251-257.
15. Creekmore TD, Eklund MK: The possibility of skeletal anchorage. *J Clin Orthod* 1993;17:266-269.
16. Kanomi R: Mini-implant for orthodontic anchorage. *J Clin Orthod* 1997;31:763-767.
17. Melsen B, Petersen JK, Costa A: Zygoma ligatures: an alternative form of maxillary anchorage. *J Clin Orthod* 1998;32:154-158.
18. Umemori M, Sugawara J, Mitani H, et al: Skeletal anchorage system for open-bite correction. *Am J Orthod Dentofacial Orthop* 1999;115:166-174.
19. Block MS, Hoffman DR: A new device for absolute anchorage for orthodontics. *Am J Orthod Dentofacial Orthop* 1995;3:251-258.
20. Celenza F, Hochman MN: Absolute anchorage in orthodontics: direct and indirect implant-assisted modalities. *J Clin Orthod* 2000;34:397-402.
21. Daskalogiannakis J: *Glossary of orthodontic terms*. Leipzig: Quintessence Publishing, 2000.
22. Higuchi KW, Slack JM: The use of titanium fixtures for intraoral anchorage to facilitate orthodontic tooth movement. *Int J Oral Maxillofac Implants* 1991;6:338-344.
23. Wehrbein H, Merz BR, Diedrich P, Glatzmaier J: The use of palatal implants for orthodontic anchorage. Design and clinical application of the orthosystem. *Clin Oral Implants Res* 1996;7:410-416.
24. Glatzmaier J, Wehrbein H, Diedrich P: Die Entwicklung eines resorbierbaren Implantatsystems zur orthodontischen Verankerung. *Fortschritte der Kieferorthopädie* 1995;56:175-181.
25. Costa A, Raffaini M, Melsen B: Miniscrews as orthodontic anchorage: a preliminary report. *Int J Adult Orthod Orthognath Surg* 1998;13:201-209.
26. Bousquet F, Bousquet P, Mauran G, Parguel P: Use of an impacted post for anchorage. *J Clin Orthod* 1996;30:261-265.
27. De Clerck H, Geerinckx V, Siciliano S: The Zygoma Anchorage System. *J Clin Orthod* 2002;36:455-459.
28. Schnelle MA, Beck FM, Jaynes RM, Huja SS: A radiographic evaluation of the availability of bone for placement of miniscrews. *Angle Orthod* 2004;74:832-837.
29. Deguchi T, Nasu M, Murakami K, et al: Quantitative evaluation of cortical bone thickness with computed tomographic scanning for orthodontic implants. *Am J Orthod Dentofacial Orthop* 2006;129:e712-721.
30. Park HS, Jeong SH, Kwon OW: Factors affecting the clinical success of screw implants used as orthodontic anchorage. *Am J Orthod Dentofacial Orthop* 2006;130:18-25.
31. Lindh C, Petersson A, Klinge B: Measurements of distances related to the mandibular canal in radiographs. *Clin Oral Implants Res* 1995;6:96-103.
32. Bernhart T, Vollgruber A, Gahleitner A, et al: Alternative to the median region of the palate for placement of an orthodontic implant. *Clin Oral Implants Res* 2000;11:595-601.
33. Schiel HJ, Klein J, Widmer B: Das enossle Implantat als kieferorthopädisches Verankerungselement. *Zeitschrift für Zahnärztliche Implantologie* 1996;12:183-188.
34. Wehrbein H, Merz BR, Diedrich P: Palatal bone support for orthodontic implant anchorage—a clinical and radiological study. *Eur J Orthod* 1999;21:65-70.
35. Crismani AG, Bernhart T, Tangl S, et al: Nasal cavity perforation by palatal implants: false-positive records on the lateral cephalogram. *Int J Oral Maxillofac Implants* 2005;20:267-273.
36. Suzuki EY, Buranastidporn B: An adjustable surgical guide for miniscrew placement. *J Clin Orthod* 2005;39:588-590.
37. Cousley RR, Parberry DJ: Surgical stents for accurate miniscrew insertion. *J Clin Orthod* 2006;40:412-417.
38. Bae SM, Park HS, Kyung HM, et al: Clinical application of micro-implant anchorage. *J Clin Orthod* 2002;36:298-302.
39. Maino BG, Bednar J, Pagin P, Mura P: The spider screw for skeletal anchorage. *J Clin Orthod* 2003;37:90-97.
40. Björk A, Skieller V: Growth of the maxilla in three dimensions as revealed radiographically by the implant method. *Br J Orthod* 1997;4:53-64.

41. Asscherickx K, Hanssens JL, Wehrbein H, Sabzevar MM: Orthodontic anchorage implants inserted in the median palatal suture and normal transverse maxillary growth in growing dogs: a biometric and radiographic study. *Angle Orthod* 2005;75: 826-831.
42. Bernhart T, Freudenthaler J, Dortbudak O, et al: Short epithetic implants for orthodontic anchorage in the paramedian region of the palate—a clinical study. *Clin Oral Implants Res* 2001;12: 624-631.
43. Thilander B: Basic mechanisms in craniofacial growth. *Acta Orthop Scand* 1991;53:144-151.
44. Friberg B, Jemt T, Lekholm U: Early failures in 4,641 consecutively placed Brånemark dental implants: a study from stage 1 surgery to the connection of completed prostheses. *Int J Oral Maxillofac Implants* 1991;6:142-146.
45. Lioubavina-Hack N, Lang NP, Karring T: Significance of primary stability for osseointegration of dental implants. *Clin Oral Implants Res* 2006;17:244-250.
46. Berglundh T, Abrahamsson I, Lang NP, Lindhe J: De novo alveolar bone formation adjacent to endosseous implants. *Clin Oral Implants Res* 2003;14:251-262.
47. Trisi P, Rebaudi A: Progressive bone adaptation of titanium implants during and after orthodontic load in humans. *Int J Period Restor Dent* 2003;22:31-43.
48. Keles A, Erverdi N, Sezen S: Bodily distalization of molars with absolute anchorage. *Angle Orthod* 2003;73:471-482.
49. Crismani AG, Bernhart T, Bantleon H-P, Cope JB: Palatal implants: the Straumann orthosystem. *Semin Orthod* 2005;11: 16-23.
50. Crismani AG, Bernhart T, Bantleon H-P, Kucher G: An innovative adhesive procedure for connecting transpalatal arches with palatal implants. *Eur J Orthod* 2005;27:226-230.
51. Calandriello R, Tomatis M, Rangert B: Immediate functional loading of Brånemark Systems implants with enhanced initial stability: a prospective 1 to 2 year clinical & radiographic study. *Clin Implant Dent Rel Res* 2003;5(Suppl 1):10-20.
52. Rocci A, Martignoni M, Burgos PM, et al: Histology of retrieved immediately and early loaded oxidized implants: light microscopic observations after 5 to 9 months of loading in the posterior mandible. *Clin Implant Dent Rel Res* 2003;5(Suppl 1):88-98.
53. Bischof M, Nedir R, Szmukler-Moncler S, et al: Implant stability measurement of delayed and immediately loaded implants during healing. *Clin Oral Implants Res* 2004;15:529-539.
54. Gallucci GO, Bernard JP, Bertosa M, Belser UC: Immediate loading with fixed screw retained provisional restorations in edentulous jaws: the pickup technique. *Int J Oral Maxillofac Implants* 2004;19:524-533.
55. Glauser R, Sennerby L, Meredith N, et al: Resonance frequency analysis of implants subjected to immediate or early functional occlusal loading. Successful vs. failing implants. *Clin Oral Implants Res* 2004;15:428-434.
56. Jaffin RA, Kumar A, Berman CL: Immediate loading of dental implants in the completely edentulous maxilla: a clinical report. *Int J Oral Maxillofac Implants* 2004;19:721-730.
57. Crismani AG, Bernhart T, Schwarz K, et al: Ninety percent success in palatal implants loaded 1 week after placement: a clinical evaluation by resonance frequency analysis. *Clin Oral Implants Res* 2006;17:445-450.
58. Ohashi E, Pecho OE, Moron M, Lagravere MO: Implant vs. screw loading protocols in orthodontics. *Angle Orthod* 2006;76:721-727.
59. Dalstra M, Cattaneo PM, Melsen B: Load transfer of mini screws for orthodontic anchorage. *Orthodontics* 2005;1:53-62.
60. Büchter A, Wiechmann D, Koerdt S, et al: Load-related implant reaction of mini-implants used for orthodontic anchorage. *Clin Oral Implants Res* 2005;16:473-479.
61. Büchter A, Wiechmann D, Gaertner C, et al: Load-related bone modeling at the interface of orthodontic micro-implants. *Clin Oral Implants Res* 2006;17:714-722.
62. Melsen B, Verna C: Miniscrew Implants: The Aarhus Anchorage System. *Semin Orthod* 2005;11:24-31.
63. Albrektsson T, Brånemark PI, Hansson HA, Lindstrom J: Osseointegrated titanium implants. Requirements for ensuring a long-lasting, direct bone-to-implant anchorage in man. *Acta Orthop Scand* 1991;52:155-170.
64. Zarb GA, Albrektsson T: Osseointegration: a requiem for periodontal ligament? *Int J Period Restor Dent* 1991;11:88-91.
65. Wehrbein H, Merz BR, Hämmerle CH, Lang NP: Bone-to-implant contact of orthodontic implants in humans subjected to horizontal loading. *Clin Oral Implants Res* 1998;9:348-353.
66. Nyström E, Kahnberg KE, Gunne J: Bone grafts and Brånemark implants in the treatment of the severely resorbed maxilla: a 2-year longitudinal study. *Int J Oral Maxillofac Implants* 1993;8:45-53.
67. Liou EJW, Pai BCJ, Lin JCY: Do miniscrews remain stationary under orthodontic forces? *Am J Orthod Dentofacial Orthop* 2004;126:42-47.
68. Deguchi T, Takano-Yamamoto T, Kanomi R, et al: The use of small titanium screws for orthodontic anchorage. *J Dent Res* 2003;82:377-381.
69. Bantleon HP, Bernhart T, Crismani AG, Zachrisson BJ: Stable orthodontic anchorage with palatal osseointegrated implants. *World J Orthod* 2002;3:109-116.
70. Männchen R, Schätzle M: Success rates of palatal orthodontic implants. A retrospective cohort study. *Clin Oral Implants Res* (accepted).
71. Berglundh T, Persson L, Klinge B: A systematic review of the incidence of biological and technical complications in implant dentistry reported in prospective longitudinal studies of at least 5 years. *J Clin Periodontol* 2002;29:197-202.
72. Pjetursson BE, Brägger U, Lang NP, Zwahlen M. Comparison of survival and complication rates of tooth-supported fixed dental prostheses (FDPs) and implant-supported fixed dental prostheses and single crowns (SCs). *Clin Oral Implants Res* 2007;18(Suppl 3):73-85.

Oral Hygiene: Possible Problems and Complications

CHAPTER 20

Frank Tsung-Ju Hsieh • David A. Covell, Jr.

"First, do no harm" is a fundamental guiding principle in medicine and dentistry. All too often orthodontists are confronted with having to consider this principle with a patient who develops poor oral hygiene partway through the orthodontic treatment. Clearly the placement of orthodontic brackets, wires, etc. creates a challenging environment for maintaining good oral hygiene. While there are measures that can be used to maintain or improve a patient's hygiene, these may not always be effective for reasons most often related to patient compliance. If unaddressed, the accumulation of bacterial plaque associated with poor hygiene may lead to demineralization of enamel and the appearance of white spot lesions, an early sign of caries formation. In addition, the bacteria growing on the teeth and orthodontic appliance will cause inflammation of the gingival tissues, a process demonstrated by enlargement or overgrowth of interdental papillae and gingival margins. Although gingivitis is reversible in most individuals, there are situations in which patients are particularly prone to gingival overgrowth (e.g., caused by genetic variations in the response of gingival tissue or side effects of medications needed for systemic health). For these patients, resumption of good oral hygiene may be inadequate, making other procedures necessary to restore normal gingival architecture. Lastly, with increasing numbers of adults seeking orthodontic treatment, more patients will have had or will need periodontal treatment prior to orthodontics, and the orthodontist will be confronted with coordinating the timing of orthodontic treatment following periodontal therapy. The questions that follow relate to the areas briefly described above and should be useful for the appreciation of some aspects of the relationship between orthodontics and periodontology.

1. What are evidence-based recommendations regarding the most effective means of preventing white spot lesions in orthodontic patients?

Systematic reviews have concluded that toothpastes with fluoride concentrations of 1500 to 5000 ppm demonstrate greater preventive effects for white spot lesion formation than those with a concentration of 1000 ppm.[1,2] In addition, supplemental use of a brush-on gel with 5000 ppm fluoride once a day has more of a preventive effect than conventional fluoride toothpaste alone.[3] The use of a polymeric tooth coating[4] or sealant[5] on the tooth surface around the brackets has been shown to have little impact on demineralization.

2. Do mouth rinses impact gingivitis?

A number of oral rinses and dentifrices have been tested in clinical trials.[6] One standard for proving the efficacy of these products for the treatment of gingivitis was implemented by the American Dental Association (ADA). The ADA Seal of Acceptance is given to a product that reduces plaque and demonstrates effective reduction of gingival inflammation over a period of at least 6 months. The agent must also be safe and not induce adverse side effects. Several products have been given the ADA Seal of Acceptance for the control of gingivitis. In one of the products the active ingredients are thymol, menthol, eucalyptol, and methyl salicylate.[7] Active ingredients in other products are chlorhexidine digluconate and triclosan.[7]

Side effects of chlorhexidine digluconate include tooth and tongue staining, increased calculus deposits, bitter taste, mouth and throat irritation, mouth sores (ulcers), coated tongue, and changes in taste of food and beverages.

If properly used, the addition of a topical antiplaque agent to a gingivitis treatment regimen for patients with deficient plaque control will likely result in the reduction of gingivitis.[8] However, experimental evidence indicates that penetration of topically applied agents into the gingival crevice is minimal.[9] Therefore, these agents are useful for the control of supragingival, but not subgingival, plaque. Among individuals who do not demonstrate excellent oral hygiene, supragingival irrigation with or without medicaments may reduce gingival inflammation beyond that normally achieved by toothbrushing alone. This effect is likely due in part to the flushing out of subgingival bacteria.[10]

3. Is oral hygiene better using a power toothbrush compared with a manual toothbrush?

Powered brushes have been defined as toothbrushes with a mechanical movement of the brush head. Powered brushes have been divided into six groups depending on their mode of action[11]:

1. **Side-to-side action:** brush head moves laterally with a side-to-side motion.
2. **Circular:** brush head rotates in one direction only.
3. **Rotation oscillation:** brush head rotates in one direction and then the other.
4. **Counter oscillation:** adjacent tufts of bristles (usually 6–10) rotate in one direction and then the other, independently. Each tuft rotates in the opposite direction to that adjacent to it.
5. **Ultrasonic:** brush bristles vibrate at ultrasonic frequencies (i.e., above 20 kHz).
6. **Unknown action:** indicates a brush action that the reviewers were unable to establish from either the trial report or the manufacturers.

Numerous clinical trials have compared manual and powered toothbrushes for their effectiveness in improving oral health, and the results are often conflicting.[11] Recent systematic reviews by the Cochrane Oral Health Group have summarized this information and provided unbiased conclusions.[12] Powered brushes reduced plaque and gingivitis at least as effectively as manual brushing. Rotation oscillation powered brushes showed statistically significant reductions of plaque and gingivitis in both the short[13] and long term.[12,13] No solid evidence was found for a higher efficacy of sonic brushes.

The systematic reviews just described used studies of general populations and were not orthodontic specific.[12,13] There is a clear need for long-term trials on the efficacy of powered brushes in the orthodontic patient population. From existing studies it can be concluded that compared with a manual toothbrush, orthodontic patients using a powered toothbrush will show a slight, but significant, reduction of bleeding on probing.[14] No conclusions can be made concerning which type of powered brush works best.[14]

4. Which oral prophylaxis technique is better for orthodontic patients: air-powder polishing system or rubber cup and pumice technique?

The conventional rubber cup prophylaxis (RCP) and the air powder polishing (APP) system (Prophy Jet) are both effective professional techniques for plaque and stain removal without detrimental effects on tooth structure and gingival tissues when used correctly.[15-17] The APP system uses a jet formed by a mixture of air, powder, and water to remove dental plaque, soft deposits and surface stains from pits, grooves, interproximal spaces, and smooth surfaces of the teeth. Barnes and associates[18] showed that the use of the APP system in orthodontic patients neither affected the composite resin or zinc-phosphate cement used to secure brackets and bands, nor caused any damage to arch wires or other appliances. Ramaglia and colleagues[19] used a split-mouth experimental design to compare the efficacy and efficiency of the APP system with the RCP technique. Significant reductions in the plaque index were found after either APP or RCP. APP was somewhat more efficient, requiring significantly less time to remove dental plaque and staining.

5. Are there ways to prevent periodontal complications during orthodontic treatment?

The use of steel rather than elastic ligatures has been recommended on brackets, including tooth-colored ("esthetic") brackets, because elastomeric rings have been shown to attract significantly more plaque than steel ligatures.[20] Use of self-ligating brackets may have a similar effect as steel ligation, but this has yet to be documented. In addition, bonded brackets are preferable to bands as demonstrated during orthodontic treatment of adults where molars with bonded brackets showed less plaque accumulation, gingivitis, and loss of attachment interproximally than did those with bands.[20-22]

It is evident in adults with a reduced but healthy periodontium that orthodontic tooth movement can be performed without further periodontal deterioration.[23-25] After a 4- to 6-month observation period following periodontal treatment, a careful clinical examination and recording of the periodontal status is necessary before orthodontic treatment is initiated. Professional scaling may be especially indicated during active intrusion of elongated maxillary incisors when new attachment is desired[26,27] since orthodontic intrusion may shift supragingival plaque to a subgingival location.[28,29] Should efforts aimed at maintaining excellent-to-good oral hygiene prove unsuccessful, termination of orthodontic treatment (appliance removal) has been recommended.[30]

6. When can orthodontic treatment be started on a patient who has been treated for periodontitis?

Following active periodontal treatment, patients in the maintenance phase of periodontal therapy should be observed for 4 to 6 months before initiating orthodontic treatment. This provides time for full expression of the benefits of the periodontal therapy and for monitoring of the patient's oral hygiene and motivation.[31] Once orthodontic treatment is started, periodontal maintenance should be scheduled at shorter intervals, in many instances with the patient being seen as frequently for periodontal maintenance as for orthodontic appliance adjustments (i.e., every 4–6 weeks).[32]

7. Are patients who have been previously treated for periodontal disease more likely to lose periodontal attachment if they receive orthodontic treatment?

Tooth movement in adults with reduced but healthy periodontium does not result in further significant loss of attachment.[33] However, adults with teeth that do not have healthy periodontal tissues may experience further breakdown and tooth loss because of abscesses during orthodontic treatment.[33] In patients (mostly adults) with active periodontitis (that is, plaque-infected deep pockets evidenced by bleeding on probing), orthodontic tooth movement may accelerate the disease process, even when good oral hygiene is practiced.[34-38]

8. Is orthodontic treatment a risk factor for gingival recession?

Gingival recession is frequently seen in teeth that are positioned labially relative to the supporting alveolus, irrespective of a history of orthodontic treatment. The most important etiologic factor in gingival recession relates to the reduced thickness of the soft tissue and bone, especially on the labial surface of labially prominent teeth.[39-43] This thin soft tissue and/or bone is a predisposing factor for gingival recession.[40] In fact, vertical loss of buccal or labial bone (dehiscence) is a prerequisite for recession.[40] Other common factors in the development of recession are age and trauma, the latter caused, for example, by improper tooth brushing or gingival lesions associated with bacterial plaque.[41]

There is evidence to suggest that the "zone" or apico-coronal height of keratinized tissue is not related to gingival recession, whereas the thickness of the keratinized tissue is an important factor. A long-term study of a non-orthodontic population has shown that the incidence of recession in areas without keratinized tissue is no greater than that found in areas with a wide expanse of keratinized tissue.[43] In contrast, orthodontic tooth movement in a labial direction in areas of thin labial tissue can result in bone dehiscence, creating an environment in which plaque and/or toothbrush trauma may cause sudden recession.[44-50] If thick gingival tissue is present in these areas, gingival recession is less likely to occur.[44,45,48-50] Thus, there is general agreement that thin labial tissue should be augmented before labial orthodontic tooth movement is begun.[44,45,48-50] It is interesting to note that for a labially positioned tooth and dehiscence, bone may form and gingival thickness increase when the tooth is moved lingually.[51-53]

In regard to the relationship between rapid maxillary expansion procedures and gingival recession, Graber and Vanarsdall[44] note that if the maxillary expansion is performed after the midpalatine suture begins to fuse (after approximately 14–16 years of age), there is a greater risk later in life of recession of the buccal gingival tissue of the maxillary premolars and molars.

9. What is the best way to manage patients predisposed to gingival overgrowth during orthodontic treatment?

There are many causes of *gingival overgrowth,* a term now favored by periodontists instead of *"gingival hyperplasia."* In many patients, proper oral hygiene is sufficient to achieve normal, healthy gingiva. In some situations, however, gingival overgrowth is drug induced or can be a manifestation of a genetic disorder. The latter may exist as an isolated abnormality or as part of a syndrome. If orthodontic treatment is needed in patients with gingival overgrowth, both orthodontic and periodontal factors should be considered. For example, in a case report of extreme hereditary gingival fibromatosis, the patient was treated periodontally prior to orthodontic treatment by removal of all gingival excess using flaps and gingivectomies.[54] After a follow-up period, orthodontic treatment was started with fixed appliances. Monthly periodontal check-ups (scaling and polishing) were scheduled to control the gingival inflammation. After the orthodontic treatment, permanent retention was applied, followed again by a complete gingivectomy in both the maxilla and mandible.

Gingival overgrowth occurs in about 50% of persons taking phenytoin (Dilantin).[55-59] Lesions may involve the interproximal spaces and become so extensive that the teeth are displaced and their crowns covered. Gingival enlargement is also seen in several blood dyscrasias. This form of gingival dysplasia is seen in acute monocytic, lymphocytic, or myelocytic leukemia. Thrombocytopenia and thrombocytopathy can also cause gingival enlargement and spontaneous bleeding. In some individuals, gingival enlargement progresses rapidly into destructive periodontal disease as a result of an altered immune response of the gingiva to the bacterial plaque. A slowly progressive fibrous enlargement of the maxillary and mandibular gingiva is a feature of idiopathic fibrous hyperplasia of the gingiva.

Characteristically, this massive gingival enlargement may cover the tooth surfaces and displace the teeth, and although the cause of the disease is unknown, there appears to be a genetic predisposition.[60,61]

Depending on home care and the relationship between the gingival tissue and the crown of the tooth, gingival hyperplasia is frequently reversible, especially after orthodontic appliances have been removed.[62] Alternatively, Graber and Vanarsdall[63] suggest that some patients may benefit from the removal of excessive gingival tissue around the crowns of the teeth, which may add to the stability of the orthodontic correction.

10. What is the relationship of periodontal regeneration procedures and orthodontic tooth movement?

Guided tissue regeneration (GTR) facilitates repair of alveolar ridge defects through the use of barriers (resorbable or nonresorbable), with or without bone grafting. Several case presentations have demonstrated that following repair of osseous defects with GTR, orthodontic tooth movement can be accomplished without adverse effects on periodontal support.[64-67] For example, following tooth movement, new bone and clinical attachment formed by GTR were found to be stable for up to 6 years.[67] In these cases, tooth movement was initiated after radiographic confirmation that the defects had been filled with bone at 5 to more than 11 months following GTR.[65-67]

Although we were unable to find more rigorous clinical studies that investigated an appropriate time to wait between GTR and the start of orthodontic tooth movement, animal studies using dogs have demonstrated that orthodontic tooth movement can be started as early as 2 months following GTR.[68] This delay was thought necessary to prevent mechanical tooth movement from interfering with the healing process of the periodontal tissues, such as accelerating membrane absorption.[68] The period of 60 days was based on previous animal studies evaluating periodontal regeneration from 60 to 90 days after treatment, where advanced healing of the periodontal tissues was found after 60 days.[68-71] Treatment of Class II furcation lesions in a dog model demonstrated that a 60-day delay in orthodontic movement did not interfere with healing or adversely impact the amount of bone regenerated by the regenerative periodontal techniques.[68,70,72,73] It should be noted that the bone remodeling cycle (sigma) in dogs is 3 months, whereas it is 4.25 months for humans,[74] thus healing to a comparable level will likely take longer in humans.

It can be concluded that in a healthy environment, orthodontic tooth movement does not adversely impact periodontal results achieved with GTR. Additional research is needed to improve our knowledge regarding how soon orthodontic treatment can follow GTR without adversely impacting the repair process. Extrapolating from animal studies, an appropriate time may turn out to be 3 to 4 months, similar to that recommended following other periodontal surgical procedures.

REFERENCES

1. Derks A, Katsarosa C, Frencken JE, et al: Caries-inhibiting effect of preventive measures during orthodontic treatment with fixed appliances. *Caries Res* 2004;38:413-420.
2. D'Agostino RB, Cancro LP, Fischman S: Effects of anticaries dentifrices on orthodontic subjects. *Comp Con Educ Dent* 1988;11:S384-S389.
3. Alexander SA, Ripa LW: Effects of self-applied topical fluoride preparations in orthodontic patients. *Angle Orthod* 2000;70:424-430.
4. Fornell AC, Sköld-Larsson K, Hallgren A, et al: Effect of a hydrophobic tooth coating on gingival health, mutans streptococci, and enamel demineralization in adolescents with fixed orthodontic appliances. *Acta Odontol Scand* 2002;60:37-41.
5. Wenderoth CJ, Weinstein M, Borislow AJ: Effectiveness of a fluoride-releasing sealant in reducing decalcification during orthodontic treatment. *Am J Orthod Dentofacial Orthop* 1999;116:629-634.
6. Hancock EB: Prevention. *Ann Periodont* 1996;1:223-249.
7. Mandel ID: Antimicrobial mouthrinses: overview and update. *J Am Dent Assoc* 1994;125(Suppl 2):2S-10S.
8. Brecx M, Brownstone E, MacDonald L, et al: Efficacy of Listerine, Meridol, and chlorhexidine as supplements to regular tooth-cleaning measures. *J Clin Periodontol* 1992;19:202-207.
9. Pitcher GR, Newman HN, Strahan JD: Access to subgingival plaque by disclosing agents using mouthrinsing and direct irrigation. *J Clin Periodontol* 1980;7:300-308.
10. The American Academy of Periodontology: *The Role of Supra- and Subgingival Irrigation in the Treatment of Periodontal Diseases (position paper)*, Chicago: The American Academy of Periodontology; April 1995.
11. Davies RM: Manual versus powered toothbrushes: what is the evidence? *Dent Update* 2006;33(3):159-162.
12. Deery C, Heanue M, Deacon S, et al: The effectiveness of manual versus powered toothbrushes for dental health: a systematic review. [Review]. *J Dent* 2004;32(3):197-211.
13. Sicilia A, Arregui I, Gallego M, et al: A systematic review of powered vs manual toothbrushes in periodontal cause-related therapy. *J Clin Periodontol* 2002;29(Suppl 3):39-54.
14. Sicilia A, Arregui I, Gallego M, et al: Home oral hygiene revisited. Options and evidence. *Oral Health Prev Dent* 2003;1 (Suppl 1):407-422.
15. Willmann DE, Norling BK, Johnson WN: A new prophylaxis instrument: effect on enamel alterations. *J Am Dent Assoc* 1980;101:923-925.
16. Weaks LM, Lescher NB, Barnes CM, Holroyd SV: Clinical evaluation of the Prophy-Jet as an instrument for routine removal of tooth stain and plaque. *J Periodontol* 1984;55:486-488.
17. Mishkin DJ, Engler WO, Javed T, et al: clinical comparison of the effect on the gingiva of the Prophy-Jet and the rubber cup and paste techniques. *J Periodontol* 1986;57:151-154.
18. Barnes CM, Russell CM, Gerbo LR, et al: Effects of an air-powder polishing system on orthodontically bracketed and banded teeth. *Am J Orthod Dentofacial Orthop* 1990;97:74-81.
19. Ramaglia L, Sbordone L, Ciaglia RN, et al: A clinical comparison of the efficacy and efficiency of two professional prophylaxis procedures in orthodontic patients. *Eur J Orthod* 1999;21:423-428.
20. Forsberg CM, Brattstrom V, Malmberg E, Nord CE: Ligature wires and elastomeric rings: Two methods of ligation, and their association with microbial colonization of *Streptococcus mutans* and *lactobacilli*. *Eur J Orthod* 1991;17:417-420.
21. Zachrisson BU: Bonding in orthodontics. In Graber TM, Vanarsdall RL Jr, editors: *Orthodontics: current principles and techniques*, edition 2. St Louis: Mosby, 1994, pp 542-626.
22. Boyd RL, Baumrind S: Periodontal considerations in the use of bonds or bands on molars in adolescents and adults. *Angle Orthod* 1992;62:117-126.
23. Boyd RL, Leggott PJ, Quinn RS, et al: Periodontal implications of orthodontic treatment in adults with reduced or normal periodontal tissues versus those of adolescents. *Am J Orthod Dentofacial Orthop* 1989;96:191-199.
24. Zachrisson BU: Periodontal changes during orthodontic treatment. In McNamara JA Jr, Ribbens KA, editors: *Orthodontic treatment and the periodontium.* Monograph 15, Craniofacial Growth Series, Center for Human Growth and Development, Ann Arbor: The University of Michigan, 1984, pp 43-65.
25. Artun J, Urbye KS: The effect of orthodontic treatment on periodontal bone support in patients with advanced loss of marginal periodontium. *Am J Orthod Dentofacial Orthop* 1988;93:143-148.
26. Melsen B, Agerbaek N, Eriksen J, Terp S: New attachment through periodontal treatment and orthodontic intrusion. *Am J Orthod Dentofacial Orthop* 1988;94:104-116.
27. Melsen B, Kragskov J: Tissue reaction to intrusion of periodontally involved teeth. In Davidovitch Z, editor: *The Biological Mechanisms of Tooth Movement and Craniofacial Adaptation.* Columbus, OH: The Ohio State University, College of Dentistry, 1992, pp 423-430.
28. Ericsson I, Thilander B, Lindhe J, Okamoto H: The effect of orthodontic tilting movements on the periodontal tissues of infected and non-infected dentitions in the dog. *J Clin Periodontol* 1977;4:115-127.
29. Ericsson I, Thilander B, Lindhe J: Periodontal condition after orthodontic tooth movements in the dog. *Angle Orthod* 1978;48:210-218.
30. Machen DE: Periodontal evaluation and updates: Don't abdicate your duty to diagnose and supervise. *Am J Orthod Dentofacial Orthop* 1990;98:84-85.
31. Zachrisson BU: Clinical implications of recent orthodontic-periodontic research findings. *Semin Orthod* 1996;2:4-12.
32. Proffit WR, Fields HW Jr: Special considerations in comprehensive treatment of adults. In Rudolph P, editor: *Contemporary orthodontics.* St Louis: Mosby, 2000, p 658.
33. Boyd RL, Leggott PJ, Quinn RS, et al: Periodontal implications of orthodontic treatment in adults with reduced or normal periodontal tissues versus those of adolescents. *Am J Orthod Dentofacial Orthop* 1989;96:191-198.
34. Artun J, Osterberg SK: Periodontal status of teeth facing extraction sites long-term after orthodontic treatment. *J Periodontol* 1987;58:24-29.

35. Thilander B: Infrabony pockets and reduced alveolar bone height in relation to orthodontic therapy. *Semin Orthod* 1996;2:55-61.
36. Ericsson I, Thilander B, Lindhe J: Periodontal condition after orthodontic tooth movements in the dog. *Angle Orthod* 1978;48:210-218.
37. Ericsson I, Thilander B, Lindhe J, Okamoto H: The effect of orthodontic tilting movements on the periodontal tissues of infected and non-infected dentitions in dogs. *J Clin Periodontol* 1977;4:278-293.
38. Zachrisson BU, Alnaes L: Periodontal condition in orthodontically treated and untreated individuals. I. Loss of attachment, gingival pocket depth and clinical crown height. *Angle Orthod* 1973;43:402-411.
39. Bernimoulin JP, Curiloviec Z: Gingival recession and tooth mobility. *J Clin Periodontol* 1977;4:107-114.
40. Maynard JG, Ochsenbein LD: Mucogingival problems, prevalence and therapy in children. *J Periodontol* 1975;46:543-552.
41. Vanarsdall RL, Corn H: Soft-tissue management of labially positioned unerupted teeth. *Am J Orthod* 1977;72:53-64.
42. Wennström JL: The significance of the width and thickness of the gingiva in orthodontic treatment. *Dtsch Zahnarztl Z* 1990;45:136-141.
43. Wennström JL: Mucogingival surgery. In Lang NP, Karring T, editors: *Proceedings of the 1st European Workshop on Clinical Periodontology*. Berlin: Quintessence, 1994:113-209.
44. Graber TM, Vanarsdall RL: *Orthodontics: current principles and techniques*, edition 2. St Louis: Mosby, 1994, pp 719-749.
45. Wennström JL: Mucogingival considerations in orthodontic treatment. *Semin Orthod* 1996;2:46-54.
46. Årtun J, Osterberg SK, Kokich VG: Long-term effect of thin interdental alveolar bone on periodontal health after orthodontic treatment. *J Periodontol* 1986;57:341-346.
47. Årtun J, Krogstad O: Periodontal status of mandibular incisors following excessive proclination: a study in adults with surgically treated mandibular prognathism. *Am J Orthod Dentofacial Orthop* 1997;91:225-232.
48. Coatoam GW, Behrents RG, Bissada NF: The width of keratinized gingiva during orthodontic treatment: its significance and impact on periodontal status. *J Periodontol* 1981;52:307-313.
49. Foushee DG, Moriarty JD, Simpson DM: Effects of mandibular orthognathic treatment on mucogingival tissue. *J Periodontol* 1985;56:727-733.
50. Maynard JG: The rationale for mucogingival therapy in the child and adolescent. *Int J Period Restor Dent* 1987;7:37-51.
51. Karring T, Numan S, Thilander B, Magnusson I: Bone regeneration in orthodontically produced alveolar bone dehiscences. *J Periodont Res* 1982;17:309-315.
52. Steiner GG, Pearson JK, Ainamo J: Changes of the marginal periodontium as a result of labial tooth movement in monkeys. *J Periodontol* 1981;52:314-320.
53. Wennstrom JL, Lindhe J, Sinclair F, Thilander B: Some periodontal tissue reactions to orthodontic tooth movement in monkeys. *J Clin Periodontol* 1987;14:121-129.
54. Clocheret K, Dekeyser C, Carels C, Willems G: Idiopathic gingival hyperplasia and orthodontic treatment: a case report. *J Orthod* 2003;30:13-19.
55. Stinnett E, Rodu B, Grizzle WE: New developments in understanding phenytoin-induced gingival hyperplasia. *J Am Dent Assoc* 1987;114:814-816.
56. Dooley G, Vasan N: Dilantin hyperplasia: a review of the literature. *J NZ Soc Periodontol* 1989;68:19-21.
57. Hall WB: Dilantin hyperplasia: a preventable lesion. *Compendium* 1990 (Suppl);14:S502-505.
58. Hassell TM, Hefti AF: Drug-induced gingival overgrowth: old problem, new problem. *Crit Rev Oral Biol Med* 1991;2:103-137.
59. Hancock RH, Swan RH: Nifedipine-induced gingival overgrowth. Report of a case treated by controlling plaque. *J Clin Periodontol* 1992;19:12-14.
60. Salinas CF: Orodental findings and genetic disorders. *Birth Defects* 1982;18:79-120.
61. Shapiro SD, Jorgenson RJ: Heterogeneity in genetic disorders that affect the orifices. *Birth Defects* 1983;19:155-166.
62. Sanders NL: Evidence-based care in orthodontics and periodontics: a review of the literature. *J Am Dent Assoc* 1999;130:521-527.
63. Graber TM, Vanarsdall RL: *Orthodontics: current principles and techniques*, edition 2. St Louis: Mosby, 1994, pp 719-749.
64. Diedrich PR: Guided tissue regeneration associated with orthodontic therapy. *Semin Orthod* 1996;2:39-45.
65. Nemcovsky CE, Zubery Y, Artzi Z, Lieberman MA: Orthodontic tooth movement following guided tissue regeneration: Report of three cases. *Int J Adult Orthod Orthognath Surg* 1996;11:347-355.
66. Stelzel MJ, Flores-de-Jacoby L: Guided tissue regeneration in a combined periodontal and orthodontic treatment: A case report. *Int J Periodontics Restor Dent* 1998;18:189-195.
67. Aguirre-Zorzano LA, Bayona JM, Remolina A, et al: Post-orthodontic stability of the new attachment achieved by guided tissue regeneration following orthodontic movement: Report of 2 cases. *Quintessence Int* 1999;30:769-774.
68. da Silva VC, Cirelli CC, Ribeiro FS, et al: Orthodontic movement after periodontal regeneration of class II furcation: a pilot study in dogs. *J Clin Periodontol* 2006;33:440-448.
69. Caffesse RG, Dominguez LE, Nasjleti CE, et al: Furcation defects in dogs treated by guided tissue regeneration (GTR). *J Periodontol* 1990;61:45-50.
70. Cirelli JA, Marcantonio E Jr, Adriana R, et al: Evaluation of anionic collagen membranes in the treatment of class II furcation lesions: a histometric analysis in dogs. *Biomaterials* 1997;18:1227-1234.
71. Araujo MG, Carmagnola D, Berglundh T, et al: Orthodontic movement in bone defects augmented with Bio-Oss. An experimental study in dogs. *J Clin Periodontol* 2001;28:73-80.
72. Machtei EE, Schallhorn RG: Successful regeneration of mandibular class II furcation defects. *Intl J Period Rest Dent* 1995;15: 146-167.
73. Houser BE, Mellonig JT, Brunsvold MA, et al: Clinical evaluation of an organic bovine bone xenograft with a bioabsorbable collagen barrier in the treatment of molar furcation defects. *Intl J Period Rest Dent* 2001;21:161-169.
74. Roberts WE, Turley PK, Brezniak N, Fielder PJ: Bone physiology and metabolism. *CA Dent Assoc J* 1987;15:54-61.

CHAPTER 21

Orthodontics and Craniofacial Deformities

Kirt E. Simmons

The treatment of patients affected by clefting and craniofacial anomalies can be both extremely rewarding and incredibly frustrating, owing to the myriad difficulties involved and the often long duration of treatment required. Care of these patients calls upon all the orthodontist's skills and knowledge necessary to treat everyday children and adults, as well as additional skills and knowledge related to the unique challenges these patients often present. These challenges can include differences in psychological states of the patients and their parents, abnormalities of dental number, size, morphology, position, eruptive potential, etc., as well as similar abnormalities of the facial and jaw components. Concomitant medical conditions can also affect the treatment options, provision of care, and potential outcomes. The following chapter is dedicated to the practitioners willing to commit to the persistence, patience, and unique demands required by these patients.

1. What is the most common craniofacial deformity?

The most common craniofacial deformity is orofacial clefting, which affects all populations. Approximately 1 in 500–700 births will have some form of orofacial clefting: cleft of the lip, palate, or some combination of both.[1] These clefts may be complete or incomplete, involve one or both sides, be isolated (i.e., non-syndromic), or be part of a more general syndrome (in about 20% of cases); they are variable in their distortions of the affected tissues and subsequent clinical presentations.

2. What are the common types of facial clefts?

- Cleft lip only, which may be unilateral or bilateral and may or may not involve the maxillary alveolus.
- Cleft palate only, which can vary from a submucous cleft of the palate (overtly it appears intact but the muscle and/or bone of the palate are deficient) to a complete cleft of the palate, even involving the alveolus.
  - **U**nilateral cleft lip and palate
  - **B**ilateral cleft lip and palate
  - **E**ach of these can be further subdivided into complete (in which the cleft extends completely through the lip and/or palate) or incomplete (in which some portion of the structure is not cleft) clefts.

3. When might cleft-affected patients be treated orthodontically/orthopedically?

Effective treatment of this type requires a specialized knowledge of these patients' unique features and typically involves several periods of time at various ages. Because of the intensive nature of orthodontic therapy, performing it in stages is preferable to long-term continuous treatment. The potential treatment stages to be considered are based on four developmental stages: infancy, primary dentition, mixed dentition, and permanent dentition. Orthodontic treatment will often be provided at several of these developmental stages.

4. What is "presurgical orthopedics"?

Orthopedic treatment of cleft-affected infants provided prior to any surgical lip or palate procedures, or presurgical orthopedics, was once routinely accepted as a necessary practice because of the dramatically distorted appearance of the maxilla at birth (Fig. 21-1). Orthopedic alignment of maxillary segments, followed by bone grafting at the time of lip and/or palate closure, was proposed to allow normal function, growth, and development.[2] However, this early surgery was ultimately shown to affect future growth and development negatively,[3,4] as compared with the relatively normal development observed in untreated adults.[5]

Although still controversial, presurgical orthopedic treatment with appliances addresses excessive maxillary distortion, especially in cases of bilateral cleft. Pin- or screw-retained "jackscrew" type or spring-loaded appliances (Fig. 21-2, *A* and *B*) can be used to expand posterior segments. Retraction of the premaxillary segments can be achieved with an additional screw component, with elastic bands between the premaxillary segment and the posterior portion, or by extraoral elastic traction across the premaxilla (Fig. 21-2, *C*), either alone or in conjunction with an active posterior expansion appliance or passive posterior "molding" appliance. At some craniofacial centers, preliminary surgical procedures are performed

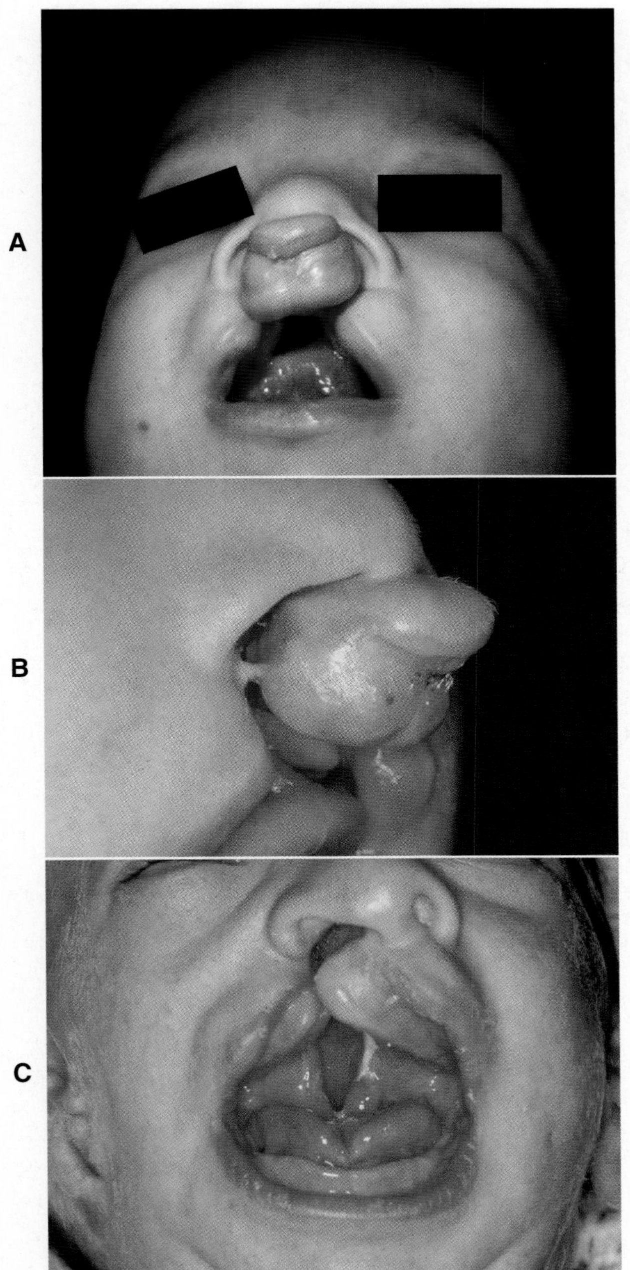

FIG 21-1 **A** and **B,** Unrepaired complete clefts of the lip and palate. Bilateral; note the posterior arch collapse, the protrusive premaxilla, short columella, and separation of the lip segments. **C,** Unilateral; note the distorted alveolar segments.

following expansion, including lip adhesion, wherein elastic force of the healing lip retracts the premaxilla.

Today, at some centers advocating early orthopedic treatment, primary alveolar bone grafting or periosteoplasty is performed at the same time as lip closure, to provide a better arch form, fewer fistulae, and decreased need for secondary bone grafting. Treatment choice must be determined by balancing the potential iatrogenic risks of presurgical expansion (e.g., damage to tooth buds, aspiration of materials, anesthetic and surgical procedural risks) with the positive benefits of treatment outcomes.[5-8] The most recent addition to presurgical orthopedics is a modification of these earlier techniques to include a nasal stent and taping to mold the cleft nose and columella.[9] Immediate surgical results are quite positive, but the long-term effects are unknown at this time.

5. What orthodontic treatment may be indicated for cleft-affected patients in the primary dentition?

Depending upon developmental milestones, surgical closure of the palate is performed between 9 and 18 months of age, leaving a cleft of the maxillary alveolus and buccal and/or lingual fistulae. Orthodontic treatment during this phase is relatively rare, involving treatment of deleterious habits, functional shifts, or space loss after premature tooth loss. Fixed or removable habit appliances can be used to address digit habits and to correct crossbites (Fig. 21-3).

Crossbite interference should be eliminated to prevent consequent unfavorable jaw growth, particularly if the patient has a functional shift of the mandible for intercuspation. Usually, selective reduction of the interfering teeth suffices, but some cases require orthodontic expansion, which may involve anterior and/or posterior expansion as well as long-term retention. However, if the maxilla has no bony continuity across the palate or alveolus, the corrected crossbite should be retained until secondary bone grafting provides that continuity.

Patients should be monitored for dental and overall development during this phase. In short-statured patients especially, delayed dental development may be due to growth hormone deficiency, because clefting is often associated with other midline defects, including pituitary and cardiovascular anomalies.

6. What orthodontic treatment may be indicated for cleft-affected patients in the mixed dentition?

EVALUATION OF NEEDS/TREATMENT PLANNING

Orthodontic evaluation and the development of long-term treatment objectives are needed at the start of this phase because of relatively rapid changes, as well as the developing social and self-awareness of the patient.[10] Assessment will involve standard orthodontic records, as well as selected periapical and/or occlusal radiographs to assess missing or supernumerary teeth and/or bone quantity and anatomy in the cleft site.

Most patients with cleft alveoli have a posterior crossbite and malaligned maxillary incisors at this stage. The collapse of the maxillary segments, especially in bilateral cases, can be severe (Fig. 21-4). These patients will need expansion of the collapsed maxillary segment(s) and/or elimination of traumatic occlusion in preparation for alveolar bone grafting. Bone grafting is ideally performed when root formation of the erupting adjacent lateral incisor or canine is one half to two thirds complete[11,12] so that complete eruption of the adjacent tooth, with its accompanying periodontal attachment, will inhibit

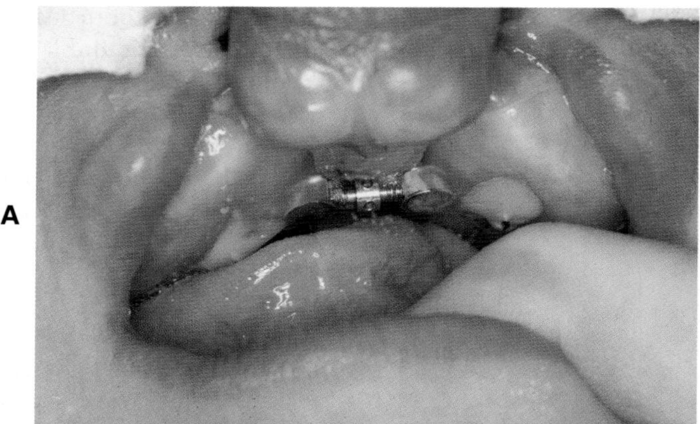

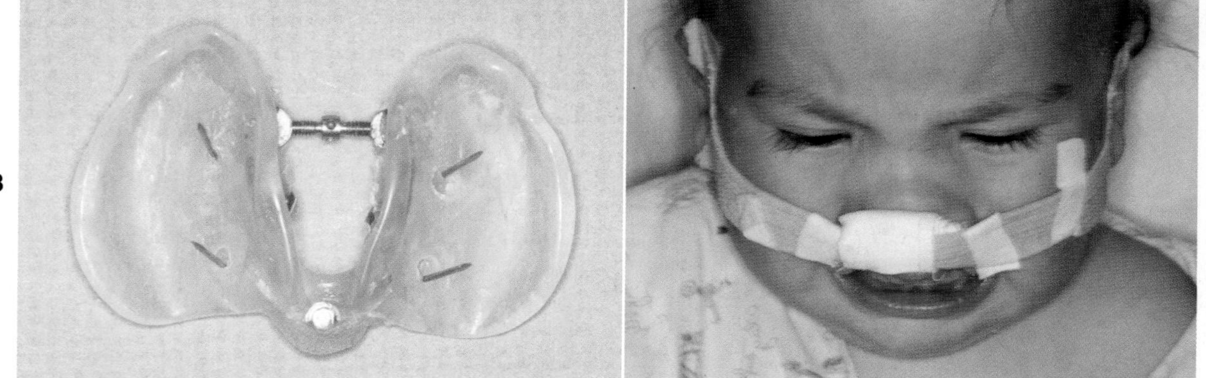

FIG 21-2 **A,** An infant orthopedic expansion appliance using a midpalatal screw (jackscrew) and posterior hinge to expand the anterior portion of the lateral palatal shelves to allow retraction of the premaxilla. **B,** Palatal side of appliance. Note the stainless-steel "staples" that are driven into the palate to maintain the appliance. **C,** An extraoral elastic traction band placed across the premaxilla to provide retraction following expansion of the posterior segments.

further bone resorption of the graft.[11,13] Although these teeth generally erupt spontaneously, it is occasionally necessary to uncover them surgically and induce eruption via orthodontic traction.[11]

ELIMINATION OF TRAUMATIC OCCLUSION

A stable maxilla is necessary for bone graft healing. Thus, traumatic occlusion of teeth in the cleft region should be eliminated, when possible, through alignment of the offending (usually maxillary incisor) teeth. Great care must be used to prevent moving the roots into the cleft site, and adequate retention is recommended to allow reformation of the cortical bone along the root prior to surgical exposure. It is often best to delay orthodontic alignment until after the graft because commonly there is only a thin layer of bone along the cleft side of the roots of adjacent teeth (Fig. 21-5, *A*). Denudation of roots during grafting can result in periodontal defects, ankylosis, root resorption, and/or decreased alveolar bone mass upon healing. If traumatic occlusion cannot be eliminated prior to graft placement, a full-time bite splint can prevent traumatic occlusion while the graft heals.

PRE-GRAFT EXPANSION

The amount and timing of pre-graft expansion should be planned in consultation with the surgeon. Whereas expansion is valuable before bone grafting to optimize surgical access, segments must not be expanded beyond the limits of surgical closure. The ideal expansion would provide coordinated maxillary and mandibular arch forms. If this interferes with the graft prognosis, three options are posed: delay the graft until adolescence and unite the segments with orthognathic or distraction surgery; perform the graft with little or no expansion and attempt expansion later (which may require surgical assistance); or accept the crossbite. If the patient is expected to need orthognathic maxillary advancement later, less expansion is indicated. Delaying the graft until adolescence may negatively affect the eruption or orthodontic movement of adjacent teeth, which could cause periodontal defects, caries, and social stigmata. In unilateral cleft-affected patients, further expansion is fairly predictable after alveolar bone grafting, although arch form may be compromised. However, post-graft expansion is less predictable in the bilateral situation, with the increased scarring and lack of a functional maxillary midline suture.

There are several appliance designs that can be used for expansion: fixed-spring appliances (e.g., quad-helix, W-arch or combinations; see Fig. 21-5, *A*); removable appliances with jackscrew devices or wire springs (Fig. 21-5, *B*); or fixed jackscrew devices (e.g., "fan" appliance; Fig. 21-5, *C*). Bilateral clefts with a posteriorly displaced premaxilla may require a separate appliance first to buccalize the premaxilla (Fig. 21-6), followed by the expander (see Fig 21-5, *C*). The selection of appliances is based on several variables: the direction and extent of expansion needed, the teeth present, the expected resistance, access to the cleft area needed by the surgeon, and the compliance anticipated by the patient. Removable appliances are preferred

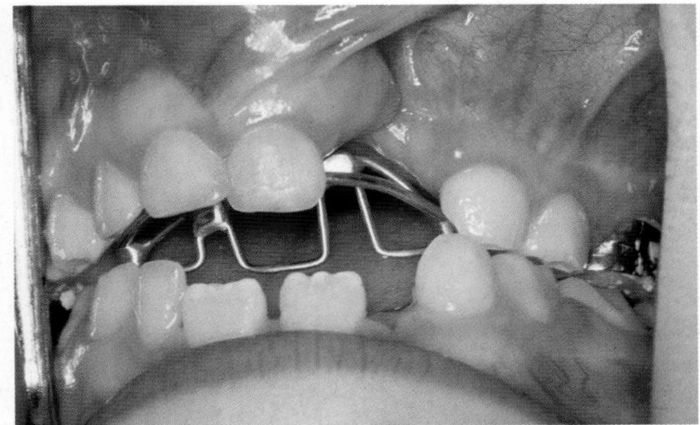

FIG 21-3 A digit-sucking appliance in a cleft-affected patient.

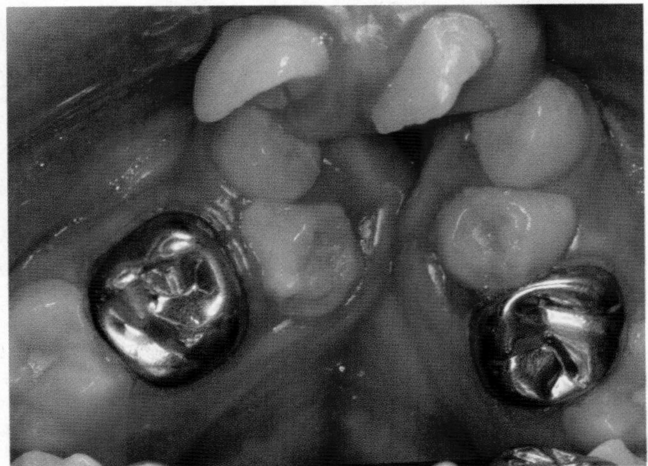

FIG 21-4 Patient with repaired bilateral cleft lip and palate exhibiting severe arch collapse of the posterior segments.

for optimal hygiene but lend themselves to compliance problems and loss. Fixed appliances cause fewer such problems, but they cause greater hygiene problems that may lead to decalcification and caries. Spring appliances apply lighter forces, under the control of the orthodontist, and the quad-helix provides lighter forces over a greater range than the W-arch. They can also be activated to expand segments differentially, which is quite useful because the lesser segment (or posterior segments in a bilateral cleft) is generally collapsed more anteriorly than posteriorly. However, repeated reactivation of spring-loaded appliances may be necessary to achieve the desired expansion. Jackscrew appliances are very rigid and generate high forces, resulting in rapid movement, but they require activation by the patient or a parent. They provide a specific amount and direction of expansion. Any fistulae present (including those unknown to the patient and/or clinician) will tend to be enlarged during the expansion. Such fistulae are generally closed at the time of the alveolar bone graft. Ideally the appliance should allow unimpeded surgical access. If it is in a position to interfere with surgery, the appliance can be modified beforehand or removed and replaced in the operating room. The

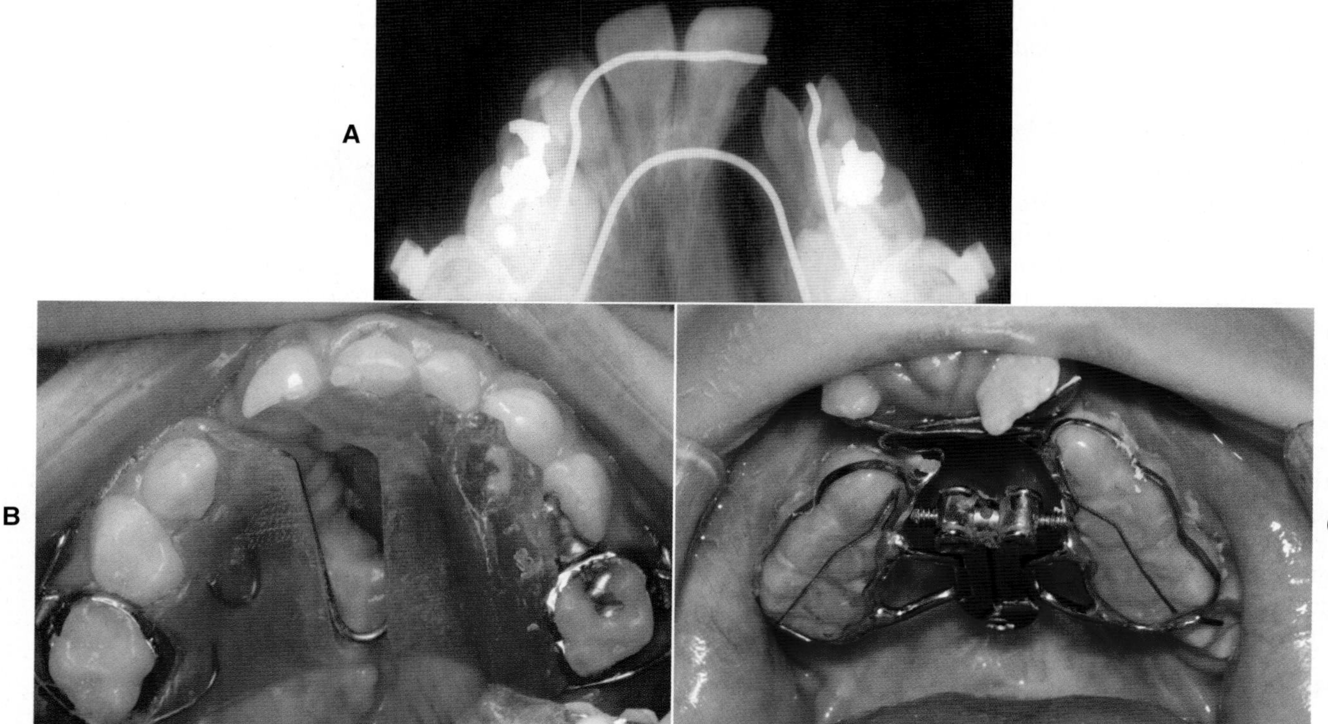

FIG 21-5 Examples of expansion appliances in cleft-affected patients. **A,** Radiograph of a "W"-arch; note the thin layer of bone on the lateral aspect of the central incisor in the cleft edge. **B,** Removable maxillary expansion appliance; note the lingual shelf of acrylic on the side of the greater segment to utilize the lower arch to reinforce anchorage and provide greater expansion of the lesser segment. Inverted "W" stainless-steel wire spring provides for expansion anteriorly. **C,** Bonded "fan" appliance in a patient with bilateral cleft lip and palate. The appliance uses posterior occlusal coverage to prevent traumatic occlusion of the incisors, since the premaxilla is flared by the lingual wires. Note that this appliance preferentially expands the anterior portion of the collapsed palatal shelves.

appliance should be conducive to good oral hygiene in order to prevent bone graft failure.[14] For proper graft healing, expansion should be maintained for 4 to 6 months after surgery, either by retaining the passive expansion appliance or by replacing it with a removable acrylic retainer or fixed lingual arch (Fig. 21-7). With complete bilateral clefting, it is important to stabilize a mobile premaxilla through the time that the graft is incorporated into the host bone.[14] This will require 6 weeks to 6 months, depending on graft size, tissue stretch and/or scarring, occlusal stability, and individual bone and soft-tissue healing capacity. A full-time maxillary splint or heavy labial or lingual fixed appliance can provide this stability.

An alternative approach advocates alveolar bone grafting at a younger age (5–7 years) followed by orthodontic stimulation of the graft by rapid expansion with a fixed-expansion (e.g., jackscrew type) appliance (see Fig. 21-5, *C*).[15] Proponents of this method claim shorter orthodontic treatment time and prevention of maxillary horizontal hypoplasia. In theory, rapid expansion could elicit an effect similar to distraction osteogenesis at the cleft site. Initial maxillary incisor alignment can

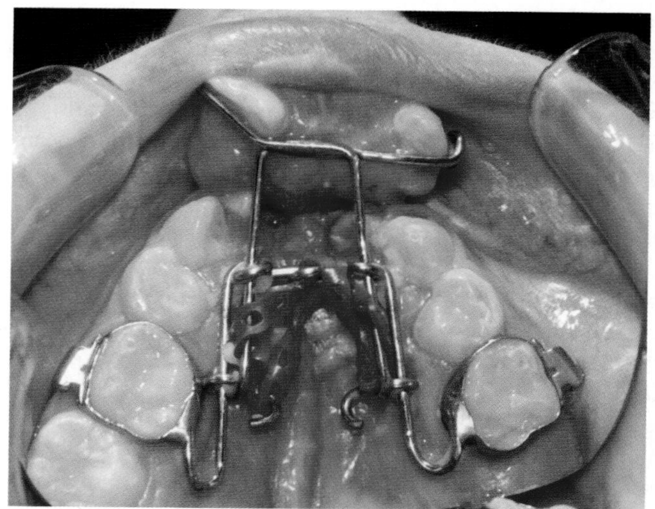

FIG 21-6 A "trombone"-style appliance uses elastic chain to advance the premaxilla out of crossbite. A separate expansion appliance is then used posteriorly followed by alveolar ridge bone grafting.

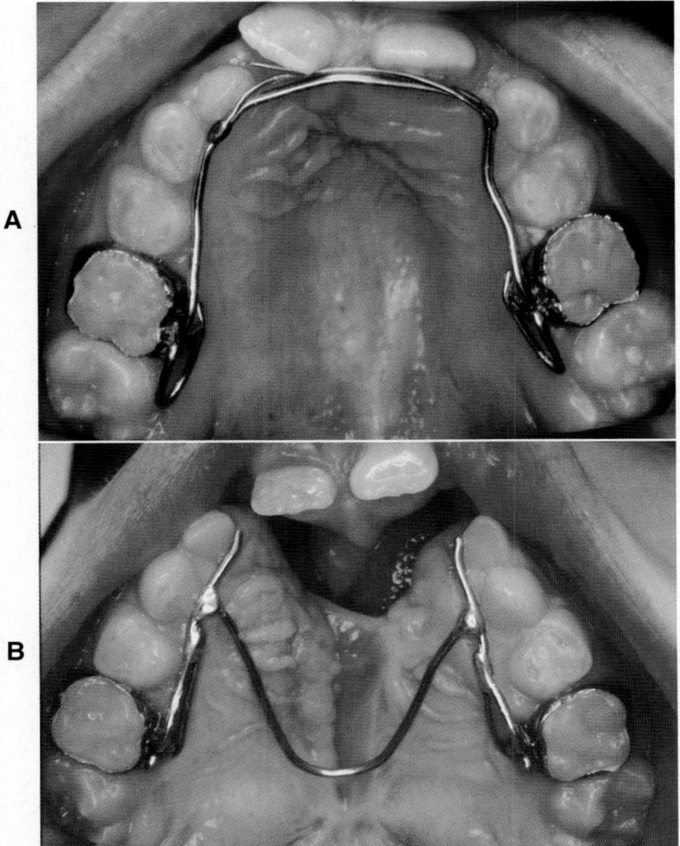

FIG 21-7 **A,** A fixed lingual arch maintains expansion after placing an alveolar bone graft and incorporating two finger springs to flare the central incisors. **B,** A modified "W" or lingual arch maintains the expansion obtained, while allowing surgical access for the alveolar bone graft.

be done with fixed orthodontic appliances immediately after the graft. Generally, the patient then takes a break from active treatment and is placed in retention. If necessary, missing or unerupted teeth may be masked with a removable acrylic retainer with plastic pontics, and a temporary bonded lingual retainer (0.0175-inch multi-strand archwire) can be used to retain spaced incisors until comprehensive orthodontic treatment is begun.

MAXILLARY PROTRACTION

Following graft stabilization and initial incisor alignment, an orthodontic assessment is indicated to evaluate the patient's pattern of maxillary and mandibular growth. Discordant monozygotic twin studies have revealed differences based on the type and severity of the cleft.[16] Growth is essentially unaffected in patients with clefts of only the lip and alveolus. Cleft palate can result only in a shorter posterior face height, a steeper mandibular plane angle, and retrognathia. Complete unilateral cleft lip and palate can lead to failure of anterior maxillary growth, resulting in posterior and inferior displacement. Patients with very flat profiles, increased face heights, and/or Class III skeletal relationships will generally exhibit a worsening of their condition with further growth. Significant skeletal deformities are often best treated with combined orthodontics and surgery, possibly in multiple stages. Young (~8 years[17-19]) patients with mild maxillary deficient clefts may benefit from orthopedic forces for maxillary protraction via bonded full occlusal coverage acrylic splints[19] or fixed banded[17-18] intraoral appliances, with extraoral protraction force applied via elastic force to a facial mask. These masks differ in their various pads, bands, and frame styles, and even include an American football-style helmet.[17-20] This treatment can effectively correct anterior crossbites and improve the prognathic profile through a limited maxillary skeletal advancement (1–3 mm), maxillary dental advancement, and counterclockwise or posterior rotation of the mandible.[17-19] The latest update to this technique uses the expansion appliance alternately to expand and constrict the maxilla repeatedly in rapid succession, followed by protraction of the lateral segments in wide bilateral clefts, to reduce the cleft gap and enhance maxillary advancement.[20]

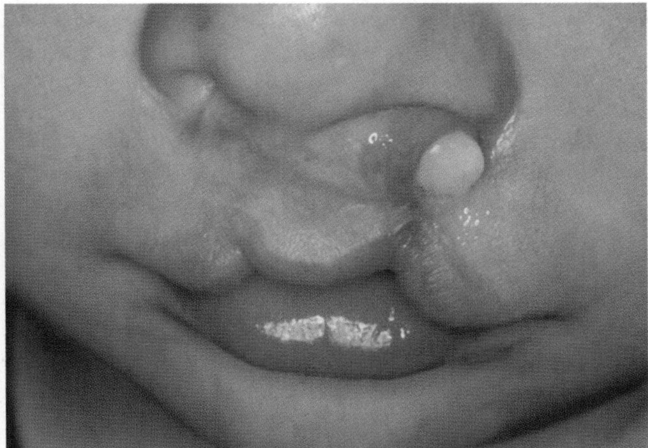

FIG 21-8 A primary canine erupted through the facial skin in a patient with repaired bilateral cleft lip and palate. Teeth in the cleft margin can also erupt into the nasal cavity.

Orthognathic surgery or distraction osteogenesis is indicated for patients with true mandibular prognathism, severe mandibular retrognathism, skeletal open bite, moderate to severe maxillary deficiency, or limited or no remaining craniofacial growth.

BILATERAL CLEFT LIP AND PALATE: UNIQUE FEATURES

Patients with complete bilateral cleft lip and palate may pose a number of challenges for the orthodontist: minimal coverage of the maxillary incisors by the upper lip, a shallow maxillary labial vestibule, a short and tight upper lip with protrusive lower lip, large fistulae, palatal webs over the maxillary molar area, missing maxillary lateral incisors, ectopically erupting teeth (Fig. 21-8) and hypoplastic or missing central incisors. These individuals also suffer from scar contracture and oral and nasal dysfunction. At this stage patients may exhibit a protrusive and mobile premaxilla, which usually contains two central incisors. Anterior crossbites are frequently observed, as are severe discrepancies between the three maxillary segments. The ideal vertical premaxillary position is difficult to assess because of common hypoplasia of the nose and/or upper lips, which can appear as vertical overdevelopment. Pregraft orthopedic movement can usually correct a truly malpositioned premaxilla.[20] The premaxilla may be repositioned laterally or intruded with a special jackscrew-type appliance,[20] or rarely it may be necessary to surgically reposition it at the time of bone grafting, although this requires great care to prevent loss of perfusion.[21] From age 4 years to maturity, forward premaxillary growth is half that of non-cleft patients, whereas mandibular growth is essentially the same.[22] Owing to initial protrusion of the premaxilla, this growth differential usually ends with an acceptable maxillary/mandibular relationship by adolescence.[22,23]

7. What orthodontic treatment may be indicated for cleft patients in the permanent dentition?

The most common problems at this point include missing, supernumerary and/or malformed teeth adjacent to the cleft area, residual maxillary constriction, displaced maxillary dental midline, frenal or periodontal abnormalities in the cleft, delayed dental development, and altered eruption patterns. Most patients with mild to moderate retrognathia can be treated with orthodontics alone, but a prognathic pattern or a severe retrognathic pattern (Fig. 21-9) requires orthognathic surgery or distraction osteogenesis.[24]

An important treatment planning consideration for many of these patients involves missing teeth, usually the lateral incisor(s). Canine substitution can be an excellent choice if the maxillary dental midline is on (or off to the non-cleft side), the canine is mesially erupted with reasonable root position and is fairly small and white, both premolars are present on the affected side, and the molar/canine relationships are Class II,. Prosthetic replacement is best when the maxillary canine is Class I or has a mesially displaced crown, but the root is still positioned distally, the maxillary midline is cleft-sided, incisors are retroclined, there are other missing teeth, and the molars are bilaterally Class I. With skeletal Class III patients, the choice also depends on whether orthognathic surgical procedures are planned. If interdental osteotomies are planned or insufficient bone exists preoperatively, some space should be left for the surgeon to close.

Prosthetic replacement of lateral incisors can be accomplished through removable prostheses, fixed partial dentures, or osseointegrated dental implants (placed following active vertical facial growth and ideally with a minimum of 7 mm of space). Children with skeletal problems (true mandibular prognathism, severe mandibular retrognathism, skeletal open bite, moderate to severe maxillary deficiency, or poor facial profiles), who will require orthognathic surgery in the long term, ideally would not begin their comprehensive orthodontic treatment until 1 to 1.5 years prior to orthognathic surgery (ideally at the completion of active craniofacial growth). This is typically at 14 to 16 years of age for females and 16 to 18 years of age for males. Growth must be followed with serial lateral cephalometric radiographs at 6- to 12-month intervals.

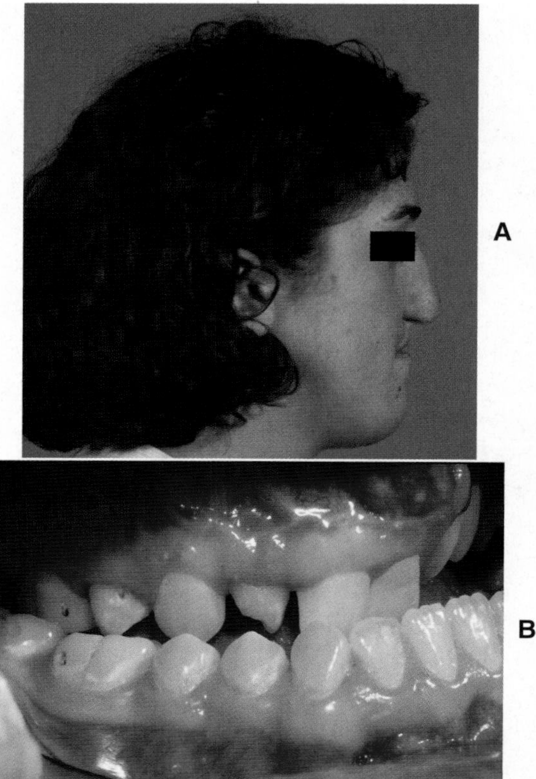

FIG 21-9 Bilateral cleft-affected patient exhibiting severe maxillary hypoplasia. **A,** Facial profile. **B,** Occlusion.

Limited treatment can address crowding, functional issues, psychosocial issues, and/or eliminate or prevent traumatic occlusion, although the benefits of such treatment must be realistically weighed against the risks of "burnout'," decalcification, root resorption, and periodontal problems.

8. What orthodontic treatment may be indicated for cleft-affected patients with significant skeletal discrepancies?

Cleft-affected patients commonly need maxillary skeletal augmentation, which may involve skeletal advancement, expansion, and vertical displacement. If there is an open bite or mandibular asymmetry, protrusion, or retrusion, the surgery may also include the mandible. The effect of these procedures on facial esthetics and functional abilities to breathe and speak must be considered with appropriate input from respective specialists.

Preoperative orthodontic treatment will involve full fixed appliances but will result in apparent "worsening" of the malocclusion, due to the removal of natural dental compensations to align the teeth properly with respect to skeletal components. Errors on the side of excessive decompensation are preferred because they allow more aggressive surgical correction. This allows minor skeletal relapses that might occur postoperatively to be managed orthodontically. Preoperative orthodontic establishment of the mandibular arch form should occur early, which will involve reversal of existing dental compensations by expansion of upright, lingually tipped molar crowns, and the flaring and leveling of mandibular incisors. Extractions for crowding should be carefully assessed, and actively closing or deepening the bite preoperatively should not be done for patients who originally presented with an open bite or minimal overbite. Instead, the open bite should be allowed to persist or even open further, because the surgeon will close the bite skeletally. Extrusive posterior tooth movements should be performed preoperatively to minimize the prospect of open bite recurrence.

All surgical plans should be approved by the patient's orthodontist. Cleft-affected orthognathic surgery patients are at greater risk for maxillary relapse. To minimize this risk, the following measures should be explored: rigid fixation, overadvancement to weak Class I relationships, maxillary overexpansion, maintenance of a large (0.040-inch) expanded buccal wire postoperatively, bone grafting, postoperative extraoral traction, and maxillary strut fixation. Posteroanterior relapse should be monitored during the first 3 postoperative months via molar, canine, and incisor relationships. If relapse is present, it should be addressed with Class III elastics and/or reverse-pull headgear. The use of Class III elastics can open the bite by extruding the posterior maxillary teeth in conjunction with a vertical-pull chin cup, straight vertical-pull headgear, and/or thick posterior bite blocks. Final lip and/or nose revisions are often best accomplished after orthodontic and orthognathic surgical procedures.

9. What syndromes are associated with clefting?

There are many syndromes for which orofacial clefting is one finding. The most common of these include amnion rupture sequence, cerebro-costo-mandibular syndrome, EEC syndrome (ectrodactyly-ectodermal dysplasia-clefting syndrome), frontonasal dysplasia (median cleft face syndrome), Kabuki syndrome, Larsen syndrome, Stickler syndrome, Van der Woude syndrome, and velocardiofacial syndrome. For a complete listing, see Gorlin et al.[25]

10. What are some other relatively common craniofacial deformities an orthodontist may be called upon to treat?

- Craniosynostoses syndromes (craniofacial dysostosis syndromes), including Apert syndrome, Crouzon syndrome, Pfeiffer syndrome, Saethre-Chotzen syndrome, and Carpenter syndrome
- Branchial arch and oral-acral syndromes, including oculo-auriculo-vertebral spectrum (hemifacial microsomia, Goldenhar syndrome), mandibulofacial dysostosis (Treacher Collins syndrome), and acrofacial dysostosis (Nager acrofacial dysostosis, Nager syndrome)
- Turner syndrome and the similar Noonan syndrome and cardio-facio-cutaneous syndrome (CFC syndrome)
- Trisomy 21 syndrome (Down syndrome)
- Alcohol embryopathy (fetal alcohol syndrome), as well as embryopathies from many other common drugs (cocaine, hydantoin, retinoic acid, thalidomide, valproate, and warfarin, to name a few)
- Achondroplasia
- Cleidocranial dysplasia
- Marfan syndrome
- Silver-Russell syndrome
- Beckwith-Wiedemann syndrome (exomphalos-macroglossia-gigantism syndrome)
- Sturge-Weber syndrome
- Prader-Willi syndrome
- Peutz-Jeghers syndrome
- Ehlers-Danlos syndrome
- Neurofibromatosis
- Ectodermal dysplasias

11. What deformities are common in the oculo-auriculo-vertebral spectrum of conditions, and what orthodontic treatment may be indicated?

The most common of these are hemifacial microsomia and the more involved Goldenhar syndrome. Hemifacial microsomia, as the name suggests, involves a variable, progressive, and asymmetric deficiency, or absence, of portions of the face (Fig. 21-10). This spectrum of disorders is extremely heterogeneous with Goldenhar's syndrome, which displays similar facial deficiencies, plus epibulbar dermoids and vertebral anomalies at the severe end of the spectrum. The first and second branchial arch derivatives are affected, including the bone and neuromuscular and soft tissues. The ears may be small to nonexistent, as may be the mandibular ramus and associated muscles, often with an aberrant or missing temporomandibular joint (TMJ). The occlusal plane is tilted superiorly on the affected side, and the ear and orbit are typically displaced inferiorly. Because of the wide variability of expression in these conditions, they have been grouped into "Types" and subtypes by various authors (ranging from I–III to I–V), based on the extent of the mandibular deformity, with the higher number generally indicating increased deficiencies of the ramus.[26-29] The one significant aberration from this generality is the Harvold Type III, which indicates an ankylosis or syndesmosis of the TMJ.

Jaw function and opening is often adequate, except in ankylosed/syndesmotic cases. In these severe cases, surgical treatment is indicated as soon as is practical, to release the ankylosis and allow growth of the mandible to occur (Fig. 21-11). In addition, some of these children will have had tracheostomies, and release of the ankylosis and/or advancement of the mandible are indicated to decannulate these children prior to school age. Ideally primary teeth will be present to allow the placement of an appliance to protract the mandible and provide for physiotherapy (i.e., opening exercises with assistance) to prevent reankylosis and loss of function. A later surgery to reconstruct the ramus and TMJ, potentially including distraction osteogenesis, will be likely.

In the more common nonankylosed types, treatment is also complex and involves many years of integrated therapy, best provided by a craniofacial team approach. The treatment timing and indications are dependent on the phenotypic presentations of the case. For an excellent detailed review of treatment, the reader is referred to Vargervik and Kaban.[30] In short, in cases where the TMJ is small but functional, a Bionator-type functional appliance

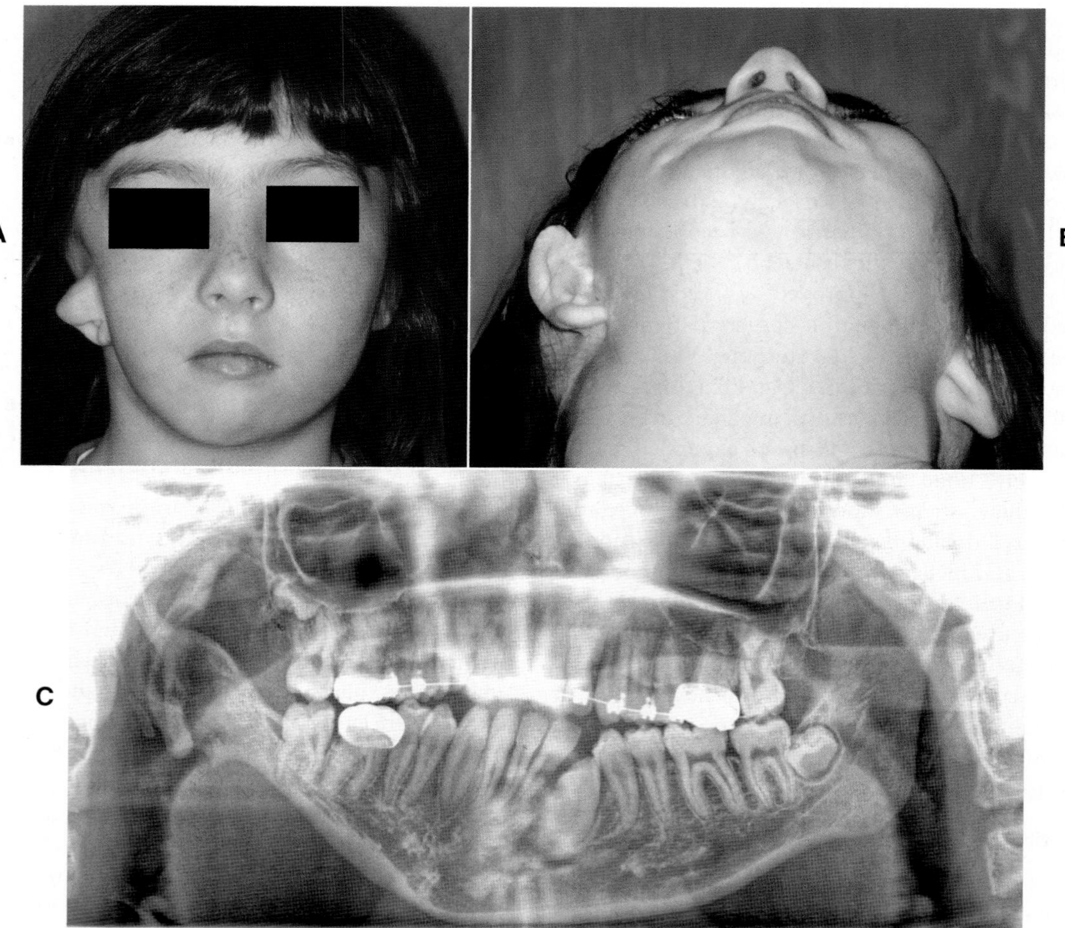

FIG 21-10 Young patient with an oculo-auriculo-vertebral disorder affecting her right side. **A** and **B,** Note the dysplastic and severely displaced ear. **C,** Note the dysplastic ramus and condyle on the affected side.

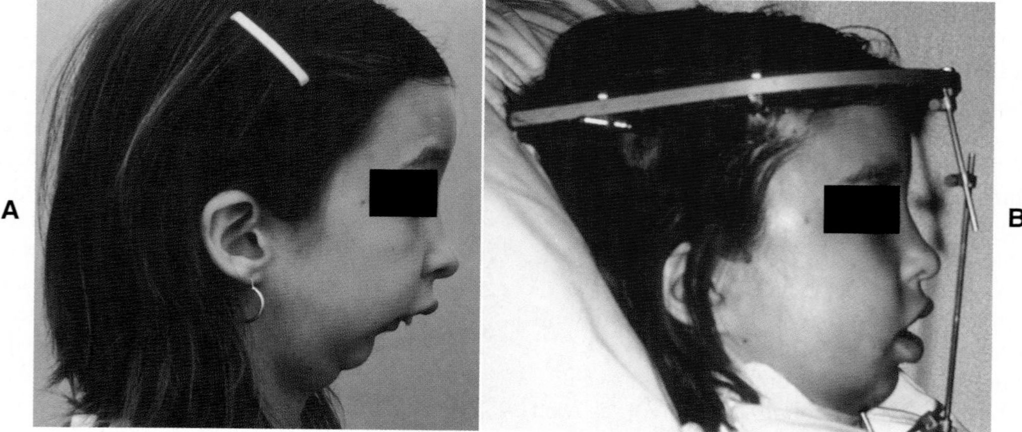

FIG 21-11 **A,** Young patient with severe retrogenia caused by ankylosis of the temporomandibular joints. **B,** Same patient after advancement of mandibular corpus and surgical reconstruction of ramus and joint.

is indicated in the mixed dentition. This asymmetric appliance advances and lowers the mandible while allowing for maxillary dental eruption on the affected side. The goals of this appliance are to relieve the occlusal cant on the affected side and stimulate downward and forward growth of the mandible on the affected side, to match that of the unaffected side. In addition, the orthodontist should manage the dental crowding and impactions often seen on the affected side. In certain cases, this treatment can eliminate the need for surgery, although good cooperation and long-term treatment are necessary. In the permanent dentition stage, orthodontic treatment will be indicated for many of these patients to prepare them for surgical correction. Alignment of the teeth and coordination of arch forms are the goals of treatment at this time. If the occlusal plane is still canted, another period of an intraoral splint, to allow active extrusion of the maxillary teeth on the affected side and leveling of the maxillary occlusal plane, can be provided if maxillary surgery is not desired or is contraindicated.

In patients having a severely aberrant condylar process, the treatment protocol is essentially the same, with surgical correction indicated for the mandible, and maxilla, if necessary. Surgical correction of the mandible, depending upon the expertise and preference of the surgeon involved, can take many forms, including rib grafts, distraction, iliac crest grafts, and calvarial grafts. Timing of surgery is somewhat controversial, with some surgeons advocating early surgery in the mixed dentition and others later in adolescence. For review of the types and timing of surgeries for these conditions, the reader is referred to Kearns et al.[31] If presurgical maxillary leveling is inadequate or not possible, postsurgical extrusion of the maxillary teeth will be indicated. The vertical correction of the mandibular ramus on the affected side will result in an open bite, which must be supported by a postsurgical splint, regardless of the surgical technique. The open bite is closed by progressive reduction of the postsurgical splint on the maxillary side, allowing eruption of the maxillary molar into occlusion first, followed by the premolars.

In the more severe cases, those lacking any condylar process and those also lacking a coronoid process, a first stage of reconstruction occurs in the mixed dentition, typically at 6 to 10 years of age. Since these patients lack a glenoid fossa and TMJ, they require construction of a fossa and pseudo-TMJ, plus construction of a condyle and ramus. Ideally the location of the new pseudo-TMJ will be as lateral and posterior as possible, and the lower borders of the mandible will be level at the time of this surgery. This will result in an open bite on the affected side, to be managed as above with a postsurgical splint and extrusion. These patients will typically require a second phase of orthodontic treatment in adolescence, followed by orthognathic surgery and/or distraction osteogenesis, as well as soft tissue augmentation (Fig. 21-12).

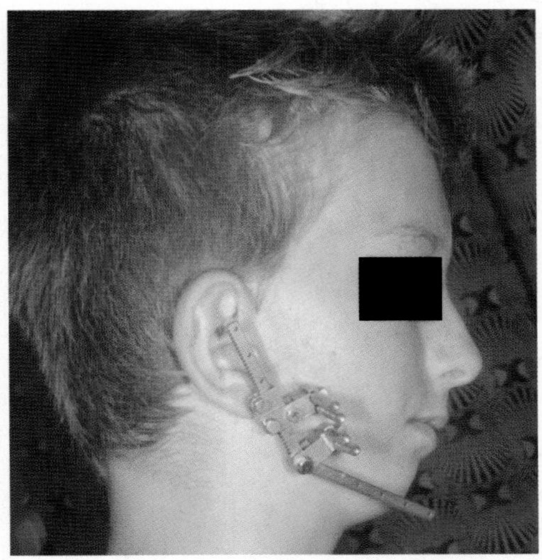

FIG 21-12 Extraoral distractor applied to a patient affected by hemifacial microsomia.

12. What deformities are common in the craniosynostoses syndromes, and what orthodontic treatment may be indicated?

Of the craniosynostoses (craniofacial dysostosis) syndromes, the most common are Apert syndrome and Crouzon syndrome. These syndromes, because of similar defects in the fibroblast growth factor receptor genes, not surprisingly share some phenotypic expressions and autosomal dominant transmission. They are both characterized by craniosynostosis and some degree of mid-facial hypoplasia with resultant relative mandibular prognathism. Apert syndrome also has symmetric syndactyly (fusing of digits) of the hands and feet, proptosis (bulging eyes), lateral palatal swellings, severe maxillary dental crowding with V-shaped arch and displaced teeth, anterior open bite, and anterior and posterior crossbites (Fig. 21-13).[25] Crouzon syndrome is similar but is characterized by shallow orbits and severe ocular proptosis. It has a more variable expression than Apert syndrome. Palatal swellings are often present but less pronounced, although the maxillary hypoplasia with dental crowding, ectopic eruption, anterior open bite, and anterior and posterior crossbites are similar. Both syndromes can exhibit a reverse curve of Spee in the lower arch.

These patients typically undergo at least three stages of reconstructive surgery: (1) release of involved cranial sutures with advancement and reshaping of the supraorbital rim within the first year, (2) Le Fort III, monobloc, or facial bipartition advancements typically at 4 to 8 years, and (3) a Le Fort I osteotomy advancement with or without genioplasty, rhinoplasty, contour bone grafting, and/or canthoplasties.[32] Orthodontic treatment usually commences following the second stage of reconstructive surgery in the mixed dentition and involves management of the dental crowding, often with extractions. Although the relative mandibular prognathism may be much improved after this second reconstructive procedure, it is important to prepare the patient and parents for its predictable return, as the mandible continues to complete its growth while the maxilla stays essentially unchanged. The orthodontist should monitor facial growth with yearly cephalometric films or 3D-CTs and begin the final stage of orthodontic preparation in anticipation of the completion of facial growth, at which time the final maxillary advancement will be performed to correct the maxillary hypoplasia. These orthodontic procedures are typical of preparation

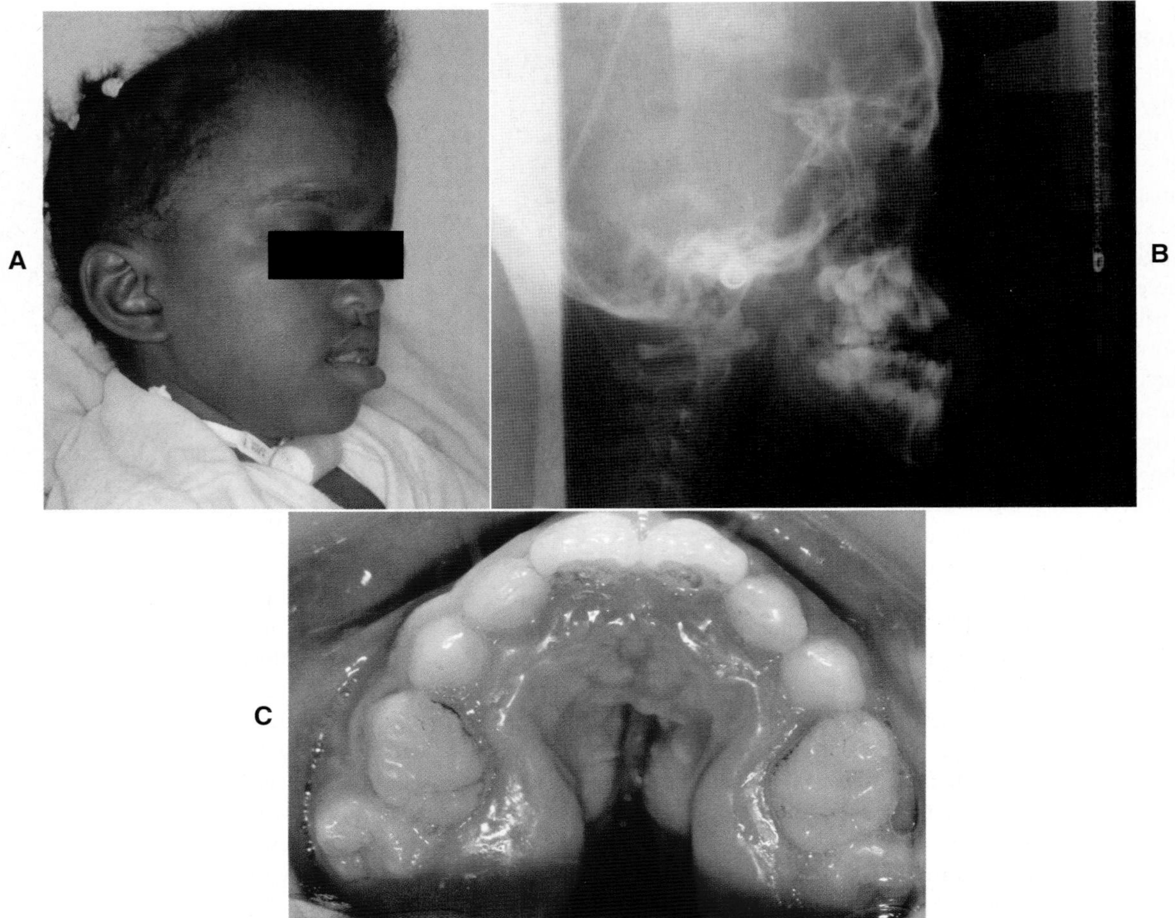

FIG 21-13 A patient with Apert syndrome. **A** and **B,** Note the midface deficiency. **C,** Palatal swellings, "V-"shaped arch, and severe crowding.

for orthognathic surgery, common to maxillary deficient patients, including alignment and coordination of arches.

13. What deformities are common in mandibulofacial dysostosis (Treacher Collins syndrome), and what orthodontic treatment may be indicated?

This syndrome, with autosomal dominant inheritance and variable expressivity, involves the derivatives of the first and second pharyngeal arch, groove, and pouch.[25] The deformities are bilateral, but not necessarily symmetric, and include ear deformities, malar hypoplasia, and mandibular hypoplasia (Fig. 21-14). The clinical presentation is characteristic and includes malformed pinnae, often accompanied by conductive hearing loss, hypoplastic supraorbital rims and zygomas with downslanting palpebral fissures and sunken cheekbones, and a hypoplastic mandible deficient in the ramus and body. In addition, the mandible exhibits a steep mandibular plane angle, a reverse curve of Spee, retrogenia, obtuse gonial angle, and condylar cartilage of the hyaline type rather than fibrocartilage.[25] There is no articular eminence, limited opening, and the maxilla is often small with an anterior open bite skeletal pattern and posterior vertical deficiency. Dental crowding can be severe, and cleft palate and palatopharyngeal incompetence are fairly common, as is macrostomia.

Treatment may involve early mandibular distraction to prevent tracheostomy caused by severe airway difficulties or to allow decannulation in those patients already tracheostomized. This should be reserved for these cases because of the significant potential morbidity of this technique at an early age.[33] The goals of orthodontic treatment should be to manage the crowding and eruption problems as indicated during the mixed dentition, but comprehensive orthodontic treatment should be delayed until facial skeletal growth is nearing completion. At that time orthodontic treatment should commence, in preparation for two-jaw orthognathic and/or distraction procedures.

14. What are some other common syndromes of interest to orthodontists?

Turner syndrome is a chromosomal disorder, with classically affected individuals having only a single X chromosome. These patients are phenotypically female, are of short stature with sexual infantilism, and have variable expression of somatic abnormalities. The classic somatic

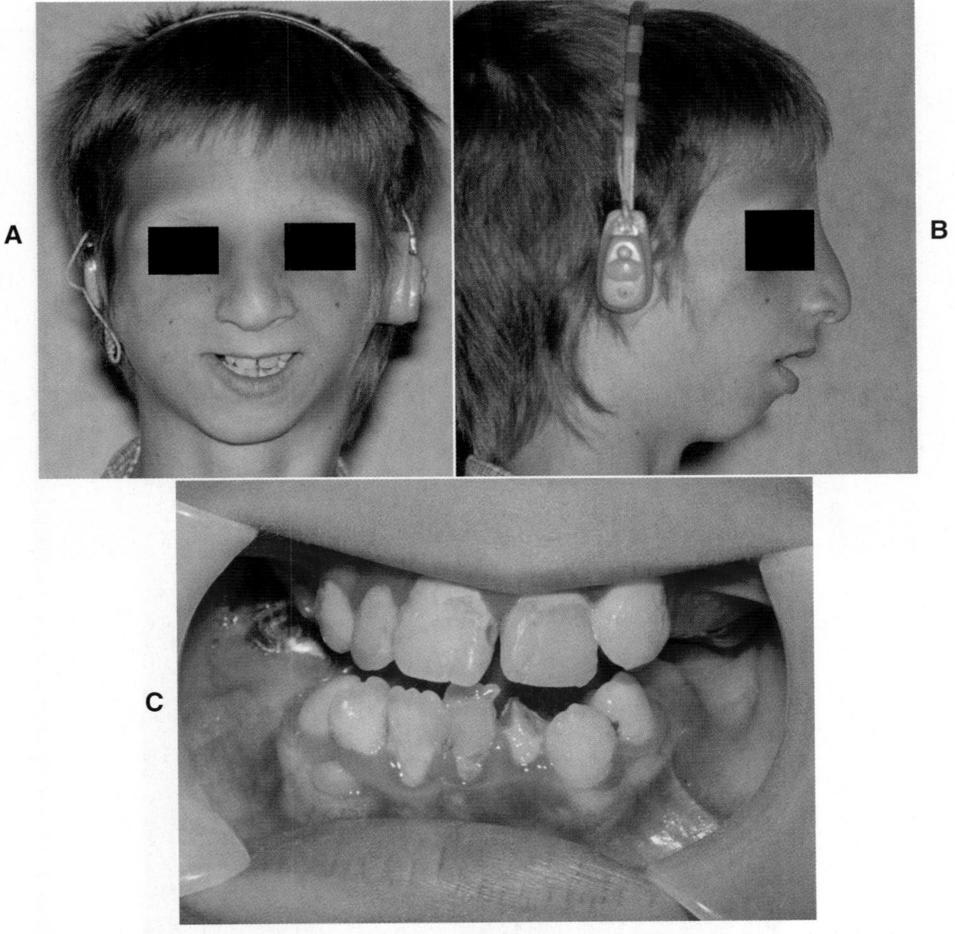

FIG 21-14 A patient with mandibulofacial dysostosis. **A** and **B,** Note the downslanting palpebral fissures, hearing aids, lack of cheekbones and relatively protrusive nose, and, **C,** anterior open bite and crowding.

abnormalities include a webbed neck, epicanthal folds, shield neck, cardiovascular abnormalities, abnormal ears, and low hairline (Fig. 21-15, *A* and *B*).[25] Dental and facial abnormalities include advanced dental age, small teeth, short roots, lateral palatal bulges, a short cranial base, and maxillary and mandibular retrognathia (Fig. 21-15, *C*).[34] From an orthodontic viewpoint, this syndrome is of interest because in mild form, these patients are often not diagnosed until puberty, when they fail to go through menarche. An astute orthodontist may be able to refer these patients at an earlier age, allowing an early diagnosis. In addition, when treating these patients, it is wise to keep in mind the high proportion with cardiovascular anomalies and the tendency for short roots and root resorption. Currently most of these patients undergo growth hormone therapy once diagnosed and eventually sex hormone therapy as well, which can have definite effects on craniofacial growth. For this reason it is wise to consult with the patient's endocrinologist regarding treatment timing and to consider the differential effect of sex and growth hormones on mandibular, versus maxillary, growth.

Another chromosomal disorder, trisomy 21 (Down) syndrome, is the most common malformation syndrome, having an incidence of about 1 in 650 live births.[25] These patients are typically short, with hypotonia, upslanting palpebral fissures, short neck, and mental retardation (Fig. 21-16, *A*). Orofacially these patients have a flat facial profile due to midface hypoplasia, a characteristic open mouth posture with protruding tongue, hypoplastic sinuses, and delayed and irregular dental eruption (Fig. 21-16, *B*). They also commonly have cardiovascular anomalies, a high incidence of periodontal disease (purportedly caused by immune system compromises and oral respiration) and sleep apnea, fissures of the tongue, missing teeth, and anomalous teeth.[35] An anterior open bite, posterior crossbite, and spaced mandibular incisors with reverse overjet are often manifest, as a result of the midface hypoplasia and anterior tongue posture. Early (6 months of age, ideally) functional therapy, consisting of manual therapy, in conjunction with removable or fixed appliances that contain acrylic bumps on the facial to stimulate the upper lip and an oval midline "bead" for the tongue to "play" with, has been advocated to improve the hypotonia of the lips and tongue

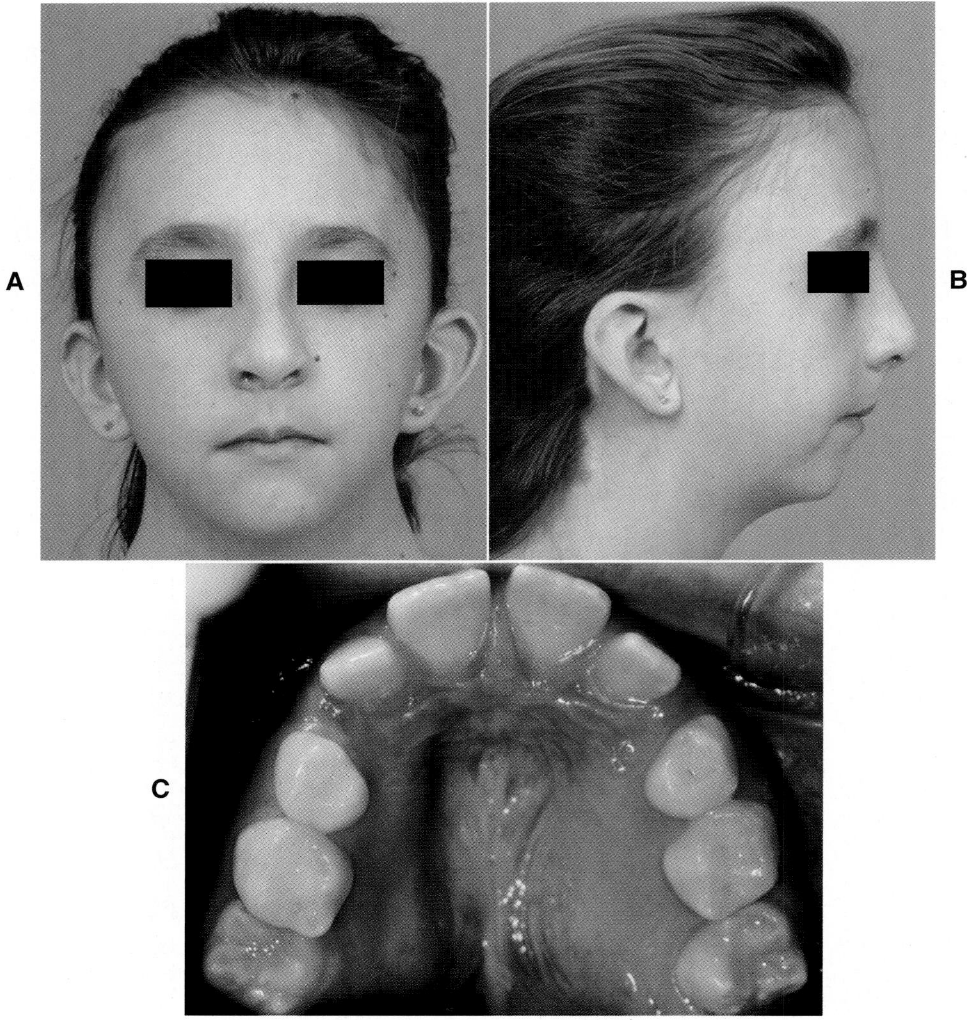

FIG 21-15 A patient with Turner syndrome. **A** and **B,** Note the low-set unusual ears, webbed neck, low hairline and retrognathia, and, **C,** lateral palatal bulges.

and prevent some of the typical sequelae of the chronic open mouth posture.[36]

Because of their constellation of facial and dental problems, these patients are clearly candidates for orthodontic care. Although access to orthodontic care for these patients is often difficult for a variety of reasons, including financial and transportation, orthodontists should not arbitrarily preclude these patients from their practice.[37] Although the basic treatment goals of these patients should not be altered, provision of care should involve some modifications specific to these individuals. Staged or multiphase treatment is often beneficial, as are shorter, morning appointments with limited procedures and additional time set aside, since these patients require extra patience on the part of the orthodontist and assistant. Parents and/or siblings can often be very helpful in attaining compliance, and it is imperative to actively involve them in home care of the appliances. The high incidence of cardiovascular problems, sleep apnea, and periodontal disease must be taken into account when deciding on treatment therapies. Sleep apnea therapies may be contraconducive to certain orthodontic treatments (such as oral-nasal positive airway pressure masks and reverse-pull headgear), whereas certain orthodontic/orthognathic therapies (such as maxillary expansion and maxillo-mandibular advancement) may have a positive effect on sleep apnea. Therefore, it is important to identify these patients, refer them for an evaluation if sleep apnea is suspected but has not been diagnosed, and consult with the physician treating them to develop a coordinated treatment plan. In the office all procedures should be carefully explained and demonstrated to the patient and parent. Every effort should be made to become "friends" with the patient first and develop a trusting relationship prior to instituting treatment. In addition, keeping appointments and procedures "fun" and providing rewards is important. These patients generally have a happy, friendly demeanor once their trust is gained and can make very good patients, although they can be obstinate at times and easily distracted (not always a liability).

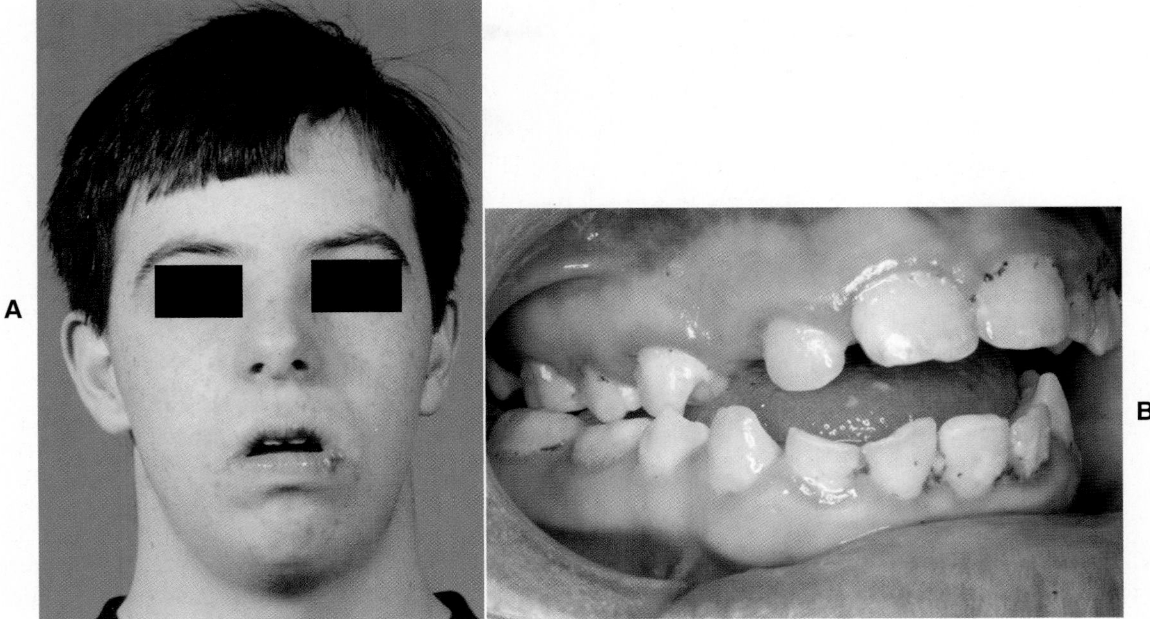

FIG 21-16 A young man with Trisomy 21 (Down) syndrome. **A,** Note the open mouth posture and hypotonia. **B,** Classic anterior open bite, marginal gingivitis, and retained food.

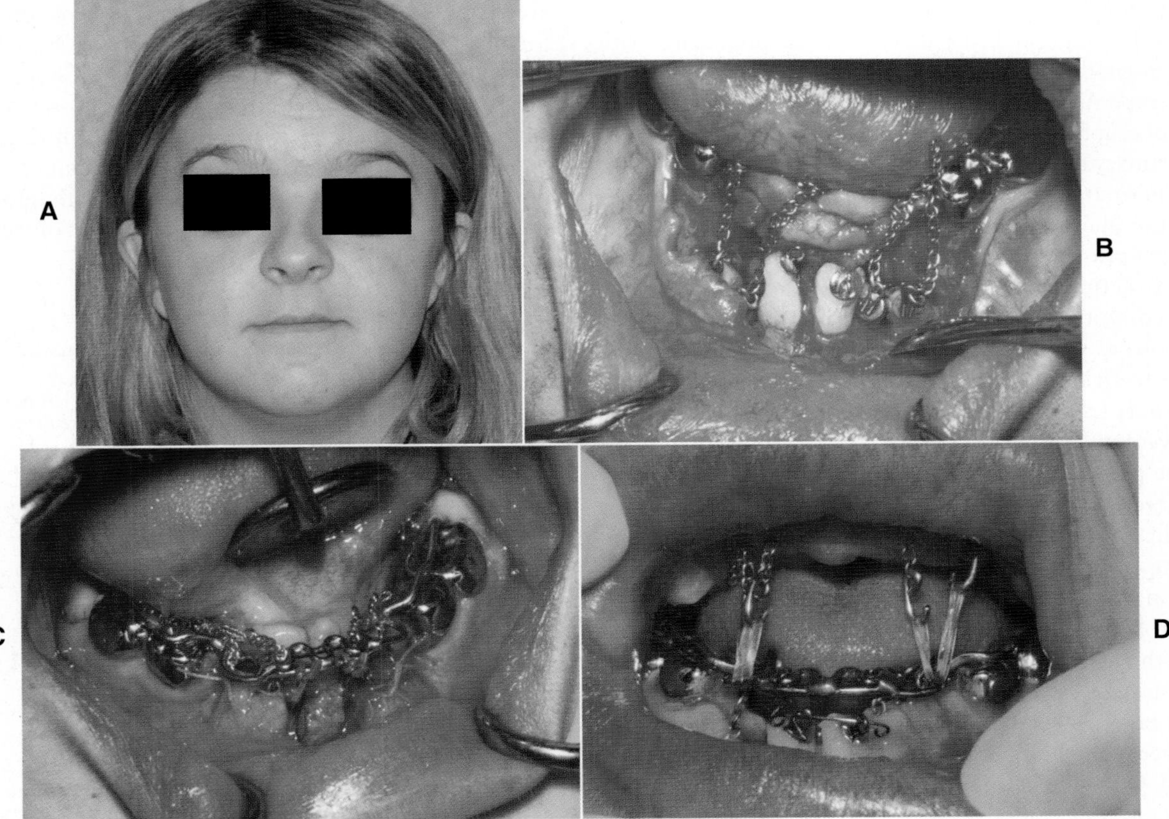

FIG 21-17 Cleidocranial dysplasia. **A,** Note the midface deficiency and broad face. **B,** Unerupted incisors bonded with pads and gold chains. **C,** Fixed eruptive appliance supported by first molars and primary molars with openings for chain to pass through. Elastic thread is tied to chains to apply eruptive force. **D,** Chains on upper unerupted incisors with hooks bent onto the chains to allow interarch elastics to be placed.

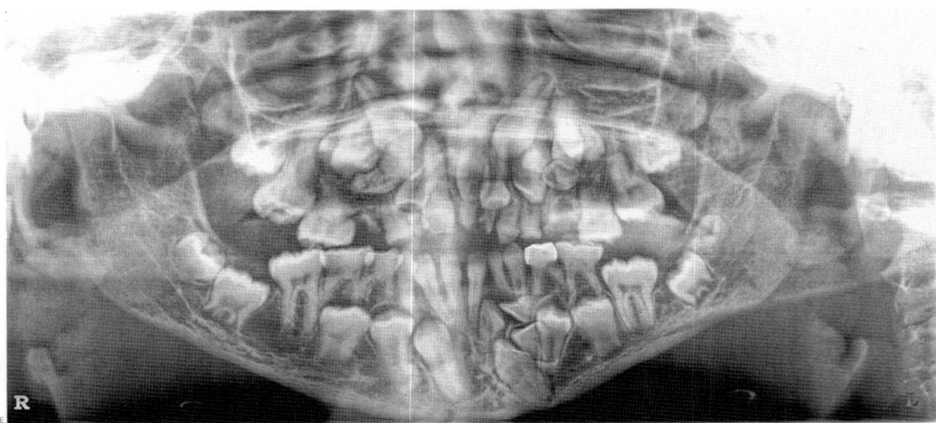

FIG 21-18 Panoramic film of a patient with cleidocranial dysplasia. Note the failure of eruption and multiple, tightly packed supernumerary teeth.

Finally, cleidocranial dysplasia (dysostosis) is an interesting syndrome with autosomal dominant inheritance. These patients are short with a broad skull, pronounced biparietal and frontal bossing, depressed nasal bridge, hypertelorism (wide-set eyes), hypoplasia of the maxilla and zygomas with a short cranial base, and deficiency of the clavicles (allowing many patients to approximate their shoulders and resulting in a drooped shoulder appearance) (Fig. 21-17, *A*).[25] Orally they present with a high arched palate, deficient premaxilla with relative prognathism caused by normal mandibular length, multiple supernumerary teeth, multiple crown deformities, and lack of eruption of the permanent teeth.[25]

The primary teeth erupt normally but often resorb poorly, and the permanent molars usually erupt, as well as occasionally the incisors, but the premolars and canines rarely erupt.[38] Eruption of the permanent teeth is not induced by simple extraction of the primary teeth.[39] Supernumerary teeth are common, especially in the maxillary incisor and canine regions as well as in the mandibular premolar regions, and these teeth are often dysplastic with dilacerated and deformed roots (possibly caused by severe spatial restrictions in the alveolus).[40] Assisted eruption of the unerupted teeth should be planned carefully, in stages using the remaining primary teeth and erupted permanent teeth as anchorage, if possible.[41] A typical plan would involve extraction of any remaining primary incisors with uncovering and bonding of traction hooks or chains to the unerupted incisors (Fig. 21-17, *B*). Fixed appliances on the remaining primary posterior teeth and permanent first molars can be used to place eruptive archwires (Fig. 21-17, *C*). Alternatively, a reciprocal anchorage concept can be used with the patient placing elastics between the maxillary and mandibular teeth (Fig. 21-17, *D*). Once the permanent incisors are erupted roughly into contact, they can be bonded with fixed appliances, the primary molars and canines extracted, supernumerary teeth removed, and traction hooks or chains placed on the permanent premolars and canines. The permanent molars and incisors can then support the eruptive archwires to these teeth, although it may still be helpful to use interarch vertical elastics. Because of the great number of supernumerary teeth present and close proximity of some of the teeth (Fig. 21-18) desirable to keep, this stage may require more than one surgical uncovering and placement of traction appliances. Second molars may also benefit from uncovering and placement of eruptive forces. Once all the permanent teeth are erupted, they are aligned, the arches coordinated, and, for many of these patients, a maxillary Le Fort I advancement and inferior displacement will be necessary. This complex treatment often requires a long duration with multiple surgeries and challenges in eating/speech during the treatment. It is a disservice to the patient and families involved not to ensure that they are comfortable with and willing to undergo these challenges prior to initiation of treatment.

REFERENCES

1. World Health Organization: Available at: www.who.int/genomics/anomalies/en/. Accessed August 27, 2007.
2. Latham RA: Orthopedic advancement of the cleft maxillary segment: a preliminary report. *Cleft Palate J* 1980;17:227-233.
3. Graber TM: Craniofacial morphology in cleft palate and cleft lip deformities. *Surg Gynecol Obstetr* 1949;88:359-369.
4. Berkowitz S: Timing of cleft palate closure — age should not be the sole determinant. *J Cranio Genet Dev Biol* 1985;(Suppl 1): 69-83.
5. Mestre JC, DeJesus J, Subtelny JD: Unoperated oral clefts at maturation. *Angle Orthod* 1960;30:78-85.
6. Millard DR, Berkowitz S, Latham RA, Wolfe SA: A discussion of presurgical orthodontics in patients with clefts. *Cleft Palate J* 1988;25:403-412.
7. Huddart AG: An evaluation of pre-surgical treatment. *Br J Orthod* 1973;1:21-25.
8. Subtelny JD: Orthodontic principles in treatment of cleft lip and palate. In Bardach J, Morris HL, editors: *Multidisciplinary management of cleft lip and palate.* Philadelphia: WB Saunders, 1990, pp 615-636.
9. Grayson BH, Cutting CB: Presurgical nasoalveolar orthopedic molding in primary correction of the nose, lip, and alveolus of infants born with unilateral and bilateral clefts. *Cleft Palate Craniofac J* 2001;38(3):193-198.

10. Moore RN: Orthodontic management of the patient with cleft lip and palate. *Ear Nose Throat J* 1986;65:46-58.
11. El Deeb M, Messer LB, Lehnert MW, et al: Canine eruption into grafted bone in maxillary alveolar cleft defects. *Cleft Palate J* 1982;19:9-16.
12. Hall HD, Werther JR: Conventional alveolar cleft bone grafting. *Oral Maxillofac Surg Clin North Am* 1991;3:609-616.
13. Bergland O, Semb G, Abyholm FE: Elimination of residual alveolar cleft by secondary bone grafting and subsequent orthodontic treatment. *Cleft Palate J* 1986;23:175-205.
14. Vig KWL, Turvey TA: Orthodontic–surgical interaction in the management of cleft lip and palate. *Clin Plast Surg* 1985;12:735-748.
15. Boyne PJ: Bone grafting in the osseous reconstruction of alveolar and palatal clefts. *Oral Maxillofac Surg Clin North Am* 1991;3:589-597.
16. Simmons KE, Johnston MC: Craniofacial morphology of monozygotic twins discordant for clefts of the lip and/or palate. In preparation.
17. Verdon P. *Utilisation raisonnée du masque orthopédique facial.* Orthodontie, Tours, 1989.
18. Tindlund RS, Per Rygh, Boe OE: protraction of the upper jaw in cleft lip and palate patients during the deciduous and mixed dentition periods in comparison with normal growth and development. *Cleft Palate Craniofacial J* 1993;30:182-194.
19. Tindlund RS, Rygh P: Maxillary protraction: different effects on facial morphology in unilateral and bilateral cleft lip and palate patients. *Cleft Palate Craniofac J* 1993;30:208-221.
20. Buschang PH, Porter C, Genecov E, et al: Face mask therapy of preadolescents with unilateral cleft lip and palate. *Angle Orthod* 1994;64:145-150.
21. Vig KWL, Turvey TA, Fonseca RJ: Orthodontic and surgical considerations in bone grafting in the cleft maxilla and palate. In Turvey TA, Vig KWL, Fonseca RJ, editors: *Facial clefts and craniosynostosis: principles and management.* Philadelphia: WB Saunders, 1996, pp 396-440.
22. Vargervik K: Growth characteristics of the premaxilla and orthodontic treatment principles in bilateral cleft lip and palate. *Cleft Palate J* 1983;20:289-302.
23. Friede H, Pruzansky S: Longitudinal study of growth in bilateral cleft lip and palate from infancy to adolescence. *Plast Reconstr Surg* 1972;49:392-403.
24. Ross RB: Treatment variables affecting facial growth in complete unilateral cleft lip and palate. *Cleft Palate J* 1987;24:3-77.
25. Gorlin RJ, Cohen MM, Hennekam RCM, editors: *Syndromes of the head and neck,* edition 4. Oxford Monographs on Medical Genetics: no. 42, New York: Oxford University Press, 2001.
26. Pruzansky S: Not all dwarfed mandibles are alike. *Birth Defects* 1969;1:120-129.
27. Harvold EP, Vargervik K, Chierici G, editors: *Treatment of hemifacial microsomia.* New York: Alan R. Liss, 1983.
28. Kaban LB, Mulliken JB, Murray JE: Three-dimensional approach to analysis and treatment of hemifacial microsomia. *Cleft Palate J* 1986;18:90-99.
29. Kaban LB, Moses ML, Mulliken JB: Surgical correction of hemifacial microsomia in the growing child. *Plast Reconstr Surg* 1988;82:9-19.
30. Vargervik K, Kaban LB: Hemifacial microsomia I. Diagnosis and management. In Bell WH, editor: *Modern practice in orthognathic and reconstructive surgery,* volume 2. Philadelphia: WB Saunders, 1992, pp 1533-1560.
31. Kearns G, Padwa BL, Kaban LB: Hemifacial microsomia: The disorder and its surgical management. In Booth PW, Schendel SA, Hausemen J-E, editors: *Maxillofacial surgery,* volume 2. Philadelphia: Elsevier, 2007, pp 918-946.
32. Posnick JC, Mühling J: Surgical treatment of craniofacial dysostosis syndrome and single-suture synostosis. In Booth PW, Schendel SA, Hausemen J-E, editors: *Maxillofacial surgery,* volume 2, edition 2. Philadelphia: Elsevier, 2007, pp 876-900.
33. Koppel DA, Moos KF: Treacher Collins syndrome. In Booth PW, Schendel SA, Hausemen J-E, editors. *Maxillofacial surgery,* volume 2, edition 2. Philadelphia: Elsevier; 2007, pp 947-958.
34. Simmons KE: Growth hormone and craniofacial changes: Preliminary data from studies in Turner's syndrome. *Pediatrics* 1999;104(Suppl):1021-1024.
35. Pilcher ES: Dental care for the patient with Down syndrome. *Down Synd Res Pract* 1998;5:111-116.
36. Hoyer H, Limbrock GJ: Orofacial regulation therapy in children with Down syndrome, using the methods and appliances of Castillo-Morales. *ASDC J Dent Child* 1990;57:442-444.
37. Musich DR: Orthodontic intervention and patients with Down syndrome. The role of inclusion, technology and leadership. *Angle Orthod* 2006;76:734-735.
38. Jensen BL, Kreiborg S: Development of the dentition in cleidocranial dysplasia. *J Oral Pathol* 1990;19:89-93.
39. Winter GR: Dental conditions in cleidocranial dysostosis. *Am J Orthodont* 1943;29:61-89.
40. Richardson A, Deussen FF: Facial and dental anomalies in cleidocranial dysplasia: A study of 17 cases. *Int J Paediatr Dent* 1994;4:225-231.
41. Daskalogiannakis J, Piedade L, Lindholm TC, et al: Cleidocranial dysplasia: 2 generations of management. *J Can Dent Assoc* 2006;72:337-342.

CHAPTER 22

Temporomandibular Disorders

Peter M. Greco

Temporomandibular disorders (TMDs) involve musculoskeletal pain disorders and functional disharmony of the masticatory system. TMD is one subcategory of orofacial pain that includes intracranial pain, headache, neuropathic pain, intraoral pain, and all other pains associated with the head and neck.[1] The preliminary role of the dental practitioner is to discern whether the patient's clinical presentation reveals a diagnosis of pathology or dysfunction that is within the realm of dental treatment and/or if the clinical diagnosis requires allied medical collaboration for effective management. Once the problem has been verified to be within the realm of dental therapy, the clinician must identify the source of the problem and treat accordingly. Often the originating source and symptomatic site of the pain are incongruous, which differs from conventional dental diagnosis. Unless the primary site from which the pain emanates is addressed by therapy, control of the problem will remain elusive.[2] Hence, history and examination are critical to diagnosis, but also unlike most dental diagnoses, the importance of the patient's history of the disorder is far more indicative than presenting signs. Keen diagnostic skills in the treatment of TMD are the key to successful management, as TMD is often a combination of etiologies rather than a single anatomical or functional disharmony. Combination of etiologies often complicates successful treatment and can frustrate the clinician and patient.

Many diagnostic systems and algorithms of TMD have been proposed since otolaryngologist James Costen first published his findings in 1934. Costen[3] described a small group of patients with ear/sinus symptoms in conjunction with functional disturbance of the temporomandibular joints (TMJs). Okeson[2] has emphasized the importance of determining whether the presenting signs or symptoms are truly emanating from the region of complaint or whether the symptoms originate from a distant site by virtue of interaction of nerve fibers that coalesce in the upper spinal cord and brain stem. He applied the terms *primary pain* and *secondary* or *heterotopic pain* to these two phenomena, respectively. Successful delineation of primary and secondary pain can mean the difference between treatment success and failure, since quality treatment can unequivocally fail if applied to the incorrect site or misdiagnosed clinical situation. Consider a patient experiencing left-sided mandibular pain as a result of a myocardial infarction who is treated via delivery of a maxillary splint, which provides a perfect mutually protected occlusal scheme. The infarct remains of fatal potential despite apparent harmony of the masticatory system.

TMDs can be classified into several subcategories[2]:

- **Masticatory disorders** including protective co-contraction, persistent local muscular soreness, myofascial or trigger-point pain, myospasm, chronic myositis, and fibromyalgia. These disorders predominate in frequency and are each managed differently.
- **Dysfunction of the joint complex itself** including disc displacements, disc/condyle/fossa incompatibilities including adhesions, and subluxation/dislocation. These problems may require surgical co-therapy and can often be anatomically documented by modern imaging techniques.
- **Inflammatory conditions** including capsulitis, synovitis, retrodiscitis, arthroses, and posttraumatic sequelae. Many are self-resolving and require little therapeutic management if diagnosed correctly.
- **Hypomobility** including ankylosis, muscle dysfunction, and anatomical impedance ranging in need from continued surveillance to initiation of collaborative care with multiple co-therapists.
- **Growth disorders** including congenital bone and muscle disorders.

Accurate diagnosis and classification are critical to proper management to determine therapeutic modalities and to assess the need for involvement of allied specialists. For example, as chronicity of TMD increases, so do the number of therapists needed for effective management given increasing difficulty in management. In general, dental practitioners are most effective at managing acute muscle problems but require increased collaboration to provide effective care as joint involvement and chronicity increases.

The intent of this chapter is to address the most common questions pertaining to TMD that arise in dental practice. Hence, the approach to these questions is intended to be practical and applicable to routine care delivery.

1. When is treatment indicated for TMD?

The presence of joint sounds is insufficient reason to implement therapy. Consequently, the persistence of joint sounds alone is an inadequate criterion for success or failure of therapy. *Pain* and/or *loss of function* are the hallmarks of need for treatment.[2] As other weight-bearing joints of the body emit joint sounds during function, the TMJs are no exception. Thus, signs and symptoms of TMJ dysfunction are common but well tolerated and are often ignored by the patient. Although statistics vary, Dolwick and Dimitriulis[4] report that 60% to 70% of the population display at least one sign of TMD and 25% display at least one symptom. It is more often seen in females than males. Furthermore, TMD is a phenomenon most commonly noted during the patient's reproductive years with peak frequency between the ages of 25 and 44 years, and only 0.7% by age 65. Hence, it is logical to infer that signs and symptoms self-resolve without or in spite of therapy. This phenomenon has been termed *regression to the means* and occurs frequently in nature.[2]

Disc position is also not critically related to the success or failure of treatment. A recent study has shown that although approximately 75% of those who have undergone arthroscopic surgery for difficulties in opening may have improvement with significant pain reduction, subsequent MRI imaging of the joints of these patients has demonstrated no true change in disc position.[5] Condylar position and occlusion may not be highly correlated. A recent investigation has revealed that there is a significant difference in the occlusal position of asymptomatic patients when comparing maximum intercuspation to condylar-dictated occlusion within the same patient.[6]

2. What is the role of occlusal disharmony in TMD?

Multiple investigations have indicated that malocclusion and functional disharmony have little role in the etiology of TMD. A review of the literature reveals that most studies exploring this topic are retrospective rather than prospective, and many are viewpoint in nature rather than evidence based. In a recent article involving questionnaire format and multivariate regression analyses of 4290 adults examined for TMD, there was no significant relationship to occlusal factors with respect to temporomandibular symptoms.[7] This finding is the norm rather than the exception.

There has been one non-treated clinical population that may have a predisposed profile for TMD. Pullinger et al.[8] observed that there was a significantly high probability of nonreducing disc displacement in growing patients with unilateral posterior crossbite. These authors attributed this tendency toward adaptation of mandibular position, which may account for the condylar displacement. Thilander[9] also recommended early correction of posterior crossbite to resolve facial asymmetry, normalize muscle activity, and avoid disc displacement resulting from asymmetric skeletal form. A later study[7] using a small subject size determined that pretreatment asymmetric joint spaces and asymmetric mandibles resolved by maxillary expansion, thus supporting early correction of posterior crossbite.

There is also insufficient evidence to indicate that occlusal adjustment is effective treatment for TMD unless there is a single tooth in hyperocclusion or is severely mobile.[7,8,10]

Okeson[2] has introduced the term *orthopedic stability* to describe the simultaneous relationship between condyles that are seated in a musculoskeletally stable position as the teeth are in maximum intercuspation. If the position of the teeth prevents superior-anterior seating of the condyles and the complex is loaded by trauma or parafunction, the loading will occur in an unstable joint relationship. This is called *orthopedic instability*. The joints, muscles, or teeth are adversely affected. Although many patients demonstrate orthopedic instability, the key factors in the development of symptoms are loading and host susceptibility. There are multiple methods of loading unstable joints inclusive of trauma and parafunction. Host susceptibility remains an elusive factor but may include gender, history, or emotional factors.

3. When are occlusal splints indicated in therapy, and when are alternative forms of management of TMD appropriate?

Some authors advocate the use of splints to diagnostically determine the position of the condyle prior to orthodontic correction or prosthetic rehabilitation.[11-14] The additional intent is to induce muscle relaxation to allow condylar seating in a physiologic position regardless of the occlusion (Figs. 22-1 and 22-2).

Okeson[2] recommends occlusal splints to address symptoms of orthopedic instability. Orthopedic instability is the lack of simultaneous superior-anterior condylar seating with the teeth in maximum intercuspation, concurrent with relaxation of the closing musculature. The intent of splint therapy is to provide a functional occlusion that is reversible or modifiable, and to concurrently interrupt destructive force patterns on the muscles and joints. Muscular symptoms are more prevalent than intracapsular disharmonies, and often surface when an unstable musculoskeletal system is loaded by parafunction resulting from emotional stress, habitual bruxing, or deep pain input. Multiple authors have substantiated the efficacy of splint therapy for the reduction of muscular symptoms.[15-18] Occlusal splints may also have a role in therapy when the overwhelming symptomatology and final diagnosis is that of intracapsular dysfunction without predominance of muscle symptoms.[19]

The design of the splint should provide orthopedic stability, albeit artificial. Efficacy of the full-coverage repositioning splint that reproduces a mutually protected occlusal scheme has been supported by evidence–based investigation. Although a number of splint designs are available, the clinician should choose the design that best suits clinical objectives. Thus, if the goal of splint therapy is to provide posterior contact with anterior disclusion in excursions, the superior repositioning splint or stabilization splint is appropriate. Supportive therapy such as physical therapy, pharmacologic management, thermal therapy, and other less conventional modalities are also used effectively, but precise diagnosis is necessary for appropriate therapeutic prescription.

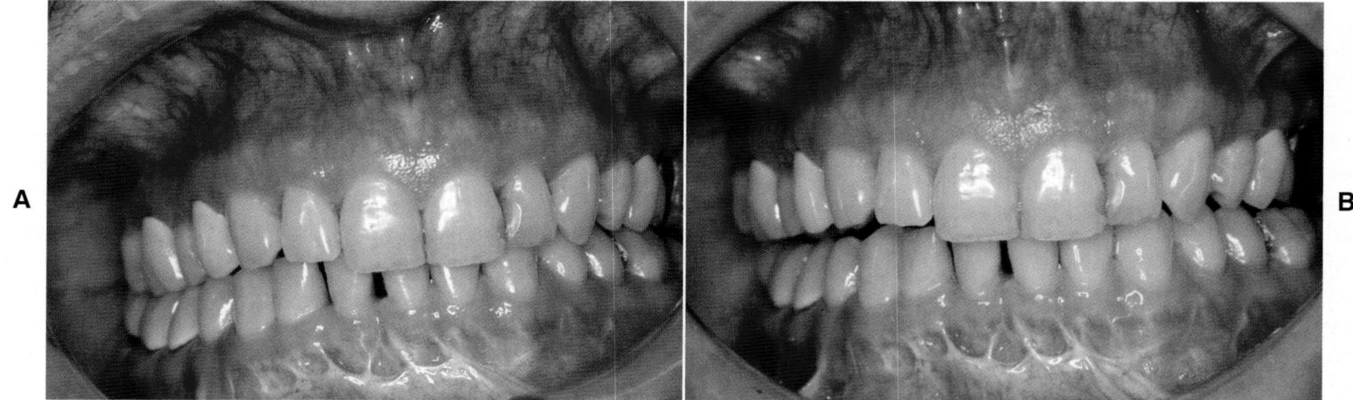

FIG 22-1 **A,** Patient with orthopedic instability and joint pain with local muscle soreness. **B,** Patient after 2 months of maxillary splint wear with condyles now seated properly.

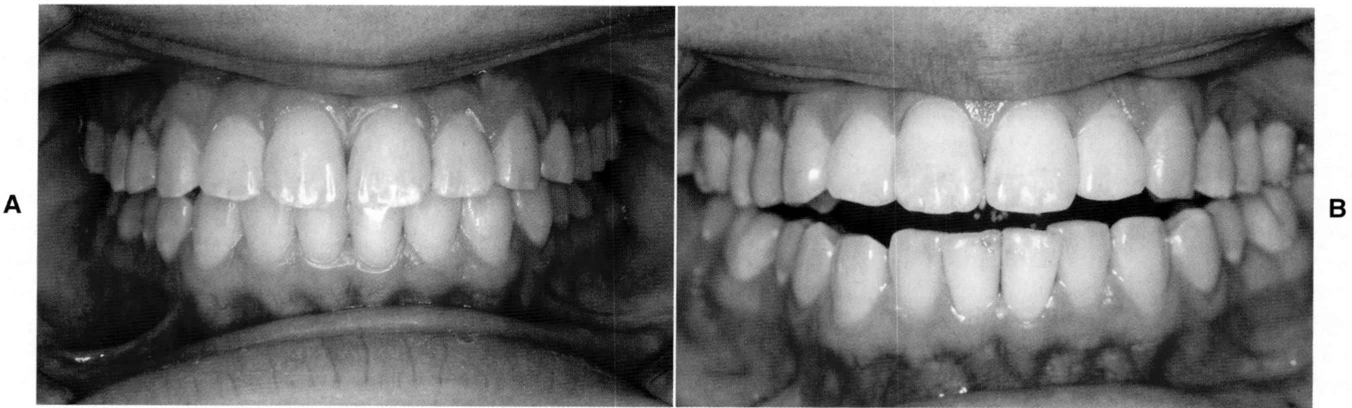

FIG 22-2 **A,** Patient with TMD secondary to a habitual intercuspal position that distracted condyles from the fossa. **B,** Patient after 6 weeks of splint therapy allowed the musculature to provide condylar seating.

4. What are the commonly used pharmacologic modalities for management of TMD?

Pharmacologic intervention for the treatment of TMD can be categorized into seven broad categories:

1. **Centrally acting muscle relaxants.** These drugs are actually interneuronal blocking agents acting at the spinal cord level and brain stem. They decrease muscular activity by inhibiting neurotransmission and are usually administered at bedtime to decrease the possibility of interference with patient lifestyle because of undesirable side effects such as vertigo or drowsiness. They may also be helpful in inducing effective stages of sleep, which is critical to management of TMD. Examples include chlorzoxazone (Parafon Forte), carisoprodol (Soma), and cyclobenzaprine (Flexeril).
2. **Anxiolytics.** Most commonly used are benzodiazepines, which provide an antianxiety effect but are often incorrectly prescribed for muscle relaxation. They are helpful in management of insomnia associated with TMD, but studies have shown that their effect on skeletal muscle relaxation is no greater than that of a placebo. Hence, these agents are helpful as an adjunct to skeletal muscle relaxation. Examples are diazepam (Valium), clonazepam (Klonopin), alprazolam (Xanax), hydroxyzine pamoate (Vistaril), and lorazepam (Ativan).
3. **Barbiturates.** These are often combined with analgesics to enhance pain relief in conjunction with the anxiolytic/muscle relaxant effect of the barbiturate. They are useful for tension-type headache. Barbiturates have serious side effects including general depression, as well as decreased excitability of cardiovascular, respiratory, and gastrointestinal systems. Sleep disturbances can occur with barbiturate use, and drug disposition tolerance can also develop as increased hepatic metabolism leads to the need of increased quantity of the drug to maintain tissue concentrations. Drug dependence, paradoxical reactions (especially in the elderly), and other physical side effects can occur. A commonly prescribed barbiturate is butabarbital, which is combined with caffeine and acetaminophen in Fioricet. The clinician needs to be very careful in prescribing this class of medications for TMD.
4. **Tricyclic antidepressants.** These are used in doses that are lower than those used for treatment of depression. They act by inhibiting the reuptake of serotonin and norepinephrine. An example is amitriptyline (Elavil) administered in doses

of 10 to 20 mg/day at bedtime, compared with 75 to 150 mg for depression. Side effects include drowsiness, xerostomia, urinary retention, blurred vision, ventricular arrhythmias, and/or postural hypotension.

5. **Opiate and nonopiate analgesics.** Nonopiate analgesics include NSAIDs and acetaminophen, the latter of which has no antiinflammatory properties and does not affect platelet aggregation. An effective regimen of NSAID dosage is 600 mg of ibuprofen three times a day at mealtimes for 1 week. This drug carries very little abuse potential but has many contraindications that are often overlooked. In the case of NSAIDs, such contraindications include intolerance in asthmatics. Nonopiates should be used with caution or avoided in allergic patients; those with hepatic or renal dysfunction, anemia, bleeding tendencies, cardiac failure, pregnancy; the elderly; or those with GI ulceration. COX-2 inhibitors are contraindicated in patients with sulfonamide allergies. Drug interactions include anticoagulants, alpha and beta blockers, thiazide and furosemide diuretics, ACE inhibitors, fluconazole (antifungal preparations), lithium, and methotrexate.
6. **Corticosteroids.** Used only locally via injection rather than systemically because of significant side effects. Corticosteroids can be destructive to joints when used repeatedly.
7. **Local anesthetics.** These are applied either diagnostically or therapeutically. Regional blocks are helpful to determine if pain is primary or secondary. Trigger point injections can be effective in the control of myofascial pain. Both short- and long-acting agents are available.
8. **Botulinum toxin.** Botulinum toxin A is a neurotoxin that prevents the release of acetylcholine at the motor end plates.[20] The toxin is injected into muscles undergoing refractory myospasm in order to produce muscle paralysis of approximately 3 months. Given the temporary nature of such therapy, the use of botulinum toxin is considered to be palliative rather than definitive, but it remains a treatment option should other therapeutic measures fail.

The clinician should thoroughly understand the pharmacologic properties of prescribed/administered medications and inform the patient of their possible side effects.

5. What are the contemporary imaging modalities used in TMD diagnosis?

Many articles have been written regarding imaging protocol. In patients without medical contraindication, nondynamic evaluation of soft tissue structures such as the disc is best accomplished by MRI evaluation, whereas hard structures such as bone and cartilage are best visualized by radiographic techniques.[21] Panoramic radiographs or conventional radiographs do not contribute to diagnostic accuracy beyond the diagnosis gleaned from history and physical examination alone.[22] Arthrography is reserved for observation of disc form, location, and joint dynamics as inferred by observation of contrast injection into the upper and/or lower joint spaces.[2] New modalities of cone beam computerized technology are effective in assessment of size, morphology, and position of the condyles but are inadequate for evaluation of musculature or disc morphology.[23-25] Imaging is therefore not indicated in suspected masticatory muscle disorders, nor in short-term inflammatory disease such as synovitis, capsulitis, or retrodiscitis.

6. What is the role of surgery in TMD management?

According to Dolwick,[4] surgery is unequivocally the therapy of choice to address the less common TMJ disorders such as ankylosis, neoplasm, growth disorders, and unmanageable dislocation. When the clinical evaluation and patient's response to conservative therapy (pharmacologic management, splint therapy, physical therapy, etc.) is unsuccessful, surgery should be considered based on presenting levels of pain and dysfunction. It is absolutely essential to verify that the TMJ is the primary site of pain rather than a heterotopic site as defined previously by Okeson.[2] Although open joint surgery may still have application in the surgeon's armamentarium, the overwhelming majority of surgery now appears to be arthrocentesis (joint lavage) and arthroscopy (lavage, adhesion release, and visualization). The latter allows tissue reduction procedures (partial or complete diskectomy, arthrotomy, and condylectomy) during arthroscopy if indicated. Numerous recent studies have demonstrated the efficacy of arthrocentesis for conditions of closed lock and osteoarthritic joints.[27-31] The reported success rate of surgery varies, but it is well established that the success rate decreases as the number of previous surgeries rises.[4] It has been reported that a near zero prognosis of successful surgery is expected if the patient has undergone two or more previous unsuccessful surgeries. As is true of treatment of TMD in general, there is no question that case selection is as important as clinical technique in TMJ surgery.

7. What is the relationship between orthodontic therapy and TMD?

This question has been extensively investigated by an evidence-based approach as summarized in an excellent review article by McNamara.[32] Twenty-one papers spanning 1980 through 1995 were reviewed, with sample sizes ranging from 22 to 462 patients per study. In summary of the multiple articles reviewed, there is little basis that orthodontic treatment affects the prognosis of TMD either positively or negatively, except in the possible case of unilateral posterior crossbite in the growing patient as previously mentioned in this chapter.

It has been stated that an elevated host susceptibility and orthopedic instability in conjunction with joint loading, especially during parafunction, can initiate or exacerbate TMD.[2] Orthodontic patients with a previous history of TMD may also be at higher risk for recurrence during treatment, especially in patients undergoing active orthodontic therapy where occlusal interferences emerge during the course of correction.[33]

The presiding consensus is that orthodontic treatment is not an effective primary treatment modality for patients with TMD, nor does orthodontic therapy predispose patients to TMD.[34] As Okeson aptly states: "The clinician who only evaluates the occlusion is likely missing as much as the clinician who never evaluates the occlusion."[2]

SUMMARY

The identification and treatment of TMD can be as rewarding as it can be frustrating. Careful diagnosis gleaned via history and confirmed by clinical examination with imaging when indicated is key to successful treatment. This approach will also indicate the need for allied specialty collaboration. Treatment should always begin conservatively and involve a clear, succinct yet informative explanation of the patient's diagnosis and treatment plan to enlist involvement of the patient in his or her rehabilitation.

ACKNOWLEDGMENT

Special thanks to Dr. Jeffrey P. Okeson for his review of this manuscript as well as for his special role in guidance and instruction of the principles of management of TMD. His contributions to dentistry and to the specialty of orthodontics have been invaluable.

REFERENCES

1. Okeson JP: Diagnostic classification of orofacial pain disorders. In *Orofacial pain: guidelines for assessment, diagnosis, and management.* Chicago: Quintessence Publishing, 1996.
2. Okeson JP: Functional neuroanatomy and physiology of the masticatory system. In *Management of temporomandibular disorders and occlusion.* St Louis: Mosby, 2003.
3. Costen JB: Syndrome of ear and sinus symptoms dependent upon disturbed function of the temporomandibular joint. *Ann Otol Rhin Laryng* 1934;43:1.
4. Dolwick MF, Dimitriulis G: Is there a role for temporomandibular surgery? *Br J Oral Maxillofac Surg* 1994;3:307-313.
5. Ohnuki T, Fukuda M, Iino M, Takahashi T: Magnetic resonance evaluation of the disk before and after arthroscopic surgery for TM disorders. *Oral Surg Oral Med Oral Path* 2003;96(Aug): 141-148.
6. Cordray FE: Three-dimensional analysis of models articulated in the seated condylar position from a deprogrammed asymptomatic population: a prospective study. Part I. *Am J Orthod Dentofacial Orthop* 2006;129:619-630.
7. Tsukiyama Y, Baba K, Clark GT: An evidence-based assessment of occlusal adjustment as a treatment for TM disorders. *J Pros Dent* 2001;86(July):57-66.
8. Pullinger AG, Seligman DA, Gorbein A: A multiple regression analysis of the risk and relative odds of temporomandibular disorders as a function of common occlusal features. *J Dent Res* 1993;72:968-979.
9. Thilander B: Temporomandibular joint problems in children. In Carlson DS, McNamara JA, Ribbens KA, editors: *Developmental aspects of temporomandibular disorders.* Ann Arbor: University of Michigan Press, 1985.
10. Huang G: Occlusal adjustment for treating and preventing TM disorders. *Am J Orthod Dentofacial Orthop* 2004;126(2):138-139.
11. Roth RH: Functional occlusion for the orthodontist. *J Clin Orthop* 1981;XV;1:32-51.
12. Roth RH: Functional occlusion for the orthodontist—part II. *J Clin Orthop* 1981;XV;2:100-121.
13. Williamson EH, Evans DL, Barton WA, Williams BH: The effect of biteplane use on terminal hinge axis location. *Angle Orthod* 1977;47:25-33.
14. Williamson EH, Steinke RM, Morse PK, Swift TR: Centric relation: a comparison of muscle determined position and operator guidance. *Am J Orthod* 1980;77:133-145.
15. Kuttila M, Le Bell Y, Savolainen-Niemi E, et al: Efficiency of occlusal appliance therapy in secondary otalgia and TM disorders. *Acta Odontol Scand* 2002;60(4):248-254.
16. Ekberg E, Vallon D, Nilner M: The efficacy of appliance a therapy in patients with TM disorders of mainly myogenic origin: A randomized, controlled short term trial. *J Orofac Pain* 2003;17(2):133-139.
17. Roark AL, Glaros AG, O'Mahoney M: Effects of interocclusal appliances on EMG activity during parafunctional tooth contact. *J Rehabil* 2003;30:573-577.
18. Greco PM, Vanarsdall RL: An evaluation of anterior temporalis and masseter muscle activity in appliance therapy. *Angle Orthod* 1999;69:141-146.
19. Schmitter M, Zahran M, Duc JM, et al: Conservative therapy in patients with anterior disc displacement without reduction using 2 common splints: a randomized clinical trial. *J Oral Maxillofac Surg* 2005;63:1295-1303.
20. Jankovic J, Brin MF: Therapeutic uses of botulinum toxin, *N Engl J Med* 1991; 324:1186-1194.
21. Styles C, Whyte A: MRI assessment in the assessment of internal derangement of pain within the TM joint: A pictorial essay. *Br J Oral Maxillofac Surg* 2002;40:220-228.
22. Epstein JB, Caldwell J, Black G: The utility of panoramic imaging of the TMJ in patients with TM disorders. *Oral Surg Oral Med Oral Path* 2001;92:236-239.
23. Brooks SL, Brand JW, Gibbs SJ, et al: Imaging of the temporomandibular joint: position paper of the American Academy of Oral and Maxillofacial Radiology. *Oral Surg Oral Med Oral Path* 1997;83(5):609-618.
24. Cevidanes LHS, Styner MA, Proffit WR: Image analysis in superimposition of 3-dimensional cone-beam computed tomography models. *Am J Orthod Dentofacial Orthop* 2006;129(5):611-618.
25. Chirani RA, Jacq JJ, Meriot P, Roux C: Temporomandibular joint: A methodology of magnetic resonance imaging 3-D reconstruction. *Oral Surg Oral Med Oral Path* 2004;97:756-761.
26. Kawamata A, Fujishita M, Kuniteru N, et al: Three dimensional computed tomography of postsurgical condylar displacement after mandibular osteotomy. *Oral Surg Oral Med Oral Path* 1998;85:371-376.
27. Nitzan DW, Price A: The use of arthrocentesis for the treatment of osteoarthritic TMJ's. *J Oral Maxillofac Surg* 2001;59(10): 1154-1159.
28. Yura S, Totsuka Y, Yoshikawa T, Inoue N: Can arthrocentesis release intracapsular adhesions? Arthroscopic Findings before and after irrigation under sufficient hydraulic pressure. *J Oral Maxillofac Surg* 2003;61:1253-1256.
29. Nitzan DW: TMJ "open lock" versus condylar dislocation: signs and symptoms, imaging treatment and pathogenesis. *J Oral Maxillofac Surg* 2002;60(May):506-511.
30. Emshoff R, Rudisch A, Bosch R, Strobl H: Prognostic indicators of the outcome of arthrocentesis; a short term follow-up study. *Oral Surg Oral Med Oral Path* 2003;96(July):12-18.
31. Gesch D, Bernhardt O, Mack F, et al: Association of malocclusion and functional occlusion with subjective symptoms of TMD in adult: Results of the study of health in Pomerania (SHIP). *Angle Orthod* 2005;75(2):183-190.
32. McNamara J: Orthodontic treatment and temporomandibular disorders. *Oral Surg Oral Med Oral Path* 1997;83(1):107-117.
33. Le Bell Y, Niemi PM, Jamsa T, et al: Subjective reactions to intervention with artificial interferences in subjects with and without a history of temporomandibular disorders. *Acta Odontol Scand* 2006;64(1):59-63.
34. Conti A, Freitas M, Conti P, et al: Relationship between signs and symptoms of TM disorders and orthodontic treatment: a cross sectional study. *Angle Orthod* 2003;73(4):411-417.

Retention in Orthodontics

CHAPTER 23

Jeryl D. English • Hitesh Kapadia

Comprehensive orthodontic therapy requires that treatment goals be established during the time of treatment planning. Begin treatment with the end in mind. These goals should include patient esthetics, improved occlusal function, and long-term retention. Little et al.[1] states that the only way to ensure continued satisfactory alignment after treatment is by the use of fixed or removable retention for life. Therefore, instability or a tendency toward relapse should be anticipated. Patients should be advised of the potential for relapse prior to treatment and of the need to stay in long-term retention.

Orthodontists should work to produce an occlusion that is functionally efficient, esthetic, and healthy. Long-term retention helps to ensure stability of the dentition. Interdigitation of the posterior occlusion plays a significant role in the control of anteroposterior and vertical facial growth and is an important factor in jaw relationships.[2] Numerous authors have stated that good intercuspation and occlusal contacts may be the key to a stable orthodontic result.[3-8]

Many of the current concepts in occlusion are derived from a benchmark study by Andrews[9] to determine the keys to normal occlusion. Criteria for inclusion of these nonorthodontic patients in the study were a pleasing appearance, straight teeth, and a good bite that would not benefit from orthodontic treatment. In these individuals, Andrews found six keys in their normal occlusions:

1. Molar relationships
2. Crown angulation
3. Crown inclination
4. No rotations
5. No spaces
6. Flat occlusal plane

It has long been the goal of orthodontists to treat their patients using these six keys as guides for establishing a normal occlusion that is esthetic and with good occlusal function. Many of these keys were included in the Objective Grading System developed by the American Board of Orthodontics (ABO) in the mid-'90s.

In an effort to enhance the reliability of the ABO examiners and provide the candidates with a tool to assess the adequacy of their finished orthodontic results, the Board has established an Objective Grading System to evaluate the final dental casts and panoramic radiographs.[10] The Directors of the ABO developed this grading system for assessing occlusal and radiographic results of orthodontic treatment. Using this system, orthodontists can grade their treated cases to determine if they are producing excellent clinical results.

1. What is retention?

Retention is the last phase of orthodontic treatment and one of the most important, where teeth are held in an esthetic and functional position.[11,12] Retention of the corrected malocclusion is just as important as the diagnosis, treatment plan, and actual orthodontic treatment to correct the patient's malocclusion. Planning for retention should be done prior to any orthodontic treatment for each individual case. The type of retention should be determined at the beginning of treatment as well as any procedures to help retain the final functional and esthetic occlusion.

2. Why is retention necessary?

The need for retention is important to maintain the stability of the occlusion achieved by the orthodontist and patient.[13] Without stability, the esthetic and functional result may relapse. The improvements achieved from long and painstaking treatment may be lost because of relapse after the orthodontic appliances are removed. Teeth that have been moved orthodontically have an inherent tendency to return to their original malocclusion positions.

3. What are the general factors affecting stability?

Throughout the orthodontic literature, many factors have been discussed concerning stability of the orthodontic treatment result.[14,15] Three factors are consistently mentioned as to why retention is necessary to maintain the orthodontic correction:

1. The time needed for the gingival and periodontal ligament fibers to reorganize.
2. Growth, especially mandibular growth, may alter the orthodontic correction.
3. Soft-tissue pressure from the oral musculature may lead to a relapse tendency.

4. Why is growth a consideration in retention?

The nature and duration of retention depends on the patient's maturational status and on anticipated future growth.[16] Growth produces occlusal changes in all three skeletal dimensions. The transverse dimension is completed first and has a lesser effect on the occlusion than the vertical and anteroposterior dimensions. However, if a patient has had transverse expansion, there is a degree of rebound even in the transverse dimension. Ideally, an adolescent patient should wear orthodontic retainers indefinitely; however, at a minimum, the retainers must be worn until growth is completed in adulthood. Even adults show some craniofacial remodeling that can cause alteration of the occlusion. In orthodontics, we are dealing with a living, dynamic system of growth. Throughout our life, orthodontic retention will help to minimize the changes in our occlusion. Therefore, retention should be considered for life if the occlusal alignment is to be maintained.

5. What are retention considerations in extraction and nonextraction cases?

There is not a specific retention philosophy for extraction cases and another for nonextraction cases. The orthodontist decides on the individual's retention plan at the beginning of treatment when the diagnostic records are used to establish the patient's treatment plan. By following this plan, it will be possible to achieve an esthetic and functional occlusion.

Edwards[16] has shown that in extraction cases, excess gingival tissue forms as the adjacent teeth are moved toward one another in closing the extraction site. This excess gingival tissue should be surgically removed to prevent relapse.

6. What are retention considerations in Class II cases?

Skeletal Class II malocclusions are corrected in two ways: restricting maxillary growth with headgear appliances, or using a functional appliance such as a Herbst or Twin Block. Class II elastics are also used, but this may cause proclining and flaring of the lower incisors. If proclined, the lower incisor will upright and crowd because of lip pressure once retention is removed. To overcome these relapse tendencies, discontinue Class II elastics at least 2 months prior to debonding. Overcorrection of the Class II treatment is recommended due to differential jaw growth resulting in long-term relapse.

This relapse tendency can be controlled by continuing to wear a headgear at night or using a functional appliance such as a Bionator to hold the occlusal relationship.[15] Obviously, this type of retention is for the patient with a more severe skeletal problem initially.

7. What are retention considerations in Class III cases?

Early correction of skeletal Class III malocclusions in the mixed dentition using a palatal expander and protraction facemask is useful for altering the skeletal components.[17,18] It is more successful in deep bite cases than in open bite cases, since the mandibular plane angle and anterior facial length will increase. Retaining the correction can be frustrating because of continued mandibular growth, which is difficult to control. Correction of true Class III malocclusions in adults caused by maxillary hypoplasia, mandibular prognathism, or a combination of the two most often requires orthognathic surgical correction. A gnathologic positioner is a useful retainer in mild Class III malocclusions. Use of chin caps to restrict mandibular growth is not very effective.

8. What are retention considerations in open bite cases?

An open bite malocclusion may be dental or skeletal in nature. A dental open bite may be caused by depression of the incisors because of a habit such as thumb- or finger-sucking or poor tongue posture. A good cephalometric value to differentiate between a dental and skeletal open bite is incision-stomion; dental open bites have intruded maxillary incisors whereas skeletal open bites have a normal incisor position. The open bite must be accurately diagnosed and treated if relapse is to be prevented.

In skeletal open bite, incisors are in a normal position, but the posterior teeth have elongated. Controlling the eruption of the maxillary molar with high-pull headgears and a transpalatal bar with a midline acrylic palatal button 4 mm off of the palate is useful to control extrusion. If correction of severe open bite is not started in the mixed dentition, it will most likely require orthognathic surgery in late adolescence or adulthood. The skeletal open bite phenotype is easily diagnosed in the early mixed dentition.

9. What are the considerations in deep bite cases?

Deep bites are common in certain malocclusions such as Class II division 2 and are caused by overeruption of the maxillary incisors, mandibular incisors, or both. Once the deep bite is corrected, it must be controlled in retention or it is likely to relapse.[19,20] Retention is accomplished with a maxillary removable retainer with a bite plate, which the lower incisors and cuspids will contact if the bite begins to deepen. The appliance should not cause the posterior teeth to disocclude. This retainer should be worn at night until the late teens or early 20s to maintain occlusal stability.

10. What are the indications for bonded lingual retainers?

Fixed orthodontic retainers are usually wires bonded to the lingual surface of the mandible anterior teeth for esthetics and prolonged retention.[21,22] These may be fabricated directly in the mouth or indirectly from an accurate stone model. The bonded retainer is placed in the patient's mouth and secured with a light cured composite resin. The fixed retainer is useful to retain the mandibular canine-to-canine region, and a bonded retainer is more esthetic than a banded retainer. The fixed bonded retainer is also used to maintain corrected midline diastema and to maintain pontic or implant space. It is also useful for maintaining the vertical position of teeth extruded into the arch such as palatally

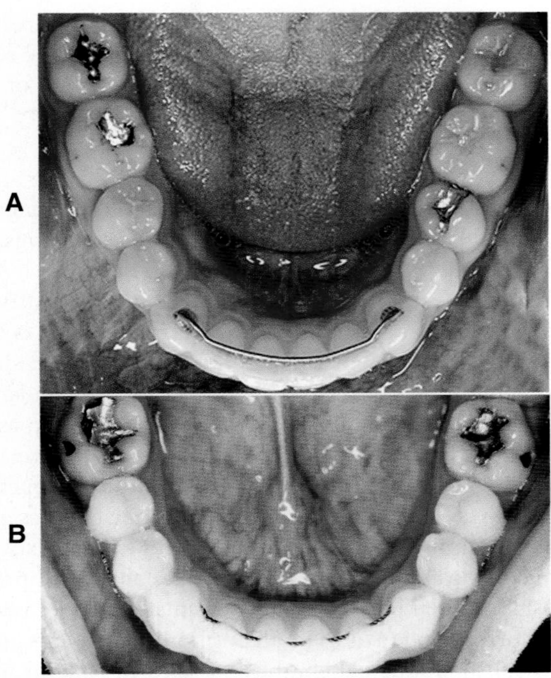

FIG 23-1 Mandibular bonded retainer. **A,** Cuspid to cuspid. **B,** Bonded to every tooth.

impacted cuspids. In most instances the retainer wire is bonded to the terminal teeth (canines) of the retainers (Fig. 23-1, *A*) and not bonded to every tooth. Fixed retainers make interproximal hygiene procedures more difficult. However, with good flossing procedures, these fixed bonded retainers could be left in place until adulthood or indefinitely if needed. It is important that the general dentist not remove the bonded lingual retainer without consultation with the orthodontist, since the teeth may relapse. Today more orthodontists are bonding a 0.0195-twisted wire to every tooth from cuspid to cuspid (Fig. 23-1, *B*). This increases stability and is possible due to improvements in the composite material.

11. What are the indications for removable retainers?

Removable retainers are effective for retention against intra-arch relapse. These retainers are made of stainless-steel wire and acrylic (Fig. 23-2).

The four basic components are the clasps, the anterior retainer wire, the acrylic body, and any auxiliaries added to the retainer. They should be fabricated from an accurate stone cast. The labial bow provides the orthodontist the ability to control the anterior teeth.

Retention clasps are necessary for the retainer to stay firmly in place. The Hawley retainer is the most common removable retainer and the type of retainer used to control a deep bite, as a bite plane is easily added. A lower Hawley retainer is much more difficult to insert because of undercuts in the premolar and molar region. A bonded lingual retainer is more suitable for the mandibular arch.

A second major removable retainer is the wrap-around retainer (Fig. 23-3). It firmly holds each tooth in position and is excellent for maintaining space closure after extractions. There are no wires across the occlusion, so there are no occlusal interferences. Wrap-around retainers are more difficult to fabricate and are therefore more expensive than regular Hawley retainers.

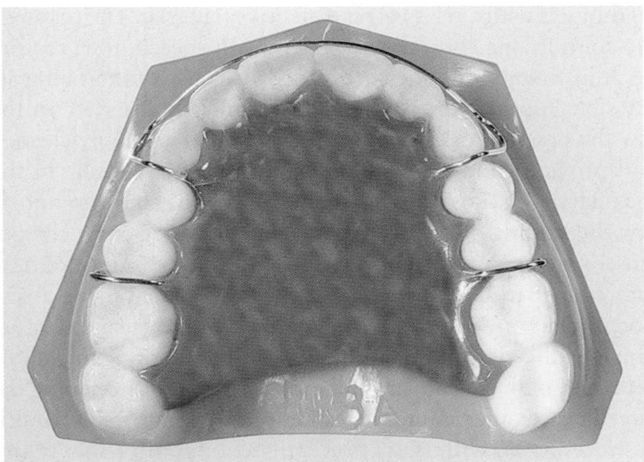

FIG 23-2 Maxillary Hawley retainer. (Courtesy of AOA Orthodontic Appliances, Sturtevant, WI.)

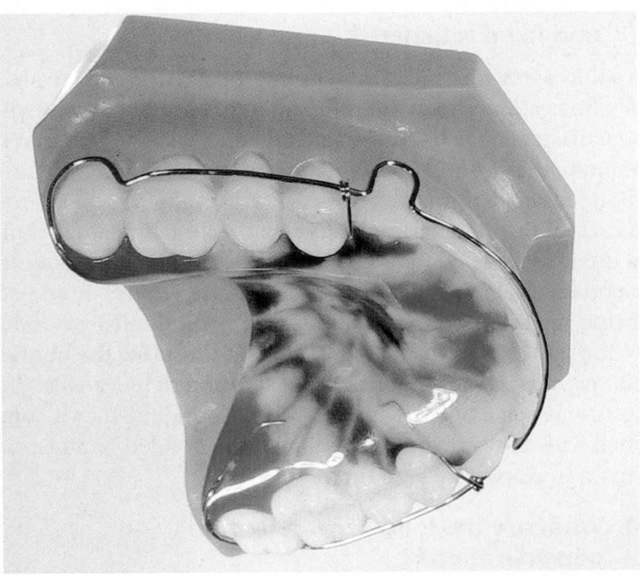

FIG 23-3 Maxillary wrap-around retainer. (Courtesy of AOA Orthodontic Appliances, Sturtevant, WI.)

12. What are the indications for vacuum-formed retainers?

With the development of clear, thin thermoplastic materials, vacuum-formed retainers have become very popular with many orthodontists in the last few years.[23] Vacuum-formed retainers have many advantages over wire and acrylic for many orthodontic patients requiring removable retainers. These retainers are fabricated on a dental study cast in approximately

30 minutes with a relatively inexpensive material. The retainers are comfortable and rarely interfere with speech, they require no adjustments, and they are esthetic because of their almost-invisible appearance. The retainer is typically inserted on the day the braces are removed. These retainers are easily cleaned and provide good stability of the occlusion, especially in the maxillary arch. Possible disadvantages are that they do not allow the settling of the occlusion, and since they cover the occlusal surfaces, masticatory forces can cause wear and require the retainer to be remade. Some have advocated using a sectional vacuum-formed retainer from cuspid to cuspid. Unfortunately, this type of retention over the long term would allow extrusion of the premolars and molars, potentially opening the bite. This retainer is simple, esthetic, and comfortable, and it has received an enthusiastic reception from both patients and orthodontists. In addition, the vacuum-forced retainer offers a perfect vehicle for transporting bleach to patients' teeth after completion of orthodontic treatment.

13. Are there indications for combining removable and fixed retainers?

In adult cases with generalized spacing, a palatal bonded retainer may be necessary to avoid re-opening of spaces. In cases with large diastemata, a bonded palatal retainer may be required to maintain the closure. In cases with a palatally impacted canine, a bonded retainer may be necessary to prevent vertical relapse. In each of the three examples, a vacuum-forced retainer could be used over the bonded retainer to help prevent breakage of the bonded retainer caused by occlusal interference or contact during biting. It is important for the orthodontist to evaluate the patient's overbite and overjet and to place the bonded retainer as gingival as possible to avoid interference with bite closure. When a properly placed lingual-bond retainer is combined with a vacuum-forced retainer, the bonded retainer can remain in place for a long time.

14. What are the long-term retention considerations?

Orthodontic retention should be continued until craniofacial growth is essentially completed in the early 20s.[24] Late mandibular growth is the greatest contributor to mandibular incisor crowding; therefore, retention is certainly a requirement for all orthodontic patients. It is commonly recommended that all patients have a retention maintenance phase for at least 1 year. After that, the patient will be seen only if there are difficulties with the retainer (e.g., if it is broken, bent, or lost). It is important that the orthodontist establish a retention protocol for each patient during the initial diagnosis and treatment planning phase. Most orthodontists use a removable retainer in the maxillary arch. As most of the relapse occurs in the first 6 months following bracket removal, the maxillary retainer is worn fulltime for 6 months. After the first 6 months, the patient can go to night wear only and gradually reduce this if no pressure areas are noted when seating the retainer. Eventually, the maxillary retainer may not be needed. The lower retainer is usually a bonded-lingual retainer, which should be left in place at least until early adulthood. Removal of this retainer should be done only after the orthodontist is consulted. Some retainers may stay for a lifetime. The answer to the question of long-term stability is long-term retention.

15. When are positioners used as retainers?

A tooth positioner is an excellent retainer in certain malocclusions, although it is more commonly used as a finishing appliance.[25,26] (Fig. 23-4).

It has the advantages of massaging the gingival tissues, and it is not subject to breakage as acrylic retainers are. It is bulky and typically is worn 2 to 4 hours per day. Positioners do not retain rotations or incisor irregularities as well as standard retainers. Positioners maintain the occlusal relationship as well as the intra-arch tooth positions. They are excellent retainers for Class II and Class III malocclusions as well as for open bite malocclusions. The optimum positioner is one that has an articulator mounting that records the patient's hinge axis. This gnathologic positioner is more expensive, but it will prevent the posterior open bite that results when a positioner is made to an incorrect hinge axis. A tooth positioner is not appropriate for every orthodontic patient, but for selected patients, it can be an excellent finishing appliance and retainer.

16. Are spring retainers useful for retreatment of mandibular incisor crowding?

Recrowding of mandibular incisors is the indication for a spring aligner to correct incisor position. If late mandibular growth is the cause of the crowding, it may be necessary to reduce the interproximal width of the incisors. The interproximal enamel can be removed with thin discs in a handpiece called air rotor stripping (ARS) or with abrasive strips. This enamel reduction must be performed cautiously to remove only 0.25 mm per side on the incisors. If the recrowding is only 2 to 3 mm, this can be corrected with the spring retainer. First, the interproximal reduction is completed followed by topical fluoride, and then an impression is taken for a study cast. The anterior teeth are sectioned and reset into proper alignment. The spring aligner is fabricated and seated in the patient's mouth. Once the teeth move into alignment, the "active" spring retainer now becomes a passive retainer. Most orthodontists find that it is actually much faster and easier to replace brackets on the anterior teeth and realign rather than using a spring retainer.

17. What are the indications for circumferential supracrestal fibrotomy (CSF)?

CSF is a surgical excision of the free gingival fibers and transseptal fibers to reduce rotational relapse. Surgery to cut the supracrestal elastic fibers is necessary because rotational relapse is caused by the network of elastic supracrestal gingival fibers returning to their original position. This surgical technique was developed by Edwards and includes infiltration with a local anesthetic followed by a circumferential incision around the tooth to the crest of alveolar bone.[27-31] These surgical cuts are made after a previously rotated tooth is orthodontically moved

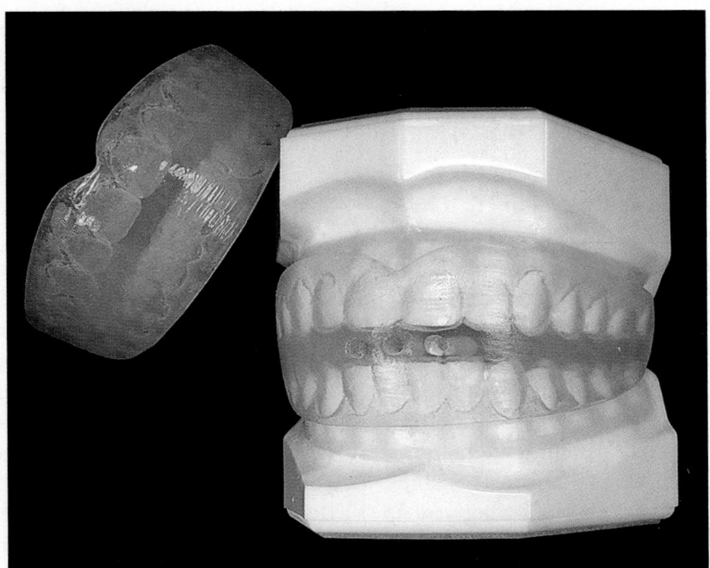

FIG 23-4 Silicone tooth positioner. (Courtesy of AOA Orthodontic Appliances, Sturtevant, WI.)

to its ideal position within the arch. There is minor discomfort after the procedure, but no periodontal pack is necessary. In most cases, it is done by the orthodontist near the end of the finishing phase of treatment. The most important consideration is to retain the tooth in its ideal position while gingival healing occurs. Some orthodontists prefer to perform the CSF after the braces have been removed, but retainers must be inserted immediately to prevent the tooth from rotating back to its original position. This procedure is indicated for a severely rotated tooth, and it is not appropriate for crowding of teeth without rotations.

18. What are the indications for a frenectomy?

A frenectomy is the surgical removal or repositioning of a frenum and is performed to enhance the stability of a corrected diastema.[32] A maxillary midline diastema is caused by insertion of the labial frenum, which is a band of heavy fibrous tissues between the central incisors. When the cause of the diastema is a prominent labial frenum, the frenectomy should be performed after orthodontic alignment and space closure, but prior to the removal of the orthodontic appliances. The major point in a frenectomy being successful is removal of the interdental fibrous tissue. It is not necessary to remove a large portion of the frenum itself. The scar tissue will stabilize the teeth and help to prevent the diastema from returning. This procedure should not be performed until the diastema is closed or the scar tissue will prevent closure. It is difficult to maintain space closure after correcting a diastema, so a lingual-bonded retainer is indicated to keep the space closed. In addition, many children in middle to late mixed dentition demonstrate diastemas of approximately 2 mm. This diastema will normally close with the eruption of the maxillary canines and does not require a frenectomy.

19. What is relapse?

Relapse is the change in tooth position toward the former location following active orthodontic treatment. Teeth are in a stable position because of the equilibrium of forces of chewing, swallowing, tongue, and cheek movements. There is a balance between the internal and external oral musculature. If a tooth is moved, this equilibrium is altered and it must be reestablished to prevent relapse. New fiber and hard tissue formation is dependent on retention. The gingival fiber networks must reorganize to accommodate the new tooth positions. Immediately after orthodontic appliances are removed, the teeth are unstable to occlusal and soft tissue pressures.[13] This is the reason every patient must be placed in orthodontic retainers for a minimum of 6 months to reestablish the equilibrium. Very few cases require minimal or no retention. If the posttreatment dentition starts developing mandibular incisor irregularities, reduction of the incisor width by slenderizing can certainly help. Usually, only minimal tooth structure has to be removed if the incisor root apices have been adequately spaced. Routine cases require retention appliances until the decision to extract or retain the third molars is determined, and the growth process is nearly completed in the early 20s.

20. What is the role of the third molars and relapse?

It is unclear what role the third molars play in the severity of late mandibular crowding. The etiology of late crowding of the mandibular arch is multifactorial and is associated with the amount and direction of late mandibular growth. There is a controversy of the relative merits of extraction of third molars to alleviate mandibular anterior crowding.[33,34] Most authors feel that the extraction of third molars for the purpose of preventing mandibular anterior relapse is not justified.

21. What is the Objective Grading System used by the American Board of Orthodontics (ABO)?

In the mid 1990s, the American Board of Orthodontics began investigating methods of making the clinical examination more objective. Because a major emphasis has always been placed on the final occlusion, the first efforts were directed at developing an objective method of evaluating the dental casts and intraoral radiographs. At the 1995 ABO Clinical Examination, 100 cases were evaluated. A series of 15 criteria were measured on each of the final dental casts and panoramic radiographs. The data showed that the majority of the inadequacies in the final results occurred in 7 of the 15 criteria (alignment, marginal ridges, buccolingual inclination, overjet, occlusal relationships, occlusal contacts, and root angulation). The following year in another field test, 300 sets of final dental casts and panoramic radiographs were evaluated by a subcommittee of four directors. Again, the majority of the inadequacies in the final results occurred in the same seven categories, but the committee had difficulty establishing adequate interexaminer reliability. Therefore, the subcommittee recommended that a measuring instrument be developed to make the measuring process more reliable. In 1997, a third field test was performed with the modified scoring system and the addition of an instrument to measure the various criteria more accurately. Based on the collective and cumulative results of extensive field tests, the Board decided to officially initiate the use of this Objective Grading System for candidates for the Clinical Examination.[10] The seven criteria are:

1. **Alignment:** In the anterior region, the incisal edges and lingual surfaces of the axillary anterior teeth and the incisal edges and labial-incisal surfaces of the mandibular anterior teeth were chosen as the guide to assess anterior alignment. In the maxillary posterior region, the mesiodistal central groove of the premolars and molars is used to assess adequacy of alignment.
2. **Marginal Ridges:** Marginal ridges are used to assess proper vertical positioning of the posterior teeth. Based on the four field tests, the most common mistakes in marginal ridge alignment occurred between the maxillary first and second molars. The second most common problem area was between the mandibular first and second molars.
3. **Buccolingual Inclination:** In order to establish proper occlusion in maximum intercuspation and avoid balancing interferences, there should not be a significant difference between the heights of the buccal and lingual cusps of the maxillary and mandibular molars and premolars.
4. **Occlusal Relationship:** Occlusal contacts are measured to assess the adequacy of the posterior occlusion. Again, a major objective of orthodontic treatment is to establish maximum intercuspation of opposing teeth. Therefore, the functioning cusps are used to assess the adequacy of this criterion (i.e., the buccal cusps of the mandibular molars and premolars and the lingual cusps of the maxillary molars and premolars).
5. **Overjet:** Overjet is used to assess the relative transverse relationship of the posterior teeth and the anteroposterior relationship of the anterior teeth.
6. **Interproximal Contacts:** Interproximal contacts are used to determine if all spaces within the dental arch have been closed. Persistent spaces between teeth after orthodontic therapy are not only unesthetic, but can lead to food impaction.
7. **Root angulation:** Root angulation is used to assess how well the roots of the teeth have been positioned relative to one another. Although the panoramic radiograph is not the perfect record for evaluating root angulation, it is probably the best means possible for making this assessment.

The Directors of the ABO spent countless hours developing this system for assessing the occlusal and radiographic results of orthodontic treatment. The usefulness of this system depends not only on its objectivity, but more importantly on the validity and reliability of the measurements. After repeated comparison of both objective and subjective systems, the Directors are confident that the "cut-off" score to pass this portion of the clinical examination is valid. Today, candidates must grade their own results before the clinical examination. Candidates will know if their results will pass the CCRE portion of the clinical examination. Furthermore, diplomates may use this scoring system at anytime in their orthodontic career to determine if they are producing "Board quality" results. The Board hopes that this method of self-evaluation will help to improve the quality of orthodontic care in the future.

REFERENCES

1. Little RM, Riedel RA, Artun J: An evaluation of changes in mandibular anterior alignment from 10 to 20 years postretention. *Am J Orthod Dentofacial Orthop* 1988;93:423.
2. Ostyn JM, Maltha JC, van't Hof MA, van der Linden FP: The role of interdigitation in the sagittal growth of the maxillomandibular complex of *Macaca fascicularis*. *Am J Orthod Dentofacial Orthop* 1996;109:71-78.
3. Tweed CS: Indications for the extraction of teeth in orthodontic procedures. *Am J Orthod* 1944;30:405-428.
4. Huckaba GW: The physiologic vasis of relapse. *Am J Orthod* 1952;38:335-350.
5. Schudy GF: Posttreatment craniofacial growth: its implications in orthodontic treatment. *Am J Orthod* 1974;65:39-57.
6. Fotis B, Melsen B, Williams S: Posttreatment changes of skeletal morphology following treatment aimed at restriction of maxillary growth. *Am J Orthod* 1985;88:288-296.
7. Harris EF, Vaden JL, Dunn KL, Behrents RG: Effects of patient age on postorthodontic stability of the mandibular arch. *Eur J Orthod* 1994;105:25-34.
8. Parkinson CE, Buschang PH, Behrents RG, et al: A new method of evaluating posterior occlusion and relation to posttreatment occlusal changes. *Am J Orthod Dentofacial Orthop* 2001;120:503-512.
9. Andrews LF: The six keys to normal occlusion. *Am J Orthod* 1972;62:296-309.
10. Casko JF, et al: Objective grading system for dental casts and panoramic radiograph. *Am J Orthod Dentofacial Orthop* 1998;114:590-599.
11. Blake M, Bibby K: Retention and stability: a review of the literature. *Am J Orthod Dentofacial Orthop* 1998;114:299-306.

12. Kaplan H: The logic of modern retention appliances. *Am J Orthod Dentofacial Orthop* 1988;93:325-337.
13. Sandowsky C: Long-term stability following orthodontic therapy. In Burstone CJ, Nanda R, editors. *Retention and stability in orthodontics.* Philadelphia: WB Saunders, 1993, pp 107-113.
14. Reitan K: Principles of retention and avoidance of treatment relapse. *Am J Orthod* 1969;55:776-790.
15. Nanda RS, Nanda SK: Considerations of dentofacial growth in long-term retention and stability: is active retention needed? *Am J Orthod Dentofacial Orthop* 1992;101:297-302.
16. Edwards J: The prevention of relapse in extraction cases. *Am J Orthod* 1971;160:128-140.
17. McNamara JA: An orthopedic approach to the treatment of Class III malocclusion in young patients. *J Clin Orthod* 1987;21:598-608.
18. Kulbersh VP, Berger J, Kersten G: Effects of protraction mechanics on the midface. *Am J Orthod Dentofacial Orthop* 1998;114:484-491.
19. Lewis P: Correction of deep overbite: A report of three cases. *Am J Orthod* 1987;91:342-345.
20. Kim TW, Little RM: Postretention assessment of deep overbite correction in Class II division 2 malocclusion. *Angle Orthod* 1999;69(2):175-186.
21. Espen HD, Zachrisson BU: Long-term experience with direct bonded lingual retainers. *J Clin Orthod* 1991;10:619-630.
22. Orchin JD: Permanent lingual bonded retainer. *J Clin Orthod* 1991;24:229-231.
23. Sheridan JJ, LeDoux W, McMinn R: Essix retainers: fabrication and supervision for permanent retention. *J Clin Orthod* 1993;27:37-45.
24. Zachrisson BU: Important aspects of long-term stability. *J Clin Orthod* 1971;9:563-583.
25. Kesling HD: The philosophy of the tooth positioning appliance. *Am J Orthod* 1945;31:297-304.
26. Carano A, Bowman SJ: Short-term intensive use of the tooth positioner in case finishing. *J Clin Orthod* 2002;36(4):216-219.
27. Edwards J: A surgical procedure to eliminate rotational relapse. *Am J Orthod* 1970;57:35-40.
28. Edward J: A long-term prospective evaluation of the circumferential supracrestal fiberotomy alleviating orthodontic relapse. *Am J Orthod* 1988;93:380-387.
29. Edwards J: The prevention of t relapse in extraction cases. *Am J Orthod* 1970;60:128-140.
30. Boose L: Fiberotomy and reproximation without lower retention, nine years in retrospect: Part I. *Angle Orthod* 1980;50:88-97.
31. Boose L: Fiberotomy and reproximation without lower retention, nine years in retrospect: Part II. *Angle Orthod* 1980;50:169-178.
32. Edwards JG: The diastema, the frenum, the frenectomy: a clinical study. *Am J Orthod* 1977;71:489-508.
33. Richardson ME: The role of the third molar in the cause of lower arch crowding: a review. *Am J Orthod Dentofacial Orthop* 1989;95(1):79-83.
34. Ades A, Joondeph D: A long-term study of the relationship of third molars to mandibular dental arch changes. *Am J Orthod Dentofacial Orthop* 1990;97:323-335.

CHAPTER

24

Soft-Tissue Diode Laser Surgery in Orthodontics

Angela Marie Tran • Jeryl D. English • Sam A. Winkelmann

Contemporary orthodontics continues to merge with modern-day technology and the growing focus on dental esthetics in today's culture. One of the main treatment goals of orthodontics has been the ability to produce an esthetic smile in a timely manner. In previous years, orthodontists have been limited in what they could do to improve treatment outcomes by the lack of technology and knowledge. In recent years, the advent of the soft-tissue diode laser has made several soft tissue procedures easily accessible and doable for orthodontists. Several advantages of the diode laser include: ease of use, the ability to maintain a hemostatic environment, minimal discomfort for the patient, ability to cut only soft tissues (not hard tissues), and sutures being unnecessary for proper wound healing. These advantages have encouraged several orthodontists to perform their own minor soft-tissue procedures, allowing the orthodontist to finish cases much more efficiently and to a higher esthetic standard. Slowly erupting teeth and gingival overgrowth that have previously lengthened treatment time can now be readily handled by the orthodontist with the use of a diode laser. Unaesthetic gingival contours and margins can now be routinely managed along with incisal recontouring in order to produce a most esthetic treatment result. Several soft-tissue procedures along with their indications and methods will be addressed in this chapter.

1. What soft-tissue procedures using a laser should an orthodontist consider?

Orthodontists continually strive to find methods to enhance treatment results and reduce treatment time. The advent of soft tissue lasers allows the orthodontist to have more control over factors that previously could impede treatment time and compromise treatment results. Several clinical instances exist where the use of a soft-tissue laser would be beneficial to both the orthodontist and the patient: gingival recontouring, aphthous ulcer management, expedition of tooth eruption, removal of operculae, and frenectomies.[1-4]

Removal of soft tissue with the laser is useful for gingival recontouring in orthodontics for esthetic, health, and time reasons. Gingival reshaping for uneven gingival margins, improving tooth proportionality, and improving a gummy smile can greatly enhance the esthetic treatment outcome. Gingival recontouring is also indicated in patients with poor hygiene where inflamed gingiva, pseudopockets, and difficulty brushing and flossing are present.[3,4] Excessive gingival tissue can often prevent the orthodontist from placing brackets in an ideal position. The removal of this gingival tissue permits the orthodontist to bond a bracket to the tooth in the desired position in a timely manner.[3,4]

Aphthous ulcers can be very uncomfortable and painful for the patient (Fig. 24-1). Traditionally, salt water rinses, topical anesthetic, and tetracycline would be prescribed to alleviate the symptoms.[3] The orthodontist now has the ability to lase the aphthous ulcer, thus relieving the patient of pain almost immediately. The laser is activated for 30 seconds at a very low wattage and kept at a distance of 1 to 2 mm away from the lesion.[3,4] Aphthous ulcers generally take up to 14 days to heal, but with laser surgery, the ulcers can heal within 1 day after treatment. The laser wound that replaces the ulcer is nonpainful and allows the patient to have a faster and more comfortable recovery.[3,4]

Soft tissues can sometimes cover a tooth and impede its eruption into the arch. The soft tissue laser can be used to remove overlying tissue so that the orthodontist can bond a bracket and begin moving the tooth immediately.[3,4]

Orthodontists sometimes find themselves waiting to band second molars when an operculum is present. The soft tissue laser can remove opercula so that the orthodontist can band the second molars and keep treatment on track.[4]

Patients who present with a large diastema often have a low frenum that contributes to the excessive spacing. After orthodontically closing the space, it is often recommended to perform a frenectomy to help stabilize the space closure. The soft-tissue laser makes frenectomy procedures easier to manage, minimal in discomfort, and hemostatic.

2. What type of laser should be used in orthodontics?

A laser is made up of a monochromatic light that travels through a tube that collimates the light energy. A protective shield encircles the light, allowing the laser to be released only

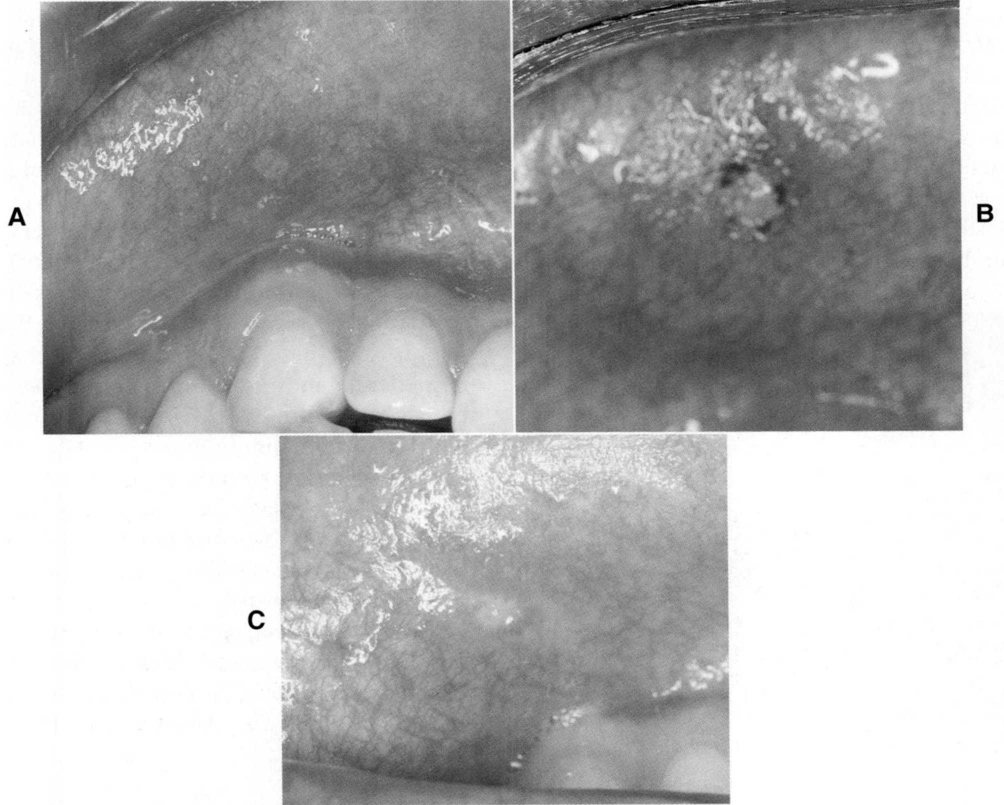

FIG 24-1 Aphthous ulcer (before and after). **A,** Aphthous ulcer before laser surgery. **B,** Aphthous ulcer immediately after laser surgery. **C,** Aphthous ulcer 1 week after laser surgery.

at the tip and not through the sides.[2] This exposed energy can be controlled by the operator through the power adjustment. The laser cuts the tissue through *ablation,* where the energy is absorbed in the cells and is immediately subjected to heating, welding, coagulation, protein denaturization, drying vaporization, and carbonization.[2] It is recommended that the laser deliver its energy in a pulsed mode, which allows intermittent cooling, less tissue damage, and less discomfort.[2]

Three main types of lasers are used in dentistry: the CO_2, erbium, and diode laser. The CO_2 laser can be difficult to use because the tip does not directly contact the surgical site; instead, it must be used at a slight distance and a delay is present from when the incision is made to when it can be seen.[2] The erbium laser has a very high wavelength and is effective in soft tissue removal; however, it does not control bleeding well.[2] The last type of laser is the diode laser, where the light energy is absorbed by the melanin of the cells[2] (Fig. 24-2). This allows the diode laser to control bleeding exceptionally well at the surgical site. The laser tip gently contacts the surgical site, allowing the operator to have tactile feedback.[2] Other advantages of the diode include its manageable size, its ability to cut only soft tissues and not hard tissues, low cost, and the fact that these procedures typically require only a topical anesthetic.[2] The laser cauterizes the surgical site while cutting so that a periodontal dressing is not necessary for healing.

3. What is the indication and technique for soft-tissue laser surgery for gingival recontouring?

The principles of cosmetic dentistry must be incorporated into orthodontic treatment in order to optimize the esthetic results.[1] Orthodontists routinely evaluate the smile line, smile arc, and tooth and gingival proportions. The orthodontist should understand the esthetic concepts of tooth proportionality, contacts, embrasures, and gingival characteristics before using laser surgery for gingival removal. The ideal maxillary central incisor should be approximately 66% to 80% width compared with height.[1] It is important to assess if a tooth disproportion is due to a short clinical crown height, gingival overgrowth, or delayed passive eruption.[1] Depending on the cause of disproportion, waiting for eruption, gingival recontouring, or dental restorations may be the optimal solution.[1] Other important esthetic concepts include the placement of contact points and embrasures. As teeth move from the midline to posterior, contact points should progress apically and embrasures should become larger.[1] Gingival esthetics also plays an important role in the success of a treatment outcome. The gingival shape (the curvature of the gingival margin of the tooth) of the mandibular incisors and maxillary laterals should have a symmetrical half-oval or half-circular shape; therefore, their gingival zenith should be located within their longitudinal axis.[1] The gingival shape of the maxillary centrals and canines is elliptical, resulting in a gingival zenith that is distal to the longitudinal axis.[1]

The orthodontist can find numerous occasions to use gingival recontouring to improve treatment results. When initially evaluating a patient for orthodontic care, the orthodontist carefully evaluates the casts and patient to determine ideal bracket placement. Most orthodontists will use the incisal edge of the teeth to determine bracket placement height. Orthodontists often find that they are unable to ideally place a bracket because of gingival overgrowth or delayed passive eruption. In these instances, it would be very helpful for the orthodontist to be able to remove any excess gingival tissue in order to place the brackets in an ideal position rather than waiting for eruption or referring the patient to a periodontist to have the teeth uncovered.[3,4]

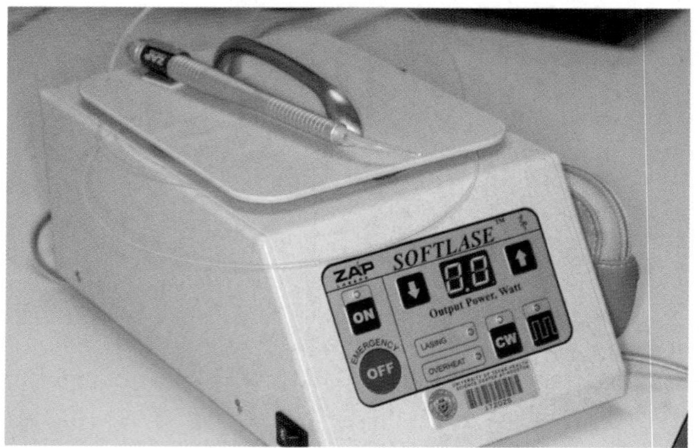

FIG 24-2 Diode laser (ZAP Softlase).

Gingival recontouring can also be very helpful in aiding patients with poor oral hygiene. Patients often have marginal to poor oral hygiene that can cause inflammation and pseudopocket formation of the gingiva. These pseudopockets can exacerbate the inflammatory process by impeding the patient's ability to thoroughly brush and floss around the teeth and gingiva.[3,4] Gingival recontouring can help to reduce this inflammation and thus allow the patient to access more areas to keep the gingivitis under control. Closing large extraction spaces can also cause redundant tissue to appear, especially in conjunction with poor oral hygiene.[3] Removal of this tissue allows the patient to keep these areas under hygienic control.

As orthodontists begin to incorporate more cosmetic dentistry into their treatment plans, gingival recontouring proves to be extremely useful in finishing a case to a better esthetic outcome (Fig. 24-3). Patients may have uneven gingival

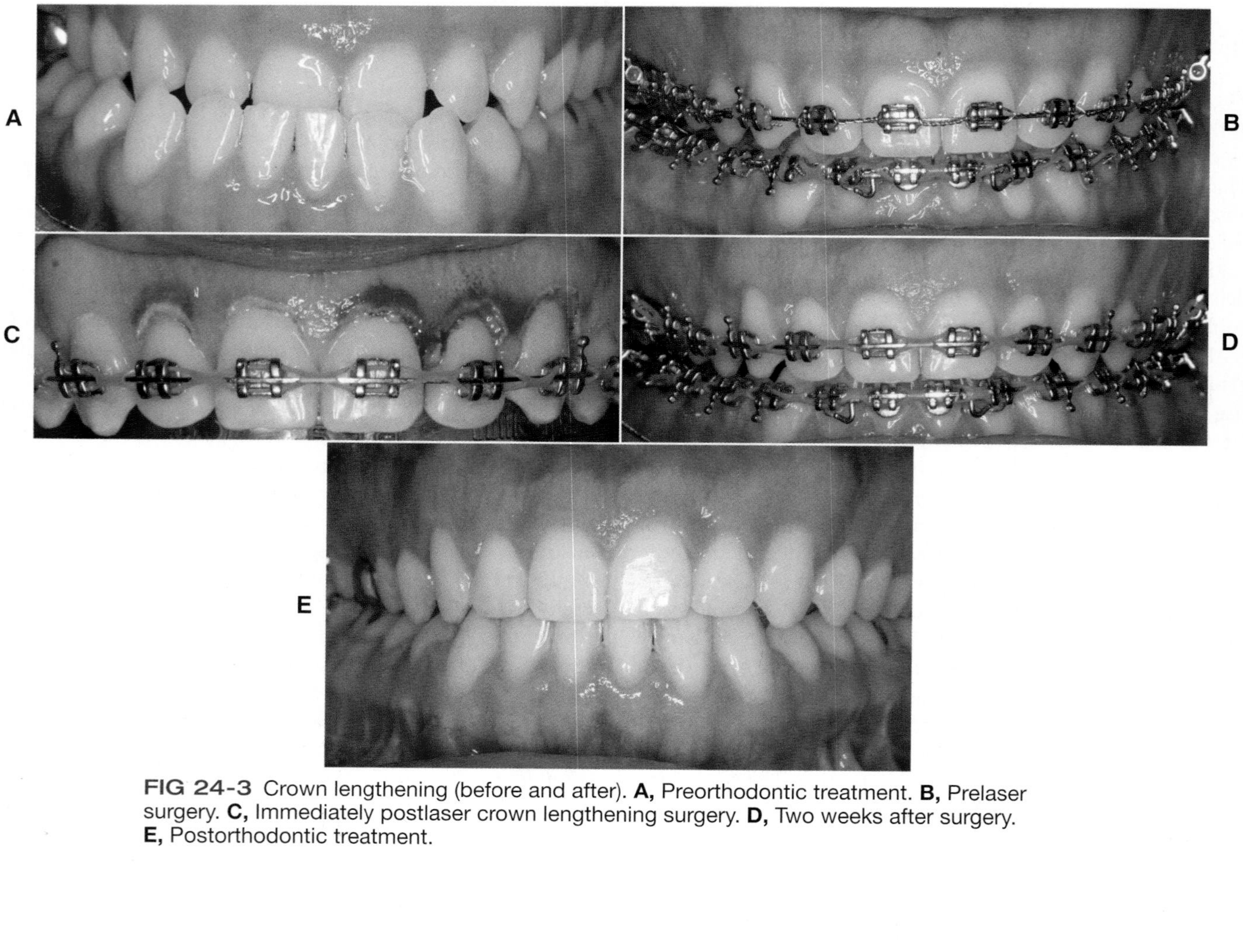

FIG 24-3 Crown lengthening (before and after). **A,** Preorthodontic treatment. **B,** Prelaser surgery. **C,** Immediately postlaser crown lengthening surgery. **D,** Two weeks after surgery. **E,** Postorthodontic treatment.

margins, gingival inflammation, or poor crown width-to-height ratios that result in a less-than-optimal treatment result. The soft-tissue laser allows orthodontists to improve tooth proportionality and gingival shape and contour in accordance to the smile arc and smile line of the individual patient.[1,2,4]

When performing a gingivectomy, apply topical anesthetic and use a probe to mark height guides, leaving 1 mm of sulcus when finished. Hold the laser tip perpendicular to the tissue at the gingival margin and use a continuous wave stroke to remove the tissue surface one layer at a time. After the ideal contours are achieved, clean the area with a microbrush or cotton ball with 3% hydrogen peroxide.[5]

4. What is the indication and technique for soft-tissue laser surgery for a frenectomy?

Patients who present with a large diastema often have a low frenum that can contribute to the excessive spacing. Orthodontists will treat the diastema by closing the space and then stabilizing it with fixed or removable retention in addition to a frenectomy. The soft-tissue laser makes performing a frenectomy much more comfortable for the patient. The healing process is less painful, no sutures or dressings are needed, and bleeding is highly controlled. As the frenum heals in its new position, the scar tissue can help to maintain the space closure (Fig. 24-4).

The technique for performing a frenectomy includes first placing topical anesthetic at the surgical site. Hold the upper lip and lightly pull the lip forward until the frenum is taut. Lase the frenum horizontally approximately 3 mm from the frenum base and use light, continuous waves until the lip is released, leaving a V-shaped crater approximately 1 inch wide. Continue to lase deep enough to prevent reattachment and then smooth the remaining tissue at the base of the frenum. Clean the surgical site with 3% hydrogen peroxide on a cotton ball.[5] Another technique, the diamond-release frenectomy, involves pulling the upper lip taut, lasing the sides of the V-shaped frenum, and then lasing the base of the frenum, which creates a "diamond"-shaped surgical site.

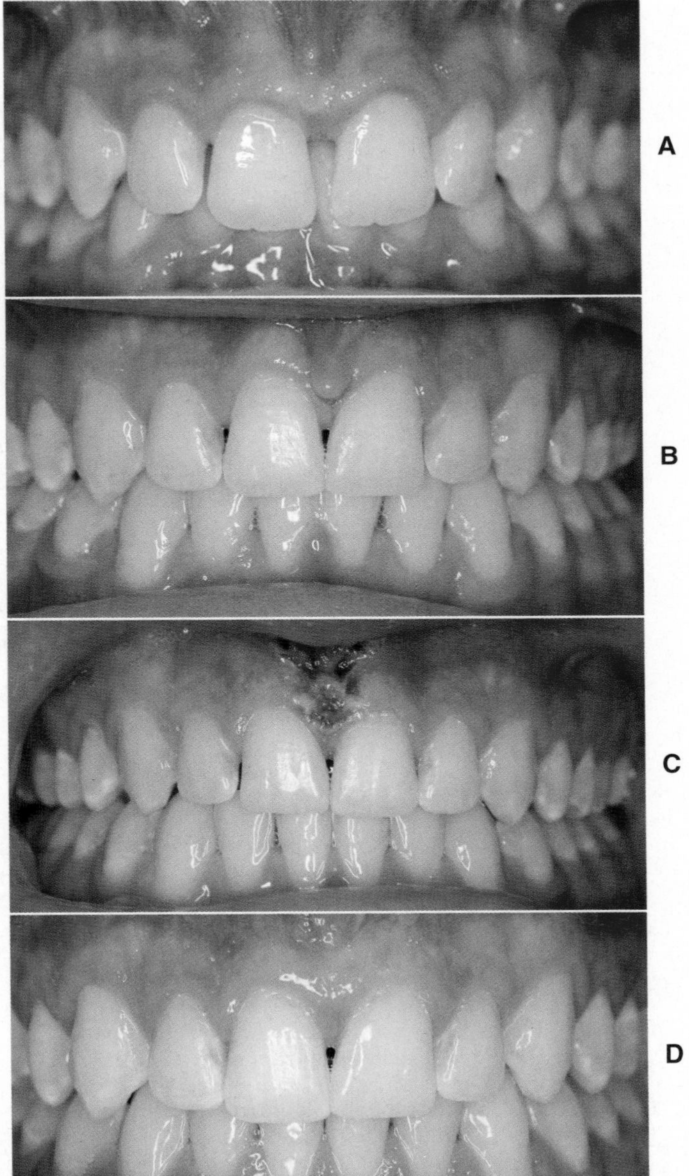

FIG 24-4 Frenectomy (before and after). **A,** Initial malocclusion with diastema. **B,** Postorthodontic treatment and prelaser surgery. **C,** Immediately after laser frenectomy surgery. **D,** One month after surgery.

5. What is the indication and procedure used with a soft-tissue laser to uncover impacted teeth?

Orthodontic treatment can sometimes be slowed drastically by waiting on an impacted tooth to erupt through soft tissue.[3] Traditionally, patients would be referred to a periodontist so that the tooth could be exposed and a bond and chain could be placed for orthodontic traction; however, thick tissue covering the tooth can still impede the tooth from finally erupting into the arch, especially palatal tissue. The soft-tissue laser can be used to remove thick tissue so that the tooth can continue to be moved into the arch without hindrance. Sometimes the impacted tooth is nearly erupted into the mouth; however, a thin layer of tissue still covers its surface.[3] In these cases the laser can be used to remove the overlying tissue so that the orthodontist can bond an attachment to the tooth and begin moving it into the arch immediately (Fig. 24-5).[3]

When lasing tissue overlying a tooth, the operator must adjust the power as needed according to the tissue thickness. After applying topical anesthetic, probe the surgical site to locate the tooth and mark the attached tissue. Carefully remove the tissue with light, continuous waves until the underlying tooth is exposed. After exposure, wipe the area with 3% hydrogen peroxide with a microbrush or cotton roll. A bond can be placed immediately after tissue removal.[5]

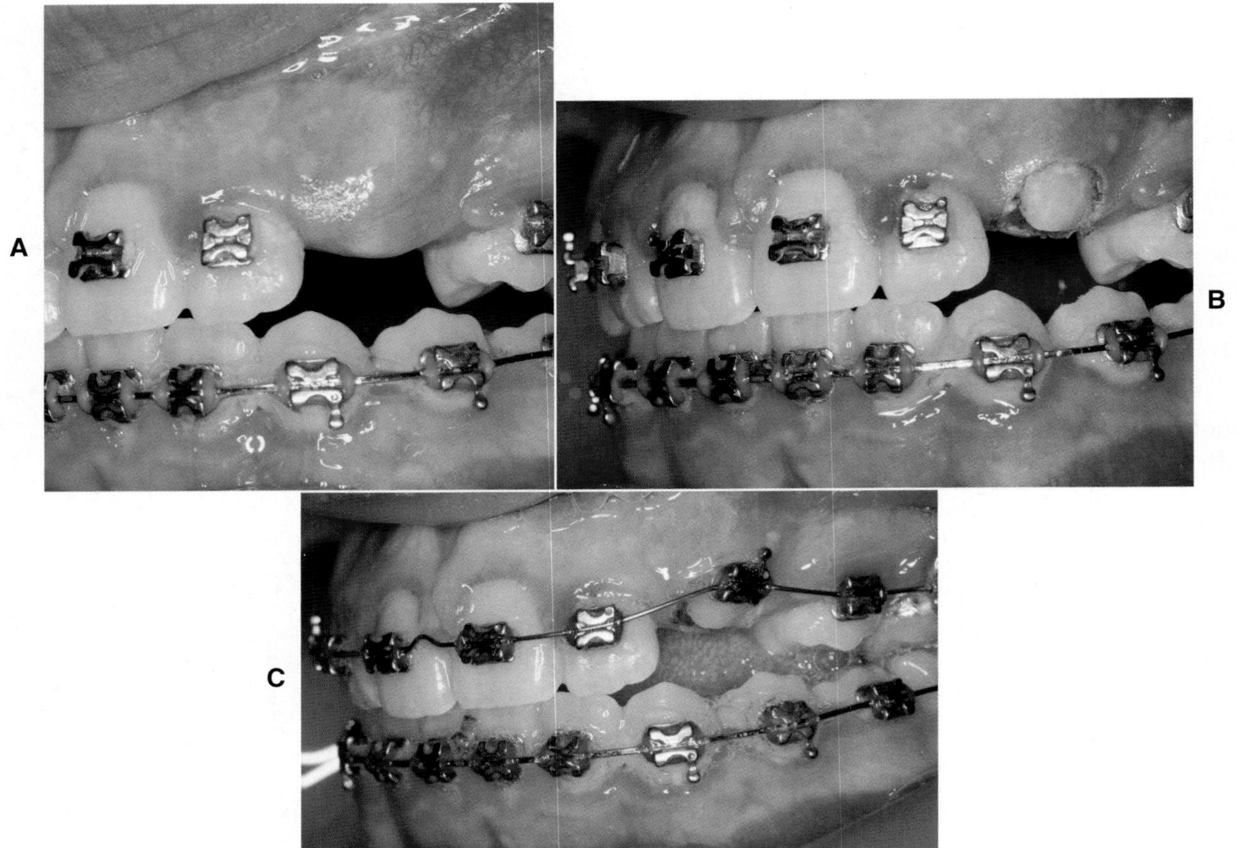

FIG 24-5 Uncovering of an impacted canine. **A,** Impacted canine before laser surgery. **B,** Canine immediately after laser surgery. **C,** Postsurgery orthodontic activation.

REFERENCES

1. Sarver DM: Principles of cosmetic dentistry in orthodontics. 1. Shape and proportionality of anterior teeth. *Am J Orthod Dentofacial Orthop* 2004;126:749-753.
2. Sarver DM, Yanosky MR: Principles of cosmetic dentistry in orthodontics. 2. Soft tissue laser technology and cosmetic gingival contouring. *Am J Orthod Dentofacial Orthop* 2005;127:85-90.
3. Sarver DM, Yanosky MR: Principles of cosmetic dentistry in orthodontics: Part 3. Laser treatments for tooth eruption and soft tissue problems. *Am J Orthod Dentofacial Orthop* 2005;127:262-264.
4. Yanosky MR: The soft-tissue laser: managing treatment and enhancing aesthetics. Available at: OrthodonticProductsOnline.com, August 2006.
5. ZAP lasers.Orthodontic laser procedures guide. Available at: www.zaplasers.com.

Secrets in Computer-Aided Surgical Simulation for Complex Cranio-Maxillofacial Surgery

CHAPTER 25

James J. Xia • Jaime Gateno • John F. Teichgraeber

Cranio-maxillofacial (CMF) surgery is an encompassing term that involves the treatment of diseases, injuries, and deformities of the skull and face. CMF deformities can be either congenital or acquired and include dentofacial deformities, congenital deformities, defects after tumor ablation, posttraumatic defects, and deformities of the temporomandibular joint (TMJ). CMF surgery requires extensive presurgical planning because of the complex nature of three-dimensional (3D) anatomy of the skull and face.

1. How many patients with CMF deformities are in the United States?

In the United States, it is estimated that 17 million individuals aged 12 to 50 years (18% of this population) have malocclusions that are severe enough to warrant surgical correction.[1-4] In addition, congenital anomalies of the CMF skeleton affect a large number of children. The most common congenital anomalies include cleft lip and palate (over 3.6 in 1000 live births[5]), craniosynostosis (343–476 per 1 million live births[6]), and hemifacial microsomia (1 per 5600 live births[5]). A majority of these patients will require surgery. Additional CMF deformities also occur after tumor ablation and trauma. Treatment for head and neck tumors often result in significant deformities that require reconstruction.[7,8] The incidence of head and neck cancer is 9.7 per 100,000 Americans. This translates into 28,000 new patients every year, which does not include patients with benign tumors who also may require surgery.[9] It is reported that nonfatal injuries from trauma affect 28 million Americans (10% of the population) annually,[10] with 37% suffering injuries involving the head and face.[11] A significant number of these patients will also require surgical treatment. Finally, 5% to 15% of the population is reported to have symptoms of TMJ disorders, with peak prevalence in young adults (20–40 years of age).[12,13] Although the majority of these patients do not need surgical treatment, patients with TMJ ankylosis, severe rheumatoid arthritis, or osteoarthritis may require TMJ reconstruction. It is estimated that about 3000 prosthetic joint replacements are performed each year,[14] as well as a similar number of autogenous reconstructions.

2. What are the current planning methods for CMF surgery?

CMF surgery requires extensive presurgical planning because of the complex nature of 3D anatomy of the skull and face. The current methods used to plan CMF surgery vary according to the type of surgery being planned but are not much different from the methods that are used to plan simple orthognathic surgery.

In general, current surgical planning methods for complex CMF deformities involve the following steps. The first step is to gather data and quantify the deformity from many different sources, including physical examination and anthropometric measurement, medical photographs, medical imaging studies (cephalometric radiographs and analysis, computed tomography [CT], etc.), and plaster dental models when the surgery involves the jaws. The second step is to simulate the surgery, including prediction tracings, plaster dental model surgery, or CT-based physical model surgery. The last step in surgical planning is to create a way of transferring the surgical plan to the patient at the time of the surgery. This is usually done by creating surgical splints, templates, measurements of the bone movements, or visual "clues."

3. Why are the current planning methods often not adequate for planning complex CMF surgery?

ISSUES WITH TWO-DIMENSIONAL PREDICTION TRACINGS

The CMF surgery is usually simulated using prediction tracings. The tracings are made from the cephalometric radiograph by outlining the bones and soft tissues onto an acetate paper.[15,16] The outlines of the bones to be moved are drawn on additional sheets of acetate paper. The surgical simulation is completed by moving the bone tracings to the desired position. The prediction tracings can also be completed by computerized software.

A significant drawback of prediction tracing is that it is two-dimensional (2D).[17-20] Patients' 3D anatomic structures are compressed at the mid-sagittal plane to a 2D cephalometric radiograph. It also creates a significant overlap of right and left structures. Prediction tracings may be clinically acceptable if the patient has only anteroposterior (AP) or vertical deformity. However, with this technique, it is impossible to simulate surgery in the three dimensions, which is essential in patients with 3D problems (i.e., asymmetries).[21,22] Another problem with prediction tracings is that they portray the dentition as a 2D image.[21,23] For this reason, surgeries that involve the dentition should also be simulated on plaster dental models that have been mounted on an articulator.[15,16,24]

ISSUES WITH CT MODELS

Three-dimensional CT scans have been successfully used to visualize and quantify the patient's condition. However, they have not been successfully used for surgical simulation because of two major reasons. First, the CT does not render the teeth with the accuracy that is necessary for surgical simulation.[21,23] Also, raw CT data are presented by a sequence of 2D cross-sectional images of the volume-of-interest, layer by layer. During the 3D reconstruction, the missing data between adjacent layers are reconstructed by mathematical algorithms (e.g., *Marching Cubes*[25]). Currently, the most precise 3D CT scanners scan at a minimum slice thickness of 0.625 mm. At this thickness, although they are adequate for bony structures, they are not capable of accurately reproducing the teeth to the degree that is necessary for surgical planning. The occlusion between maxillary and mandibular teeth requires a high degree of precision. Even a 0.5 mm error may cause malocclusion. Furthermore, it is very difficult, if not impossible, to remove artifacts, which is the scattering caused by orthodontic brackets or dental metallic restorations. Because of these limitations, surgeries that involve the teeth are still simulated on plaster dental models.[15,16,24]

With the fast development of cone-beam CT technology, the scanning slice thickness is reduced to 0.2 mm. It also has a better control on the artifacts. Radiation exposure to the patients has been significantly reduced. The cone-beam CT scanner has become a favorite gadget for orthodontists and dentists. However, in the treatment of complex CMF deformity, the surgeons want to see the "true" replica of CMF bones. The images from cone-beam CT have relatively lower contrast compared with regular medical CT images. This makes the segmentation process (to separate the bones from soft tissue on the CT image) rather difficult. After 3D reconstruction, it is common to observe that the anterior walls of the maxillary sinus or orbital floors are "mystically" missing on the 3D model. Although the artifacts produced by cone-beam CT are minimal, the rendition of the teeth is still inappropriate for simulating the final occlusion or for making the surgical splints.

ISSUES WITH CT-BASED PHYSICAL MODELS

Another means of simulating surgery is to use CT-based physical models produced by rapid prototyping techniques (e.g., stereolithography apparatus [SLA] models). Even though these models are useful, they have a number of disadvantages. One disadvantage is that in cases involving the occlusion, the teeth are not accurate enough for precise surgical simulation. This is because the CT image data, from which the models are built, are unable to accurately render the teeth and are also subject to artifacts. An additional plaster dental model surgery is still necessary to establish a new dental occlusion and to fabricate surgical splints. Another disadvantage is that it is impossible to simulate different surgeries on a single model. Once the model is cut, it is impossible to undo the cut.

ISSUES WITH PLASTER DENTAL MODEL SURGERY

Surgeries that involve the teeth are also simulated on plaster dental models.[15,16,24] The purpose of this step is to establish a new dental occlusion and to fabricate surgical splints. The splint helps the surgeon establish the desired relationship between maxilla and mandible. A drawback of plaster dental models is that they do not depict the surrounding bony structures.[23,26] Therefore, it is impossible for the surgeon to visualize the skeletal changes that occur during model surgery, which is critical in the treatment of complex CMF deformities. Finally, there are two major issues regarding the use of plaster dental model surgery.

Issues with Face-Bow Transfer

The ability of the surgeon to transfer the desired surgical plan to the patient during orthognathic surgery depends mainly on the accuracy of the surgical splint. The fabrication of an accurate splint requires that the models be mounted to replicate the position of the patient's dentition. However, Ellis et al.[24] demonstrated a significant difference between the inclination of the occlusal plane on the mounted models and the actual occlusal plane as measured on the cephalograms. Another study[27] shows that the average occlusal plane inclination using the SAM Anatomical Face-Bow was 7.8 ± 4.2 degrees, statistically significant greater than the actual. The mean occlusal plane inclination of the models obtained using the Erickson Surgical Face-Bow was 4.4 ± 2.2 degrees statistically significant greater than the actual.

The advantage of using models that are accurately oriented to Frankfort horizontal becomes evident once the implications of using inaccurately mounted models are understood. Fig. 25-1 illustrates the results of using inaccurate models to fabricate an intermediate splint. Fig. 25-1, *A*, depicts the cephalometric tracing of a hypothetical patient with mandibular prognathism and maxillary hypoplasia. The surgical plan for this patient calls for a 10 mm maxillary advancement and a 4 mm mandibular setback. In this case, the axis-orbital plane (face-bow) is 12 degrees off the Frankfort horizontal. Fig. 25-1, *A*, depicts the articulator on which the models have been mounted using the conventional system. The occlusal plane inclination of the mounted models (Fig. 25-1, *B*) is 12 degrees greater than that on the cephalometric tracing (see Fig. 25-1, *A*). In Fig. 25-1, *C*, the maxillary model has been advanced 10 mm forward, and the intermediate splint has been fabricated. Fig. 25-1, *D*, depicts the planned position for the maxilla and the actual position of the maxilla at the time of surgery. In this hypothetical case, the position of the maxilla at surgery is 1.5 mm behind the planned position, producing a maxillary advancement of only 8.5 mm, or 15% less than desired.

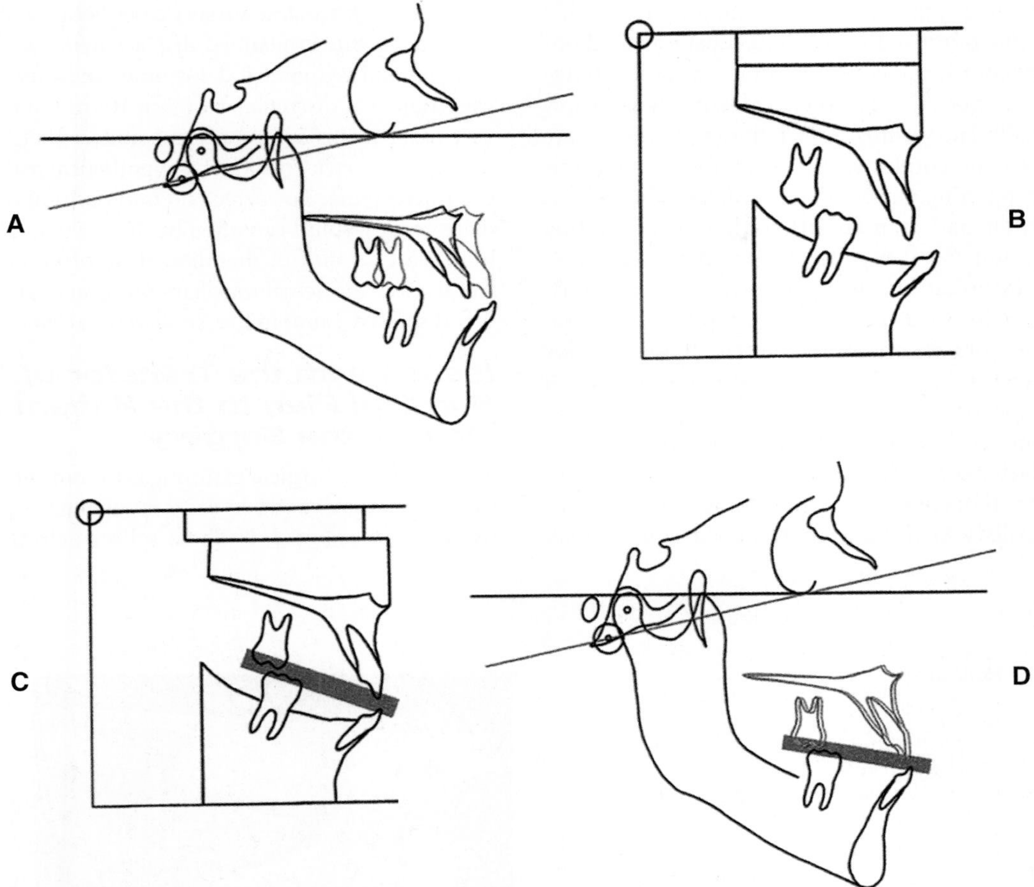

FIG 25–1 Face-bow transfer in a hypothetical patient. **A,** Prediction tracing in a hypothetical patient. The horizontal line in black is Frankfort horizontal. The red line is the axis-orbital plane, which is 12 degrees off Frankfort horizontal. The plan calls for a 10 mm maxillary advancement (blue line). **B,** The models mounted on an articulator. Note that the occlusal plane inclination of the mounted models is 12 degrees steeper than the actual occlusal plane. **C,** Model surgery. The maxillary model has been advanced 10 mm, and the intermediate splint (red) has been fabricated. **D,** The maxillary position at surgery. The blue outline represents the desired position for the maxilla. The red outline represents the actual position at surgery. Note that the actual position is 1.5 mm behind the desired position.

In order to solve this problem, researchers and clinicians have developed various techniques. Ellis et al.[24] developed a modified mounting technique used with Hanau articular. Gateno et al.[27] also developed face-bow transferring technique used with SAM articulator that takes the individual anatomic variations among subjects into consideration.

Issues with Mandibular Autorotation

Predictable outcomes in double-jaw surgery depend on precisely positioning the maxilla. This is important, not only because an ideal maxillary position is necessary to achieve good mid-facial aesthetics, but also because the ultimate position for the mandible depends on it.

The first step in double-jaw surgery is to place an external reference marker (e.g., a K-wire or a screw) in the nasal bones. The vertical distance between this marker and the edges of the maxillary incisors is recorded. This measurement will help establish the correct vertical position for the maxilla. In double-jaw surgery, the maxilla is usually cut first. In order to position the maxilla at the time of the surgery, surgeons use an intermediate surgical splint that determines the AP and transverse position of the maxilla as well as any desired rotations in space. The intermediate splint is temporarily placed between the osteotomized maxilla and the mandible, and the teeth are wired in this position. The vertical position of the maxilla is then determined by autorotating the maxillo-mandibular complex to a predetermined vertical position, using the pre-determined distance between nasal marker and incisor edges as reference. Once the maxilla is in place, the dental fixation is released and the mandible is osteotomized and positioned according to the position of the maxilla. The splint is fabricated prior to surgery using plaster dental models, which have been mounted on an articulator. Articulators are mechanical devices that simulate the movement of the mandible. They are based on the principle that during opening and closing of the mandible in its most retruded position (centric relation), the condyles rotate around a hinge axis (hinge axis theory).[28-32] However, recent studies show that during mandibular opening, translation and rotation are always continuous and combined.[33-35] Even for the first millimeter of mouth opening, the condyles actually follow a path (combined rotation and translation), rather than rotating around a single point.[30,36,37] Because the mandible also slides forward during autorotation, the maxillo-mandibular complex will also move forward accordingly. Unfortunately, current dental articulators are unable to simulate these complex movements. Therefore, traditional surgical planning, which uses semiadjustable articulators to simulate surgery and fabricate the intermediate surgical splint, frequently results in unplanned displacement of the maxilla in the AP dimension.

Clinically, the authors have noted that although the amount of unplanned maxillary AP displacement can be relatively small in simple orthognathic surgery cases because of limited surgical movement, this unplanned displacement can be significant in complex and asymmetric deformities. In patients with hemifacial microsomia, a discrepancy of 5 to 10 mm in the occlusal plane (occlusal cant) is commonly encountered. Fig. 25-2, *A*, depicts the cephalometric tracing of a hypothetical patient with hemifacial microsomia. To correct a 6 mm occlusal cant, the intermediate surgical splint can often be thicker than 20 mm and result in at least 20 mm of mandibular autorotation (Fig. 25-2, *B*). In this case, the actual maxillary position after surgery is anteriorly displaced 5 mm in the AP direction (Fig. 25-2, *C*).

Issues with the Transfer of the Surgical Plan to the Patient at the Time of the Surgery

The last step in surgical planning is to transfer the surgical plan to the operating room. In cases involving the jaws, this is done using dental splints.[15,16] These splints help the surgeon place

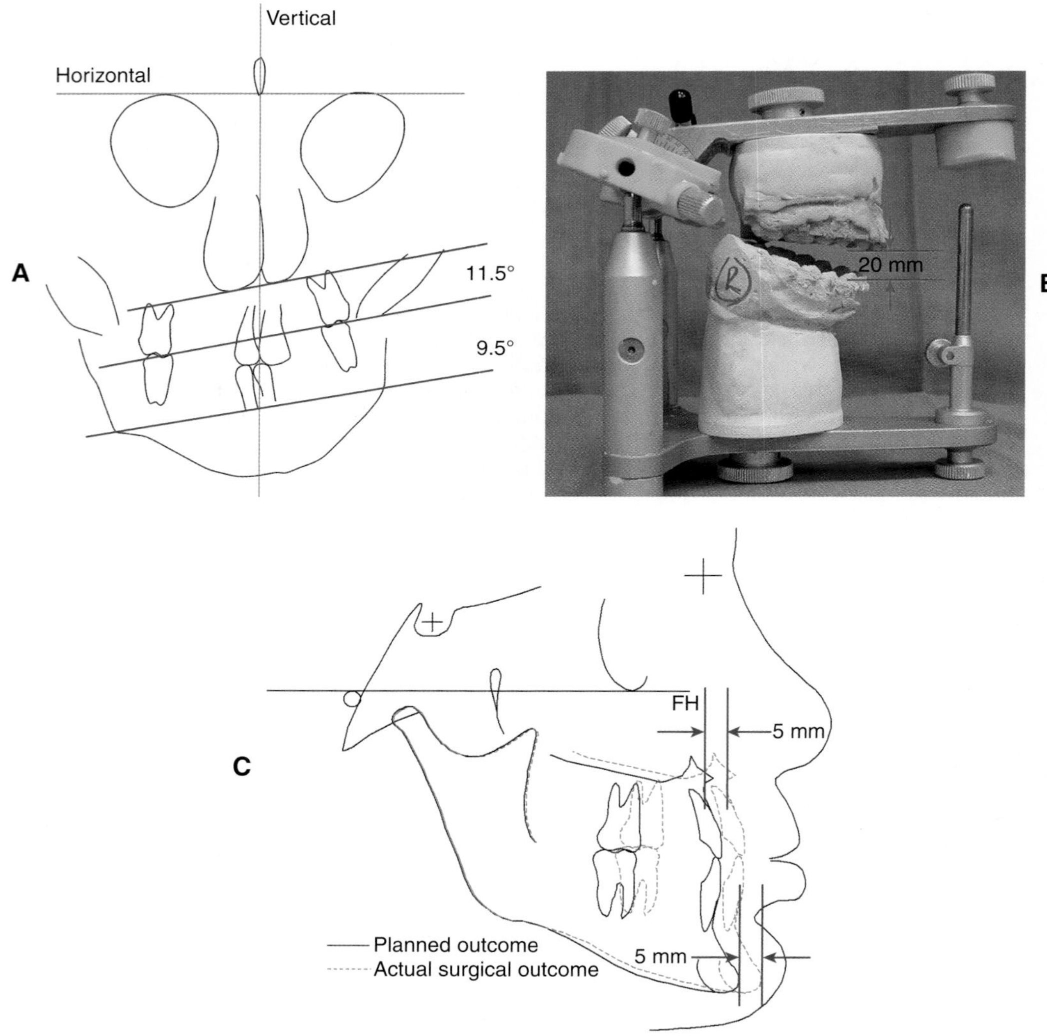

FIG 25-2 A hypothetical patient with hemifacial microsomia. **A,** Cephalometric tracing of a hemifacial microsomia case. **B,** Autorotate the mandible in order to correct the cant and make an intermediate splint. **C,** Unplanned 5 mm maxillary and mandibular advancement. The solid black line represents the desired maxillary position; the red dotted line represents the actual outcome with unplanned 5 mm anterior displacement.

the jaws in the desired position. However, for the craniofacial cases that do not involve dentitions (e.g., orbital osteotomies, cranial vault reshaping), surgeons currently do not have an accurate method of transferring the plan to the operating room. Certain measurements taken during the planning process can be used to guide surgery, but most commonly the placement of the bones in the desired position is more an art than a science.

HOW TO SOLVE THESE ISSUES?

The success of CMF surgery depends not only on the surgical techniques, but also upon an accurate surgical plan. Because of the problems mentioned previously, it is evident that the current methods used to plan CMF surgery are often inadequate. In addition, in many cases these methods are known to produce unwanted outcomes. Moreover, the whole planning process is time consuming.[38] An experienced surgeon frequently spends 4 to 6 hours to complete the surgical plan and to fabricate the splints. Finally, the cost of planning a complex case, both in time and in resources, can be fairly high.[38]

The need to improve the current surgical planning methods has led researchers to develop a more sophisticated planning method for CMF surgery (i.e., computer-aided surgical simulation [CASS]). CASS has wide applications in maxillofacial surgery,[19,39-44] craniofacial surgery,[20,45] trauma, and distraction osteogenesis.[20,46-50] Using CASS, surgeons can perform "virtual surgery" and create a 3D prediction of the patient's surgical outcomes as if they are performing surgery in the operating room.

4. What are the basic steps of CASS to plan a CMF surgery?

There are four major steps in the CASS. The first step of the CASS is to create 3D computer models of volume-of-interest. The second step is to quantify the deformity using 3D and 2D measurements. The third step is to simulate the surgery in the computer. The final step of the CASS is to transfer the computer surgical plan to the patient.

5. How do you create a computer model that is adequate for planning a CMF surgery?

If the surgery does not involve teeth, the conventional 3D CT model can be used for surgical planning. However, if the surgery involves teeth, as mentioned previously, the conventional CT model does not present the teeth accurately to the degree that is necessary for surgical planning. Therefore, a composite skull model[17,21,51] is required. This model simultaneously displays an accurate rendition of both the bony structures and the teeth.

In order to create a composite skull model, a bite-jig is first created (Fig. 25-3, *A*). It is used to relate the upper and lower dental casts to each other and to support a set of fiducial markers, which are used to register the digital dental models to the 3D CT skull model. To facilitate the fabrication of the jig, self-curing methyl methacrylate material is directly placed between the maxillary and mandibular teeth to create a bite registration in centric relation. Each jig incorporates four fiducial marker supporters, which are placed buccal to the lateral incisors and second premolars. The supporters are arranged in various planes in order to maximize the accuracy of the registration. A set of CT-compatible fiducial markers is inserted into the supporters at the time of the CT scanning so they can be captured without scattering by the CT scanner (see Fig. 25-3, *A*). After the bite-jig is created, a CT scan of the patient's craniofacial skeleton is obtained while the patient is biting on the bite-jig (Fig. 25-3, *B* and *C*). Thereafter, the digital dental models are created by scanning the plaster dental models in a very high resolution scanner (0.15 mm or more accurate) (Fig. 25-3, *D* and *E*). Using the fiducial markers, the "bad" teeth on the CT

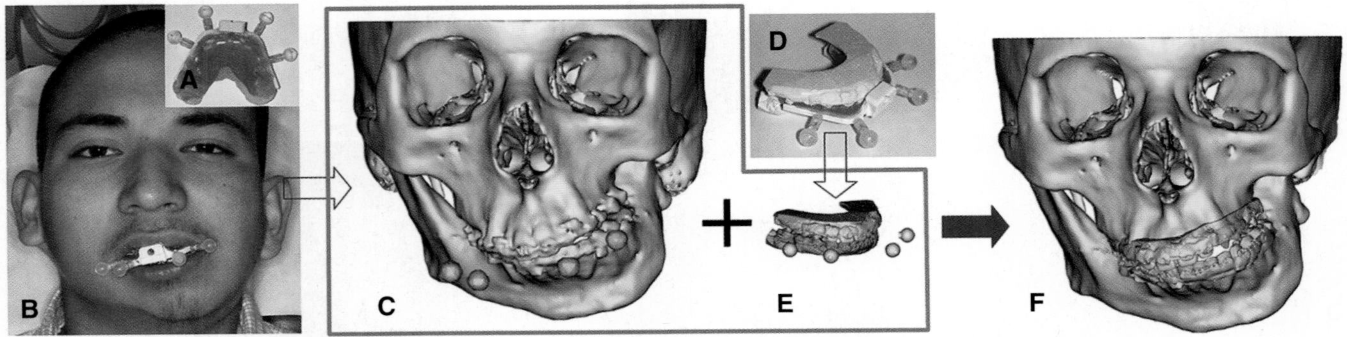

FIG 25-3 The creation of the computerized composite skull model. **A,** Bite-jig was created with fiducial CT/MRI-compatible fiducial markers. **B,** The patient was biting on the bite-jig with fiducial markers during CT scan. **C,** Three separate but correlated computer models were reconstructed: a midface model, a mandibular model, and a four-fiducial-marker model. **D,** The bite-jig with fiducial markers was placed between the upper and lower plaster dental models during the scanning process. **E,** Three separate but correlated computer models were also reconstructed: an upper digital dental model, a lower digital dental model, and a four-fiducial-marker model. **F,** The computerized composite skull model simultaneously displayed an accurate rendition of both the bony structures and the teeth. (From Gateno J, Xia JJ, Teichgraeber JF, et al: *J Oral Maxillofac Surg* 2007;65(4):728-734.)

skull model are removed and replaced by the "good" teeth from the digital models. This results in a computerized composite skull model that simultaneously displays an accurate rendition of both the bony structures and the teeth (Fig. 25-3, *F*).

6. How do you plan the surgery using CASS techniques?

The composite skull model is initially prepared (pre-cut) to simulate various osteotomies. As an example, they may include a Le Fort I osteotomy, a sagittal split osteotomy, an inverted "L" osteotomy, or a genioplasty. After the model is prepared, the surgeon is able to move the bony segments to the desired position and rotate each bony segment around a pivot point according to quantitative guidance and the surgeon's visual judgment. Once the bony segments are in the desired location, the simulated outcomes and surgical movements are recorded. Using CASS, the surgeon is able to simulate a number of different surgical treatments in order to create the most appropriate surgical plan.

7. How do you transfer the computerized surgical plan to the patient at the time of the surgery?

The final step of the CASS is to transfer the computer surgical plan to the patient. In order to accomplish this, surgical dental splints and templates are created using computer-aided designing/computer-aided manufacturing techniques.[17,51,52] In surgeries that involve the teeth, surgical dental splints are created by a computational process after inserting a digital wafer between the maxillary and mandibular dental arches (see Fig. 25-4, *A*). In surgeries that do not involve the teeth, digital templates can be created (Fig. 25-4, *B*). They are used during surgery to help the surgeons achieve the desired results. The templates record the 3D surface geometry of the area of interest so that the template fits on the bone in a unique position. The digital splints and templates are then sent to a rapid prototyping machine to fabricate physical splints and templates (see Fig. 25-4, *C* and *D*). They can then be sterilized and used at the time of the surgery (Fig. 25-4, *E* and *F*).

In surgeries that involve bone graft, the computerized mirror-imaging technique is used to mirror image the geometry from the healthy side to the defect side. The mirrored image from the healthy side is then superimposed over the defect side (Fig. 25-5, *A*). The difference of geometries between the two sides is computed, resulting in a digital bone graft template (Fig. 25-4, *B*). Using rapid prototyping machines, the digital templates are fabricated to physical templates (Fig. 25-5, *C*) that are used during surgery to sculpt autogenous bone (Fig. 25-5, *D*) to precisely replace the missing bone (Fig. 25-5, *E*). If desired, the digital templates can also be used to directly fabricate implantable implants.

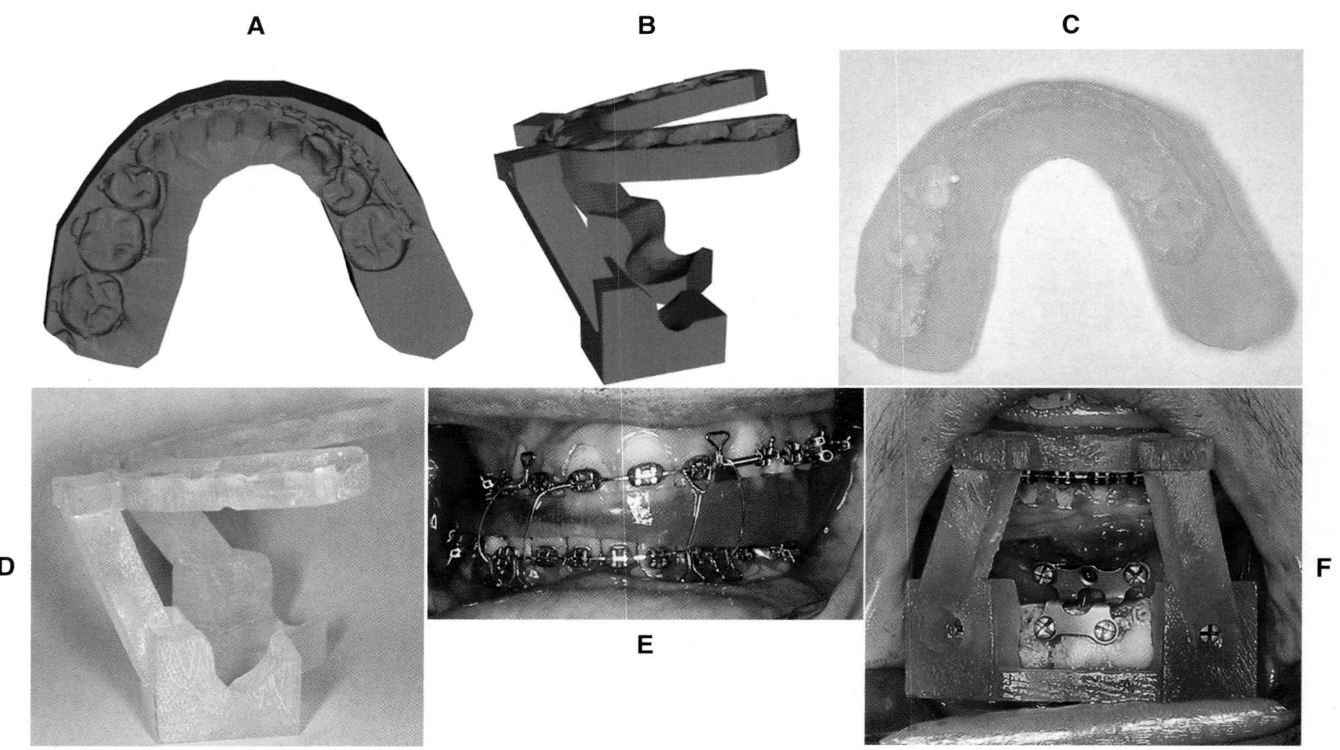

FIG 25-4 Surgical dental splints and templates are created using computer-aided designing/computer-aided manufacturing technique. **A,** Digital surgical splint. **B,** Digital chin template. **C,** Physical surgical splint. **D,** Physical chin template. **E,** The use of physical surgical splint at the time of the surgery. **F,** The use of physical chin template at the time of the surgery. (From Gateno J, Xia JJ, Teichgraeber JF, et al: *J Oral Maxillofac Surg* 2007;65(4):728-734.)

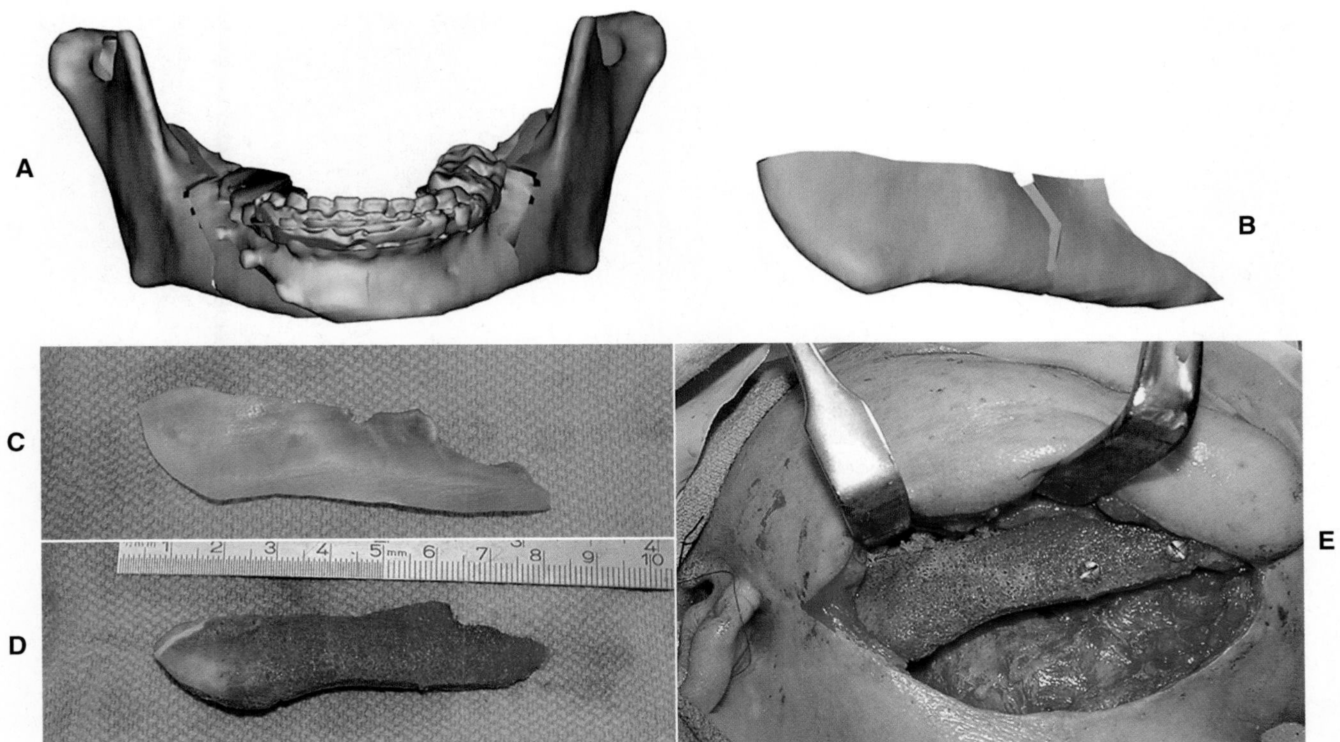

FIG 25-5 Surgical planning of onlay bone grafting. **A,** A mirror image of the unaffected side was created. It was superimposed over the affected side. **B,** A digital template that depicted the differences between the mirror image and the affected side was created. **C,** A physical form of the same template was fabricated. **D,** Autogenous bone was harvested and sculpted according to the shape of the template. **E.** The sculpted autogenous bone graft precisely replaced the missing bone. (From Gateno J, Xia JJ, Teichgraeber JF, et al: *J Oral Maxillofac Surg* 2007;65(4):728-734.)

Finally, a physical model with the planned outcome can be fabricated for pre-bending the bone plates that are used in the surgery (Fig. 25-6). This will not only improve the accuracy of the operation, but also reduce the total operative time by eliminating the need to bend these plates at the time of the surgery.

8. What is the accuracy of using the CASS method in complex CMF surgery?

Fig. 25-7 illustrates a typical patient that is best treated using CASS. The patient suffered TMJ ankylosis caused by a left ear infection at the age of 5. He was treated by arthroplasty and costochondral graft. Although the arthroplasty was successful, the costochondral graft and the left face failed to grow. The practitioner used the CASS planning method. The computer-generated surgical splints and templates were used to transfer the computerized surgical plan to the patient at the time of the surgery. The osteotomized maxilla was positioned using the computer-generated intermediate splint. The mandible and chin were then osteotomized, repositioned, and fixated by mini-plates. Bone grafts were harvested and carved according to the planned size and shape. Six-week postoperative CT scans showed the surgical plans were precisely reproduced in the operating room and the deformities were corrected as planned. The comparison chart of the patient's preoperative, planned, and postoperative outcomes are shown in Fig. 25-7.

The ideal surgical plan is the one that can be reproduced accurately in the operating room. A recent published study evaluated the accuracy of CASS in the treatment of patients with complex CMF deformities.[53] This pilot study showed, with CASS planning, that the largest linear difference between the planned and the actual postoperative outcomes was within 1.99 mm and the largest median of the linear difference was 0.85 mm. The largest angular difference between the planned and the actual postoperative outcomes was limited within 3.48 degrees and the largest median of the angular difference was 1.70 degrees.

9. What is the cost-effectiveness for using the CASS?

A recent published study compared the costs and benefits between using CASS and the current surgical planning methods for complex CMF surgery.[38] The comparison of methods applies to all CMF surgeries where the patient's condition is severe enough to undergo a CT scan and an SLA model is necessary for the surgical planning process. The study showed that CASS has lower costs in terms of surgeon time, patient time, and material costs. Specifically, total surgeon hours spent in

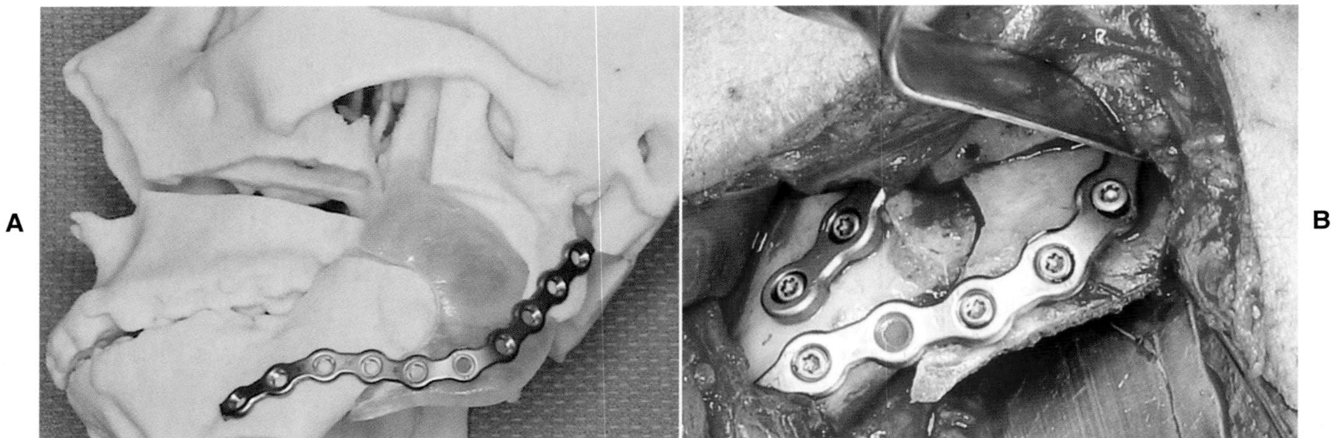

FIG 25-6 A physical model of the planned outcome is fabricated and used to pre-bend the bone plates that will be used in the surgery. **A,** Pre-bend the bone plates based on a physical model of planned outcome and bone graft. **B,** Adopt the pre-bent bone plates at the time of the surgery. (From Gateno J, Xia JJ, Teichgraeber JF, et al: *J Oral Maxillofac Surg* 2007;65(4):728-734.)

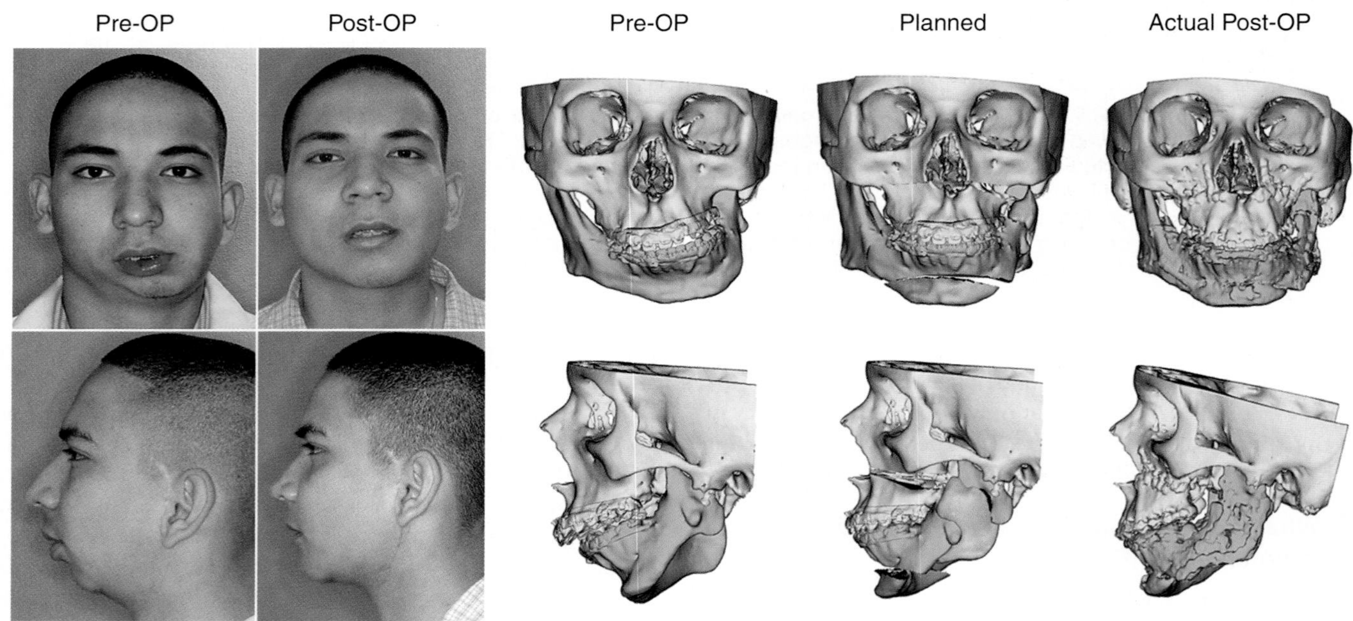

FIG 25-7 Comparison chart of a patient's preoperative, planned, and postoperative outcomes. (From Gateno J, Xia JJ, Teichgraeber JF, et al: *J Oral Maxillofac Surg* 2007;65(4):728-734.)

planning are 5.25 hours compared with 9.75 hours for current standard methods. Material and scanning costs are $1900 for CASS compared with about $3510 for standard methods. Patient time for planning is reduced from 4.75 hours to 2.25 hours with CASS. The reduction in both time and other costs remains when the upfront costs of CASS are added to the variable costs. Amortized across the 600 patients per year (1800 for the assumed 3-year life of the training and software), this adds only a few dollars and a fraction of an hour per surgery. Even in the case of a small clinic when the cost is amortized for 6 patients per year (18 patients for the assumed 3-year life of the training and software), the per-surgical costs (9.65 hours and $2456) will still favor CASS.

10. What other method can be used to transfer the computerized plan to the patient at the time of the surgery?

Surgical navigation is an alternative tool to transfer the computerized surgical plan to the patient at the time of the surgery. The navigation system is similar to a car global positioning

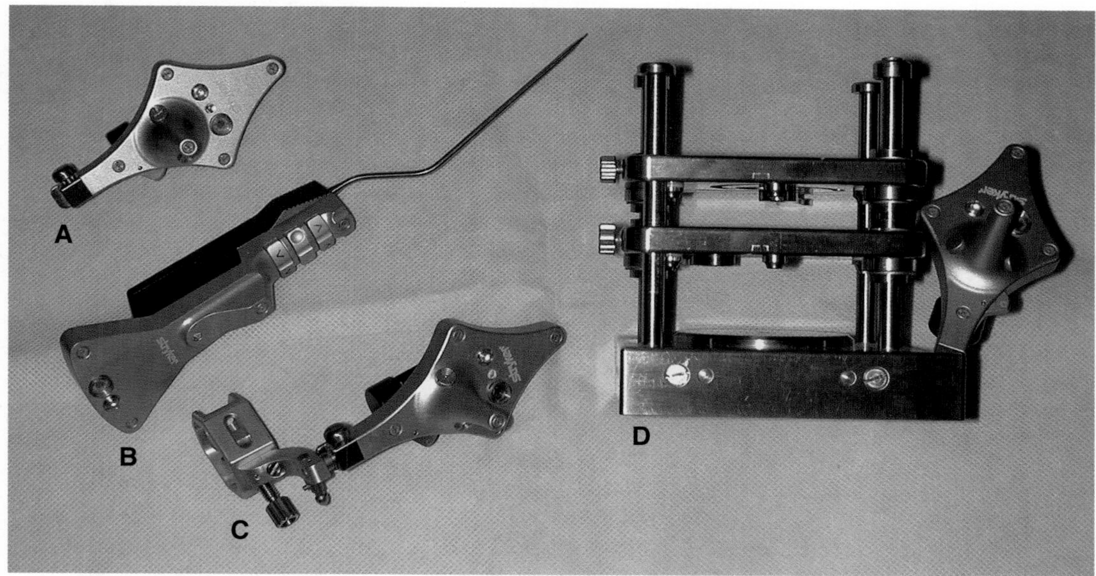

FIG 25-8 Navigation emitters consist of patient tracker *(A)*, navigation pointer *(B)*, instrument tracker *(C)*, and, calibration station *(D)*.

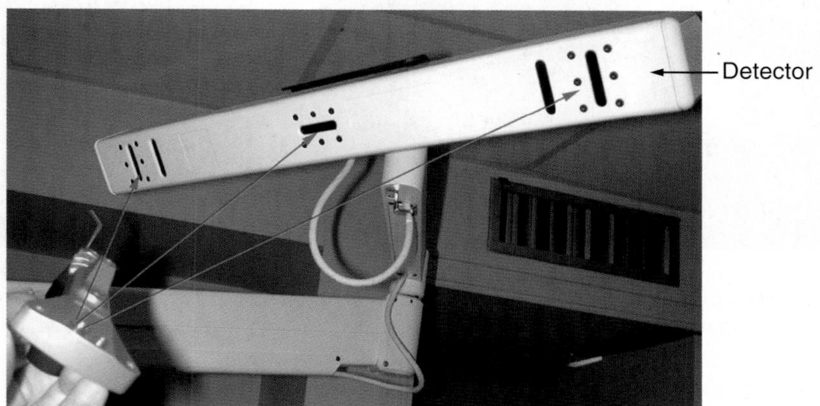

FIG 25-9 A unique link is generated between the detector and the emitters after the registration process.

system (GPS). It consists of a computer, a monitor, a set of cameras (like the satellites), and a series of navigated instruments (like the GPS handheld). The navigated instruments include a patient tracker (Fig. 25-8, *A*), a navigation pointer (Fig. 25-8, *B*), an instrument tracker (Fig. 25-8, *C*) and a calibration station (Fig. 25-8, *D*). The navigated instrument (i.e., a patient tracker mounted on the patient's skull) emits infrared signal of the *x*, *y*, and *z* coordinates to the cameras (Fig. 25-9). Once the cameras receive these signals and send them to the computer, a unique link is established between the camera and the instrument (see Fig. 25-9). Therefore, the position of the patient's head can be tracked down by the patient tracker. Equally, the position of both surgical instrument and pointer can be tracked by the instrument tracker. The calibration station (see Fig. 25-8, *D*) is a special type of the emitter. It calibrates the position of the instrument's tip to the instrument tracker. Virtually any kind of surgical instrument can be calibrated by the calibration station and instrument tracker. Finally, the monitor displays the sagittal, coronal, axial, and 3D views of the CT image, as well as the location of the navigated surgical instruments (Fig. 25-10).

This technology has been proven accurate, with a precision ranging from 0.2 to 1.1 mm.[47,54-56] Surgical navigation also offers an improved spatial representation of complex surgical environments, helping the surgeon to respect vessels, nerves, external and middle ear or middle cranial fossa.[48,57,58] However, navigation technology requires the installation of cameras and sensors followed by registration. This extra step may prolong the surgery in comparison to the use of surgical splints and templates. Another disadvantage is the cost of the navigation system. An additional staff member is also required during the surgery for the manipulation of the computer. Therefore, the indication of using surgical navigation technology is crucial. The authors reserve this technology to the surgery in which the

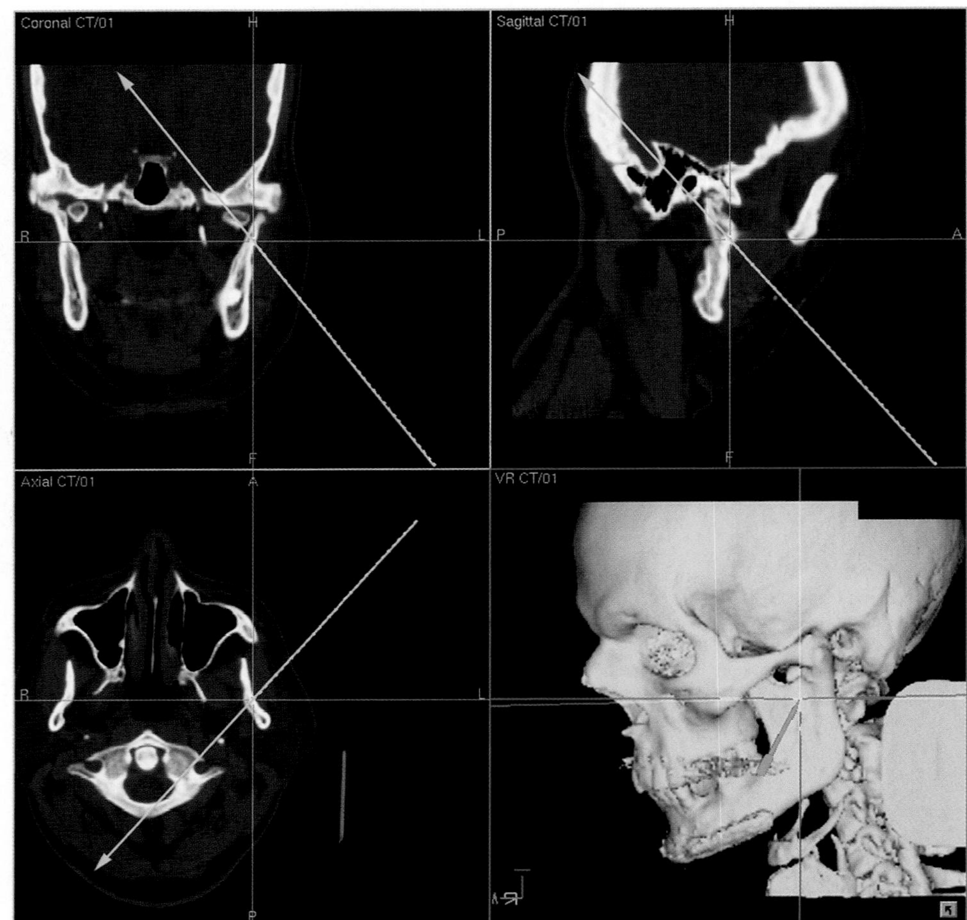

FIG 25-10 The navigation monitor displays the sagittal, coronal, axial, and 3D views of the CT image, as well as the location and trajectory of the navigated surgical instruments. The resection margins have also recorded in the navigation computer, forming a computerized surgical plan.

use of surgical splints and templates is generally not feasible. These surgeries usually involve the area that has less significant surface geometry or limited surgical exposure (i.e., reconstruction of complex post-traumatic deformities of the midface[45] or TMJ ankylosis.[17,59,60]

REFERENCES

1. National Center for Health Statistics, Third National Health and Nutrition Examination Survey (NHANES III, 1988-1994). Hyattsville, MD: National Center for Health Statistics, 1996.
2. Proffit WR, Fields HW Jr, Ackerman JL, et al: *Contemporary orthodontics,* edition 3. St Louis: Mosby, 2000.
3. Proffit WR, Phillips C, Dann CT: Who seeks surgical-orthodontic treatment? *Int J Adult Orthod Orthognath Surg* 1990;5:153.
4. Severt TR, Proffit WR: The prevalence of facial asymmetry in the dentofacial deformities population at the University of North Carolina. *Int J Adult Orthod Orthognath Surg* 1997;12:171.
5. Gorlin RJ, Cohen MM, Hennekam RCM, editors: *Syndromes of the head and neck,* edition 4. New York: Oxford University Press, 2001.
6. Cohen MM, MacLean RE: *Craniosynostosis: Diagnosis, evaluation, and management,* edition 2. New York: Oxford University Press, 2002.
7. National Center for Health Statistics, National Hospital Discharge Survey: Annual Summary with Detailed Diagnosis and Procedure Data. Vital and Health Statistics series 13, no 151. DHHS publication No.(PHS)2001-1722, Hyattsville, MD: National Center for Health Statistics, 1999.
8. American Society of Plastic Surgeons, National Plastic Surgery Statistics: Cosmetic and Reconstructive Patient Trends (2000/2001/2002). American Society of Plastic Surgeons, 2000/2001/2002.
9. Cancer Statistics Branch, Surveillance Research Program, National Cancer Institute SEER*Stat Software (www.seer.cancer.gov/seerstat), version 5.0.20. Bethesda, MD: National Cancer Institute, April, 2003.
10. WISQARS: Overall injury causes: nonfatal injuries and rates per 100,000 (2001-2002, United States). Atlanta: National Center for Injury Prevention and Control, 2003.
11. Ticknon L: *Trauma Statistics.* Minneapolis, MN: Trauma Registry, Hennepin County Medical Center, 2003.
12. NIH Office of Medical Application of Research: National Institutes of Health Technology Assessment Conference on Management of Temporomandibular Disorders, Bethesda, Maryland, April 29-May 1, 1996. Proceedings. *Oral Surg Oral Med Oral Pathol Oral Radiol Endod* 1997;83:49.
13. National Institutes of Health: Management of temporomandibular disorders. National Institutes of Health Technology Assessment Conference Statement. *J Am Dent Assoc* 1996;127:1595.

14. Cowley T: Numbers of patient undergo TMJ reconstruction annually. Personal communication, 2003.
15. Bell WH, editor: *Surgical correction of dentofacial deformities.* Philadelphia: WB Saunders, 1980.
16. Bell WH, editor: *Modern practice in orthognathic and reconstructive surgery*. Philadelphia: WB Saunders, 1992.
17. Xia JJ, Gateno J, Teichgraeber JF: Three-dimensional computer-aided surgical simulation for maxillofacial surgery. *Atlas Oral Maxillofac Surg Clin North Am* 2005;13:25.
18. Papadopoulos MA, Christou PK, Athanasiou AE, et al: Three-dimensional craniofacial reconstruction imaging. *Oral Surg Oral Med Oral Pathol Oral Radiol Endod* 2002;93:382.
19. Xia J, Ip HH, Samman N, et al: Computer-assisted three-dimensional surgical planning and simulation: 3D virtual osteotomy. *Int J Oral Maxillofac Surg* 2000;29:11.
20. Gateno J, Teichgraeber JF, Xia JJ: Three-dimensional surgical planning for maxillary and midface distraction osteogenesis. *J Craniofac Surg* 2003;14:833.
21. Gateno J, Xia J, Teichgraeber JF, et al: A new technique for the creation of a computerized composite skull model. *J Oral Maxillofac Surg* 2003;61:222.
22. Santler G: 3-D COSMOS: a new 3-D model based computerised operation simulation and navigation system. *J Maxillofac Surg* 2000;28:287.
23. Santler G: The Graz hemisphere splint: a new precise, non-invasive method of replacing the dental arch of 3D-models by plaster models. *J Craniomaxillofac Surg* 1998;26:169.
24. Ellis E 3rd, Tharanon W, Gambrell K: Accuracy of face-bow transfer: effect on surgical prediction and postsurgical result. *J Oral Maxillofac Surg* 1992;50:562.
25. Lorensen WE, Cline HE: Marching cubes: a high resolution 3D surface construction algorithm. *Comput Graph* 1987;21:163.
26. Lambrecht JT: *3D Modeling technology in oral and maxillofacial surgery.* Chicago: Quintessence, 1995, pp 61.
27. Gateno J, Forrest KK, Camp B: A comparison of 3 methods of face-bow transfer recording: implications for orthognathic surgery. *J Oral Maxillofac Surg* 2001;59:635.
28. Grant PG: Biomechanical significance of the instantaneous center of rotation: the human temporomandibular joint. *J Biomech* 1973;6:109.
29. Rubenstein LK, Strauss RA, Isaacson RJ, et al: Quantitation of rotational movements associated with surgical mandibular advancement. *Angle Orthod* 1991;61:167.
30. Rekow ED, Speidel TM, Koenig RA: Location of the mandibular center of autorotation in maxillary impaction surgery. *Am J Orthod Dentofacial Orthop* 1993;103:530.
31. Sheppard IM: The effect of the hinge axis clutches on condyle position. *J Prosthet Dent* 1958;8:260.
32. Sperry TP, Steinberg MJ, Gans BJ: Mandibular movement during autorotation as a result of maxillary impaction surgery. *Am J Orthod* 1982;81:116.
33. Nagerl H, Kubein-Meesenburg D, Fanghanel J, et al: Elements of a general theory of joints. 6. General kinematical structure of mandibular movements. *Anat Anz* 1991;173:249.
34. McMillan DR, McMillan AS: A comparison of habitual jaw movements and articulator function. *Acta Odontol Scand* 1986;44:291.
35. McMillan AS, McMillan DR, Darvell BW: Centers of rotation during jaw movements. *Acta Odontol Scand* 1989;47:323.
36. Ferrario VF, Sforza C, Miani A Jr, et al: Open-close movements in the human temporomandibular joint: does a pure rotation around the intercondylar hinge axis exist? *J Oral Rehabil* 1996;23:401.
37. Hellsing G, Hellsing E, Eliasson S: The hinge axis concept: a radiographic study of its relevance. *J Prosthet Dent* 1995;73:60.
38. Xia JJ, Phillips CV, Gateno J, et al: Cost-effectiveness analysis for computer-aided surgical simulation in complex cranio-maxillofacial surgery. *J Oral Maxillofac Surg* 2006;64:1780.
39. Altobelli DE, Kikinis R, Mulliken JB, et al: Computer-assisted three-dimensional planning in craniofacial surgery. *Plast Reconstr Surg* 1993;92:576.
40. Vannier MW, Marsh JL, Warren JO: Three dimensional CT reconstruction images for craniofacial surgical planning and evaluation. *Radiology* 1984;150:179.
41. Marsh JL, Vannier MW: The "third" dimension in craniofacial surgery. *Plast Reconstr Surg* 1983;71:759.
42. Xia J, Samman N, Yeung RW, et al: Three-dimensional virtual reality surgical planning and simulation workbench for orthognathic surgery. *Int J Adult Orthod Orthognath Surg* 2000;15:265.
43. Xia J, Samman N, Yeung RW, et al: Computer-assisted three-dimensional surgical planing and simulation. 3D soft tissue planning and prediction. *Int J Oral Maxillofac Surg* 2000;29:250.
44. Xia J, Ip HH, Samman N, et al: Three-dimensional virtual-reality surgical planning and soft-tissue prediction for orthognathic surgery. *IEEE Trans Inf Technol Biomed* 2001;5:97.
45. Westendorff C, Gulicher D, Dammann F, et al: Computer-assisted surgical treatment of orbitozygomatic fractures. *J Craniofac Surg* 2006;17:837.
46. Schicho K, Figl M, Seemann R, et al: Accuracy of treatment planning based on stereolithography in computer assisted surgery. *Med Phys* 2006;33:3408.
47. Klug C, Schicho K, Ploder O, et al: Point-to-point computer-assisted navigation for precise transfer of planned zygoma osteotomies from the stereolithographic model into reality. *J Oral Maxillofac Surg* 2006;64:550.
48. Heiland M, Habermann CR, Schmelzle R: Indications and limitations of intraoperative navigation in maxillofacial surgery. *J Oral Maxillofac Surg* 2004;62:1059.
49. Gateno J, Teichgraeber JF, Aguilar E: Computer planning for distraction osteogenesis. *Plast Reconstr Surg* 2000;105:873.
50. Gateno J, Allen ME, Teichgraeber JF, et al: An in vitro study of the accuracy of a new protocol for planning distraction osteogenesis of the mandible. *J Oral Maxillofac Surg* 2000;58:985.
51. Gateno J, Teichgraeber JF, Xia J: Method and apparatus for fabricating orthognathic surgical splints (US Patent 6,671,539). In USPTO Patent Full-Text and Image Database. U.S. Patent and Trademark Office, USA, Dec. 30, 2003.
52. Gateno J, Xia J, Teichgraeber JF, et al: The precision of computer-generated surgical splints. *J Oral Maxillofac Surg* 2003;61:814.
53. Xia JJ, Gateno J, Teichgraeber JF, et al: Accuracy of the computer-aided surgical simulation (CASS) system in the treatment of patients with complex craniomaxillofacial deformity: A pilot study. *J Oral Maxillofac Surg* 2007;65:248.
54. Marmulla R, Hilbert M, Niederdellmann H: Inherent precision of mechanical, infrared and laser-guided navigation systems for computer-assisted surgery. *J Craniomaxillofac Surg* 1997;25:192.
55. Hassfeld S, Muhling J: Navigation in maxillofacial and craniofacial surgery. *Comput Aided Surg* 1998;3:183.
56. Husstedt H, Heermann R, Becker H: Contribution of low-dose CT-scan protocols to the total positioning error in computer-assisted surgery. *Comput Aided Surg* 1999;4:275.
57. Gellrich NC, Schramm A, Hammer B, et al: Computer-assisted secondary reconstruction of unilateral posttraumatic orbital deformity. *Plast Reconstr Surg* 2002;110:1417.
58. Smith JA, Sandler NA, Ozaki WH, et al: Subjective and objective assessment of the temporalis myofascial flap in previously operated temporomandibular joints. *J Oral Maxillofac Surg* 1999;57:1058.
59. Baumann A, Schicho K, Klug C, et al: Computer-assisted navigational surgery in oral and maxillofacial surgery. *Atlas Oral Maxillofac Surg Clin North Am* 2005;13:41.
60. Malis D, Xia JJ, Gateno J, et al: New protocol for 1-stage treatment of TMJ ankylosis using surgical navigation. *J Oral Maxillofac Surg* 2007;65(9):1843.

Index

A

Page numbers followed by a b, indicate boxes; f, figures; t, tables.

D

G

H

I

J

K

L

N

O

Q

R

T

U